D0906802

GEORGE I. KAGAN, D.D.S.
I IT RESEARCH INSTITUTE
10 WEST 35TH ST., #14F3-1
CHICAGO, IL 60616-3799

CHICAGO PUBLIC LIBRARY
BUSINESS / SCIENCE / TECHNOLOGY
400 S. STATE ST   60605

GEORGE I. KAGAN, D.D.S.
IIT RESEARCH INSTITUTE
10 WEST 35TH ST., #NR3-1
CHICAGO, IL 60616-3799

Textbook of
Clinical
Perio-
dontology

Jan Lindhe

Textbook of Clinical Perio- dontology

Munksgaard

Textbook of Clinical Periodontology

Copyright © 1984 Munksgaard, Copenhagen
1st edition, 2nd printing
Previous edition copyright © 1983 Munksgaard, Copenhagen
All rights reserved

No part of this publication may be reproduced, stored
in a retrieval system, or transmitted in any form or
by any means, electronic, mechanical photocopying,
recording or otherwise without prior permission by the
copyright owner.

Cover by Lars Thorsen
Typesetting: Satsform, Åbyhøj
Reproduction: Københavns Kliché & Offset, Copenhagen
Printed in Denmark 1984 by Th. Laursen, Tønder

ISBN 87-16-09186-8

Distributed in North and South America by
W. B. Saunders Company, Philadelphia, Pennsylvania
ISBN 0-7216-1315-2

Library of Congress catalog card No. 83-51204

List of Contributors

CHICAGO PUBLIC LIBRARY
BUSINESS / SCIENCE / TECHNOLOGY
400 S. STATE ST   60605

Ainamo, Jukka, LDS, O. D., Professor and
   Chairman
Department of Periodontology
School of Dentistry
University of Helsinki
Finland

Attström, Rolf, LDS, O. D., Professor and
   Chairman
Department of Periodontology
School of Dentistry
University of Lund
Sweden

Bergenholtz, Gunnar, LDS, O. D.,
   Associate Professor and Chairman
Department of Oral Diagnosis
School of Dentistry
University of Gothenburg
Sweden

Carlsson, Jan, LDS, O. D., Professor and
   Chairman
Department of Oral Microbiology
School of Dentistry
University of Umeå
Sweden

Ericsson, Ingvar, LDS, O. D., Associate
   Professor
Department of Periodontology
School of Dentistry
University of Gothenburg
Sweden

Evers, Hans, LDS
ASTRA
Södertälje
Sweden

Frandsen, Asger, LDS, Dr. Odont.,
   Professor and Chairman
Department of Periodontology
Royal Dental College, Copenhagen
Denmark

Glantz, Per-Olof, LDS, O. D., Professor
   and Chairman
Department of Prosthetic Dentistry
School of Dentistry
University of Lund
Sweden

Hamp, Sven-Erik, LDS, O. D., Associate
   Professor and Chairman
Department of Periodontology
Linköping
Sweden

Heijl, Lars, LDS, O. D., Associate
   Professor
Department of Periodontology
School of Dentistry
University of Gothenburg
Sweden

Karring, Thorkild, LDS, Dr. Odont.,
   Professor and Chairman
Department of Periodontology
Royal Dental College, Aarhus
Denmark

Kristoffersen, Tore, LDS, Dr. Odont.,
   M. S., Professor and Chairman
Department of Periodontology
School of Dentistry
University of Bergen
Norway

Lie, Tryggve, LDS, Dr. Odont., Associate
   Professor
Department of Periodontology
School of Dentistry
University of Bergen
Norway

Lindhe, Jan, DMD, Ph. D., Professor and
   Dean
School of Dental Medicine
University of Pennsylvania
USA

Meyer, Knut, LDS, Assistant Professor
Department of Periodontology
School of Dentistry
University of Bergen
Norway

Nyman, Sture, LDS, O. D.,
    Professor
Department of Periodontology
School of Dentistry
University of Gothenburg
Sweden

Pindborg, J. J., LDS, Dr. Odont., Professor
    and Chairman
Department of Oral Pathology
Royal Dental College, Copenhagen
Denmark

Rosling, Bengt, LDS, O. D., Research
    Associate
Department of Periodontology
School of Dentistry
University of Gothenburg
Sweden

Rylander, Harald, LDS, O. D., Associate
    Professor
Department of Periodontology
School of Dentistry
University of Gothenburg
Sweden

Slots, Jörgen, LDS, Dr. Odont., Professor
Department of Oral Microbiology
School of Dentistry
University of Gothenburg
Sweden

Theilade, Jörgen, LDS, B. Sc. D., M. S.,
    Associate Professor and Chairman
Department of Electron Microscopy
Royal Dental College, Aarhus
Denmark

Thilander, Birgit, LDS, O. D., Professor
    and Chairman
Department of Orthodontics
School of Dentistry
University of Gothenburg
Sweden

Wennström, Jan, LDS, O. D., Associate
    Professor
Department of Periodontology
School of Dentistry
University of Gothenburg
Sweden

Illustrations

Berglundh, Tord, LDS
Department of Periodontology
School of Dentistry
University of Gothenburg
Sweden

Foreword

Upon reading this book – and as I sit down pen in hand, to introduce the reader to this text on Periodontology – I become literally overwhelmed by the memory of Dr. Jens Waerhaug, the father of modern periodontology, my tutor and friend. Thus, this could easily become an emotional outlet for personal affection and devotion on the part of his first student; feelings which in the reserved climate of Scandinavian collegiality were never adequately expressed while he was alive. But it will not. The man, the friend, had passed on, but the scientist, the revolutionary, the genius is very much alive in every chapter of this treatise on periodontal diseases and their treatment and prevention.

It all began with the publishing of Jens Waerhaug's dissertation *"The Gingival Pocket"* in 1952, through which he laid the intellectual foundation for an entirely new era in periodontology. This was followed by a rapid succession of experiments, designed to answer questions one by one, reflecting a delightfully imaginative mind and profound clinical perception. In this way, step by step, he unveiled the mysteries surrounding periodontal diseases.

The reaction was – reactionary, especially among authoritarians. To others of us, the novelty of the dynamic approach to the experiments and the clarity of the clinical trials opened a large window on to a realm never heretofore seen. The Scandinavian school of periodontal research was born.

Some 30 years have elapsed, but as this text bears forceful witness to, the torch has been passed on.

The reader will find that this book is somewhat traditional in its infrastructure and layout. Its uniqueness lies in the consistency of the basic paradigm from one chapter to the next and in the weight of scientific evidence brought to bear. This book affords both an intelligent synthesis and an excellent overview of the progress in the science and practicalities of modern periodontology and brings together a large amount of current experimental data compiled by the editor and the authors themselves in the context of their own clinical experience.

The problems of periodontal diseases and their clinical management are not solved. However, the authors are all committed to the idea that at the present stage of development, there is enough knowledge to formulate clinical concepts for the practical management of these diseases. The strong message that emerges is that, although the technology may not be ideal, periodontal diseases can today be prevented and treated.

At a time of an information explosion in dental literature, this text is a most refreshing example of how scientific advances can be communicated for the clinician's comprehension and use.

The style is bold without being reckless; it is provocative without being presumptuous. The word "proper" is used profusely throughout the chapters. They still make proper reading, and I propose to recommend this book for general practitioners and specialists, students and teachers, clinicians and scientists, and for anyone else interested in the transfer of basic and clinical science to patient management in periodontal diseases.

Harald Löe, D. D. S., Dr. Odont., Director, National Institute of Dental Research, National Institutes of Health, Bethesda, Maryland 20205, U. S. A.

March 1983

Preface

This *Textbook of Clinical Periodontology* was prepared with the needs of undergraduate and graduate students of dentistry in mind. It is our hope, however, that the text may be of interest and use also to general practitioners and dentists with a special interest in periodontology.

This book is divided into two parts. The first part deals with the biology of the periodontal tissues and the epidemiology, etiology and pathogenesis of periodontal disease. Special emphasis has been given to bacterial plaque as the main etiological factor in periodontal disease and to the pathogenesis of various forms of plaque associated periodontal disorders. In two separate chapters material is presented illustrating how systemic disorders may influence periodontal disease and how the periodontal tissues may become the seat of tumors of both benign and malignant character.

The second part of the book deals with the clinical management of periodontal disease; examination procedures, diagnosis, treatment planning, treatment and maintenance therapy. It was our intention to create an analytical and critical text describing the present state of clinical periodontology. Particular efforts have been made to distinguish between facts obtained from pertinent research and unsubstantiated assumptions regarding the effect of different treatment procedures often utilized in periodontal therapy.

Textbook of Clinical Periodontology is the result of the inspiring collaboration, loyalty and never failing efforts of many past and present members and close friends of the staff of the Department of Periodontology, School of Dentistry, University of Gothenburg, Sweden. During various periods of time we have had the privilege of the cooperation of research workers and clinicians from all over the world. I would not like to complete this preface without expressing our sincere appreciation to Drs. Hilding Björn (University of Lund), Harald Löe (NIDR, Bethesda), Helmut Zander (Eastman Dental Center, Rochester), Hubert Schroeder (University of Zurich), Sigmund Socransky (Forsyth Dental Center, Boston), Max Listgarten (University of Pennsylvania) and Roy Page (University of Washington) for introducing us to and guiding our work in different fields of periodontal research.

We should also like to express our sincere gratitude to Dr. Tord Berglundh who was responsible not only for editing the photographical material but also for producing most of the drawings and schematic illustrations included in the various chapters of this book.

Last but not least it is a privilege to thank the publisher and the editorial and technical staff of Munksgaard International Publishers for their generosity and their skill in handling the printing and the reproduction of our material.

The text was completed in the early Fall of 1982. Research findings published in the literature since then have added to our knowledge and understanding of periodontal disease but have not, in any significant way, altered or invalidated the conclusions made in the various chapters of this book.

Gothenburg, March 1983
Jan Lindhe

Acknowledgement

In the preparation of this *Textbook of Clinical Periodontology* illustration material has kindly been placed at our disposal by a number of distinguished research workers and clinicians. It is a pleasure for me to acknowledge the following contributors: B. Bergman, Anna-Lisa Björn, J. Egelberg, P. A. Knudsen, M. Listgarten, D. Lundgren, S. W. Meitner, P. Milleding, A. M. Polson, H. E. Schroeder, K. A. Selvig, E. Strandman, R. E. Walton, Jytte Westergaard, Jens Waerhaug, H. A. Zander.

Contents

The Anatomy of the Periodontium

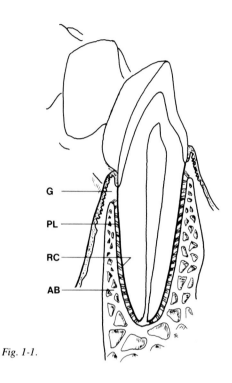

G

PL

RC

AB

Fig. 1-1.

This chapter presents a brief description of the normal features of the different tissues of the periodontium. It is assumed that the reader has prior knowledge of oral histology.

The periodontium (peri = around, odontos = tooth) comprises *the gingiva,* the *periodontal ligament,* the *root cementum* and the *alveolar bone.* The main function of the periodontium is to *attach* the tooth to the bone tissue of the jaws and to *maintain the integrity* of the surface of the masticatory mucosa of the oral cavity. The periodontium, also called *"the attachment apparatus"* or *"the supporting tissues of the teeth",* undergoes certain changes with age and is, in addition, subjected to both morphological and functional alterations. Thus, the periodontium is in a process of continuous change-associated adjustment related to aging, mastication and the oral environment.

Fig. 1-1 is a schematic drawing of a tooth with its periodontium: the *gingiva* (G), the *periodontal ligament* (PL), the *root cementum* (RC) and the *alveolar bone* (AB).

The Gingiva

Macroscopic anatomy

The oral mucosa (mucous membrane) is continuous with the skin of the lips and the mucosa of the soft palate and pharynx. The oral mucous membrane consists of (1) the *masticatory mucosa* which includes the gingiva and the covering of the hard palate, (2) the *specialized mucosa* which covers the dorsum of the tongue and (3) the *remaining* or the *lining mucosa.*

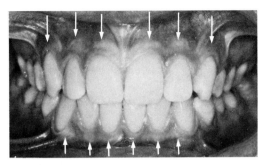

Fig. 1-2.

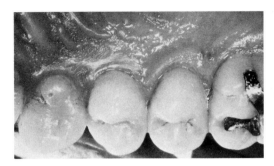

Fig. 1-3.

Fig. 1-2. The gingiva is that part of the *masticatory* mucosa which covers the alveolar process and surrounds the cervical portion of the teeth. The gingiva obtains its final shape and texture in conjunction with the eruption of the teeth.

In coronal direction the coral pink gingiva terminates in the *free gingival margin* which has a scalloped outline. In apical direction the gingiva is continuous with the loose, darker red *alveolar mucosa* (lining mucosa) from which the gingiva is separated by a usually, easily recognizable borderline called either the *mucogingival junction* (arrows) or the *mucogingival line*.

Fig. 1-3. There is no mucogingival line present in the palate since the hard palate and the maxillary alveolar process are covered by the same type of masticatory mucosa.

Fig. 1-4. Two parts of the gingiva can be differentiated:
1) the *free gingiva* (FG)
2) the *attached gingiva* (AG)

The *free gingiva* is coral pink, has a dull surface and firm consistency, and comprises the gingival tissue at the vestibular and lingual/palatal aspects of the teeth, and the *interdental gingiva* or the *interdental papillae*. On the vestibular and lingual side of the teeth, the free gingiva extends from the gingival

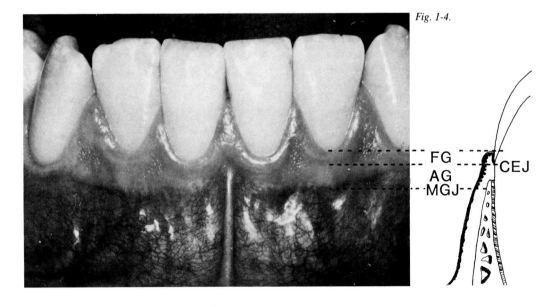

Fig. 1-4.

margin in apical direction to the *free gingival groove* which is positioned at a level corresponding to the level of the *cemento-enamel junction* (CEJ). In clinical examinations it has been observed that a free gingival groove is only present in about 30-40% of adults. The free gingival groove is often most pronounced on the vestibular aspect of the teeth, occurring most frequently in the incisor and premolar regions of the mandible, and least frequently in the mandibular molar and maxillary premolar regions (*mucogingival junction:* MGJ).

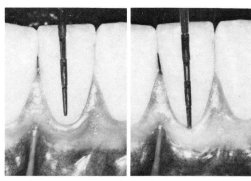

Fig. 1-5a.   Fig. 1-5b.

Fig. 1-5. The *free gingival margin* is often rounded in such a way that a small invagination or sulcus is formed between the tooth and the gingiva (Fig. 1-5a).

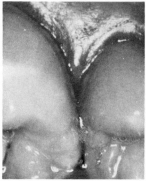

Fig. 1-6.

When a periodontal probe is inserted into this invagination and, further, apically towards the cemento-enamel junction, the gingival tissue is separated from the tooth and a *"gingival pocket"* or *"gingival crevice"* is artificially opened. Thus, in normal or *clinically healthy gingiva* there is in fact no "gingival pocket" or "gingival crevice" present but the gingiva is in close contact with the enamel surface. In the illustration to the right (Fig. 1-5b) a periodontal probe has been inserted in the tooth/gingiva interface and artificially opened a "gingival crevice" approximately to the level of the cemento-enamel junction.

After completed tooth eruption, the free gingival margin is located on the enamel surface approximately 0.5-2 mm coronal to the cemento-enamel junction.

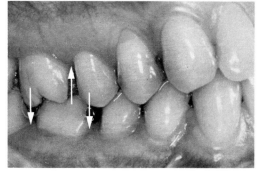

Fig. 1-7a.   Fig. 1-7b.

Fig. 1-6. The shape of the *interdental gingiva* (the *interdental papilla*) is determined by the contact relationships between the teeth, the width of the approximal tooth surfaces and the course of the cemento-enamel junction. In anterior regions of the dentition, the interdental papilla is of pyramidal form while in the molar regions, the papillae are more flattened in buccolingual direction (arrows). Due to the presence of interdental papillae, the free gingival margin follows a more or less accentuated, scalloped course through the dentition (see also Fig. 1-2.).

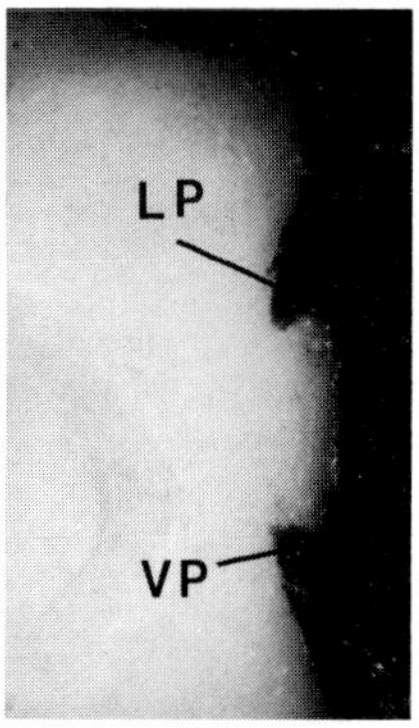

Fig. 1-7. In the premolar/molar regions of the dentition, the teeth have approximal contact surfaces (Fig. 1-7a) rather than contact points. Since the interdental papilla has a shape in conformity with the outline of the interdental contact, a concavity – *a col* – is established in the premolar and molar regions, as demonstrated in Fig. 1-7b where the distal tooth has been removed. Thus, the interdental papillae in these areas often have

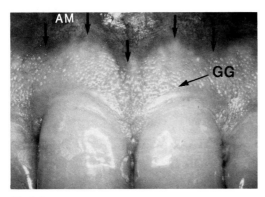

Fig. 1-8.

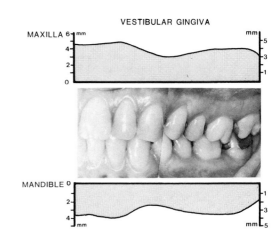

Fig. 1-9a.

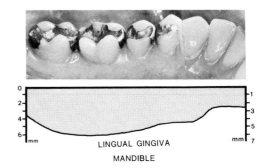

Fig. 1-9b.

one vestibular (VP) and one lingual/palatal portion (LP) separated by the col region.

Fig. 1-8. The *attached gingiva* is, in coronal direction, demarcated by the *free gingival groove* (GG), or when such a groove is not present, by a horizontal plane placed at the level of the cemento-enamel junction. The attached gingiva extends in apical direction to the mucogingival junction (arrows), where it becomes continuous with the alveolar (lining) mucosa (AM).

The attached gingiva is of firm texture, coral pink in color, and often shows a fine, surface stippling giving it the appearance of orange peel. This stippling, however, is only present in about 40% of adults.

This type of mucosa is firmly attached to the underlying alveolar bone and cementum by connective tissue fibers and is, therefore, comparatively immobile in relation to the underlying tissue. The darker red, alveolar mucosa (AM) located apical to the mucogingival junction, on the other hand, is loosely bound to the underlying bone. Therefore, in contrast to the attached gingiva, the alveolar mucosa is mobile in relation to the underlying tissue.

Fig. 1-9 describes how the width of the gingiva varies in different parts of the mouth. In the maxilla (1-9a), the vestibular gingiva is generally widest in the area of the incisors and most narrow adjacent to the premolars. In the mandible (1-9b), the gingiva on the

lingual aspect is particularly narrow in the area of the incisors and wide in the molar region. The range of variation is 1-9 mm.

Fig. 1-10 illustrates an area in the mandibular premolar region where the gingiva is

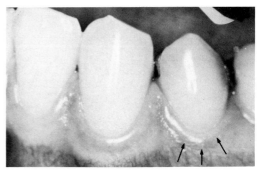

Fig. 1-10.

extremely narrow. The arrows indicate the location of the mucogingival junction.

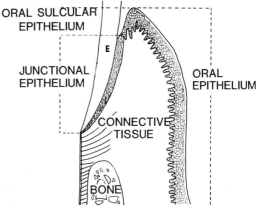

Fig. 1-12a.

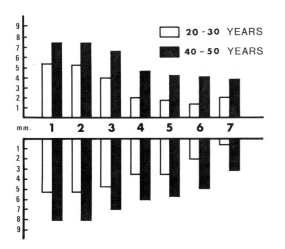

Fig. 1-11.

Fig. 1-11 depicts the result of a study in which the width of the attached gingiva was assessed and related to the age of the patients examined. It was found that the gingiva in 40-50 year olds was significantly wider than that in 20-30 year olds. This observation indicates that the width of the gingiva tends to increase with increasing age. Since the mucogingival junction remains stable throughout life in relation to the lower border of the mandible, the increasing width of the gingiva may suggest that the teeth, as a result of occlusal wear, slowly erupt throughout life.

Microscopic anatomy

The oral epithelium
Fig. 1-12a. A schematic drawing of the histological section, presented in Fig. 1-12b, describing the composition of the gingiva and the contact area between the gingiva and the enamel (E). The free gingiva comprises all tissue structures located coronal to a horizontal line placed at the level of the cemento-enamel junction (CEJ). The epithelium covering the free gingiva may be dif-

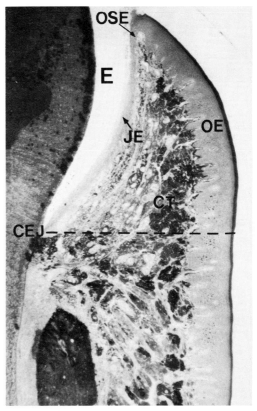

Fig. 1-12b.

ferentiated as follows:
oral epithelium (OE) which faces the oral cavity
oral sulcular epithelium (OSE) which faces the tooth without being in contact with the tooth surface

junctional epithelium (JE) which participates in the contact between the gingiva and the tooth.

The boundary between the oral epithelium (OE) and the underlying connective tissue (CT) has a wavy course. The connective tissue portions which project into the epithelium are called *connective tissue papillae* and are separated from each other by *epithelial ridges* – so-called *"rete pegs"*. In normal, non-inflamed gingiva, rete pegs and connective tissue papillae are lacking at the boundary between the junctional epithelium and its underlying connective tissue. Thus, a characteristic morphological feature of the oral epithelium and the oral sulcular epithelium is the presence of rete pegs while these structures are lacking in the junctional epithelium.

Fig. 1-13. A model of the *oral epithelium* of the gingiva after the connective tissue has been removed is presented in Fig. 1-13. The *subsurface* (i.e. the surface of the epithelium

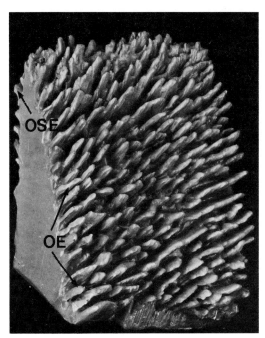

Fig. 1-14.

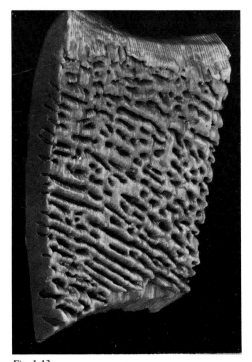

Fig. 1-13.

facing the connective tissue) of the oral epithelium exhibits several depressions corresponding to the connective tissue papillae which project into the epithelium. It can be seen that the epithelial projections, which in histological sections separate the connective tissue papillae, constitute a more continuous system of epithelial ridges.

Fig. 1-14 presents a model of the *connective tissue*, corresponding to the model of the epithelium shown in Fig. 1-13. The tooth surface is located at the left-hand side of the illustration. The epithelium is removed. Notice the connective tissue papillae which project into the space occupied by the oral epithelium (OE) and the oral sulcular epithelium (OSE).

Fig. 1-15a. A model of the outer surface of the *oral epithelium* of the attached gingiva is presented in Fig. 1-15a. The surface exhibits the minute depressions (1, 2, 3) which, when present, give the gingiva its characteristic stippled appearance (see also Fig. 1-8).

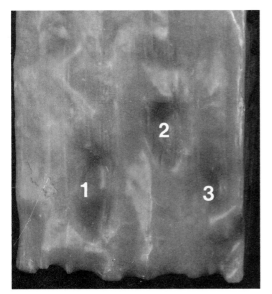

Fig. 1-15a.

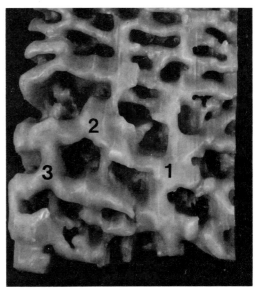

Fig. 1-15b.

Fig. 1-15b. A photograph of the *subsurface* (i.e. the surface of the epithelium facing the connective tissue) of the same model as described in Fig. 1-15a. The subsurface of the epithelium is characterized by the presence of epithelial ridges which merge at various locations (1, 2, 3). The depressions (1-3) seen on the outer surface of the epithelium (shown in Fig. 1-15a) correspond with the fusion sites 1-3 between epithelial ridges (shown in Fig. 1-15b) at the subsurface of the epithelium. Thus, the depressions on the surface of the gingiva are established at the areas of fusion between various epithelial ridges.

Fig. 1-16. A portion of the oral epithelium which covers the free gingiva is illustrated in this photomicrograph. The oral epithelium is a keratinized, stratified, squamous epithelium which on the basis of the degree to which the *keratin producing* cells are differentiated can be divided into the following cell layers:
1) *basal layer* (stratum basale or stratum germinativum)
2) *spinous cell layer* (stratum spinosum)
3) *granular cell layer* (stratum granulosum)
4) *keratinized cell layer* (stratum corneum)

It should be observed that in this section, cell nuclei are lacking in the outer cell layers. Such an epithelium is denoted *orthokeratinized.* Often, however, the cells of the stratum corneum of human, masticatory mucosal epithelium, contain remnants of the nuclei. In such case the epithelium is denoted *parakeratinized.*

Fig. 1-17. In addition to the keratin producing cells, which comprise about 90% of the

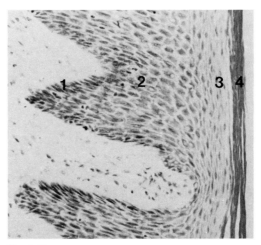

Fig. 1-16.

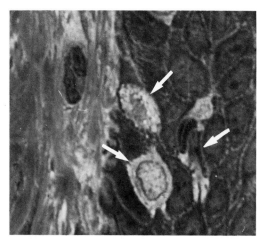

Fig. 1-17.

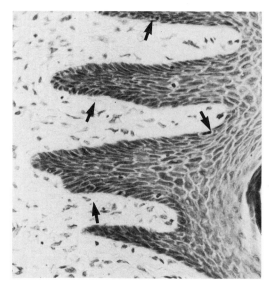

Fig. 1-18.

total cell population, the oral epithelium contains the following 3 types of cell:
1) melanocytes
2) Langerhans' cells
3) non-specific cells (i.e. cells which do not exhibit the same ultrastructural characteristics as the other 2 cell types).

All 3 cell types are stellate and have cytoplasmic extensions of various size and appearance. These cells are also called "clear cells" (arrows) since in the histological section they appear lighter than the surrounding keratin producing cells.

The photomicrograph shows 3 "clear cells" (arrows) located in the region of the stratum basale and stratum spinosum of the oral epithelium. Thus, these "clear cells" which are not producing keratin can be either melanocytes, Langerhans' cells or nonspecific cells. The melanocytes are pigment-containing cells while the Langerhans' cells are believed to play a role in the defense mechanism of the oral mucosa. It has been suggested that the Langerhans' cells react with antigens which are in the process of penetrating the epithelium. An early immunological response is initiated, inhibiting or preventing further antigen penetration of the tissue.

Fig. 1-18. The cells in the *basal layer* are either cylindrical or cuboid, and are in contact with the *basement membrane*. The basal cells possess the ability to divide, i.e. undergo mitotic cell division. The cells marked with arrows in the photomicrograph are in the process of dividing. It is in the basal layer that the epithelium is renewed and therefore this layer is also termed *stratum germinativum.*

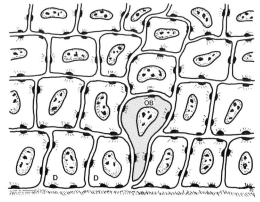

Fig. 1-19.

26

Fig. 1-19. When 2 daughter cells (D) have been formed by cell division, an adjacent "older" basal cell (OB) is pushed into the *spinous cell layer* and starts, as a keratinocyte, to traverse the epithelium. It takes approximately 1 month for a keratinocyte to reach the outer epithelial surface where it becomes desquamated from the stratum corneum. In a given time, the number of cells which divide in the basal layer equals the number of cells which become desquamated from the surface. Under normal conditions there is complete equlibrium between cell renewal and desquamation. As the basal cell migrates through the epithelium it becomes flattened and has its long axis parallel to the tissue surface.

Fig. 1-21 is an electronmicrograph (magnification × 70,000) of an area including part of a basal cell, the basement membrane and part of the adjacent connective tissue. The basal cell (BC) occupies the upper portion of the picture. Immediately beneath the basal cell an approximately 400 Å wide electron lucent zone can be seen which is called *lamina lucida* (LL). Beneath the lamina lucida an electron dense zone of approximately the same thickness can be observed. This zone is called *lamina densa* (LD). From the lamina densa so-called *anchoring fibers* (AF) project in fan-shaped fashion into the connective tissue. The anchoring fibers are approximately 1 μm in length and terminate freely in the connective tissue.

The basement membrane, that appeared as an entity under the light microscope, thus, in the electronmicrograph, appears to comprise one lamina lucida and one lamina densa with adjacent connective tissue fibers (anchoring fibers). The cell membrane of the epithelial cells facing the lamina lucida harbors a number of electron dense, thicker zones appearing at various intervals along the cell membrane. These structures are called *hemidesmosomes* (HD). The cytoplasmic *tonofilaments* (CT) in the cell converge

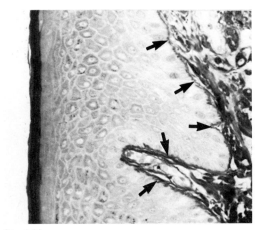

Fig. 1-20.

Fig. 1-20. The basal cells are found immediately adjacent to the connective tissue and are separated from this tissue by a *basement membrane,* probably produced by the basal cells. Under the light microscope this membrane appears as a zone approximately 1 μm wide (arrows), which reacts positively to a PAS stain (periodic acid Schiff stain). This positive reaction demonstrates that the basement membrane (arrows) contains carbohydrate (glycoproteins). The epithelial cells are surrounded by an extracellular substance which also contains protein polysaccharide complexes.

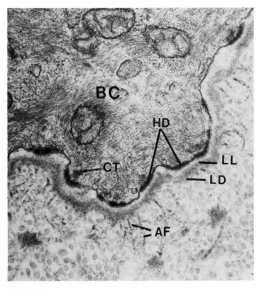

Fig. 1-21.

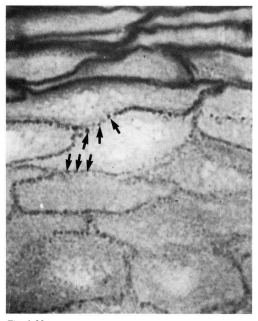

Fig. 1-22.

Stratum spinosum consists of 10-20 layers of relatively large, polyhedral cells, equipped with short cytoplasmic processes resembling spines. The cytoplasmic processes (arrows) occur at regular intervals and give the cells a prickled appearance. The cells are attached to one another by numerous "desmosomes" (pairs of hemidesmosomes) which are located between the cytoplasmic processes of adjacent cells.

Fig. 1-23 shows an area of stratum spinosum in an electron micrograph. The dark-stained structures between the individual epithelial cells represent the desmosomes (arrows). As stated above, a desmosome may be considered as 2 hemidesmosomes facing one another. The presence of a large number of desmosomes indicates that the attachment between the epithelial cells is solid. The light cell (LC) in the center of the illustration harbors no hemidesmosomes and is, therefore, not a keratinocyte but rather a "clear" cell (see also Fig. 1-17).

towards such hemidesmosomes. The hemidesmosomes are involved in the attachment of the epithelium to the underlying basement membrane.

Fig. 1-22 illustrates an area of stratum spinosum in the gingival oral epithelium.

Fig. 1-24 is a schematic drawing describing the composition of a desmosome. A desmosome consists of 2 adjoining hemidesmosomes separated by a zone containing electron dense granulated material (GM). In addition, a hemidesmosome comprises the following structural components: 1) the outer leaflets (OL) of the cell membrane of 2 adjoining cells, 2) the thick inner leaflets (IL) of the cell membranes and 3) the attachment plaques (AP) which represent granular and fibrillar material in the cytoplasm.

Fig. 1-25. As mentioned previously, the oral epithelium also contains *melanocytes* which are responsible for the production of the pigment melanin. Melanocytes are present in individuals with marked pigmentation of the oral mucosa (Indians and Negroes) as well as in individuals where no clinical signs of pigmentation can be seen. In this electron micrograph a melanocyte (MC) is present in the lower portion of the stratum spinosum. In contrast to the keratinocytes, this cell contains melanin granulae (MG) and has no

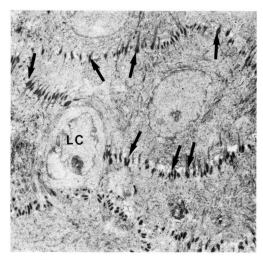

Fig. 1-23.

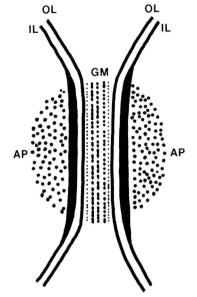

Fig. 1-24.

changes which occur during this process are indicated in this diagram of a keratinized, stratified, squamous epithelium. From the basal layer (Str. basale) to the granular layer (Str. granulosum) both the number of tonofilaments (F) in the cytoplasm and the number of desmosomes (D) increase significantly. In contrast, the number of organelles such as mitochondria (M), lamellae of rough endoplasmic reticulum (E) and Golgi complexes (G) decreases in the keratinocytes on their way from the basal layer towards the surface. In the stratum granulosum, electron dense keratohyalin

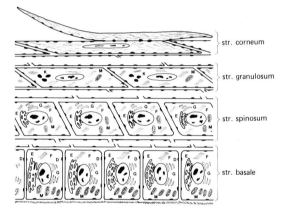

Fig. 1-26.

tonofilaments or hemidesmosomes. Note the large amount of tonofilaments in the cytoplasm of the adjacent keratinocytes.

Fig. 1-26. When traversing the epithelium from the basal layer to the epithelial surface, the keratinocytes undergo continuous differentiation and specialization. The many

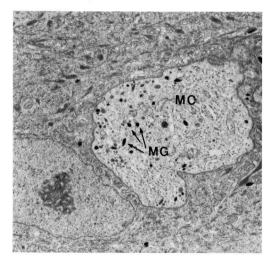

Fig. 1-25.

bodies and clusters of glycogen containing granula start to occur. Such granula are believed to be related to the synthesis of keratin.

Fig. 1-27 is a photomicrograph of the stratum granulosum and stratum corneum. Keratohyalin granula (arrows) are seen in the stratum granulosum. There is often an abrupt transition of the cells from the stratum granulosum to the stratum corneum. This is indicative of the keratinization of the cytoplasm of the keratinocyte and its conversion into an "acellular" structure bordered by a cell membrane. The cytoplasm of the cells in the stratum corneum (SC) is filled with keratin and the entire apparatus for

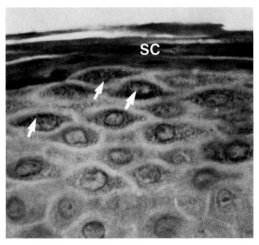

Fig. 1-27.

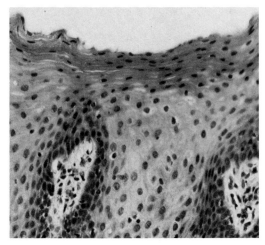

Fig. 1-28.

protein synthesis and energy production, i.e. the nucleus, the mitochondria, the endoplasmic reticulum, the Golgi complex is lost. In parakeratinized epithelia, however, the cells of the stratum corneum contain remnants of nuclei. Keratinization is considered as a process of differentiation rather than degeneration. It is a process of protein synthesis which requires energy and is dependent on functional cells, i.e. cells containing a nucleus and a normal set of organelles.

In summary:
The keratinocyte undergoes continuous differentiation on its way from the basal layer to the surface of the epithelium. Thus, once the keratinocyte has left the basement membrane it can no longer divide but maintains a capacity for production of protein (tonofilaments and keratohyalin granules). In the granular layer, the keratinocyte is deprived of its energy and protein producing apparatus (probably by enzymatic breakdown) and is abruptly converted into a keratin filled cell which from the stratum corneum is shed from the tissue surface.

Fig. 1-28 illustrates a portion of the epithelium covering the alveolar (lining) mucosa. In contrast to the epithelium of the masticatory mucosa, the lining mucosa has

no stratum corneum. Notice that cells containing nuclei can be identified in all layers, from the basal layer to the surface of the epithelium.

The dentogingival epithelium
The tissue components of the dentogingival region achieve their final structural characteristics in conjunction with the eruption of the teeth. This is illustrated in Fig. 1-29.
a) When the enamel of the tooth is fully developed, the enamel-producing cells (ameloblasts) become reduced in height, produce a basal lamina and form, together with cells from the outer enamel epithelium, the so-called *reduced enamel epithelium* (RE). The basal lamina *(epithelial attachment lamina: EAL)* lies in direct contact with the enamel; the contact between this lamina and the epithelial cells is maintained by hemidesmosomes. The reduced enamel epithelium surrounds the crown of the tooth from the moment the enamel is properly mineralized until the tooth starts to erupt.
b) As the erupting tooth approaches the oral epithelium, the cells of the outer layer of the reduced enamel epithelium, as well as the cells of the basal layer of the oral

epithelium (OE), show increased mitotic activity (arrows); the former ameloblasts do not divide. The reduced enamel epithelium is gradually tranformed during tooth eruption into a *junctional epithelium.*

c) When the tooth has penetrated into the oral cavity, the reduced enamel epithelium and the oral epithelium fuse at the incisal edge of the tooth. Large portions immediately apical to the incisal area of the enamel are then covered by a junctional epithelium (JE) containing only few layers of cells. The cervical region of the enamel, however, is still covered by ameloblasts (AB) and outer cells of the reduced enamel epithelium.

d) During the later phases of tooth eruption, all cells of the reduced enamel epithelium are transformed into a junctional epithelium. This transformed epithelium is continuous with the oral epithelium and participates in the attachment between the tooth and the gingiva. The *secondary epithelial attachment,* produced by the basal cells of the junctional epithelium, is composed of the former *epithelial attachment lamina* and the hemidesmosomes of the basal cells of this junctional epithelium.

If the free gingiva is excised after the tooth has fully erupted, a new junctional epithelium and new attachment lamina, indistinguishable from the ones found following tooth eruption, will develop during healing. The fact that this new junctional epithelium and new attachment lamina have developed from the oral epithelium indicates that the cells of the oral epithelium possess the ability to differentiate into cells of junctional epithelium, and to synthesize and secrete basal lamina material.

Fig. 1-30 is a histological section cut through the border area between the tooth and the gingiva, i.e. the dentogingival region. The enamel (E) is to the left. Towards the right follow the junctional epithelium (JE), the oral sulcular epithelium (OSE) and the oral epithelium (OE). The junctional epithelium differs morphologically from the oral sulcular epithelium and oral epithelium, while the two latter are structurally very similar. The junctional epithelium is widest in its coronal portion (about 15-20 cell layers), but becomes thinner towards the cemento-enamel junction (CEJ).

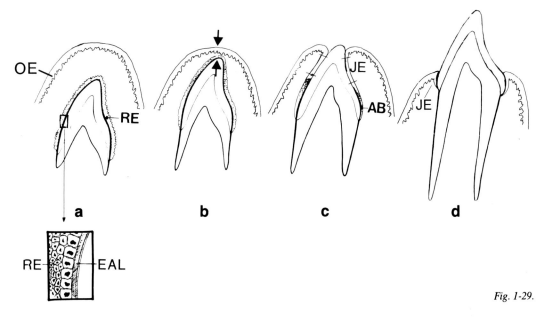

Fig. 1-29.

31

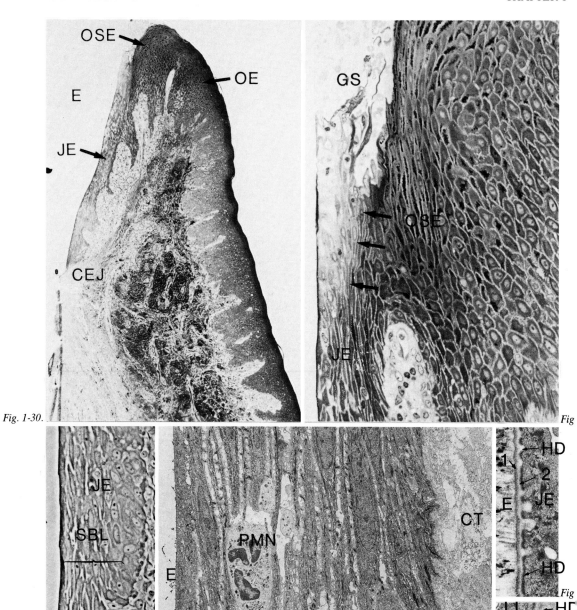

Fig. 1-30.

Fig

Fig. 1-32a.   *Fig. 1-32b.*   *Fig. 1-32d.*

Fig. 1-31. The junctional epithelium has a free surface at the bottom of the *gingival sulcus* (GS). It is from this surface that the epithelial cells of the junctional epithelium are desquamated. Like the oral sulcular epithelium and the oral epithelium, the junctional epithelium is continuously renewed through cell division in the basal layer. The cells migrate to the base of the gingival sulcus from where they are shed. The border between the junctional epithelium (JE) and the oral sulcular epithelium (OSE) is indicated by arrows. The cells of the oral sulcular epithelium are cuboid and the surface of this epithelium is keratinized.

Fig. 1-32 illustrates different characteristics of the junctional epithelium.

Fig. 1-32a shows that the cells of the junctional epithelium (JE) are arranged into one basal layer (BL) and several suprabasal layers (SBL).

Fig. 1-32b. The basal cells as well as the suprabasal cells are flattened with their long axis parallel to the tooth surface. (CT = connective tissue, E = enamel space).

There are distinct differences between the oral sulcular epithelium, the oral epithelium and the junctional epithelium:
1) the size of the cells in the junctional epithelium is, relative to the tissue volume, larger than in the oral epithelium
2) the intercellular space in the junctional epithelium is, relative to the tissue volume, comparatively wider than in the oral epithelium
3) the number of desmosomes is smaller in the junctional epithelium than in the oral epithelium.

Note the comparatively wide intercellular spaces between the oblong cells of the junctional epithelium, and the presence of 2 neutrophilic granulocytes (PMN) which are traversing the epithelium.

The framed area (A) is shown in a higher magnification in Fig. 1-32c, from which it can be seen that the basal cells of the junctional epithelium are not in direct contact with the enamel (E). Between the enamel and the epithelium (JE) one electron lucent zone (1) and one electron dense zone (2) can be seen. The electron lucent zone is in contact with the cells of the junctional epithelium (JE). These 2 zones have a structure very similar to that of the lamina densa (LD) and lamina lucida (LL) in the basement membrane area (i.e. the epithelium (JE) – connective tissue (CT) interface) described in Fig. 1-32d. Furthermore, the cell membrane of the junctional epithelial cells, both towards the enamel and the connective tissue, harbors hemidesmosomes (HD). Thus, the interface between the enamel and the junctional epithelium is similar to the interface between the epithelium and the connective tissue.

Fig. 1-33 is a schematic drawing of the most apically positioned cell in the junctional epithelium. The enamel (E) is depicted to the left in the drawing. It can be seen that the electron dense zone (2) between the junctional epithelium and the enamel can be considered as a continuation of the lamina densa (LD) in the basement membrane. Similarly, the electron lucent zone (1) can be considered as a continuation of the lamina lucida (LL). It should be noticed, however, that in variance with the epithelium connective tissue interface, there are no anchoring fibers (AF) attached to the lamina densa-like structure. However, like the basal cells adjacent to the basement membrane (at the connective tissue interface), the cells of the junctional epithelium facing the lamina lucida, harbor hemidesmosomes. Thus, the interface between the junctional epithelium and enamel is structurally very similar to the epithelium connective tissue interface, which means that the junctional epithelium is not only in contact with the enamel but is actually physically attached to the tooth via hemidesmosomes.

The connective tissue
The predominant tissue component of the

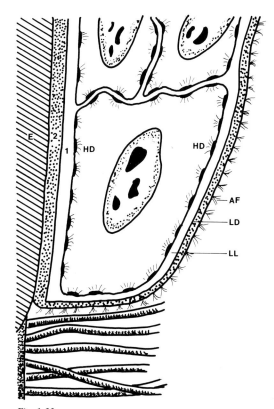

Fig. 1-33.

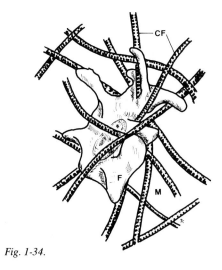

Fig. 1-34.

gingiva and periodontal ligament is the connective tissue. The major components of the
connective tissue are *collagen fibers* (around
60% of connective tissue volume), *fibroblasts* (around 5%), *vessels, nerves* and *matrix* (around 35%).

Fig. 1-34. The drawing illustrates a fibroblast
(F) residing in a network of connective tissue
fibers (CF). The intervening space is filled
with matrix (M) which constitutes the "environment" for the cell.

Cells
The different types of cell present in the connective tissue are a) fibroblasts, b) mast
cells, c) macrophages, d) neutrophilic granulocytes, e) lymphocytes and f) plasma cells.

Fig. 1-35. *The fibroblast* is the most predominant connective tissue cell (65% of the total
cell population). The fibroblast is engaged in
the production of various types of fibers
found in the connective tissue, but is also
instrumental in the synthesis of the connective tissue matrix. The fibroblast is a spindle
shaped or stellate cell. Fig. 1-35 shows part
of a fibroblast in electron microscopic magnification. The cytoplasm contains a well
developed granular endoplasmic reticulum
(E) with ribosomes. The Golgi complex (G)
is usually of considerable size and the
mitochondria (M) are large and numerous.
Furthermore, the cytoplasm contains many
fine tonofilaments (F). Adjacent to the cell
membrane, all along the periphery of the
cell, a large number of vesicles (V) can be
found.

Fig. 1-36. The *mast cell* is responsible for the
production of certain components of the
matrix. This cell also produces vasoactive
substances, which can affect the function of
the microvascular system and control the
flow of blood through the tissue. Fig. 1-36
presents a mast cell in electron microscopic
magnification. The cytoplasm is characterized by the presence of a large number of
vesicles (V) of varying size. These vesicles
contain biologically active substances such

as proteolytic enzymes, histamin and heparin. The Golgi complex (G) is well developed, while rough surface endoplasmic reticulum structures are scarce. A large number of small cytoplasmic projections, i.e. microvilli (MV), can be seen along the periphery of the cell.

Fig. 1-37. The *macrophage* has a number of different phagocytic and synthetic functions in the tissue. Fig. 1-37 shows a macrophage in electron microscopic magnification. The nucleus is characterized by numerous invaginations of varying size. A zone of electron dense chromatin condensations can be seen along the periphery of the nucleus. The Golgi complex (G) is well developed and numerous vesicles (V) of varying size are present in the cytoplasm. Rough surface endoplasmic reticulum (E) is scarce, but a certain number of free ribosomes (R) are evenly distributed in the cytoplasm. Remnants of phagocytosed material are often found in lysosomal vesicles: phagosomes (PH). In the periphery of the cell a large number of microvilli of varying size can be seen.

The macrophage as well as the mast cell is actively involved in the defense of the tissue against foreign and/or irritating substances.

Besides fibroblasts, mast cells and macrophages, the connective tissue also contains undifferentiated mesenchymal cells, the function of which is not properly understood.

The connective tissue also harbors *inflammatory cells* of various types, for example neutrophilic granulocytes, lymphocytes and plasma cells.

Fig. 1-38. The *neutrophilic granulocytes* (see Chapter 5), also called *polymorphonuclear leukocytes* (Fig. 1-38a), have a characteristic appearance. The nucleus is lobulate and numerous lysosomes (L), containing lysosomal enzymes, are found in the cytoplasm.

The *lymphocytes* (Fig. 1-38b.) are characterized by an oval to spherical nucleus containing localized areas of electron dense chromatin. The narrow border of cytoplasm

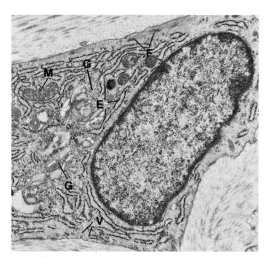

Fig. 1-35.

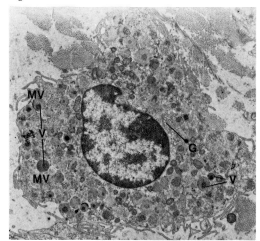

Fig. 1-36.

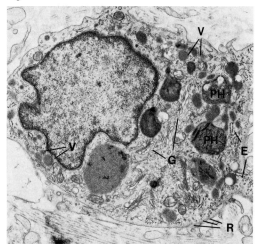

Fig. 1-37.

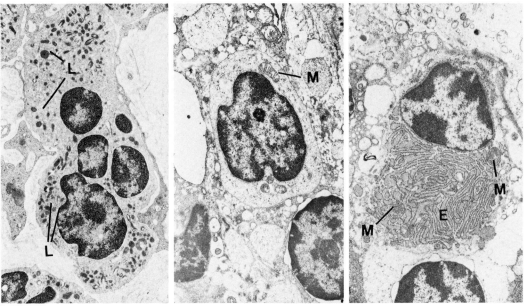

Fig. 1-38a.   *Fig. 1-38b.*   *Fig. 1-38c.*

surrounding the nucleus contains numerous free ribosomes, a few mitochondria (M) and in localized areas endoplasmic reticulum with fixed ribosomes. Lysosomes are also present in the cytoplasm.

The *plasma cells* (Fig. 1-38c) contain an eccentrically located spherical nucleus with radially deployed electron dense chromatin. Endoplasmic reticulum (E) with numerous ribosomes is found randomly distributed in the cytoplasm. In addition, the cytoplasm contains numerous mitochondria (M) and a well developed Golgi complex.

Fibers
The connective tissue fibers are produced by the fibroblasts and can be divided into: a) *collagen fibers,* b) *reticulin fibers,* c) *oxytalan fibers,* and d) *elastic fibers.*

Fig. 1-39. The *collagen fibers* predominate in the gingival connective tissue and they comprise the most essential components of the periodontium. The electron micrograph shows cross- and longitudinal sections of collagen fibers. The collagen fibers have a characteristic cross-banding with a period-

icity of 700 Å between the individual dark bands.

Fig. 1-40 illustrates some important features of the production and the compositon of col-

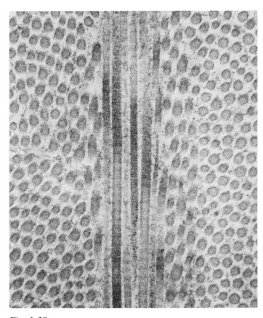

Fig. 1-39.

36

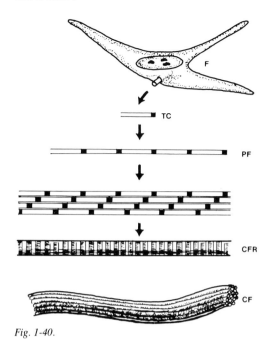

Fig. 1-40.

mately 700 Å occurs under light microscopy. The collagen fibers (CF) are bundles of collagen fibrils, aligned in such a way that the fibers also exhibit a cross-banding with a periodicity of 700 Å. In the tissue, the fibers are usually arranged in bundles. As the *collagen fibers* mature, covalent cross-links are formed between the tropocollagen molecules resulting in an age-related reduction in collagen solubility. *Cementoblasts* and *osteoblasts* also possess the ability to produce collagen.

Fig. 1-41. Reticulin fibers – as seen in this photomicrograph – exhibit argyrophilic staining properties and are numerous in the tissue adjacent to the basement membrane (arrows). However, reticulin fibers also occur in large numbers in the loose connective tissue surrounding the blood vessels.

lagen fibers. (F = fibroblast). The smallest unit, the collagen molecule, is often referred to as *tropocollagen*. A tropocollagen molecule (TC) which is seen in the upper portion of the drawing is approximately 3000 Å long and has a diameter of 15 Å. It consists of 3 polypeptide chains intertwined to form a helix. Each chain contains about 1,000 amino acids. One third of these are glycine and about 20% proline and hydroxyproline, the latter being almost only found in collagen. Tropocollagen synthesis takes place inside the fibroblasts from which the tropocollagen molecule is secreted into the extracellular space. Thus, the polymerization of tropocollagen molecules to collagen fibers takes place in the extracellular compartment. First, tropocollagen molecules are aggregated longitudinally to *protofibrils* (PF), which are subsequently laterally aggregated in parallel to *collagen fibrils* (CFR), with an overlapping of the tropocollagen molecules by about 25% of their length. Due to the fact that special refraction conditions develop after staining at the sites where the tropocollagen molecules adjoin, a cross-banding with a periodicity of approxi-

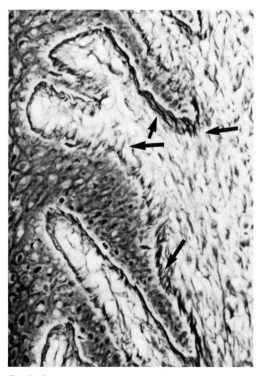

Fig. 1-41.

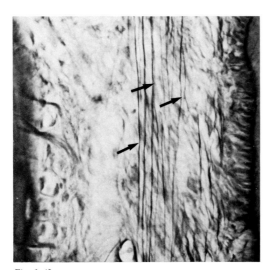

Fig. 1-42.

Thus, reticulin fibers are present at the epithelium connective tissue and the endothelium connective tissue interfaces.

Fig. 1-42. Oxytalan fibers are present in all connective tissue structures of the periodontium and seem to be composed of long thin fibrils with a diameter of approximately 150 Å. The photomicrograph illustrates them (arrows) in the periodontal ligament, where they have a course mainly parallel to the long axis of the tooth. The function of these fibers is as yet unknown.

Fig. 1-43. Elastic fibers are only present in the connective tissue of the gingiva and periodontal ligament in association with blood vessels. However, in the connective tissue of the alveolar (lining) mucosa, elastic fibers are numerous. In this photomicrograph they can be seen in the loose alveolar mucosa (arrows). The gingiva (G) seen coronal to the mucogingival junction (MGJ) contains no elastic fibers.

Fig. 1-44. Although many of the collagen fibers in the gingiva and periodontal ligament are irregularly or randomly distributed, most tend to be arranged in groups of bund-

les with a distinct orientation. According to their insertion and course in the tissue, the oriented bundles in the gingiva can be divided into the following groups:

a) *Circular fibers* (CF) are those fiber bundles which run their course in the free gingiva and encircle the tooth in a cuff- or ring-like fashion.

b) *Dentogingival* fibers (DGF) are embedded in the cementum of the supraalveolar portion of the root and project from the cementum in a fan-like configuration out into the free gingival tissue of the facial, lingual and interproximal surfaces.

c) *Dentoperiosteal fibers* (DPF) are embedded in the same portion of the cementum as the dentogingival fibers, but run their course apically over the vestibular and lingual bone crest and terminate in the tissue of the attached gingiva. In the border area between the free and attached gingiva, the epithelium often lacks support by underlying oriented collagen fiber bundles. In this area the free gingival groove (GG) is often present.

d) *Transseptal fibers* (TF), seen on the drawing to the right, extend between the supra-alveolar cementum of approximating teeth. The transseptal fibers run straight across the interdental septum

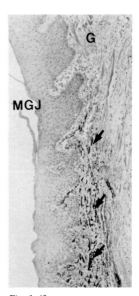

Fig. 1-43.

38

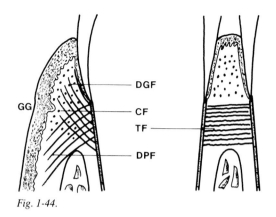

Fig. 1-44.

and are embedded in the cementum of adjacent teeth.

Fig. 1-45 illustrates in a histological section the orientation of the transseptal fiber bundles (arrows) in the supraalveolar portion of the interdental area. It should be observed that the transseptal fibers also connect the supraalveolar cementum (C) with the crest of the alveolar bone (AB). The 4 groups of collagen fiber bundles reinforce the interdental papilla and provide the resilience and tone which is necessary for maintaining its architectural form.

Matrix
The matrix of the connective tissue is first produced by the fibroblasts, although some constituents are produced by mast cells, and other components are derived from the blood. The matrix is the medium in which the connective tissue cells are embedded and is essential for the maintenance of the normal function of the connective tissue. Thus, the transportation of water, electrolytes, nutrients, metabolites, etc., to and from the individual, connective tissue cells occurs within the matrix. The main constituents of the connective tissue matrix are protein-polysaccharide macromolecules. These complexes are normally differentiated into *proteoglycans* and *glycoproteins*. The *proteoglycans* contain glycosaminoglycans as

the polysaccharide units (chondroitin sulfate etc.) which, via covalent bonds, are attached to one or more protein chains. The polysaccharide component is always predominant in the proteoglycans. The glycosaminoglycan called "hyaluronic acid" is probably not bound to protein. The *glycoproteins* also contain polysaccharides, but these macromolecules are different from glycosaminoglycans. The protein component is predominating in glycoproteins. In the macromolecules, mono- or oligosaccharides are, via covalent bonds, connected with one or more protein chains.

Fig. 1-46a. Normal function of the connective tissue depends on the presence of proteoglycans and glycosaminoglycans. The polysaccharide moiety of the proteoglycan, the glycosaminoglycans, are large, flexible, chain formed, negatively charged molecules, each of which occupies a rather large space.

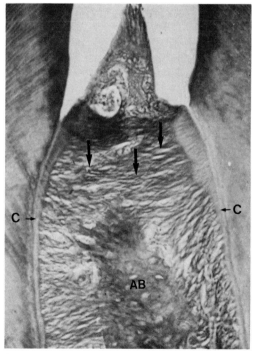

Fig. 1-45.

Fig. 1-46b. In such a space, smaller molecules, e.g. water and electrolytes, can be incorporated while larger molecules ($\mathbb{RR}$) are prevented from entering. The proteoglycans thereby regulate diffusion and fluid flow through the matrix and are important determinants for the fluid content of the tissue and the maintenance of the osmotic pressure. In other words the proteoglycans act as a molecule filter and, in addition, play an important role in the regulation of cell migration (movements) in the tissue.

Fig. 1-46c. Due to their structure and hydration, the macromolecules exert resistance towards deformation, thereby serving as regulators of the consistency of the connective tissue. If the gingiva is suppressed, the macromolecules become deformed. When the pressure is eliminated the macromolecules regain their original form. Thus, the macromolecules are of importance for the resilience of the gingiva.

Epithelial differentiation
There are many examples of the fact that during the embryonic development of vari-ous organs, a mutual inductive influence occurs between the epithelium and the connective tissue. The development of the teeth is a characteristic example of such phenomena. The connective tissue is on the one hand a determining factor for a normal development of the tooth bud while, on the other, the enamel epithelia exert a definite influence on the development of the mesenchymal components of the teeth. It has been suggested that tissue differentiation in the adult organism can be influenced by environmental factors. The skin and mucous membranes for instance often display increased keratinization and hyperplasia of the epithelium in areas which are exposed to mechanical stimulation. Thus, the tissues seem to adapt to environmental stimuli. The presence of keratinized epithelium on the masticatory mucosa has been considered to represent an adaptation to mechanical irritation released by mastication. However, research has demonstrated that the characteristic features of the epithelium in such areas are genetically determined. Some pertinent observations are reported in the following:

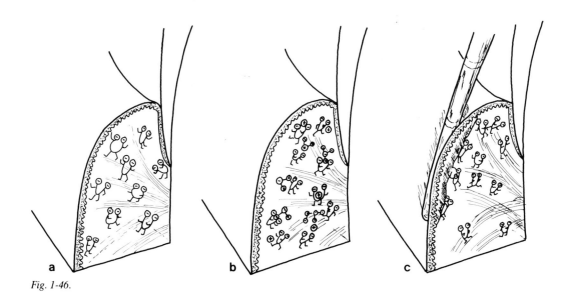

Fig. 1-46.

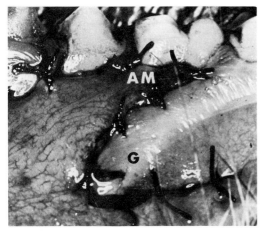

Fig. 1-47.

Fig. 1-47 shows an area in a monkey where the gingiva (G) and the alveolar mucosa (AM) have been transposed by a surgical procedure. The alveolar mucosa is placed in close contact with the teeth while the gingiva is positioned in the area of the alveolar mucosa.

Fig. 1-48 shows the same area 4 months later. Despite the fact that the transplanted gingiva (G) is movable in relation to the underlying bone, like an alveolar mucosa, it has retained its characteristic, morphological features of a masticatory mucosa. How-

ever, a narrow zone of new keratinized gingiva (NG) has regenerated between the alveolar mucosa (AM) and the teeth. The alveolar mucosa (AM) is interposed between the transplanted gingiva (G) and the newly formed gingiva (NG).

Fig. 1-49 presents a histological section cut through the transplanted gingiva seen in Fig. 1-48. Since elastic fibers are lacking in the gingival connective tissue (G), but are numerous in the connective tissue of the alveolar mucosa (AM), the transplanted tissue can readily be identified. The epithelium covering the transplanted gingival tissue exhibits a distinct keratin layer on the surface and also the configuration of the epithelium connective tissue interface (i.e. rete pegs and connective tissue papillae) is similar to that of normal nontransplanted gingiva. Thus, the heterotopically located gingival tissue has maintained its original specificity. *This observation demonstrates that the characteristics of the gingiva are genetically determined rather than being the result of functional adaptation to environmental stimuli.*

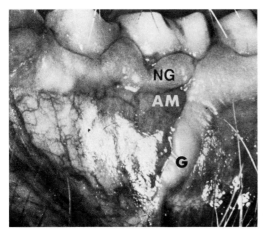

Fig. 1-48.

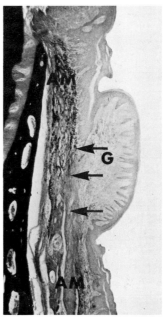

Fig. 1-49.

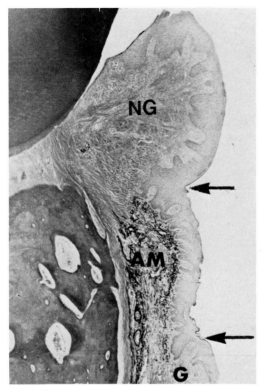

Fig. 1-50.

Fig. 1-50 shows a histological section cut through the coronal portion of the area of transplantation. The transplanted gingival tissue (G) shown in Fig. 1-49 can be seen in the lower portion of the photomicrograph. The alveolar mucosa transplant (AM) is seen between the arrows in the middle of the illustration. After surgery, the alveolar mucosa was positioned in close contact with the teeth as seen in Fig. 1-47. After healing, a narrow zone of keratinized gingiva (NG) developed coronally to the alveolar mucosa transplant (see Fig. 1-48). This new zone of gingiva (NG), seen in the upper portion of the histological section, is covered by keratinized epithelium and the connective tissue contains no dark-stained elastic fibers. In addition, it is important to notice that the junction between keratinized and nonkeratinized epithelium corresponds exactly to the junction between "elastic" and "nonelastic" connective tissue. The connective tissue

of the new gingiva has regenerated from the connective tissue of the supraalveolar area and periodontal ligament and has separated the alveolar mucosal transplant from the tooth. It is most probable that the epithelium which covers the new gingiva has migrated from the adjacent epithelium of the alveolar mucosa.

Fig. 1-51 presents a schematic drawing of the development of the new, narrow zone of keratinized gingiva (NG) seen in Figs. 1-48 and 1-50.
a) Granulation tissue has proliferated coronally along the root surface (arrow) and has separated the alveolar mucosa transplant (AM) from its contact with the tooth surface.
b) Epithelial cells have migrated from the alveolar mucosal transplant (AM) onto the newly formed gingival connective tissue. Thus, the newly formed gingiva has become covered with a keratinized epithelium (KE) which has originated from the nonkeratinized epithelium of the alveolar mucosa (AM). This implies that the newly formed gingival connective tissue (NG) possesses the ability to induce changes in the differentiation of the

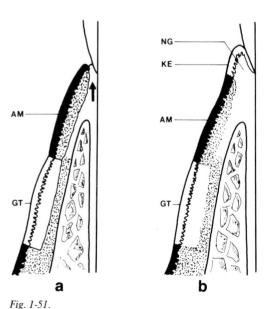

Fig. 1-51.

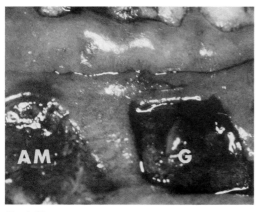

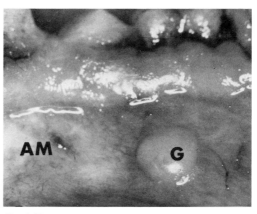

Fig. 1-52.   *Fig. 1-53.*

epithelium originating from the alveolar mucosa. This epithelium which is normally nonkeratinized, apparently, differentiates to keratinized epithelium because of stimuli arising from the newly formed gingival connective tissue. (*Gingival transplant*: GT.)

Fig. 1-52 illustrates a portion of gingival connective tissue (G) and alveolar mucosal connective tissue (AM) which, after a particular transplantation, has healed into wound areas in the alveolar mucosa. Epithelialization of these transplants can only occur through migration of epithelial cells from the surrounding alveolar mucosa.

Fig. 1-53 shows the transplanted gingival connective tissue (G) after reepithelialization. This tissue portion has attained an appearance similar to that of the normal gingiva, indicating that this connective tissue is now covered by keratinized epithelium. The transplanted connective tissue from the alveolar mucosa (AM) is covered by nonkeratinized epithelium and has the same appearance as the surrounding alveolar mucosa.

Fig. 1-54a-c presents 2 histological sections through the area of the transplanted gingival connective tissue. The section shown in Fig.1-54a is stained for elastic fibers

(arrows), the tissue in the middle which contains none is the transplanted gingival connective tissue (G). Fig. 1-54b shows an adjacent section stained with hematoxylin and eosin. By comparing a and b it can be seen that:

1) the transplanted gingival connective tissue is covered by keratinized epithelium (between arrows)
2) the epithelium-connective tissue-interface has the same wavy course (i.e. rete pegs and connective tissue papillae) as seen in normal gingiva.

The photomicrographs seen in Figs. 1-54c and 1-54d illustrate, at a higher magnification, the border area between the alveolar mucosa (AM) and the transplanted gingival connective tissue (G). Note the relationship between keratinized epithelium and "inelastic" connective tissue, and between nonkeratinized epithelium and "elastic" connective tissue (arrows). This relationship implies that the transplanted gingival connective tissue possesses the ability to alter the differentiation of epithelial cells as previously suggested (Fig. 1-51). From being nonkeratinizing cells, the cells of the epithelium of the alveolar mucosa have evidently become keratinizing cells. *This means that the specificity of the gingival epithelium is determined by genetical factors inherent in the connective tissue.*

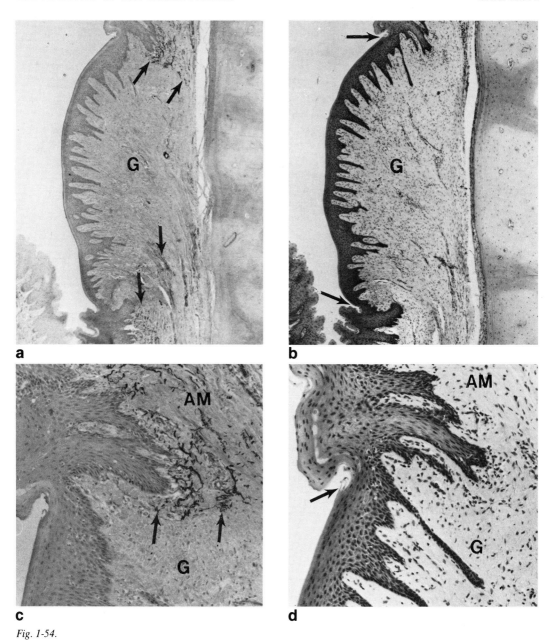

a

b

c

d

Fig. 1-54.

The periodontal ligament

The periodontal ligament is the soft connective tissue which surrounds the roots of the teeth and joins the root cementum and the alveolar bone.

Fig. 1-55 is a radiograph of a mandibular pre-molar-molar region. The periodontal ligament is included in the space between the roots (R) of the teeth and the alveolar bone (AB) which surrounds the tooth to a level approximately 1 mm apical to the cemento-

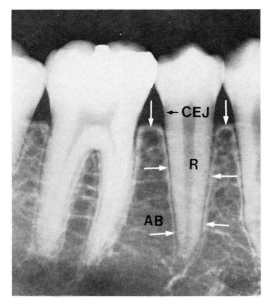

Fig. 1-55.

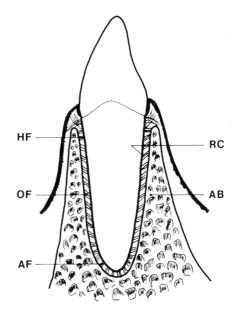

Fig. 1-56.

enamel junction (CEJ). Radiographically, 2 types of alveolar bone can be distinguished: the part of the bone which covers the alveolus and the marginal border of the alveolar process is called the *cortical bone,* and as a radiopaque line (arrows) sometimes referred to as the *"lamina dura".* The portion of the alveolar process which is delineated by the "lamina dura" is made up of *cancellous bone* which appears radiographically as a meshwork. The periodontal ligament is continuous with the supraalveolar connective tissue and communicates with the marrow space of the alveolar bone. The periodontal ligament space has the shape of an hourglass and is narrowest at the mid-root level. The width of the periodontal ligament is approximately 0.25 mm ± 50%. The presence of a periodontal ligament is essential for the mobility of the teeth. Tooth mobility is to a large extent (see Chapter 12) determined by the width, height and quality of the periodontal ligament.

Fig. 1-56 illustrates in a schematic drawing how the periodontal ligament is positioned between the alveolar bone (AB) and the root cementum (RC). The tooth is joined to the bone by bundles of collagen fibers which can be divided into the following main groups:
1) Horizontal fibers (HF)
2) Oblique fibers (OF)
3) Apical fibers (AF)

Fig. 1-57. The periodontal ligament and the root cementum develop from the loose connective tissue (the follicle) which surrounds the tooth bud. The schematic drawing depicts the various stages in the organization of the periodontal ligament which forms concomitantly with the development of root and the eruption of the tooth.
a) The tooth bud is formed in a crypt of the bone. The collagen fibers produced by the fibroblasts in the loose connective tissue of the tooth bud are, during the process of their maturation, embedded into the newly formed cementum immediately apical to the cemento-enamel junction (CEJ). The fibers fasciculate, oriented towards the coronal portion of the bone crypt. These fiber bundles will later form the *dentogingival fiber group,*

45

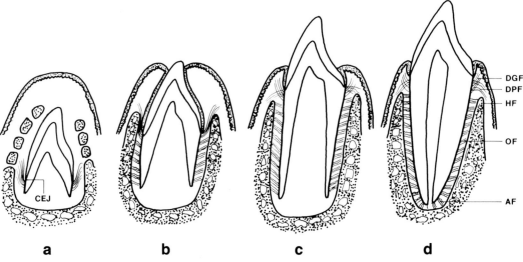

Fig. 1-57.

the *dentoperiosteal fiber group* and the *transseptal fiber group* which belong to the oriented fibers of the gingiva (see Fig. 1-44).

b) The true periodontal ligament fibers, the *principal fibers* develop in conjunction with the eruption of the tooth. First fibers can be identified which are entering the most marginal portion of the alveolar bone.

c) Later, more apically positioned bundles of oriented collagen fibers are seen.

d) The orientation of the collagen fiber bundles alters continuously during the phase of tooth eruption. First, when the tooth has reached contact in occlusion and is in proper function, the fibers of the periodontal ligament associate into groups of well oriented *dentoalveolar collagen fibers:*

1) Horizontal fibers,
2) Oblique fibers,
3) Apical fibers (see Fig. 1-56)

Fig. 1-58. This schematic drawing illustrates the development of the principal fibers of

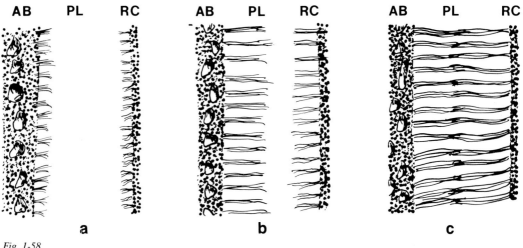

Fig. 1-58.

the periodontal ligament. The alveolar bone (AB) is seen to the left, the periodontal ligament (PL) is depicted in the center and the root cementum (RC) is seen to the right.

a) First small, fine, brush-like fibrils are detected arising from the root cementum and projecting into the PL space. The surface of the bone is, at this stage, covered by osteoblasts. From the surface of the bone only a small number of radiating, thin, collagen fibrils can be seen.

b) Later on, the number and thickness of fibers entering the bone increase. These fibers radiate towards the loose connective tissue in the mid-portion of the periodontal ligament area (PL), which contains more or less randomly oriented, collagen fibrils. The fibers originating from the cementum are still short while those entering the bone gradually become longer. The terminal portions of these fibers carry finger-like projections.

c) The fibers originating from the cementum, subsequently increase in length and thickness and fuse in the periodontal membrane space with the fibers originating from the alveolar bone. When the tooth, following eruption, reaches contact in occlusion and starts to function, the principal fibers become organized in bundles and run continuously from the bone to the cementum.

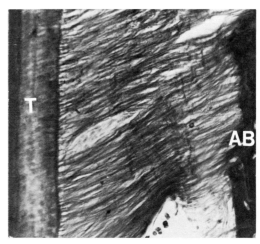

Fig. 1-59.

Fig. 1-59 illustrates how the principal fibers of the periodontal ligament run continuously from the tooth (T) to the alveolar bone (AB). The individual bundles have a slightly wavy course which allows the tooth to move within its socket – physiological mobility. The principal fibers, embedded in the cementum, have a smaller diameter but are more numerous than those embedded in the alveolar bone.

Fig. 1-60a shows the presence of small clusters of epithelial cells (arrows) in the periodontal ligament. These cells, called the *"rests of Mallassez"*, represent remnants of the *epithelial sheath of Hertwig*. The "rests of Mallassez" are situated in the periodontal

ligament at a distance of 15-75 μm from the root surface. A group of such cells is seen in a higher magnification in *Fig. 1-60b*.

Fig. 1-61. Electron microscopically it can be seen that the "rests of Mallassez" are surrounded by a basement membrane (BM) and that the cell membranes of the epithelial cells exhibit the presence of desmosomes (D) as well as hemidesmosomes (HD). The epithelial cells contain only few mitochondria and have a poorly developed, endoplas-

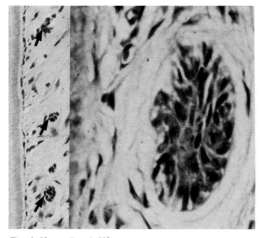

Fig. 1-60a.   Fig. 1-60b.

47

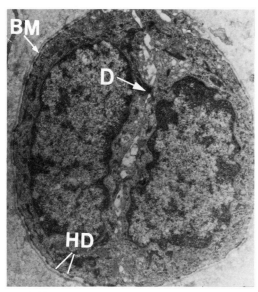

Fig. 1-61.

tooth. The "rests of Mallassez", which in ordinary histological sections appear as isolated groups of epithelial cells, form, in this specimen, a continuous network of epithelial cells surrounding the root; their function is presently unknown.

The root cementum

The cementum is a specialized calcified tissue covering the root surfaces and, occasionally, small portions of the crown of the teeth. It has many features in common with bone tissue; however, the cementum (1) contains no blood or lymph vessels, (2) has no innervation, (3) does not undergo physiological resorption and remodelling, but *is* characterized by continuing deposition throughout life. Cementum serves different functions. It attaches the periodontal ligament fibers to the root and contributes to the process of repair after damage to the root surface. Two different types of cementum are recognized:

1) *primary cementum* or *acellular cementum* which forms in conjunction with root formation and tooth eruption
2) *secondary cementum* or *cellular cementum* which forms after tooth eruption and in response to functional demands.

mic reticulum. This means that they are vital, but resting, cells with minute metabolism.

Fig. 1-62 is a photomicrograph of a periodontal ligament removed from an extracted

Fig. 1-63 shows a portion of the periodontal ligament. The root cementum (RC) which is in contact with the root dentin to the left is called the *primary cementum*. This primary cementum contains no cells and is thus also denoted *acellular cementum*. This primary or acellular cementum is formed concomitantly with the formation of the root dentin and in the presence of the epithelial sheath of Hertwig. During tooth formation the epithelial sheath of Hertwig, which lines the newly formed predentin, is broken. The epithelial cells migrate into the loose, connective tissue lateral of the tooth bud. Fibroblasts from this loose, connective tissue, occupy the area next to the predentin and produce a layer of randomly oriented, collagen fibrils which make contact with, but do not enter, the newly formed dentin. The fi-

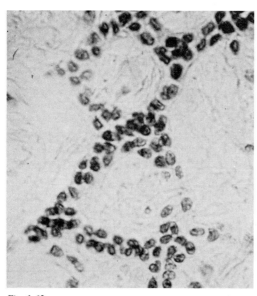

Fig. 1-62.

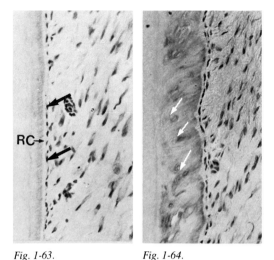

Fig. 1-63.   Fig. 1-64.

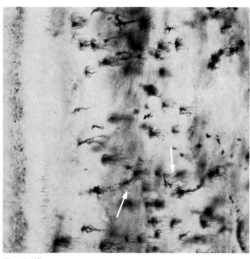

Fig. 1-65.

broblasts differentiate into cementoblasts and remain on the lateral surface of the cementoid.

Fig. 1-64 describes the structure of the *secondary cementum* which, in contrast to the primary cementum, contains cells. This structure is also called *cellular cementum.* Secondary or cellular cementum is laid down on top of the primary cementum throughout the functional period of the tooth. It is often only found on the intra-alveolar part of the root. Both cellular and acellular cementum are produced by cementoblasts. Some of these cells (arrows) become incorporated into the cementoid, subsequently calcifying to form cementum. The cells which are incorporated in the cementum are called *cementocytes.*

Fig. 1-65 illustrates how cementocytes (black cells) reside in lacunae in cellular cementum. They are linked together by cytoplasmic processes (arrows) running in canaliculi in the cementum. The cementocytes are also, via cytoplasmic processes, linked with the cementoblasts on the surface. The presence of cementocytes allows transportation of nutrients through the

cementum, and contributes to the maintenance of the vitality of this mineralized tissue.

Fig. 1-66a is a photomicrograph of a horizontal section through the periodontal ligament (PL) in an area where the root is covered with acellular cementum (AC). The portions of the principal fibers which are embedded in the root cementum and in the alveolar bone (AB) are called *Sharpey's fibers.* A major portion of the acellular cementum consists of Sharpey's fiber bundles which have become mineralized. In the photomicrograph it can be seen that these often start close to the cementodentin junction (arrows). In the acellular cementum they have a smaller diameter and are more densely packed than those in the alveolar bone. During the continuous formation of acellular cementum portions of the periodontal ligament fibers (principal fibers) adjacent to the root become embedded with mineral crystals, i.e. mineralized. Thus, the Sharpey's fibers in the cementum should be regarded as a direct continuation of the collagen fibers in the supraalveolar connective tissue and the periodontal ligament (Fig. 1-66b). The Sharpey's fibers form the so-called

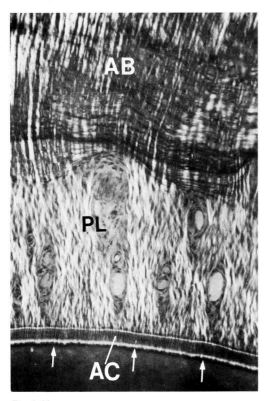

Fig. 1-66a.

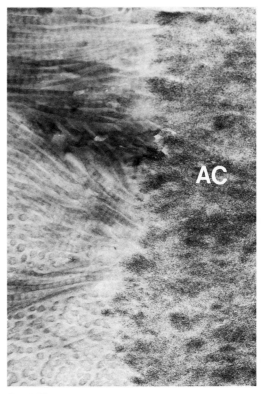

Fig. 1-67.

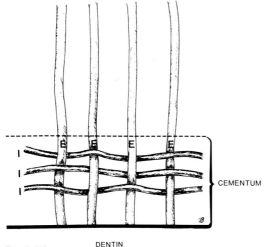

Fig. 1-66b.

extrinsic fiber system (E) of the cementum and are produced by fibroblasts in the periodontal ligament. The *intrinsic fiber system* (I) is produced by cementoblasts and is composed of fibers oriented, more or less, parallel to the long axis of the root.

Fig. 1-67 shows principal fibers entering acellular cementum (AC). The characteristic cross-banding of the collagen fibers is masked in the cementum because apatite crystals have become deposited in the fiber bundles during the process of mineralization.

Fig. 1-68. In contrast to the bone, the cementum (C) contains no nerves and no blood or lymph vessels. The cementum does not exhibit alternating periods of resorption and apposition, but increases in thickness throughout life by deposition of successive new layers of tissue. During this process of gradual apposition, the particular portion of the principal fibers which resides immediately adjacent to the root surface becomes calcified. Mineralization occurs by the deposition of hydroxyapatite crystals, first

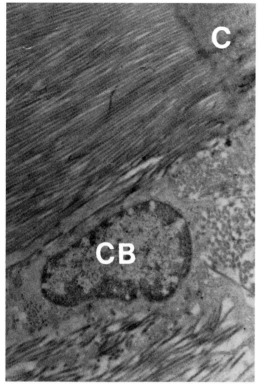

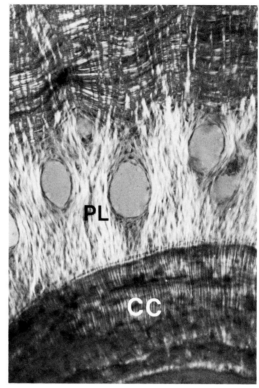

Fig. 1-68.   *Fig. 1-69.*

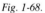

within the collagen fibers, later upon the fiber surface and finally in the interfibrillar matrix. Fig. 1-68 shows a cementoblast (CB) located near the surface of the cementum and between 2 inserting principal fiber bundles. Generally the acellular cementum is more properly mineralized than the cellular cementum. Sometimes only the periphery of the Sharpey's fibers of the *cellular cementum* is calcified, leaving an uncalcified core.

Fig. 1-69 is a photomicrograph showing a horizontal section through the periodontal ligament (PL) in an area where the root surface is covered with cellular cementum (CC). This cementum, which is formed after the termination of tooth eruption and often in response to functional demands, is densely packed with coarse collagen fibrils oriented parallel to the root surface (intrin-

sic fiber system) and Sharpey's fibers (extrinsic fibre system) which run more or less perpendicularly to the cementodentin junction. These Sharpey's fibers, which are thicker and more dispersed than those in the acellular cementum, continue as principal fibers, undisrupted from the cementum into the periodontal ligament. The cementoid on the surface increases in thickness by gradual apposition throughout life and is considerably more pronounced in the apical portion of the root than in the cervical portion where the thickness is only 20-50 μm while in the apical root portion it is often 150-250 μm.

The alveolar bone

The alveolar processes develop in conjunction with the development and eruption of the teeth and are gradually resorbed if the

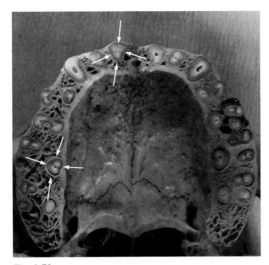

Fig. 1-70.

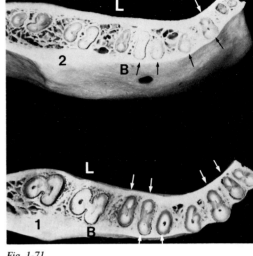

Fig. 1-71.

teeth are lost. Thus, the alveolar processes are tooth dependent structures. Together with the root cementum and the periodontal membrane fibers, the alveolar bone comprises the supporting tissue of the teeth, and distributes and resolves generated forces, e.g. mastication and other tooth contacts.

Fig. 1-70 illustrates a cross-section through the alveolar process of the maxilla at the mid-root level of the teeth. Note that the bone which covers the root surfaces is considerably thicker at the palatal than at the buccal aspect of the jaw. The walls of the sockets are lined by *compact* bone (arrows) which interproximally is connected with mainly *cancellous* bone. The cancellous bone contains bone trabeculae, the architecture and size of which are partly genetically determined and partly the result of the forces to which the teeth are exposed during function.

Fig. 1-71 shows cross-sections through the mandibular alveolar process at levels corresponding to the coronal 1) and apical 2) thirds of the roots. The compact bone lining the wall of the sockets is often continuous with the compact or *cortical* bone at the lingual (L) and buccal (B) aspects of the alveolar

process (arrows). Note how the bone on the buccal and lingual aspects of the alveolar process varies in thickness from one region to another. In the incisor and premolar regions, the cortical bone plate at the buccal aspect of the teeth is considerably thinner than at the lingual aspect. In the molar region, the bone is thicker at the buccal than at the lingual aspect.

Fig. 1-72 presents vertical sections through various regions of the mandibular dentition. The bone plate at the buccal and lingual aspects of the teeth varies considerably in thickness, e.g. from the premolar to the molar region. Note, for instance, how the presence of the oblique line (*linea obliqua*) results in a shelf-like, bone process (arrows) at the buccal aspect of the second and third molars.

Fig. 1-73 shows a section through the periodontal ligament (PL), tooth (T), and the alveolar bone (AB). The compact bone, that in a radiograph (Fig. 1-55) appears as "lamina dura" (LD), lines the tooth socket and is perforated by numerous *Volkmann's canals* (arrows) through which blood vessels and nerves pass from the alveolar bone (AB) to the periodontal ligament (PL). The layer

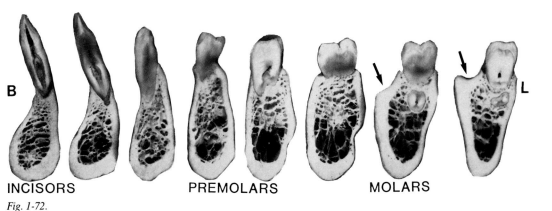

INCISORS   PREMOLARS   MOLARS

Fig. 1-72.

of bone into which the Sharpey's fiber bundles are inserted is called *"bundle bone"* and lies at the inner surface of the bony wall of the socket. Thus, from a functional point of view this "bundle bone" has many features in common with the cementum layer on the root surfaces.

Fig. 1-74. The alveolar process starts to form early in fetal life, with mineral deposition at small foci in the mesenchymal matrix surrounding the tooth buds. These small cal-

cified areas increase in size, fuse, become resorbed and remodelled until a continuous mass of bone has formed around the fully erupted teeth. The outer surface of the bone is always lined with a nonmineralized zone of tissue, an *osteoid* which in turn is covered by the *periosteum*. The periosteum contains *collagen fibers, osteoblasts* and *osteoclasts*. The marrow spaces inside the bone are lined with *endosteum* which has many features in common with the periosteum at the outer surface of the bone. The photomicrograph in

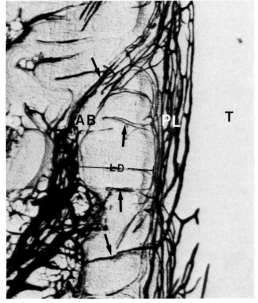

Fig. 1-73.

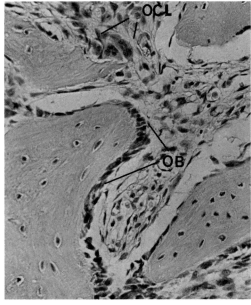

Fig. 1-74.

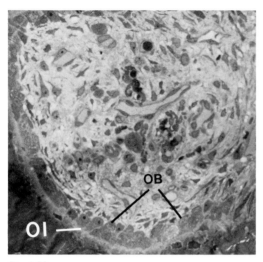

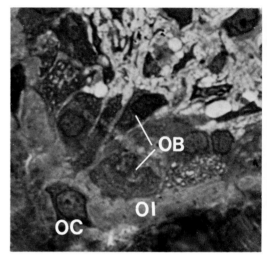

Fig. 1-75.   *Fig. 1-76.*

Fig. 1-74 illustrates the presence of bone forming osteoblasts (OB) and bone resorbing osteoclasts (OCL) in the endosteum.

Fig. 1-75. Osteoblasts and osteoclasts are present in the following areas:
1) On the surface of the bone trabeculae in cancellous bone
2) On the outer surface of cortical bone which delineates the jaws
3) In the sockets towards the periodontal membrane
4) On the inside of the cortical bone towards the marrow spaces.

In the photomicrograph of Fig 1-75 osteoblasts (OB) reside on the surface of a bone trabecula. The osteoblasts produce osteoid (OI) consisting of collagen fibers and a matrix which contains mainly glycoproteins and proteoglycans. This bone matrix or osteoid (OI) undergoes calcification by the deposition of minerals which are subsequently transformed to hydroxyapatite.

Fig. 1-76. During the process of maturation and calcification of the osteoid some of the osteoblasts (OB) are trapped in the osteoid (OI) as seen in this photomicrograph. Cells which are present in the osteoid, and later on

in the calcified bone tissue, are termed *osteocytes* (OC).

Fig. 1-77. Osteocytes (OC) resident in lacunae in calcified bone are linked to each other and to osteoblasts on the bone surface through cytoplasmic processes running in canaliculi (arrows). The drawing in *Fig. 1-78* illustrates how osteoblasts (OB) and osteocytes (OC) are linked to each other by cyto-

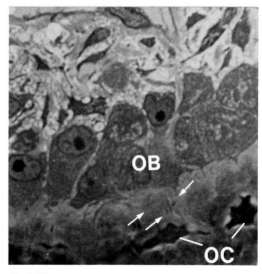

Fig. 1-77.

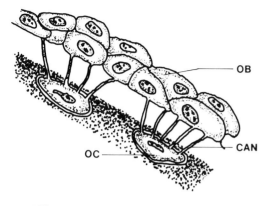

Fig. 1-78.

the bone. The surface between the osteocytes with their cytoplasmic processes on the one side, and the calcified matrix on the other, is very large. It has been calculated that the interface between cells and matrix in a cube of bone, $10 \times 10 \times 10$ cm, amounts to approximately 250 m^2. This enormous surface of exchange serves as a regulator, e.g. for the serum calcium and the serum phosphate levels via hormonal control mechanisms.

plasmic processes running in canaliculi (CAN).

Fig. 1-79 illustrates an osteocyte residing in a lacuna in the bone. The cytoplasmic processes radiate in different directions.

Fig. 1-80 illustrates how the osteocytes (OC) make contact with each other via cytoplasmic processes running in canaliculi (CAN) in

Fig. 1-81 shows a horizontal section through the alveolar bone (AB), periodontal ligament (PL) and tooth (T). The nutrition of the bone is secured by the incorporation of blood vessels in the bone tissue. These blood vessels surrounded by bone lamellae, eventually constitute the center of an *osteon* (O). The central canal (which mainly contains the blood vessel) in an osteon is called the *Haversian canal* (HC). The osteon is also called a *Haversian system*. The blood vessels in the *Haversian canals* are connected with each other by anastomoses running in the *Volkmann's canals*. The alveolar bone is continually renewed in response to functional demands. The teeth erupt and migrate in mesial direction throughout life to compensate for attrition. Such movement of the

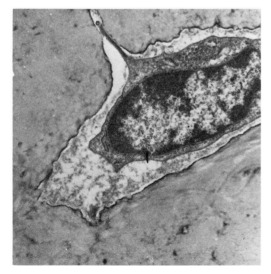

Fig. 1-79.

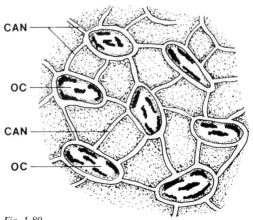

Fig. 1-80.

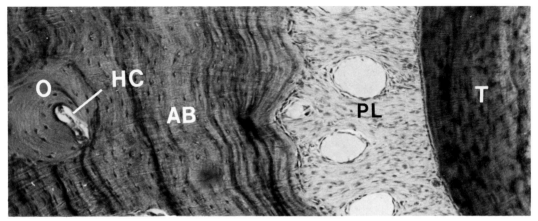

Fig. 1-81.

teeth implies remodelling of the alveolar bone. During the process of remodelling, the bone trabeculae are continuously resorbed and reformed and the cortical bone mass is dissolved and replaced by new bone. During breakdown of the cortical bone, resorption canals are formed by proliferating blood vessels. Such canals, which in their center contain a blood vessel, are subsequently refilled with new bone by the formation of lamellae arranged in concentric layers around the blood vessel. Thus, a new *Haversian system* (O), as seen in the photomicrograph, is established.

Fig. 1-82. The apposition of new bone is always associated with osteoblasts. These cells produce an osteoid which subsequently undergoes calcification. Osteolysis (i.e. breakdown of bone) is an active cellular process associated with osteoclasts, probably developed from blood monocytes. The photomicrograph demonstrates osteoclastic activity at the surface of the bone (AB) facing the periodontal ligament (PL). The osteoclasts (OCL) are multinucleated cells which frequently reside in so-called *Howship's lacunae* on the bone surface.

Fig. 1-83 shows an osteoclast (OCL) residing in a *Howship's lacuna* on the surface of the bone (B). The osteoclast resorbs organic as well as inorganic substance. The resorption occurs by the release of acid substances (lac-

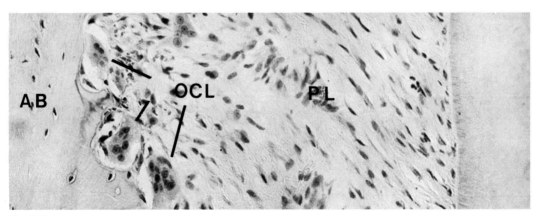

Fig. 1-82.

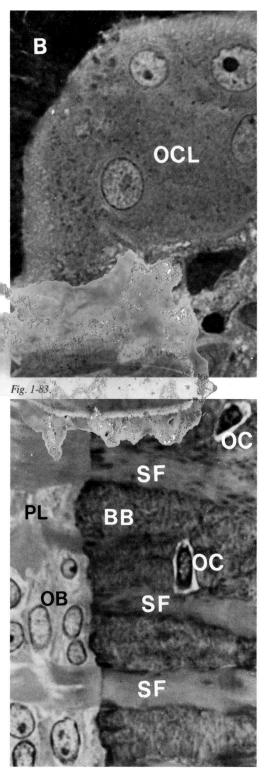

Fig. 1-83.

Fig. 1-84.

tic acid, etc.) which form an acidic environment in which the mineral salts of the bone tissue become dissolved. Remaining organic substances are eliminated by osteoclastic phagocytosis.

Fig. 1-84. Collagen fibers of the periodontal ligament (PL) are inserting in the mineralized bone which lines the wall of the tooth socket. This bone, which as previously described is called *bundle bone* (BB), has a high turnover rate. The portions of the collagen fibers which are inserted inside the bundle bone are called Sharpey's fibers (SF). These fibers are mineralized at their periphery, but often have a nonmineralized central core. The collagen fiber bundles inserting in the bundle bone generally have a larger diameter and are less numerous than the corresponding fiber bundles in the cementum on the opposite side of the periodontal ligament. Individual bundles of fibers can be followed all the way from the alveolar bone to the cementum. However, despite being in the same bundle of fibers, the collagen adjacent to the bone is always less mature than that adjacent to the cementum. The collagen on the tooth side has a low turn-over rate. Thus, while the collagen adjacent to the bone is renewed relatively fast, the collagen adjacent to the root surface is renewed slowly or not at all. Note the occurrence of osteoblasts (OB) and osteocytes (OC).

The blood supply of the periodontium

Fig. 1-85. The schematic drawing depicts the blood supply to the teeth and the periodontal tissues. The *dental artery* (a.d.) which is a branch of the *superior* or *inferior alveolar (dental) artery* (a.a.i) dismisses the *intraseptal artery* (a.i.) before it enters the tooth socket. The terminal branches of the intraseptal artery (*rami perforantes,* rr.p.) penetrate the lamina dura in canals at all levels of the socket. They anastomose in the

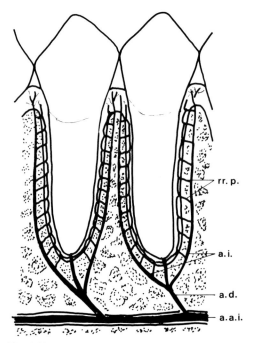

Fig. 1-85.

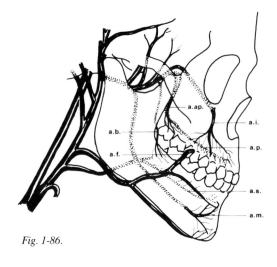

Fig. 1-86.

lary", artery) runs through the *greater palatine canal* (arrow) to the palate. As this artery runs in frontal direction it puts out branches which supply the masticatory mucosa of the palate.

Fig. 1-88. The various arteries are often considered to supply certain well defined regions of the dentition. In reality, however, there are numerous anastomoses present between the different arteries. Thus, the *entire system of blood vessels,* rather than individual groups of vessels, should be regarded as the unit supplying the soft and hard tissues of the maxilla and the mandible, e.g. in this figure there is an anastomosis (arrow) between the *facial artery* (a.f.) and the blood vessels of the mandible.

periodontal ligament space, together with blood vessels originating from the apical portion of the periodontal ligament and with other terminal branches, from the intraseptal artery (a.i.). Before the dental artery (a.d.) enters the root canal it puts out branches which supply the apical portion of the periodontal ligament.

Fig. 1-86. The gingiva receives its blood supply mainly through *supraperiosteal* blood vessels which are terminal branches of the *sub lingual artery* (a.s.), the *mental artery* (a.m.), the *buccal artery* (a.b.), the *facial artery* (a.f.), the *greater palatine artery* (a.p.), the *infra orbital artery* (a.i.) and the *posterior superior dental artery* (a.ap.).

Fig. 1-87 depicts the course of the greater palatine artery (a.p.) in a specimen of a monkey which at sacrifice was perfused with plastic. Subsequently, the soft tissue was dissolved. The greater palatine artery (a.p.) which is a terminal branch of the ascending *palatine artery* (from the *maxillary,* "internal maxil-

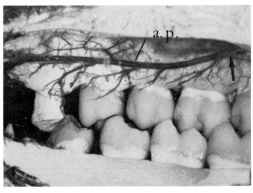

Fig. 1-87.

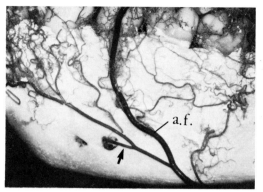

Fig. 1-88.

Fig. 1-89 illustrates a vestibular segment of the maxilla and mandible from a monkey which at sacrifice was perfused with plastic. Notice that the vestibular gingiva is supplied with blood mainly through supraperiosteal blood vessels (arrows).

Fig. 1-90. As can be seen, blood vessels (arrows) terminate at the alveolar bone crest. They originate from vessels in the periodontal ligament and contribute to the blood supply of the free gingiva.

Fig. 1-91 shows a specimen from a monkey which at the time of sacrifice was perfused with indian ink. Subsequently, the specimen was treated to make the tissue transparent (cleared specimen). To the right, the supraperiosteal blood vessels (sv) can be seen, which during their course towards the free gingiva put forth numerous branches to a subepithelial plexus (sp) located immediately beneath the oral epithelium of the free and attached gingiva. This subepithelial plexus in turn yields thin capillary loops to each of the connective tissue papillae projecting into the oral epithelium (OE). The number of such capillary loops is constant over a very long time and is not altered by application of epinephrine or histamine to the gingival margin. This implies that the blood vessels of the lateral portions of the gingiva, even under normal circumstances, are fully utilized and that the blood flow to the free gingiva is regulated entirely by velocity alterations. In the free gingiva, the supra-periosteal blood vessels (sv) anastomose with blood vessels from the periodontal ligament and the bone. To the left (in Fig. 1-91), beneath the junctional epithelium (JE), is a plexus of blood vessels termed the *dentogingival plexus* (dp). The blood vessels in this plexus have a thickness of approxi-

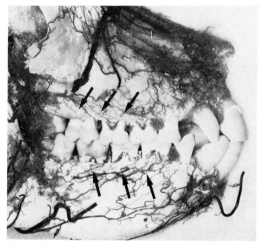

Fig. 1-89.

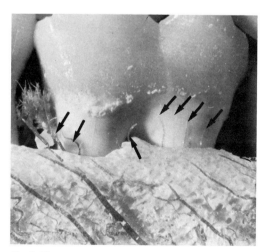

Fig. 1-90.

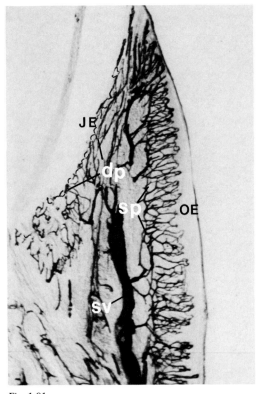

Fig. 1-91.

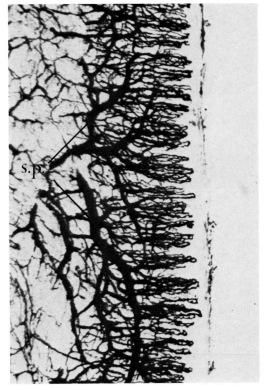

Fig. 1-92.

mately 40 μm which means that they are mainly venules. In healthy gingiva, no *capillary loops* are found in the dentogingival plexus.

Fig. 1-92. This figure illustrates how the subepithelial plexus (sp), beneath the oral epithelium of the free and attached gingiva, yields thin capillary loops to each connective tissue papilla. These capillary loops have a diameter of approximately 7 μm which means they have the size of true capillaries.

Fig. 1-93 illustrates the *dentogingival plexus* in a section cut parallel to the subsurface of the junctional epithelium. As can be seen, the dentogingival plexus consists of a fine-meshed network of blood vessels. In the upper portion of the picture, capillary loops can be detected belonging to the subepithelial plexus beneath the oral sulcular epithelium.

Fig. 1-94 is a schematic drawing of the blood supply to the free gingiva. As stated above, the main blood supply of the free gingiva is derived from the *supraperiosteal blood vessels* (sv) which in the gingiva, anastomose with blood vessels from the alveolar bone (ab) and periodontal ligament (pl). To the right in the drawing, the oral epithelium (OE) is depicted with its underlying subepithelial plexus of vessels (sp). To the left beneath the junctional epithelium (JE) the *dentogingival plexus* (dp) can be seen which, under normal conditions, is comprised of a fine-meshed network without capillary loops.

Fig. 1-95 illustrates a section prepared through a tooth (T) with its periodontium. Blood vessels (perforating rami; arrows) arising from the intraseptal artery in the alveolar bone run through canals (Volkmann's canals) in the socket wall (VC) into

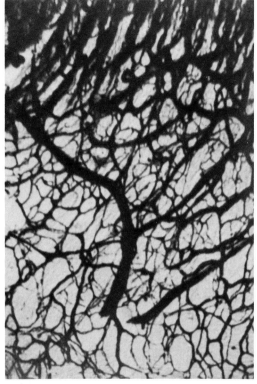

Fig. 1-93.

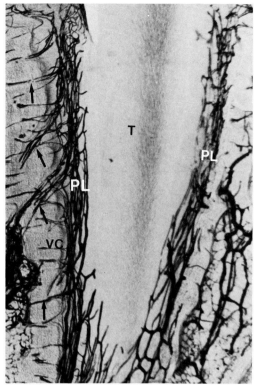

Fig. 1-95.

the periodontal ligament (PL) where they anastomose.

Fig. 1-96 shows the blood vessels in the periodontal ligament in a section cut parallel to the root surface. After entering the periodontal ligament, the blood vessels (perforating rami; arrows) anastomose and form a polyhedral network which surrounds the root like a stocking. The majority of the blood vessels in the periodontal ligament are found close to the alveolar bone. In the coronal portion of the periodontal ligament blood vessels run in coronal direction, passing the alveolar bone crest, into the free gingiva (see Fig. 1-90).

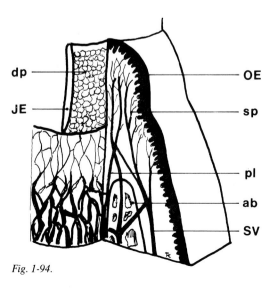

dp — — OE
JE — — sp
— pl
— ab
— SV

Fig. 1-94.

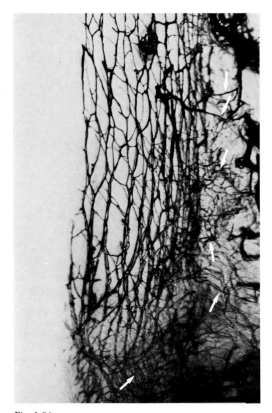

Fig. 1-96.

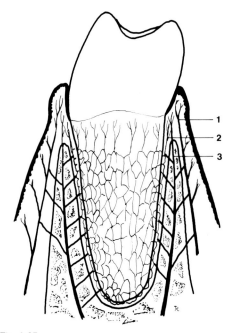

Fig. 1-97.

Fig. 1-97 is a schematic drawing of the blood supply of the periodontium. The blood vessels in the periodontal ligament form a polyhedral network surrounding the root. Note that the free gingiva receives its blood supply from 1) supraperiosteal blood vessels, 2) the blood vessels of the periodontal ligament and 3) the blood vessels of the alveolar bone.

Fig. 1-98 illustrates schematically, the so-called "extravascular" circulation through which nutrients and other substances are carried to the individual cells and metabolic products removed from the tissue. In the arterial (A) end of the capillary, to the left in the drawing, a hydraulic pressure of approximately 35 mm Hg is maintained as a result of the pumping function of the heart. Since the hydraulic pressure is higher than the osmotic pressure (OP) in the tissue (which is approximately 30 mm Hg), a transportation of substances will occur from the blood vessels to the extravascular space (ES). In the venous (V) end of the capillary system, to the right in the drawing, the hydraulic pressure has decreased to approximately 25 mm Hg (i.e. 5 mm lower than the osmotic pressure in the tissue). This allows a transportation of substances from the extravascular space to the blood vessels. Thus, the difference between the hydraulic pressure and the osmotic pressure results in a transportation of substances from the blood vessels to the

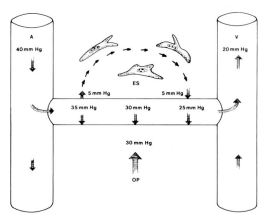

Fig. 1-98.

extravascular space in the arterial part of the capillary, while, in the venous part, a transportation of substances occurs from the extravascular space to the blood vessels. Hereby an extravascular circulation is established (arrows).

The lymphatic system of the periodontium

Fig. 1-99. The smallest lymph vessels, the *lymph capillaries,* form an extensive network in the connective tissue. The wall of the lymph capillary consists of a single layer of endothelial cells. For this reason such capillaries are difficult to identify in an ordinary histological section. The lymph is absorbed from the tissue fluid through the thin walls into the lymph capillaries. From the capillaries, the lymph passes into larger *lymph vessels* which are often in the vicinity of cor-

responding blood vessels. Before the lymph enters the blood stream it passes through one or more *lymph nodes* in which the lymph becomes filtered and supplied with lymphocytes. The lymph vessels are like veins provided with valves. The lymph from the periodontal tissues is drained to the lymph nodes of the head and the neck. The labial and lingual gingiva of the mandibular incisor region is drained to the *submental lymph nodes* (sme). The palatal gingiva of the maxilla is drained to the *deep cervical lymph nodes* (cp). The buccal gingiva of the maxilla and the buccal and lingual gingiva in the mandibular premolar-molar region are drained to *submandibular lymph nodes* (sma). Except for the third molars and mandibular incisors all teeth with their adjacent periodontal tissues are drained to the *submandibular lymph nodes* (sma). The third molars are drained to the *jugulodigastric lymph node* (jd) and the mandibular incisors to the *submental lymph nodes* (sme).

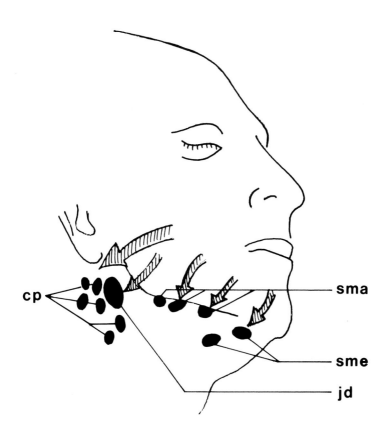

Fig. 1-99.

63

The nerves of the periodontium

Like other tissues in the body, the periodontium contains receptors which record pain, touch and pressure. The periodontal ligament, but not the gingiva, cementum and alveolar bone, also contains proprioceptors, giving information concerning movements and positions (i.e. deep sensibility). In addition to the different types of sensory receptors which belong to the somatic nervous system, nerve components are found innervating the blood vessels of the periodontium. Such nerve components belong to the autonomic nervous system. Nerves recording pain, touch, and pressure have their trophic center in the *semilunar ganglion,* while the proprioceptive nerves have the trophic center in the more centrally positioned *mesencephalic nucleus.* Both types of nerves

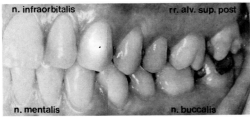

Fig. 1-100a.

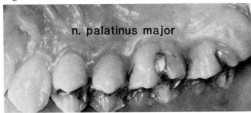

Fig. 1-100b.

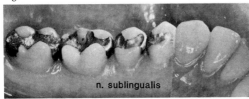

Fig. 1-100c.

are brought to the periodontium via the *trigeminal nerve* and its end branches. Due to the presence of receptors in the periodontal membrane, small forces applied on the teeth may be identified. For example, the presence of a very thin (10-30 μm) metal foil (strip) placed between the teeth during occlusion can readily be identified. It is also well known that a movement which brings the teeth of the mandible in contact with the occlusal surfaces of the maxillary teeth is arrested reflexively and altered into an opening movement if an inert particle is detected in the chew. Thus, the receptors in the periodontal ligament together with the proprioceptors in muscles and tendons, play an essential part in the regulation of chewing movements and chewing forces.

Fig. 1-100 shows the various regions of the gingiva which are innervated by end branches of the trigeminal nerve. The gingiva on the labial aspect of maxillary incisors, canines and premolars is innervated by *superior labial branches* from the *infraorbital nerve*, n. infraorbitalis (Fig. 1-100a). The buccal gingiva in the maxillary molar region is innervated by branches from the *posterior superior dental nerve*, rr. alv. sup. post. (Fig. 1-100a). The palatal gingiva is innervated by the *greater palatal nerve*, n. palatinus major (Fig. 1-100b), except for the area of the incisors which is innervated by the *long sphenopalatine nerve*, n. pterygopalatini. The lingual gingiva in the mandible is innervated by the *sublingual nerve*, n. sublingualis (Fig. 1-100c), which is an end branch of the *lingual nerve.* The gingiva at the labial aspect of mandibular incisors and canines is innervated by the *mental nerve*, n. mentalis, and the gingiva at the buccal aspect of the molars by the *buccal nerve*, n. buccalis (Fig. 1-100a). The innervation areas of these 2 nerves frequently overlap in the premolar region. The teeth in the mandible including their periodontal ligament are innervated by the *inferior alveolar nerve*, n. alveolaris inf., while the teeth in the maxilla are innervated by the *superior alveolar plexus*, n. alveolares sup.

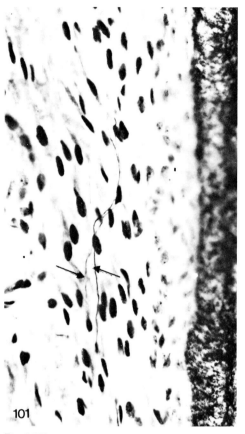

Fig. 1-101. The small nerves of the periodontium follow almost the same course as that of the blood vessels. The nerves to the gingiva run in the tissue superficial to the periosteum and put out several branches to the oral epithelium on their way towards the free gingiva. The nerves enter the periodontal membrane through the perforations (Volkmann's canals) in the socket wall. In the periodontal membrane, the nerves join larger bundles which take a course parallel to the long axis of the tooth. The photomicrograph illustrates small nerves (arrows) which have emerged from the larger bundles in order to supply certain parts of the periodontal ligament.

Fig. 1-101.

References:

Ainamo, J. & Talari, A. (1976) The increase with age of the width of attached gingiva. *Journal of Periodontal Research* **11,** 182-188.

Anderson, D. T., Hannam, A. G. & Matthews, G. (1970) Sensory mechanisms in mammalian teeth and their supporting structures. *Physiological Review* **50,** 171-195.

Carranza, F. A., Itoiz, M. E., Cabrini, R. L. & Dotto, C. A. (1966) A study of periodontal vascularization in different laboratory animals. *Journal of Periodontal Research* **1,** 120-128.

Egelberg, J. (1966) The blood vessels of the dento-gingival junction. *Journal of Periodontal Research* **1,** 163-179.

Fullmer, H. M., Sheetz, J. H. & Narkates, A. J. (1974) Oxytalan connective tissue fibers. A review. *Journal of Oral Pathology* **3,** 291-316.

Karring, T. (1973) Mitotic activity in the oral epithelium. *Journal of Periodontal Research, Suppl.* **13,** 1-47.

Karring, T., Lang, N. P. & Löe, H. (1974) The role of gingival connective tissue in determining epithelial differentiation. *Journal of Periodontal Research* **10,** 1-11.

Karring, T. & Löe, H. (1970) The three-dimensional concept of the epithelium-connective tissue boundary of gingiva. *Acta Odontologica Scandinavia* **28,** 917-933.

Karring, T., Ostergaard, E. & Löe, H. (1971) Conservation of tissue specificity after heterotopic transplantation of gingiva and alveolar mucosa. *Journal of Periodontal Research* **6,** 282-293.

Kvam, E. (1973) Topography of principal fibers.

Scandinavian Journal of Dental Research **81**, 553-557.

Listgarten, M. A. (1966) Electron microscopic study of the gingivo-dental junction of man. *American Journal of Anatomy* **119**, 147-178.

Listgarten, M. A. (1972) Normal development, structure, physiology and repair of gingival epithelium. *Oral Science Review* **1**, 3-67.

Lozdan, J. & Squier, C. A. (1969) The histology of the mucogingival junction. *Journal of Periodontal Research* **4**, 83-93.

Melcher, A. H. (1976) Biological processes in resorption, deposition and regeneration of bone. In *Periodontal Surgery, Biologic Basis and Technique,* ed. S.S. Stahl, pp. 99-120. Springfield: C. C. Thomas.

Page, R. C., Ammons, W. F., Schectman, L. R. & Dillingham, L. A. (1974) Collagen fiber bundles of the normal marginal gingiva in the marmoset. *Archives of Oral Biology* **19**, 1039-1043.

Schroeder, H. E. & Listgarten, M. A. (1971) *Fine Structure of the Developing Epithelial Attachment of Human Teeth.* 2nd ed., p. 146. Basel: Karger.

Schroeder, H. E. & Münzel-Pedrazzoli, S. (1973) Correlated morphometric and biochemical analysis of gingival tissue. Morphometric model, tissue sampling and test of stereologic procedure. *Journal of Microscopy* **99**, 301-329.

Schroeder, H. E. & Theilade, J. (1966) Electron microscopy of normal human gingival epithelium. *Journal of Periodontal Research* **1**, 95-119.

Schultz-Haudt, S. P. & Aas, E. (1962) Dynamics of the periodontal tissues. II. The connective tissue. *Odontologisk Tidsskrift* **70**, 397-428.

Selvig, K. A. (1965) The fine structure of human cementum. *Acta Odontologica Scandinavica* **23**, 423-441.

Selvig, K. A. (1968) Differences between cementum and bone tissue. *Norske Tannlaegeforenings Tidsskrift* **78**, 71-86.

Stallard, R. E. (1963) The utilization of H^3-proline by the connective tissue elements of the periodontium. *Periodontica* **1**, 185-188.

Valderhaug, J. P. & Nylen, M. U. (1966) Function of epithelial rests as suggested by their ultrastructure. *Journal of Periodontal Research* **1**, 67-78.

Epidemiology of Periodontal Disease

General principles in epidemiological research

The word epidemiology originally stands for the science of epidemics. In medicine, epidemiological methods are utilized for determining what proportion of the population, at a given time, is affected by a disease. In such studies the basic unit is the individual member of the community to be studied. With modern possibilities for automatic data processing, the results from epidemiological research have become of increasing importance in the planning and administration of health care.

Epidemiological methodology

Epidemiological research may have various objectives. One objective is to assess the treatment needs of a disease of known etiology. Especially when repeated at given time intervals, such studies can provide health care planners with valuable information about the need of manpower and other resources. Another objective may be to clarify the factors contributing to, or directly causing, the disease under study. In such cases, a simple clarification of disease prevalence is seldom sufficient. Instead, the full range of systematic epidemiological research may have to be utilized. The strategy of such an approach has been summarized by MacMahon et al. (1960) as follows:

1) *Descriptive epidemiology* – description of the distribution of disease, with comparison of its frequency in different populations and different segments of the same population.

2) *Formulation of hypotheses* – tentative theories designed to explain the observed distribution of the disease in terms of the most direct causal associations.

3) *Analytic epidemiology* – observational studies designed specifically to examine the hypotheses resulting from the descriptive studies.

4) *Experimental epidemiology* – experimental studies on human populations to stringently test those hypotheses which stand the test of observational and analytic studies.

A classic example of the utilization of the full range of epidemiological strategy in dentistry, is represented by the progressive research leading to the clarification of the role of fluorides in the frequency and prevention of dental caries. During the last few decades, the use of the same 4 stages of systematic epidemiological research has also given us our present knowledge of the directly causative and contributory factors of periodontal disease. A description of the various steps taken and achievements made in this progressive development may enhance the understanding of the need for the large variety of periodontal indices which are available in current dental literature.

Specific problems in dental epidemiology

In studies on the frequency and distribution of medical conditions such as tuberculosis, cardiac disease, etc., the number of subjects affected is given in per cent of the number of subjects examined. The problem in dentistry has been that, in many populations, practically all subjects have experienced either dental caries or periodontal disease, or both. Consequently, comparison of proportions of the population affected by these 2 oral diseases has proved to be of little value. Instead, researchers interested in the epidemiology of dental diseases have utilized individual teeth or tooth surfaces as the basic unit of examination and have analysed their data accordingly.

The simple and straightforward DMF Index for assessment of past caries experience has been successfully used since the 1930's. As a result, epidemiological data from different parts of the world is now available for those researchers and health administrators who are interested in oral health promotion, both locally and on a global basis. Already in the late 1940's Massler was concerned with the fact that there was no index system for periodontal disease, the simplicity and applicability of which could be compared with the DMF Index for past caries experience (Massler et al. 1950). To date, although some progress has been made, this concern still exists.

Epidemiology of periodontal disease

Before any periodontal indices had been developed, periodontal health was commonly classified as being good, medium or poor. This way of classifying the periodontal condition was used as late as the 1950's. Such subjective criteria did not permit results from different studies to be compared because the good ones in one group and with one examiner, could well be worse than the poor ones in another group with another examiner. The use of the criteria was strongly dependent on the interest and training of the examiner, as shown by prevalence rates for gingivitis which ranged from 8-98% in similar populations (see reviews by Schour & Massler 1947, Ramfjord 1959).

A review of currently available indices for the evaluation of periodontal health or disease reveals a confusing abundance of classification systems. Because it is difficult to choose an appropriate index from among the many which aim to measure periodontal disease and related factors, the individual investigator usually finds it laborious to perform a meaningful comparison of his own results with those of another investigator. The following review is an attempt to clarify the origin of some periodontal indices by presenting their purpose in the perspective of time. The intention is to demonstrate why so many different index systems have been considered necessary and how their use has assisted us to reach the degree of knowledge of periodontology which we have today.

Descriptive and analytic studies

The first well defined classification system for gingivitis was published by Schour & Massler (1947). These investigators examined the gingival conditions of children in post-war Italy. The essence of the PMA Index is to determine the number of (1) inflamed papillae (P), (2) gingival margins (M) and (3) areas of attached gingiva (A) at the labial surface of each anterior tooth (Fig.

Schour & Massler 1947

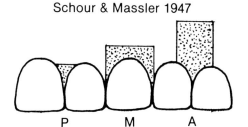

P   M   A

Fig. 2-1. Schour & Massler's PMA-index (1947) is based on recording of inflamed papillae (P), gingival margins (M) and areas of attached gingiva (A) on the facial aspects of anterior teeth.

2-1). The PMA Index was later modified by Parfitt (1957) and has been used extensively, particularly in the United States and Britain. Although limited to describe only gingivitis around anterior teeth, the PMA Index offered, for the first time, a possibility to compare prevalence and severity scores recorded from different populations.

In the 1950's WHO became interested in the assessment of periodontal disease in the Far East where caries at that time was not a major health problem. The PMA Index was inadequate for this purpose because it lacked criteria describing the amount of lost tooth attachment. A suitable instrument for the purpose was developed by Russell who published the Periodontal Index (PI) in 1956 (Fig. 2-2). In the epidemiological determination of periodontal health or disease the PI is probably the most widely used index. Its simple criteria are applied to each tooth in the mouth and scoring is performed as follows: a tooth with a healthy periodontium (0), gingivitis around only part of the tooth (1), gingivitis encircling the tooth (2), pocket formation (6) and loss of function due to excessive mobility (8). Mean PI scores for individuals and population groups have usually been used for describing the average severity of disease. It should be noted that due to the nature of its criteria the PI is a reversible scoring system, i.e. the individual can, following proper treatment, have his score lowered or reduced to 0.

In contrast to the PI, the Periodontal Disease Index (PDI) of Ramfjord (1959), when used to assess destructive disease, measures loss of tooth attachment instead of pocket depth. This particular part of the PDI includes an irreversible change which cannot be influenced by treatment. The main difference between the PI and the PDI is thus that the former records the need for treatment (periodontal disease status) while the latter scores the accumulated consequences of the disease (periodontal status). For example, with horizontal loss of alveolar bone support, the periodontal status of a given tooth would be the same before and after proper treatment.

Mainly by the use of the PI (Russell 1956), extensive data has been collected from populations all around the world. Analyses of the findings have revealed that differences in prevalence and severity of periodontal disease are associated with race, geographic area, sex, socioeconomic status, educational level, etc.

For proper understanding of the rapid development which has taken place within research on the epidemiological aspects of periodontal disease, it is important to realize that classification systems for the assessment of oral hygiene have existed for only 20 years. An oral hygiene classification was included in the PDI system (Ramfjord 1959). With the use of the better known Oral

Russell 1956

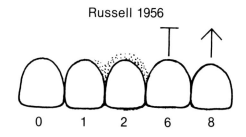

0   1   2   6   8

Fig. 2-2. Russell's Periodontal Index (PI) (1956) has been widely used for assessment of average severity of periodontal disease in large population groups. Scores 1 and 2 indicate gingivitis along part of or the total circumference of the tooth, score 6 indicates pathological pocketing and score 8 stands for loss of function due to excessive mobility.

Hygiene Index (OHI) of Greene & Vermillion (1960) it has been shown that all the apparent racial, geographic and other demographic differences in the severity of periodontal disease disappeared when disease levels were related directly to levels of oral hygiene (see reviews by Löe 1963, Scherp 1964, Waerhaug 1966). Russell himself suggested that the amount of plaque and calculus, together with the age of the group of subjects, may explain as much as 90% of their periodontal disease experience (Russell 1963).

The crude criteria of the OHI were based on 2 components: the coronal extension of plaque (Debris Index) and, likewise, the coronal extension of supragingival calculus and/or concurrent occurrence of subgingival calculus on the tooth surface (Calculus Index). A detailed description of the Oral Hygiene Index is presented in Fig. 2-3.

Greene & Vermillion 1960

Debris index (DI)

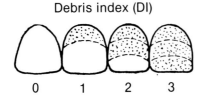

0   1   2   3

Calculus index (CI)

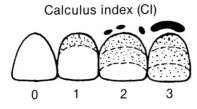

0   1   2   3

Fig. 2-3. The Oral Hygiene Index (OHI) consists of 2 separate components. The Debris Index (DI) measures coronal extension of soft deposits up to the first, second, or last third of the facial or lingual tooth surface. The Calculus Index (CI) measures the corresponding coronal extension of supragingival calculus and/or the presence of separate flecks or a continuous band of subgingival calculus. The OHI score is the sum of the DI and CI scores.

By means of descriptive and analytic studies it was possible to demonstrate that a strong positive correlation exists between increasing age and a progressive and irreversible loss of tooth attachment (Fig. 2-4). In diagrams representing disease levels of populations, the lines illustrating Russell's PI scores and the CI scores of the OHI increase in an almost parallel manner with advancing age. Up to about 40 years of age the CI score is slightly higher than the PI score. After 40 the calculus score starts to approach its maximum level whereas the periodontal disease score continues to progress (Fig. 2-4).

There are many difficulties in interpreting the results from cross-sectional epidemiological studies. One source of confusion has been the lack of correlation between plaque scores and the amount of attachment loss. The simple explanation is that all plaque indices, the debris component of the OHI included, measure only the amount of supragingival plaque. Comparisons between age groups indicate that the amount of supragingival plaque does not vary to any obvious extent with age (Fig. 2-5). A large amount of plaque on the teeth thus seems to reflect a permanent characteristic of the oral hygiene behavior of a particular individual rather than the end result of a life-long accumulation of microbial deposits. The oral hygiene level, as the concept is understood today, can not be expected to correlate to pocket formation and loss of alveolar bone. The steep ascent of the OHI scores with age (Fig. 2-5) is thus mainly due to the rapidly increasing scores for the calculus component (CI) of the OHI (Fig. 2-4).

During the past 2 decades ample evidence has accumulated of the existence of an inferior periodontal health situation in developing countries as compared with that observed in countries of the affluent western world. For example, the mean PI score of 206 Norwegian Army recruits was found to be 0.80 whereas a group of 281 University students of the same age in Ceylon scored as high as 1.14 (Waerhaug 1967). However, when the groups were reorganized according

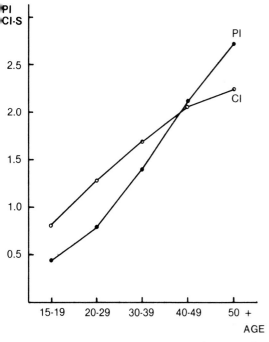

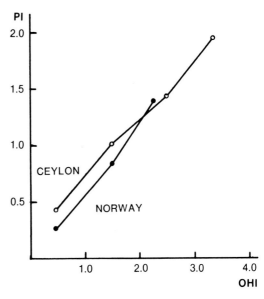

Fig. 2-4. On the population level the increase of Periodontal Index scores with age is found to correlate closely to a corresponding increase in the amount of dental calculus (Greene 1963).

Fig. 2-6. A close association between PI and OHI scores was demonstrated by Waerhaug (1967) in both Norwegian recruits ($\bar{x}$ PI = 0.80) and students of corresponding age in Ceylon ($\bar{x}$ PI = 1.14). The difference in disease level was thus due to different oral hygiene levels.

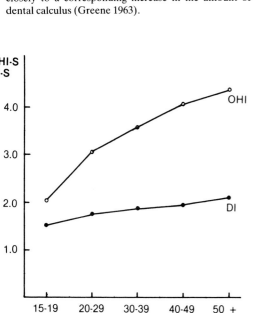

Fig. 2-5. That Oral Hygiene Index scores tend to increase with advancing age is mainly due to increasing Calculus Index scores (cf. Fig. 2-4). The Debris Index scores remain more or less constant through life (Greene 1963).

to their individual OHI and PI scores, no difference was found which could have been indicative of racial variations in tissue response to the suggested etiological agent (Fig. 2-6). Further comparisons between these 2 countries seem to confirm strongly the view that on a population level the amount of plaque and calculus found in the dentition is the discriminating factor for differences between levels of periodontal disease (Löe et al. 1978, Ånerud et al. 1979).

Experimental epidemiology

Both the OHI and its later modification OHI-S (Greene & Vermillion 1964) are rather crude indices, best suited for rapid screening of large population groups. Once the association between periodontal disease and oral hygiene had been demonstrated epidemiologically, an increasing interest in

71

experimental research and clinical trials developed. In most cases the objective of such trials was to evaluate the relative effectiveness of various therapeutic measures. For this purpose more sensitive index systems were required.

In attempts to measure the inhibition of calculus formation, the Calculus Surface Index (CSI) (Ennever et al. 1961) and the V-M Index (Volpe & Manhold 1962, Volpe et al. 1965) were developed. These indices were designed for use in clinical trials of short duration. The CSI measures the prevalence of calculus on the 4 surfaces of the 4 mandibular incisors (Fig. 2-7) and is recommended for studies of less than 8 weeks' duration, whereas the V-M Index measures the coronal extension of supragingival calculus on the lingual surfaces of the 6 mandibular anterior teeth (Fig. 2-8) and is suitable also for longer study periods (Mühlemann 1968). Both indices have been used for clinical evaluation of the effect of potential anticalculus agents (for review see Mühlemann 1968, Schroeder 1969).

In an attempt to quantify plaque removal with electric as compared to manual toothbrushes, Quigley & Hein (1962) found the criteria of the OHI too crude to differentiate between small changes in the amount of plaque. These investigators, therefore, added 2 criteria between scores 0 and 1 in the OHI system (Fig. 2-9).

At about the same time in Norway, Löe & Silness attempted to study the changes

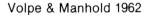
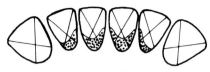

Volpe & Manhold 1962

V-M index in mm

Fig. 2-8. The V-M index was designed for assessment of the formation of supragingival calculus in long-term experiments. The amount of calculus is measured in mm along the 2 diagonal lines drawn over the lingual surface of each one of the lower anteriors. The score is expressed in mm of calculus.

occurring in the gingival tissues of pregnant women. For such a study, an index system was needed by which the most subtle changes could also be detected. The development and presentation of the Gingival Index (GI) system by Löe & Silness (1963) and the Plaque Index system (PlI) by Silness & Löe (1964) opened up a new era in experimental periodontology (Figs. 2-10a,b and 2-11).

In the PlI and GI system, separate recordings are made for the 4 smooth surfaces of each tooth. The maximum number of recordings made per subject thus increases from 28 tooth scores to $4 \times 28 = 112$ tooth surface scores. In the PlI system, the previous method of scoring the coronal extension of plaque was replaced by the assessment of plaque thickness at the gingival margin. In

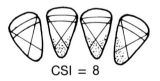

Ennever et al. 1961

CSI = 8

Fig. 2-7. The Calculus Surface Index (CSI) was designed for assessment of supragingival calculus formation during short-term experimental studies. Presence or absence of mineralized deposits is determined for the 4 surfaces of the mandibular incisors. The score per subject ranges from 0-16.

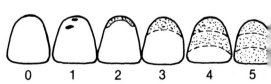

Quigley & Hein 1962

0   1   2   3   4   5

Fig. 2-9. For use in experimental studies Quigley & Hein (1962) augmented the OHI with 2 low scores between Greene & Vermillion's (1960) recordings 0 and 1.

the GI system, the extension of signs of inflammation around a part or the total circumference of the tooth (the basis of the gingivitis component of the PI) was replaced by 4 degrees of severity at each tooth surface. The scoring of signs of reversible gingival inflammation was no longer combined with an assessment of irreversible loss of tooth attachment as was the case in earlier periodontal indices. Also, the very name of the P1I system reflected the improved understanding at that time of the primarily bacterial character of the soft deposits, which earlier had commonly been denoted debris or materia alba.

By the use of the P1I and GI system it was possible to perform the well known and now classical study on "Experimental gingivitis in man" which definitely proved the direct cause and effect relationship between plaque and gingivitis (Löe et al. 1965).

The Gingival Index has later been modified with regard to the manner in which testing for bleeding tendency is performed. Originally, score 2 was given to a gingival unit if bleeding occurred after "pressure" (Löe & Silness 1963), as illustrated in Fig. 2-10a. This criterion was changed to bleeding after "probing" (Fig. 2-10b) by Löe in 1967. With both methods the probe is used for the detection of bleeding only when visible signs of inflammation are present in the marginal gingiva.

That gingivitis does not, in all cases, lead to progressive destruction of tooth attachment is a common finding in the clinic and has also been demonstrated in experimental studies (Lindhe et al. 1975). It is generally accepted, however, that dental calculus, in spite of epidemiological "evidence", is not the etiologic agent in progressive periodontal disease. The causative factor is the layer of viable microorganisms which always covers subgingival calculus deposits. The strong positive correlation which exists between the PI and CI scores in Fig. 2-4 thus results from the fact that the dental calculus is the retention factor for the subgingival plaque. For the recording of factors which contribute to gingival inflammation through plaque retention, yet another index was developed by Björby & Löe (1967). By the use of the Retention Index it became possible, on the 4

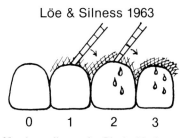

Löe & Silness 1963

0   1   2   3

Fig. 2-10a. According to the Gingival Index, severity of gingivitis is assessed separately at the 4 smooth surfaces of the tooth. Whenever the gingival margin looks inflamed, it is massaged with the side of the periodontal probe. If this massage does not result in bleeding, the unit scores 1; if bleeding occurs, score 2 is given. Ulceration and "spontaneous" bleeding scores 3.

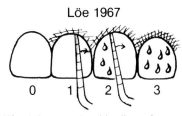

Löe 1967

0   1   2   3

Fig. 2-10b. Subsequently "bleeding after pressure" (Löe & Silness 1963, Fig. 2-10a) was replaced with "bleeding after probing" (Löe 1967). Currently presence or absence of bleeding (score 2) is determined after running a blunt probe along the soft tissue wall of the entrance of the gingival crevice.

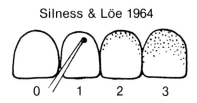

Silness & Löe 1964

0   1   2   3

Fig. 2-11. According to the Plaque Index, a tooth surface scores 0 when it is clean and 1 when it looks clean but material can be removed from its gingival third with a sharp explorer. Visible plaque scores 2 and a tooth surface covered with abundant plaque scores 3.

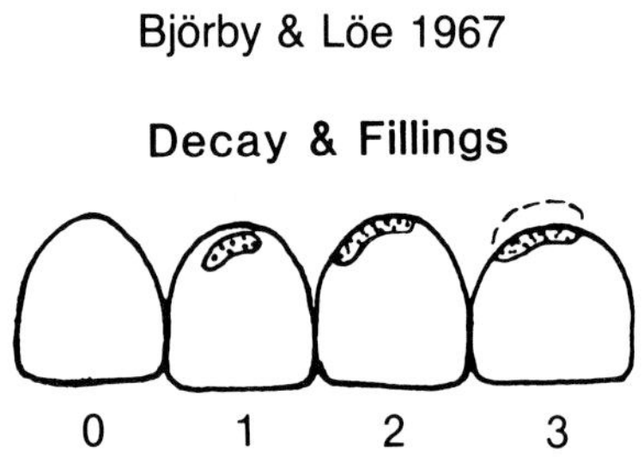

Björby & Löe 1967

Decay & Fillings

0   1   2   3

Fig. 2-12. The Retention Index has 3 components which can be used separately or combined. An open caries lesion or a defective margin of a filling or crown within the gingival third of the tooth surface is given score 1 when it does not make contact with the gingiva, score 2 when it contacts the gingival margin, and score 3 when it extends 1 mm or more beneath the gingiva.

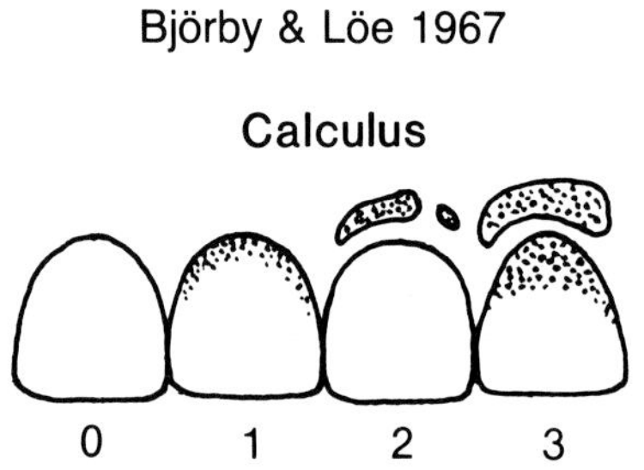

Björby & Löe 1967

Calculus

0   1   2   3

Fig. 2-13. The third component of the Retention Index measures calculus, also at the gingival margin only. A strand of mineralized material at the orifice of the pocket is given the same score as supragingival calculus (1). Subgingival calculus is given score 2 and presence of abundant calculus results in score 3 for the tooth surface.

surfaces of each tooth, to evaluate the degree of plaque retention caused by untreated carious lesions and fillings or crowns with defective gingival margins (Fig. 2-12), or by supra- or subgingivally located calculus deposits (Fig. 2-13).

In order to make the recording of the periodontal disease status complete, the Plaque Index, the Gingival Index, and the Retention Index should, according to Löe and collaborators, be augmented with measurements of pocket depth to the nearest mm (Glavind & Löe 1967).

By the end of the 1960's any previous doubts about the etiology of gingivitis and

the causes of periodontal tissue breakdown had been dispelled. In the 1970's, therefore, experimental periodontal research was directed mainly towards the clarification of the relative effects that could be obtained by different modalities for plaque control. By the use of the already available index systems it became possible to confirm more accurately the positive effect of oral hygiene measures on periodontal health, already reported by Lövdal et al. in 1961. In addition to the documentation of the preventive effect of periodontal treatment (Lightner et al. 1971, Suomi et al. 1971), the decisive role of personal oral hygiene combined with proper maintenance care in the form of regular professional cleaning of the patients' teeth was also clearly demonstrated by means of controlled longitudinal studies (Suomi et al. 1973, Ramfjord et al. 1975, Rosling et al. 1976, Axelsson & Lindhe 1981).

Individual variation

Epidemiological, clinical and laboratory research have shown, beyond doubt, that plaque and calculus are associated with gingivitis and periodontal tissue breakdown. Yet, in discussions with practising dentists, one is repeatedly told about the individual patient who has had abundant plaque, calculus and ill-fitting restorations for a lifetime, without evidence of destructive changes in the attachment apparatus. Another typical exception is the young patient with relatively good oral hygiene and advanced breakdown of the attachment of incisors and first molars. The very fact that such cases do not conform to generally accepted rules, makes them easy to remember. No doubt, both extremes exist. It should be realized, however, that they are in no way in conflict with epidemiological findings.

Epidemiological studies are expected to fulfil certain requirements. One of these is that the study group is representative of the population whose periodontal disease status is to be assessed. The requirement of representativeness means that each individual in the population should have an equal possibility to become included in the sample. Another requirement is that the sample is sufficient in size so that the effect of the exceptional case is eliminated. A simple example would be a study for determining whether men are taller than women. It is possible that the first woman measured is found to be taller than all the men and the other women in the sample. Only measurement of a large group of people will eventually eliminate the effect of this one giant lady, and thus give the expected result, i.e. that men *on an average* seem to be slightly taller than women.

In the individual patient, the degree of periodontal disease is not determined by the microbial plaque alone. The so-called "individual host response", which contains a number of immunological and other systemic components, is also of marked importance. According to the Plaque Principle the following equations can be used to simplify the relation between plaque and periodontal disease:

$$Gingivitis = \frac{Plaque}{Host\ response}$$

$$Periodontitis = Age \times \frac{Plaque}{Host\ response}$$

These equations indicate that a difference in quantity or quality of plaque results in different amounts of disease only when the host response is constant. On the other hand, similar amounts and compositions of bacterial deposits can develop more or less dramatic signs of gingivitis depending on individual differences in the tissue reaction of the host. For example, it has been shown in clinical trials that the deciduous dentition is extremely resistant to plaque (Mackler & Crawford 1973, Matsson 1978).

In the case of destructive periodontal disease, the duration of plaque irritation is an additional factor to be considered. Each individual seems to have a characteristic equilibrium between plaque irritation and host response. If this equilibrium is negative,

sooner or later periodontal disease will develop. In order to assess the host response of an individual it is, therefore, not sufficient to determine the amount or quality of the plaque or various plaque retentive elements. The additional explaining factor is the age of the patient. Loss of one third of the tooth attachment may indicate a fair host response if the patient is 50 years or older, whereas the same situation would be alarming in an individual aged 15-20 years.

The presence of a varying host response to plaque accumulation was already noted by Löe et al. (1965) in their experimental gingivitis study. All test subjects started the experiment with clean teeth and healthy gingivae. However, when all oral hygiene measures were disbanded, some subjects reached Gingival Index score 1.0 in 10 days and others in 21 days.

Indeed, it should be understood that correlations calculated from epidemiological studies can only indicate that *on an average* there seems to be a strong positive or negative association between a potential etiologic factor and the disease under study. Russell's argument, for instance, that 90% of all periodontal disease can be explained by oral hygiene and age, is valid only on a population level or in population groups which are large enough to eliminate the effect of variation between individuals (Fig. 2-14).

During recent years research in microbiology has indicated that the composition of supra- and subgingival plaque may be of decisive importance in the development of periodontal disease. Such a claim is difficult to confirm or reject by means of epidemiological research. The problem is similar to that of isolating the causative factor when a window is broken by throwing a stone: it is difficult to judge whether it was the weight of the stone or the weakness of the glass which caused the end result. In the field of dermatology it is well known that it is the susceptibility of the individual patient, rather than the presence of pathogenic fungi *per se,* which determines whether or not a dermatitis develops. The possibility thus remains that the presence of a certain type of

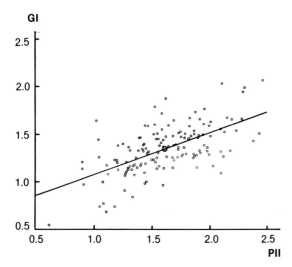

Fig. 2-14. The scatter diagram is based on the individual PlI and GI scores of 154 young adult males. Within the group the positive correlation between PlI and GI is quite high (r = 0.62). However, there are individuals with high GI and low PlI scores and vice versa (Ainamo 1970).

the 700 subjects with "worst periodontal disease status" was larger than the corresponding figure for all the remaining 2800 subjects.

The presentation of the data in this way certainly gives better information for use in treatment planning than do either average severity scores or simple prevalence rates.

In the identification of high susceptibility groups several different approaches can be utilized. Traditionally, on the basis of early epidemiological studies on large populations, the main interest has been to determine oral hygiene levels, i.e. quantification of the etiologic factor. Especially in preventive programs, plaque has thus been considered equal to early gingivitis. According to the study on young Finnish males (Fig. 2-15) a more realistic approach may be to assess susceptibility on the basis of already existing signs of pathology, such as bleeding ten-

bacterial flora in periodontal disease is the result, rather than the cause, of disease.

Identification of risk groups

Considering the fact that there are individuals who show minor or no signs of irreversible periodontal breakdown after life-long exposure to irritation from dental plaque, it seems important to try to utilize epidemiological methods to identify individuals with an unfavorable host response, i.e. individuals who are susceptible to periodontal disease.

In a recent survey of 3500 Finnish Army recruits, pockets with a depth of 4 mm or more were found in 11%, whereas a total of 73% of the recruits demonstrated gingival bleeding around one or more of the 14 teeth probed in the right half of the jaw (Ainamo et al. 1980). In a more detailed analysis, the group was organized into 10 subgroups of equal size according to increasing numbers of teeth involved in the disease process (Fig. 2-15). It then became evident that the number of teeth with bleeding gingivae in

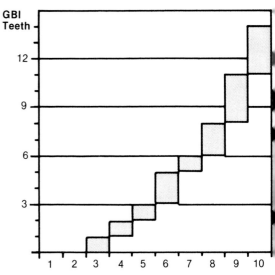

Fig. 2-15. A total of 3344 Finnish recruits was organized according to increasing gingival bleeding tendency in the right sides of the jaws. The group was then divided into 10 subgroups of equal size (deciles). The 3 first deciles were practically free of bleeding whereas in the worst 20% (deciles 9 and 10) bleeding occurred after gentle probing around 8-14 of the 14 teeth examined (Ainamo et al. 1980).

dency, subgingival calculus and early loss of alveolar bone. Assessment of disease rather than of a potentially pathogenic microbiota is common practice also in the medical profession.

As bacterial plaque seems to explain only part of the periodontal disease status, one can only hope that future research will result in possibilities to determine also those indirect systemic factors which influence the individual's host response. By means of biochemical, cytological and immunological tests it may one day be possible to reliably identify those individuals who are most likely to become affected by periodontal disease and give priority to such individuals in programs aimed at prevention.

Assessment of treatment needs

In many areas of the world, in spite of the present knowledge of the etiology and pathogenesis of periodontal disease, various barriers still seem to exist which obstruct the implementation of prevention and treatment of this disease. In a number of countries this difficulty can partly be explained by the late introduction of periodontics in the dental curriculum. Older dentists may, thus, have had no formal training in periodontics. The general public may be ignorant of the possibility of obtaining treatment and lack motivation to accept it. Another main reason, however, is probably related to the still existing lack of a simple and rapid scoring system for determining periodontal treatment needs, already pursued by Massler in 1950.

Some sporadic efforts have been made to create simplified indices for scoring periodontal disease indicators (Ainamo & Bay 1975, Ainamo & Ainamo 1978) and for assessing treatment needs in a given population (Bellini & Gjermo 1973, Johansen et al. 1973, Oliver 1977). Such efforts have been welcomed by practising dentists and public dental health administrators. For practising

dentists the assessment of different severities of disease on 4 surfaces of each tooth may not always be the most meaningful way of clinical charting.

Dichotomous scoring

During the very productive years of periodontal research in the 1960's, the trend was to develop increasingly sensitive index systems for the clarification of the etiology and pathogenesis of periodontal disease. During the 1970's considerable emphasis was put on improving the possibilities for the dental practitioner to implement the acquired knowledge, mainly by efforts to resimplify the scoring systems. Instead of scoring severity per tooth surface, recording of the presence or absence of symptoms at each tooth was suggested by Ainamo & Bay (1975) and Ainamo & Ainamo (1978) for a number of periodontal disease indicators. Dichotomous scoring was adopted for epidemiological purposes by the WHO (1978) and found suitable for use also in clinical trials (Ainamo et al. 1977).

The Periodontal Treatment Need System (PTNS)

The Periodontal Treatment Need System, introduced by Johansen et al. (1973), represented an entirely new approach to determination of treatment needs. The system allows a fairly accurate assessment of the amount and type of periodontal treatment required by the individual patient. The assessment can be made in only 1-3 min.

According to the PTNS, the dentition is divided into 4 quadrants. For each quadrant assessments are made to determine whether the worst affected tooth would require periodontal surgery, scaling, or improved personal oral hygiene. Only the worst condition is recorded since, for example, a quadrant requiring surgical therapy would also need scaling, and a patient having either one of these two treatment needs would also need instructions for improved oral hygiene.

JOHANSEN ET AL   1973 (PTNS)

a   OH EDUCATION

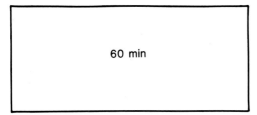

b   SCALING

30 min	30 min
30 min	30 min

c   SURGERY

60 min	60 min
60 min	60 min

Fig. 2-16. According to assessments using the Periodontal Treatment Need System (PTNS: Johansen et al. 1973), the average time required for treatment of adult patients is 60 min for oral hygiene instruction, including follow-ups and reinstruction, and 30 min for scaling and 60 min for surgery per quadrant of the dentition.

The next step in the development of the PTNS was to assess the time required for delivering the 3 different types of treatment (Johansen et al. 1973). Treatment time is thus used as a common denominator for all 3 categories of treatment. In a group of 42 periodontal patients the average time required was 60 min per quadrant for surgery, 30 min per quadrant for scaling, and 60 min per person for improving personal oral hygiene to an acceptable level (Fig. 2-16).

Although the PTNS is both rapid and easy to use, it does not seem to have gained much attention. The method is more informative in the screening of adult patients (Bellini & Gjermo 1973) than in the assessment of early treatment needs in children and adolescents.

The Periodontal Screening Examination (PSE)

The Periodontal Screening Examination represents another type of approach for determining treatment needs. The method was introduced by Oliver in 1977 and has gained a relatively wide use, e.g. by practising dentists, particularly in the United States. The PSE involves assessment of probing depth at the mesiobuccal and distobuccal line angle of each remaining tooth. Bleeding after probing and probing depths of 0-3 mm, 4-5 mm, and 6 mm or more, are the indicators of the actual treatment need.

The PTNS and the PSE both give direct indications whether the patient can be taken care of by the dental hygienist, whether treatment should be delivered by the examining general practitioner or, whether the services of a specialist periodontist are required. For such purposes the PTNS would seem more reliable than the PSE. Through the examination of all surfaces of all teeth *all* patients with at least one 6 mm or deeper pocket will be identified even when only 1 score per quadrant is recorded (PTNS). The PSE, though it records 2 surfaces of each tooth, still harbors the inherent shortcoming of all partial scoring systems; in this case a single deep pocket on the lingual aspect of a tooth is inevitably overlooked. It has recently been demonstrated that partial indices give a fair to good estimate of average periodontal disease severity levels in population groups but fail to identify a number of individual patients with localized periodontal disease of the more advanced type (Ainamo & Ainamo 1982).

The Community Periodontal Index of Treatment Needs (CPITN)

In 1977 the development of an international method for assessment of periodontal treatment needs was initiated by the Oral Health Unit of the World Health Organization. After 5 years of intensive work, close collaboration with the FDI (Federation Dentaire Internationale), and extensive field testing in a number of countries all around the world, the resulting recommendation for the use of the Community Periodontal Index of Treatment Needs (CPITN) was eventually published (Ainamo et al. 1982).

The CPITN is a combination of the dichotomous scoring principle, the treatment need assessment used in the PTNS, and the division of the full dentition into 6 segments as suggested by O'Leary (1967). Instead of quadrants, sextants are thus used as basic units of examination for and recording of treatment needs (Fig. 2-17). For a sextant to qualify for recording, it must contain at least 2 functioning teeth. The observations made from only 1 remaining tooth are included in the recording for the adjoining sextant.

Only 1 recording is given to each sextant. In developing countries with low experience of dental caries and reparative treatment, loss of tooth attachment may proceed rather evenly in all areas of the dentition. In such cases, the sextant recording may be determined after examination of the first and second molars in the posterior, and 1 central incisor in the anterior, sextants. This selection of 10 index teeth is recommended for use in epidemiological surveys (Fig. 2-17, Alternative I) although the results thus obtained may overestimate periodontal treatment needs in young individuals and may, as with the use of the PSE, fail to identify an occasional adult subject with localized advanced breakdown of the periodontium.

In adult inhabitants of western, industrialized countries advanced periodontal breakdown is often observed at only one or a limited number of sites. To ensure that all

WHO 1983 (CPITN)

ALTERNATIVE I. EPIDEMIOLOGY

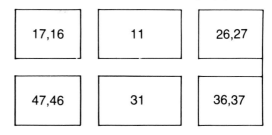

ALTERNATIVE II. TREATMENT

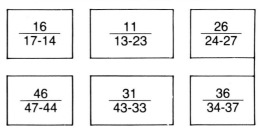

Fig. 2-17. For scoring according to the Community Periodontal Index of Treatment Needs (CPITN) the dentition is divided into six segments (sextants). Each sextant is given one code number, regardless of number of teeth examined. In epidemiological surveys (Alternative I) the code number may be based on the examination of 10 index teeth, whereas for treatment purposes (Alternative II) the code number is given after examination of 6 index teeth in children and adolescents (above the horizontal line) and after examination of all teeth in each sextant in subjects aged 20 years or older (below the horizontal line) (Ainamo 1983).

subjects in need of treatment for advanced periodontitis in such populations are identified, the examination of all teeth in the sextant is recommended (Fig. 2-17, Alternative II, below the horizontal line).

In subjects under the age of 20 from industrialized countries it is fairly uncommon to find loss of attachment around other teeth if the first molars and/or incisors are not affected. In determining the periodontal treatment needs in such children and adolescents it is, therefore, recommended to restrict the examination to 6 index teeth (Fig. 2-17, Alternative II, above the horizontal line). The second molars included in the

79

WHO 1982

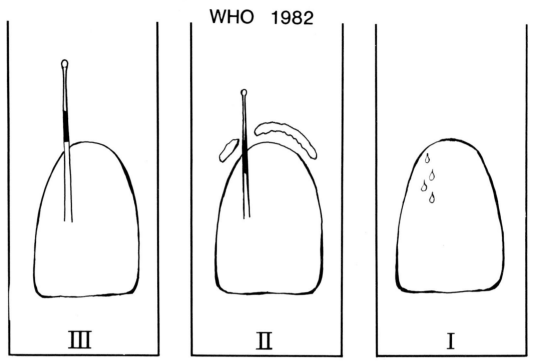

Fig. 2-18. Classification of treatment needs according to the CPITN. Complex treatment (III) is required when the color coded area (3.5-5.5 mm) of the WHO probe disappears underneath the gingival margin. The finding of a 6 mm or deeper pocket is recorded by giving code 4 to the sextant. Scaling (II) is indicated if the deepest pocket is 4 or 5 mm (code 3) or if supra- or subgingival calculus or defective margins of fillings or crowns (code 2) are found. If no pockets or plaque retentions are observed but bleeding occurs after probing, code 1 is given to the sextant. The corresponding treatment need is oral hygiene instruction (I).

epidemiological alternative are deleted because of their tendency to give false positives with regard to deep pockets during the eruptive stage of these teeth (Ainamo 1983). False pockets may also occur in adults, e.g. between the distal surface of the second molar and a hyperplastic retromolar pad.

For further simplification of the examination, a special WHO periodontal probe was developed. The probe has a "ball point", 0.5 mm in diameter, for easy detection of subgingival calculus and to decrease the risk of over-measurement of pocket depth (Fig. 2-18). The force used at probing should not exceed that corresponding to 20-25 g. The color coded area extends from 3.5 to 5.5 mm:

Code 4 is given to the sextant if at one or

more teeth the color coded area of the WHO probe disappears into the inflamed pocket indicating pocket depth of 6 mm or more. Such a sextant requires "complex treatment", i.e. either deep scaling, curettage or surgical intervention. In most cases the patient would be referred to a specialist periodontist for treatment.

Code 3 is given to the sextant if the color coded area of the probe remains partially visible when inserted into the deepest pocket. Pocket depth is now 4 or 5 mm and treatment of the sextant can be managed with thorough scaling and proper oral hygiene.

Code 2 is assigned to the sextant if there are no pocket depths exceeding 3 mm (colored area remains totally visible) but dental calculus or other plaque retentions are seen at, or recognized underneath, the gingival margin. The treatment need for code 2 is the same as for code 3, scaling and improved oral hygiene.

Code 1 is given to a sextant when there are no pockets and no calculus or overhangs of fillings but bleeding occurs after gentle probing of one or more pockets. A maximum score of 1 indicates that the patient only needs instructions for improved oral hygiene.

As shown in Fig. 2-19, only the highest code number per sextant is recorded. The need for complex treatment (code 4) thus includes also the needs for scaling and oral hygiene instruction, and codes 3 and 2, correspondingly, always require improved oral hygiene in addition to scaling.

Recording of the CPITN codes can be performed in only 1-3 min. The method is, thus,

TYPE OF TREATMENT	TYPE OF TREATMENT			
	III	II	I	0
III + II + I	6	+	+	0
	5	1	+	0
	4	2	+	0
	3	3	+	0
	2	4	+	0
	1	5	+	0
II + I	0	6	+	0
	0	5	1	0
	0	4	2	0
	0	3	3	0
	0	2	4	0
	0	1	5	0
I	0	0	6	0
	0	0	5	1
	0	0	4	2
	0	0	3	3
	0	0	2	4
	0	0	1	5
0	0	0	0	6

Fig. 2-20. Possibilities of classifying groups of subjects according to the CPITN. The first 6 combinations involve the need for both complex treatment (III), scaling (II), and oral hygiene instruction (I). The next group of 6 combinations is in need of scaling (II) and oral hygiene instruction (I). Oral hygiene instruction only (I) is required in the third group. The last line indicates total health (0) which would be a relatively rare finding in the beginning of the 1980's.

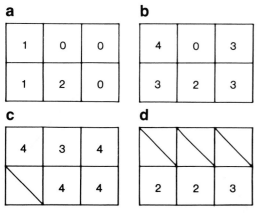

Fig. 2-19. Examples of CPITN recordings. Case a needs scaling in the mandibular anterior sextant and oral hygiene instructions for elimination of the bleeding also in the right side posterior sextants. In case b complex treatment is needed in 1 and scaling in all but 1 sextant. If this is a young patient the possibility of juvenile periodontitis should be considered. Case c needs complex treatment in 4 sextants and scaling in all but the edentulous mandibular right sextant. In case d the maxilla is edentulous (or only 1 tooth remains). The lower jaw requires scaling in all 3 sextants. In addition, cases b, c and d all require oral hygiene instruction as well

practical for preliminary assessment of the need for periodontal treatment during initial screening of the oral health status of a new patient. On the basis of the 6 code numbers, the patient can be referred to a hygienist or a specialist for detailed recording of disease status. After treatment, the CPITN is again useful for monitoring of the maintenance of periodontal health.

In epidemiological research, earlier index systems have usually described disease status by average scores for a given population. Such data (see Fig. 2-4) gives no information about the proportion of the population affected. The CPITN is designed to indicate directly what percentage of a given age group requires complex treatment, scaling, or oral hygiene instructions (Fig. 2-20). For treatment planning it is also essential to know whether 4 deep pockets in a dentition are located all in one (Fig. 2-19b) or in 4 different sextants (Fig. 2-19c).

With the CPITN, it is not meaningful to use the various code numbers for calculating average scores for individuals or population groups. As with the PTNS (Johansen et al. 1973), the possibility exists with the CPITN to use the separately calculated treatment time per sextant and per type of treatment as a common denominator for assessment of the total amount of treatment required.

Current and future trends

The epidemiology of periodontal disease is a relatively young science. Research conducted during the last few decades indicates that periodontal disease is one of the most common plagues of mankind. The direct causal association between bacterial colonization on the tooth surface and the inflammatory destruction of tooth attachment has been clearly demonstrated. The rate of destruction has further been found to vary considerably from one subject to another, depending mainly on individual differences in tissue response to the bacterial irritation.

Although, from a practical point of view the etiology of periodontal disease has been clarified, this does not mean that research in the area of periodontal epidemiology has become redundant. For the interested researcher, epidemiological methodology offers fascinating possibilities for solving periodontal problems also in the future. Further work is badly needed in the area of simple charting of periodontal disease status, assessment of treatment needs, and identification of high risk groups. The main challenge for the 1980's is to determine how to utilize all the acquired knowledge for the benefit of the population. At the same time, epidemiological research on microbiological aspects and host response factors is only in its infancy. And finally, epidemiological methods will continue to be required for the monitoring of periodontal health, and for the evaluation of the effect of various preventive and therapeutic programs and procedures.

References

Ainamo, J. (1970) Concomitant periodontal disease and dental caries in young adult males. *Proceedings of the Finnish Dental Society* **66**, 303-366.

Ainamo, J. (1983) Assessment of periodontal treatment needs. Adaptation of the WHO Community Periodontal Index of Treatment Needs (CPITN) to European conditions. In *Public Health Aspects of Periodontal Disease in Europe*, ed. Frandsen, A. Berlin: Quintessenz Verlag. In press.

Ainamo, J. & Ainamo, A. (1978) Development of oral health during dental studies in India and Finland. *International Dental Journal* **28**, 427-433.

Ainamo, J. & Ainamo, A. (1982) Partial indices as depictors of periodontal disease status and treatment needs. *Journal of Dental Research* **61**, Abstr., 221.

Ainamo, J., Ankkuriniemi, O. & Parviainen, K. (1980) The prevalence of caries and periodontal disease in the same subjects. In *The Borderland between Caries and Periodontal Disease. II*, ed. Lehner, T. & Cimasoni, G., pp. 9-29. Academic Press, London-Toronto-Sydney, Grune & Stratton, New York-San Fransisco.

Ainamo, J., Barmes, D., Beagrie, G., Cutress, T., Martin, J. & Sardo-Infirri, J. (1982) Development of the World Health Organization (WHO) Community Periodontal Index of

Treatment Needs (CPITN). *International Dental Journal* **32**, 281-291.

Ainamo, J. & Bay, I. (1975) Problems and proposals for recording gingivitis and plaque. *International Dental Journal* **25**, 229-235.

Ainamo, J., Sjöblom, M., Ainamo, A. & Tiainen, L. (1977) Growth of plaque while chewing sucrose and sorbitol flavoured gum. *Journal of Clinical Periodontology* **4**, 151-160.

Ånerud, Å., Löe, H., Boysen, H. & Smith, M. (1979) The natural history of periodontal disease in man. Changes in gingival health and oral hygiene before 40 years of age. *Journal of Periodontal Research* **14**, 526-540.

Axelsson, P. & Lindhe, J. (1981) The significance of maintenance care in the treatment of periodontal disease. *Journal of Clinical Periodontology* **8**, 281-294.

Bellini, H. T. & Gjermo, P. (1973) Application of the Periodontal Treatment Need System (PTNS) in a group of Norwegian industrial employees. *Community Dentistry and Oral Epidemiology* **1**, 22-29.

Björby, A. & Löe, H. (1967) The relative significance of different local factors in the initiation and development of periodontal inflammation. *Journal of Periodontal Research* **2**, Abstr., 76-77.

Ennever, J., Sturzenberger, O. P. & Radike, A. W. (1961) The Calculus Surface Index method for scoring clinical calculus studies. *Journal of Periodontology* **32**, 54-57.

Glavind, L. & Löe, H. (1967) Errors in the clinical assessment of periodontal destruction. *Journal of Periodontal Research* **2**, 180-184.

Greene, J. C. (1963) Oral hygiene and periodontal disease. *American Journal of Public Health* **53**, 913-922.

Greene, J. C. & Vermillion, J. R. (1960) The Oral Hygiene Index: A method for classifying oral hygiene status. *Journal of American Dental Association* **61**, 172-179.

Greene, J. C. & Vermillion, J. R. (1964) The simplified oral hygiene index. *Journal of American Dental Association* **68**, 7-13.

Johansen, J. R., Gjermo, P. & Bellini, H. T. (1973) A system to classify the need for periodontal treatment. *Acta Odontologica Scandinavica* **31**, 297-305.

Lightner, L. M., O'Leary, T. J., Drake, R. B.,

Crump, P. P. & Allen, M. F. (1971) Preventive periodontic treatment procedures: results after 46 months. *Journal of Periodontology* **42**, 555-561.

Lindhe, J., Hamp, S. E. & Löe, H. (1975) Plaque-induced periodontal disease in beagle dogs. *Journal of Periodontal Research* **10**, 243-255.

Löe, H. (1963) Epidemiology of periodontal disease. *Odontologisk Tidsskrift* **71**, 479-503.

Löe, H. (1967) The Gingival Index, the Plaque Index and the Retention Index systems. *Journal of Periodontology* **38**, 610-616.

Löe, H., Ånerud, Å., Boysen, H. & Smith, M. (1978) The natural history of periodontal disease in man. Study design and baseline data. *Journal of Periodontal Research* **13**, 550-562.

Löe, H. & Silness, J. (1963) Periodontal disease in pregnancy. I. Prevalence and severity. *Acta Odontologica Scandinavica* **21**, 533-551.

Löe, H., Theilade, E. & Jensen, S. B. (1965) Experimental gingivitis in man. *Journal of Periodontology* **36**, 177-187.

Lövdal, A., Arno, A., Schei, O. & Waerhaug, J. (1961) Combined effect of subgingival scaling and controlled oral hygiene on the incidence of gingivitis. *Acta Odontologica Scandinavica* **19**, 537-555.

Mackler, S. B. & Crawford, J. J. (1973) Plaque development and gingivitis in the primary dentition. *Journal of Periodontology* **44**, 18-24.

MacMahon, B., Pugh, T. F. & Ipsen, J. (1960) *Epidemiologic Methods*. Boston: Little and Brown.

Massler, M., Schour, I. & Chopra, B. (1950) Occurrence of gingivitis in suburban Chicago school children. *Journal of Periodontology* **21**, 146-164.

Matsson, L. (1978) Development of gingivitis in pre-school children and young adults. *Journal of Clinical Periodontology* **5**, 24-34.

Mühlemann, H. R. (1968) *In vivo* measurements of dental calculus. *Annals of the New York Academy of Sciences* **153**, 164-196.

O'Leary, T. J. (1967) The periodontal screening examination. *Journal of Periodontology* **38**, 617-624.

Oliver, R. C. (1977) Patient evaluation. *International Dental Journal* **27**, 103-106.

Parfitt, G. J. (1957) A five year longitudinal study

of the gingival condition of a group of children in England. *Journal of Periodontology* **26**, 26-32.

Quigley, G. A. & Hein, J. W. (1962) Comparative cleansing efficiency of manual and power brushing. *Journal of the American Dental Association* **65**, 26-29.

Ramfjord, S. P. (1959) Indices for prevalence and incidence of periodontal disease. *Journal of Periodontology* **30**, 51-59.

Ramfjord, S. P., Knowles, J. W., Nissle, R. R., Burgett, F. G. & Shick, R. A. (1975) Results following three modalities of periodontal therapy. *Journal of Periodontology* **46**, 522-526.

Rosling, B., Nyman, S., Lindhe, J. & Jern, B. (1976) The healing potential of the periodontal tissues following different techniques of periodontal surgery in plaque-free dentitions. A 2 year clinical study. *Journal of Clinical Periodontology* **3**, 233-250.

Russell, A. L. (1956) A system of classification and scoring for prevalence surveys of periodontal disease. *Journal of Dental Research* **35**, 350-359.

Russell, A. L. (1963) International nutrition surveys: A summary of preliminary dental findings. *Journal of Dental Research* **42**, 232-244.

Schour, I. & Massler, M. (1947) Gingival disease in postwar Italy (1945). I. Prevalence of gingivitis in various age groups. *Journal of the American Dental Association* **35**, 475-482.

Schroeder, H. E. (1969) *Formation and Inhibition of Dental Calculus.* Berne and Stuttgart: Hans Huber Publishers.

Scherp, H. W. (1964) Current concepts in periodontal disease research: epidemiological contributions. *Journal of the American Dental Association* **68**, 667-675.

Silness, J. & Löe, H. (1964) Periodontal disease in pregnancy. II. Correlation between oral hygiene and periodontal condition. *Acta Odontologica Scandinavica* **24**, 747-759.

Suomi, J. D., Greene, J. C., Vermillion, J. R., Doyle, J., Chang, J. J. & Leatherwood, E. C. (1971) The effect of controlled oral hygiene procedures on the progression of periodontal disease in adults: results after third and final year. *Journal of Periodontology* **42**, 152-160.

Suomi, J. D., Smith, L. W., Chang, J. J. & Barbano, J. P. (1973) Study on the effect of different prophylaxis frequencies on the periodontium of young adults. *Journal of Periodontology* **44**, 406-410.

Volpe, A. R. & Manhold, J. H. (1962) A method of evaluating the effectiveness of potential calculus inhibiting agents. *New York State Dental Journal* **28**, 289-290.

Volpe, A. R., Manhold, J. H. & Hazen, S. P. (1965) *In vivo* calculus assessment. I. A method and its examiner reproducibility. *Journal of Periodontology* **36**, 292-298.

Waerhaug, J. (1966) Epidemiology of periodontal disease. In *Workshop in Periodontics,* ed. Ramfjord, S. P., Kerr, D. A., Ash, M. M., pp. 179-211, Michigan: Ann Arbor.

Waerhaug, J. (1967) Prevalence of periodontal disease in Ceylon. Association with age, sex, oral hygiene, socioeconomic factors, vitamin deficiences, malnutrition, betel and tobacco consumption and ethnic group. *Acta Odontologica Scandinavica* **25**, 205-231.

WHO (1978) *Epidemiology, Etiology and Prevention of Periodontal Diseases.* Geneva: Technical Report Series 621.

CHAPTER 3

Dental Plaque and Dental Calculus

Introduction

Proper oral hygiene has for centuries been recommended in dental textbooks as a preventive measure against dental diseases. However, the significance of dental deposits for the development of periodontal disease lacked scientific basis until the middle of this century, when well designed epidemiological studies were performed (e.g. Lövdal et al. 1958, Greene 1960, 1963, Greene & Vermillion 1960, Ramfjord 1961, Löe 1963, Russell 1963, Wærhaug 1971). From such surveys it is now established that the presence of dental deposits, whether mineralized or not, is undoubtedly the most important factor in the development of periodontal disease (WHO 1961).

Final evidence for this statement was presented as a result of clinical studies in which gingivitis was experimentally initiated by the abolition of oral hygiene procedures (Löe et al. 1965, Theilade et al. 1966). When a correct regime of oral hygiene was reinstituted, gingival inflammation resolved within a week, restoring gingival health.

The transition from gingivitis to destructive periodontal disease has not been demonstrated experimentally in man. However, in dogs gingivitis develops as the result of plaque accumulation (Egelberg 1965a) and if it is allowed to continue for a sufficiently long period, permanent destruction of the supporting tissues of the teeth occurs typical of human periodontal disease (Saxe et al. 1967, Lindhe et al. 1973). These results indicate that destructive periodontal disease may develop from longstanding gingivitis, and thus support the conclusions drawn from epidemiologic studies.

Additional evidence for the role of dental deposits in the development of periodontal disease in man, has been derived from studies in which the progression of periodontal disease has been markedly retarded by the introduction of correct oral hygiene measures (e.g. Lövdal et al. 1961, Suomi et al. 1971, Ramfjord et al. 1973, Knowles et al. 1979). In highly motivated individuals correct plaque control may practically arrest the progression of periodontal disease (Lindhe & Axelsson 1973, Axelsson & Lindhe 1974, 1981, Söderholm 1979) and following therapy induce considerable bone repair in patients who have lost bony support due to periodontal disease (Rosling et al. 1976). Thus, there is excellent reason for the interest, developed over the last 25 years, in the subject of dental deposits.

Unfortunately, the successful plaque preventive measures available today are time consuming for the individual as well as for the dental profession. It is therefore unlikely that a significant proportion of the population of the world will benefit from the available knowledge of plaque control in this century. Less demanding plaque control methods are sought and a better understanding of the nature of dental deposits is essential for the development of safe alternative inhibitors of plaque and calculus formation.

Dental plaque

Definition and classification of dental plaque

Dental plaque may be defined as bacterial aggregations on the teeth or other solid oral structures (Dawes et al. 1963, Egelberg 1970, Kelstrup & Theilade 1974, Theilade 1977).

However, this definition is not employed universally although, for clinical purposes, it seems adequate and simple. Another definition distinguishes dental plaque from materia alba, the latter comprising the soft white material consisting of bacterial aggregations, leukocytes and desquamated oral epithelial cells accumulating in an unclean mouth at the surface of plaque or teeth (WHO 1961, Mühlemann & Schroeder 1964). According to this definition the differentiation between dental plaque and materia alba is determined by the strength of the adherence of the deposit. If it is removed by the mechanical action of a strong water spray, the material is termed materia alba; if it withstands the water spray, it is called dental plaque. The distinction between these two types of bacterial accumulation is of questionable value and is often impractical to use clinically. Hence, the term dental plaque will be used in this chapter to designate both types of bacterial aggregations on the solid surfaces in the mouth.

Plaque in the dentogingival region is of primary concern to the therapist dealing with periodontal disease. Dentogingival plaque may arbitrarily be classified as supragingival plaque deposited on the clinical crowns of teeth, and subgingival plaque located in the gingival sulcus or the periodontal pocket. Of course this classification of dentogingival plaque is only precise at a given moment, as the separating border between the two types of plaque, i.e. the gingival margin, may shift coronally due to swelling of the gingival tissues, or it may migrate apically as a result of gingival recession. If this shift in the position of the gingival margin occurs, the classification of the plaque located between the previous and the new location of the gingival margin is automatically changed. However, in spite of the theoretical inaccuracies of the classification, its value in practice is well documented.

Clinical appearance and distribution of plaque

Supragingival plaque is clinically detectable once it has reached a certain thickness and then it appears as a whitish, yellowish layer primarily along the gingival margins of the teeth (Fig. 3-1). Plaque may be difficult to identify if it is present in small quantities (Fig. 3-2). In this case its presence may be ascertained by scraping the tooth surface along the gingival margin with the end of a probe or by using a disclosing solution (Fig. 3-3). This may be a conventional dye, staining the plaque or a fluorescent dye which can be demonstrated by illumination with ultraviolet light (Hefferren et al. 1971, Lang et al. 1972).

Subgingivally situated plaque cannot be diagnosed directly *in situ*. And since subgingival plaque is normally present in thin layers, it is not possible to diagnose such deposits by clinical inspection. Plaque may form anywhere on solid structures in the mouth, if the site is protected from the normal mechanical cleaning action of the tongue, the cheeks and the lips. Plaque deposits are, thus, regularly present in the fissures of the occlusal surfaces, in pits and ir-

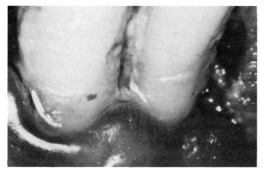

Fig. 3-1. Supragingival plaque of a thickness which makes it clinically visible. The interproximal space between the two teeth is completely occupied by plaque.

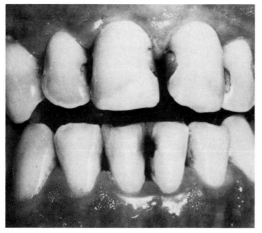

Fig. 3-2. No visible plaque is apparent.

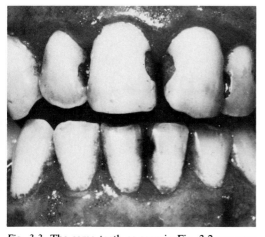

Fig. 3-3. The same teeth as seen in Fig. 3-2 are now stained with a disclosing solution, revealing plaque along the gingival margin of the mandibulary incisors and cuspids. Similarly plaque is present on the ill-fitting restorations of the approximal surfaces of the maxillary incisors.

regularities, even on the smooth tooth surfaces, on fillings and artificial crowns and especially along ill-fitting restorations, on orthodontic bands and on removable orthodontic appliances and dentures.

Composition of dental plaque

The easiest way to get information on the composition of dental plaque is to remove a small sample from the tooth surface, transfer it to a microscope slide and stain it with a bacterial stain (Fig. 3-4). Examination of the preparation in a microscope with transillumination will reveal a multitude of bacteria of different morphological forms. Some host cells will also be present, either epithelial cells from the desquamated oral epithelia or blood cells, primarily polymorphonuclear leukocytes.

Well established plaque may contain microorganisms other than bacteria. Mycoplasms have been demonstrated, and small numbers of yeasts and protozoa may also be present (Burnett & Schuster 1978). In spite of the fact that plaque has often previously been considered as food debris, at least by the lay public, recognizable dietary remains are infrequently encountered in dental plaque.

Microbiology of dental plaque

In 1 mm^3 of dental plaque weighing about 1 mg, more than 10^8 bacteria may be counted. A multitude of different species of microorganisms is present and it is not currently possible to identify them all. Studies of the microbial composition of gingival plaque have been performed ever since it was discovered that specific organisms were the cause of many diseases affecting mankind. Such studies will continue for the foreseeable future as improved methods become available for culturing and identifying the individual species present. There are still microorganisms in the mouth (such as spirochetes) for which the available culturing techniques are insufficient. This means

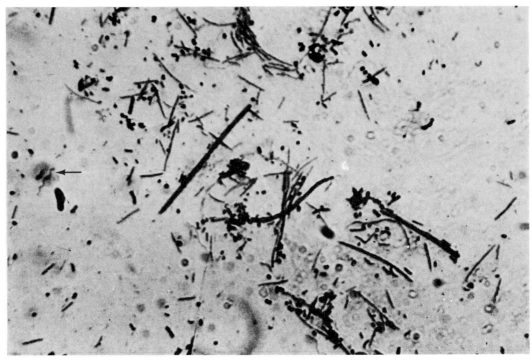

Fig. 3-4. Gram stained smear of old human supragingival plaque. Cocci constitute a relatively small proportion of the bacterial flora. Filamentous organisms predominate, and a spirochete is present in the field (arrow).

that such microorganisms cannot be adequately studied. Other types, though culturable, cannot be correctly determined because of lacking taxonomic data and reference strains essential for the final identification of the bacterial species. However, certain patterns of microbial composition of plaque at different sites in the mouth have become evident. Apparently, the characteristic environment of each location favors development of a certain microbial community.

Supragingival plaque

In an investigation called "Experimental gingivitis in man" (Löe et al. 1965, Theilade et al. 1966), the oral hygiene of a group of dental students was improved during several weeks of intensive instruction in the use of toothbrush and toothpicks. This resulted in a very low occurrence of plaque and excellent gingival conditions. Then, all oral hygiene measures were withdrawn allowing plaque to reaccumulate along the gingival margin. After 2-3 weeks, all subjects had developed gingivitis. During the experimental period plaque samples were obtained at regular intervals and subjected to a bacteriological examination of Gram stained smears. The bacteria present in the samples were classified according to their Gram reaction and morphology. The results of this analysis were tabulated as the percentage distribution of the various types of microorganisms.

At commencement, with healthy gingivae, very few bacteria were present on the cervical surfaces of the teeth. The removable deposit was dominated by desquamated epithelial cells on or between which few bacteria could be seen. Of these, about 90% were Gram positive cocci and rods, the remainder primarily Gram negative. When all oral hygiene measures were withdrawn, the simple bacterial plaque composition changed drastically. During the first phase of plaque development comprising the initial 2 days of the experiment, not only the number of all types of bacteria increased, but their proportional distribution changed as well. Gram negative cocci and rods now comprised a greater proportion of the flora. The second phase of plaque development, days 3 and 4, was characterized by a proliferation of fusobacteria and filamentous bacteria. During the third phase, days 5-9, spirilla and spirochetes appeared, so that the complex flora seen in old plaque had become established. After about 7 days, the various groups of bacteria had proliferated to the extent that the Gram positive cocci and rods, which initially predominated, now constituted only 50% of the complex flora. During the remaining period up to 3 weeks, no further major changes in the bacterial distribution occurred (Fig. 3-5).

A more detailed classification of the bacteria present in early stages of supragingival plaque development is slowly becoming available from cultural studies (Rönström et al. 1977, Socransky et al. 1977, Theilade et al. 1982), and is in accordance with the initially reported observations. It is now apparent that the very early flora, 3-8 h after proper tooth cleaning, is dominated by streptococci. Most of these have been identified as *Streptococcus mitior*, while *Streptococcus sanguis* and *Streptococcus milleri* are present in smaller numbers. *Streptococcus mutans*, to which an important role in plaque formation is often ascribed, is either absent or present only in very low numbers. Gram positive rods constitute a small proportion of this early flora, primarily *Actinomyces viscosus* and *Actinomyces naeslundii*. Furthermore, during this initial formative stage, the microorganisms adhere very loosely to the tooth surface, so that a spray of water will remove most of them (Theilade & Mikkelsen 1972, Brecx et al. 1981). As previously mentioned, some authors do not consider such loose deposits as plaque and recommend that material that

may be removed by a water-spray be termed materia alba. However, as even loosely adhering bacteria may eventually become irreversibly attached to the tooth, and are therefore potential determinants of the composition of the plaque established at a later stage, the interest in the early bacterial populations is justified, regardless of the term ascribed to this deposit.

It is not until after 24 h without cleaning that a clinically demonstrable layer of plaque has formed. The number of microorganisms adhering to the tooth at this time represents

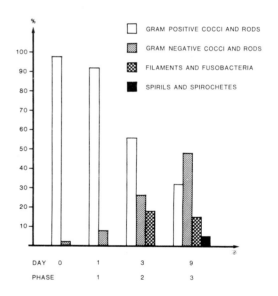

Fig. 3-5. Percentage distribution of different types of organisms on the mesial surface of the lower left premolar in a particular human subject at days 0, 1, 3, and 9 of experimental gingivitis. In the first phase of the plaque development, represented by day 1, the relative number of Gram negative cocci and rods increases. In the second phase, represented by day 3, the percentage of Gram negative cocci and rods further increases and fusobacteria and filamentous bacteria appear. In the third phase, represented by day 9, the Gram negative cocci and rods have augmented again in relative number, and in addition spirils and spirochetes are present. In contrast Gram positive cocci and rods constitute a continuously decreasing proportion of the plaque during plaque development. Based on results presented by Theilade et al. (1966).

the net balance between (1) previously attached bacteria which have subsequently been detached and rinsed away by the salivary flow, (2) those which have become irreversibly adherent and started to multiply, and finally (3) bacteria arriving later from the saliva to the site where they are trapped and aggregated to those already there. Recent studies indicate that multiplication of initially adhering microorganisms accounts for a major portion of the increased number of bacteria collected on the tooth after 24 h (Brecx 1979, Ørstavik & Ruangsri 1979, Rönström 1979, Brecx et al. 1983). It has been estimated that during this first day of plaque formation the mean generation time, that is the time it takes for the bacteria to double their number, is about 3 h (Socransky et al. 1977, Brecx et al. 1983). This means that 1 microorganism during the first 24 h period may multiply to a total of 256 microorganisms. A large number of these are detached and lost in saliva which is constantly swallowed. Saliva thus has an important rinsing effect, but is unfortunately insufficient to prevent plaque formation.

After the first day of plaque growth the flora becomes increasingly more complex. The proportion of streptococci decreases to 45% at 24 h while Gram negative anaerobic cocci (Veillonella) rapidly increase to about 20%. Facultative and obligate anaerobic species of Actinomyces also become more prominent constituting about 25% after 3 days. Gram negative anaerobic rods make up about 5% of the cultivable flora after 3 days (Theilade et al. 1982 a). These recent data are in accordance with earlier published data from developing supragingival plaque (Ritz 1967, Socransky et al. 1977).

During the following 3 weeks of undisturbed plaque formation the relative proportions of the various types of bacteria in the cultivable flora continue to change (Syed & Loesche 1978). The Gram positive cocci decrease in relative numbers particularly because the Gram positive rods increase, especially due to the appearance of a high proportion of Actinomyces israelii. Among

the Gram negative bacteria, Veillonella is the most prominent organism while rods such as Bacteroides and Fusobacterium still constitute small proportions. Although the details of the complex bacterial composition of older plaque are far from complete, the general trend is clear. As the dentogingival plaque layer increases in thickness, the millieu changes to favor anaerobic microorganisms and an increasing number of Gram negative rods may now grow, especially in the deeper layers next to the tooth (Ritz 1969). The changed growth condition may be influenced by the concomitantly developing inflammation in the gingiva, resulting in a marked increase in the flow of gingival exudate which contains a number of growth factors not readily available in saliva. Additional nutrition is also provided by microbial symbiosis and through the death and disruption (lysis) of microorganisms in the plaque. After 3 weeks of plaque growth significant numbers of plaque bacteria are no longer viable (Theilade & Theilade 1970).

Subgingival plaque
Colonization of the gingival sulcus and the subsequently developing periodontal pocket most frequently starts from an already occurring deposit of supragingival plaque. Thus, the bacterial composition of subgingival plaque is partly influenced by that existing in the adjacent portion of the supragingival bacterial deposit.

However, the subgingival environment will influence the growth conditions of this area. The access to the oral cavity is limited which favors anaerobic development. Nutrients are readily available from the gingival exudate, the volume of which is increased as a result of inflammation in the gingiva. Detachment of already established microorganisms is limited due to the protecting gingival tissues, making it possible for organisms without special adhesion mechanisms to survive. On the other hand, the possibility for arrival of additional salivary bacteria is limited or impossible. These factors may explain why the bacterial composition of subgingival plaque is different from that of the adjacent supragingival plaque.

In patients, who have suffered from mild to moderate gingivitis for at least 2-3 months, streptococci only account for around 25% of the microbial flora of subgingival plaque. *Streptococcus mitis* and *S. sanguis* are predominant species. Approximately another 25% of the subgingival bacteria is comprised of various *Actinomyces* species. Gram negative anaerobic rods contribute a further 25% of the subgingival flora with *Fusobacterium, Bacteroides, Selenomonas,* and *Campylobacter* prominent (Slots et al. 1978).

Since spirochetes are not readily cultured, they are not represented in this account of the predominantly cultivable flora. However, their presence may be ascertained by darkfield microscopy, and may constitute up to 2% in gingival sulci at sites characterized as relatively healthy (Listgarten & Helldén 1978).

In advanced periodontal disease with pathologically deepened pockets along the root surface, the flora of subgingival deposits is somewhat different. The cultivable microbiota is dominated by up to 90% of anaerobic microorganisms. The Gram negative bacteria, almost exclusively rods, constitute 75% of these, *Bacteroides melaninogenicus* and *Fusobacterium nucleatum* are prominent (Crawford et al. 1975, Slots 1977). Again, the spirochetes have not been included in this account, but darkfield microscopy reveals that in the deep pockets of advanced periodontal disease they comprise 40-50% of the flora.

In a special form of periodontal disease in young patients, termed juvenile periodontitis, the subgingival flora is strikingly different from that described above. The cultivable flora has the same overall characteristics as other deep pockets, such as the predominance of anaerobic bacteria of which the Gram negative rods constitute up to 60%. These, however, comprise species different from those found in deep pockets in older patients (Slots 1976). Also total counts

by darkfield microscopy have revealed that in juvenile periodontitis sites, spirochetes only accounted for about 7% of the flora (Liljenberg & Lindhe 1980). Thus, in juvenile periodontitis, the proportion of spirochetes is intermediate between that found in mild gingivitis and that of advanced periodontal disease.

From this review of the subgingival microbial flora of the gingival crevice in health and disease certain general trends become apparent. As disease progresses the proportion of the Gram positive cocci and rods, such as streptococci and *Actinomyces,* decreases, while the Gram negative rods increase drastically, as do the anaerobic bacteria (Fig. 3-6).

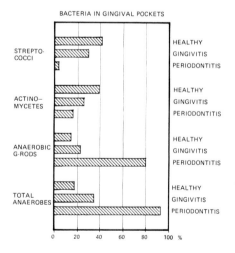

Fig. 3-6. Percentage predominantly cultivable bacteria in gingival sulci of patients with healthy gingiva and moderate gingivitis, and in periodontal pockets from patients with advanced marginal periodontitis. As periodontal disease progresses the relative numbers of Gram positive organisms such as streptococci and Actinomycetes decrease at the expense of anaerobic bacteria, particularly Gram negative rods. Based on results from Slots (1976, 1977) and from Slots et al. (1978).

Structure of dental plaque

Supragingival plaque

Supragingival plaque has been examined in a multitude of studies by light and electron microscopy to gain information on its internal structure (Mühlemann & Schneider 1959, Turesky et al. 1961, Theilade 1964, Frank & Brendel 1966, Leach & Saxton 1966, Frank & Houver 1970, Schroeder & De Boever 1970, Theilade & Theilade 1970, Eastcott & Stallard 1973, Saxton 1973, Rönström et al. 1975, Tinanoff & Gross 1976, Lie 1978).

The introduction of the electron microscope in dental research was a significant development for studies of dental plaque, both because the size of many bacteria approaches the ultimate resolving power of the light microscope, and because the resins used for embedding allowed for sections thinner than the smallest bacterial dimension. Hereby the substructure of plaque could be identified. Simultaneously, advances in biochemistry made it possible to interpret the structural details revealed by electron microscopy.

In studies of the internal details of plaque, samples are required in which the deposits are kept in their original relation to the surface on which they have formed. This may be accomplished by removing the deposits with the tooth. If plaque of known age is the object of study, the tooth surfaces are cleaned at a predetermined time before removal (McDougall 1963, Frank & Houver 1970, Schroeder & De Boever 1970). If the removal of the tooth on which the plaque is located becomes impractical, pieces of natural teeth or artificial surfaces may be attached to solid structures in the mouth and removed after a given interval. This method of plaque collection was used at the beginning of the century by Black (1911), who used a glass slide attached to his upper denture as a substrate for the developing plaque. The systematic use of artificial surfaces for collection of plaque was reintroduced during the 1950's. Thin plastic foils of Mylar® were attached to lower incisor teeth for known periods after which they were removed for histologic, histochemical and electron microscopic examination of the deposited material (Mandel et al. 1957, Mühleman & Schneider 1959, Zander et al. 1960, Schroeder 1963, Theilade 1964). Later other types of plastic materials, such as Westopal®, Epon®, Araldite® and spray plast, have been employed for this purpose (Berthold et al. 1971, Kandarkar 1973, Lie 1975, Listgarten et al. 1975, Rönström et al. 1975). Results from several such studies indicate that plaque formed on natural or artificial surfaces does not differ significantly in structure or microbiology (Hazen 1960, Berthold et al. 1971, Nyvad et al. 1982, Theilade et al. 1982 a & b), indicating that at least some of the principal mechanisms involved in plaque formation are unrelated to the nature of the solid surface colonized. However, there are small but important differences in the chemical composition of the first layer of organic material formed on these artificial surfaces compared with that formed on natural tooth surfaces (Sönju & Rölla 1973, Sönju & Glantz 1975, Öste et al. 1980). Tooth surfaces, enamel as well as exposed cementum, are normally covered by a thin acquired pellicle of glycoproteins (Figs. 3-7, 3-9, 3-10). If removed, e.g. by mechanical instrumentation, it reforms within minutes. The pellicle is believed to play an active part in the selective adherence of bacteria to the tooth surface. For details of the proposed mechanisms, see Chapter 4.

The first cellular material adhering to the pellicle on the tooth surface or other solid surfaces consists of coccal bacteria with small numbers of epithelial cells and polymorphonuclear leukocytes (Fig. 3-8). The bacteria are either encountered on or within the pellicle as single organisms or as aggregates of microorganisms (Figs. 3-11, 3-14). Larger numbers of microorganisms may be carried to the tooth surface by epithelial cells (Figs. 3-12, 3-13).

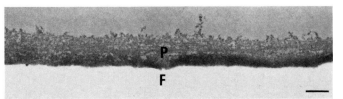

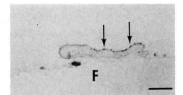

Fig. 3-7. Thin sections of pellicle (P) deposited within minutes on a Mylar film (F) attached to the buccal surface of a premolar. Magnification X 6 000. Bar: 1 μm.

Fig. 3-8. Semithin section of deposit collected on plastic film (F) applied to the buccal surface of a premolar during a 4 h period. A thin layer of pellicle material covers the plastic film and an adhering epithelial cell is covered by coccal bacteria (arrows). Magnification X 615. Bar: 10 μm.

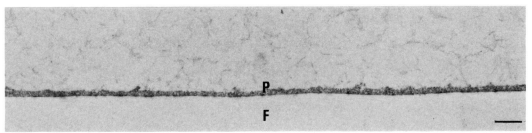

Fig. 3-9

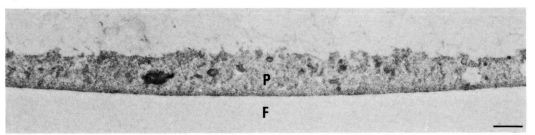

Figs. 3-9 & 3-10. Thin section of pellicle (P) deposited on plastic film (F) applied to the buccal surface of a premolar during a 4 h period. Magnification X 14 000. Bar: 0.5 μm.

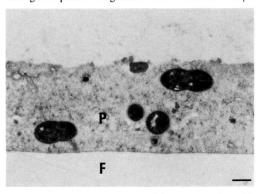

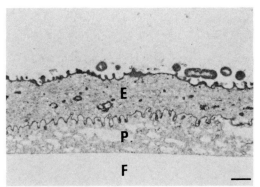

Fig. 3-11. Thin section of pellicle (P) collected within 4 h on a plastic film (F) applied to the buccal surface of a premolar. Within the pellicle material 4 microorganisms are deposited. Magnification X 10 000. Bar: 0.5 μm.

Fig. 3-12. Thin section of pellicle (P) formed on plastic film (F) applied to the buccal surface of a premolar during a 4 h period. An epithelial cell (E) carrying a few bacteria on its surface is adhering to the pellicle material. Magnification X 5 000. Bar: 1 μm.

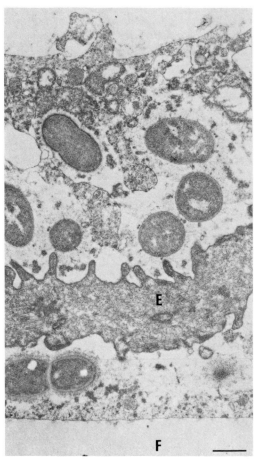

Fig. 3-13. Thin section of 4 h old plaque formed on plastic film (F) containing bacteria and an epithelial cell (E). Magnification X 17 000. Bar: 0.5 μm.

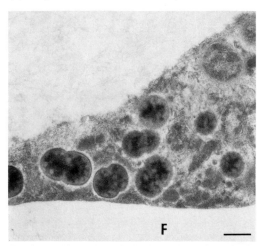

Fig. 3-14. Thin section of 8 h plaque formed on plastic film (F) containing an aggregate of bacteria. Magnification X 16 500. Bar: 0.5 μm.

The number of bacteria found on the surface a few hours after cleaning depends on the procedures applied to the sample before examination, the reason being that adherence to the solid surface is initially very weak. If no special precautions are taken during the preparatory processing, the early deposits are easily lost (Brecx et al. 1981). Apparently the adherence of microorganisms to solid surfaces takes place in 2 steps: (1) a reversible phase in which the bacteria adhere loosely, and later (2) irreversible phase during which their adherence becomes consolidated (Marshall et al. 1971, Gibbons & van Houte 1975). Another factor which may modify the number of bacteria in early plaque deposits is the presence of gingivitis, which increases the plaque formation rate so that the more complex bacterial composition is attained earlier (Saxton 1973, Hillam & Hull 1977, Brecx et al. 1980). Plaque growth may also be initiated by microorganisms harbored in minute irregularities in which they are protected from the natural cleaning of the tooth surface.

During the first few hours bacteria, that resist detachment from the pellicle, may start to proliferate and form small colonies of morphologically similar organisms (Fig. 3-15). However, since other types of organisms may also proliferate in an adjacent region, the pellicle becomes easily populated by a mixture of different microorganisms (Fig. 3-16). In addition, some organisms seem able to grow between already established colonies (Fig. 3-17), and, finally, it is likely that clumps of organisms of different species become attached to the tooth surface or to the already attached microorganisms. Such clumps will also produce mixed colonies when they proliferate. Therefore, the overall impression of plaque composition after a few days is characterized by complexity. At this time it also becomes evident that different types of organisms may benefit from each other. One example is the corncob configurations resulting from the growth of cocci on the surface of a filamentous microorganism (Listgarten, et al. 1973). Another feature of older plaque is the pre-

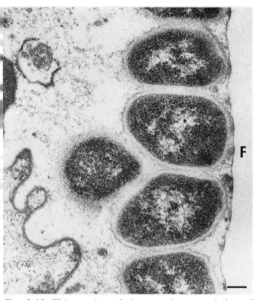

Fig. 3-15. Thin section of plaque colony consisting of morphologically similar bacteria deposited on plastic film (F) applied to the buccal surface of a premolar during an 8 h period. Magnification X 33 000. Bar: 0.2 μm.

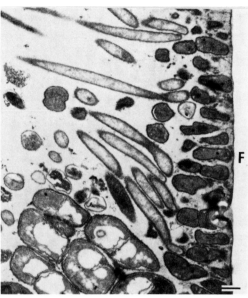

Fig. 3-16. Thin section of plaque colony containing different types of bacteria formed on Mylar film (F) during a 3 day period. Magnification X 9 100. Bar: 0.5 μm.

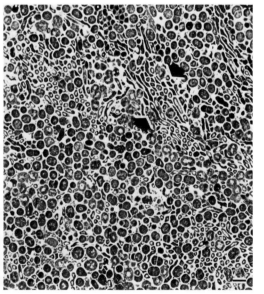

Fig. 3-17. Thin section of 3 day old plaque. The predominant organisms appear to be cocci and rods into which strands of filamentous organisms grow (arrows). Magnification X 2 800. Bar: 1 μm.

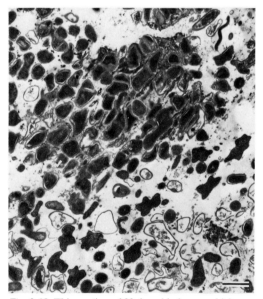

Fig. 3-18. Thin section of 23 day old plaque, which contains a considerable number of dead or lysed bacteria as evidenced by partly or completely empty bacterial cell walls termed ghosts. A spirochete is seen in the upper right corner of the illustration. Magnification X 5 800. Bar: 1 μm.

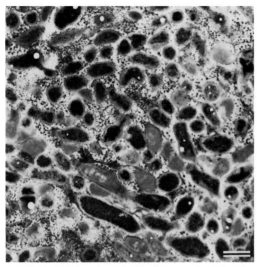

Fig. 3-19. Thin section of old plaque stained for the demonstration of polysaccharides by reacting them with electron dense material appearing dark in the illustration. Many bacteria contain large amounts of intracellular polysaccharide, and the intermicrobial matrix contains extracellular polysaccharides. Magnification X 6 600. Bar: 1 μm.

sence of dead and lysed bacteria (Fig. 3-18) which may provide additional nutrients to the still viable bacteria in the neighborhood (Theilade & Theilade 1970).

The material present between the bacteria in dental plaque is called the intermicrobial matrix and accounts for approx. 25% of the plaque volume. Three sources may contribute to the intermicrobial matrix: the plaque microorganisms, the saliva, and the gingival exudate.

The bacterial metabolism may release various end products. Some bacteria may produce various extracellular carbohydrate polymers, serving as energy storage or as anchoring material to secure their retention in plaque (Fig. 3-19). Degenerating or dead bacteria may also contribute to the intermicrobial matrix. Different bacterial species often have distinctly different metabolic pathways and capacity to synthesize extracellular material. The intermicrobial matrix in plaque, therefore, varies consider-

ably from region to region. A fibrillar component is often seen in the matrix between Gram positive cocci (Fig. 3-20), and is in accordance with the fact that several oral streptococci synthesize levans and glucans from dietary sucrose. In other regions, the matrix appears granular or homogeneous (Fig. 3-21). In parts of the plaque with the presence of Gram negative organisms, the intermicrobial matrix is regularly characterized by the presence of small vesicles surrounded by a trilaminar membrane, which is similar in structure to that of the outer envelope of the cell wall of the Gram negative microorganisms (Fig. 3-22). Such vesicles probably contain endotoxins (Hofstad et al. 1972).

It must be remembered, however, that the transmission electron microscope does not reveal all organic components of the intermicrobial matrix and the more soluble constituents may be lost during the procedures required prior to sectioning and examination of the plaque sample. Biochemical techniques may be used to identify such compounds (Silvermann & Kleinberg 1967, Krembel et al. 1969, Kleinberg 1970, Hotz et al. 1972, Rölla et al. 1975, Bowen 1976). Such studies indicate that proteins and carbohydrates constitute the bulk of the organic material while lipids appear in much lower amounts. However, studies are few in which bacteria and intermicrobial matrix have been analysed separately, and thus the total compositional nature of the matrix is still far from being finally established. Some of the proteins in the matrix are altered salivary glycoproteins, probably partly degraded by the microorganisms utilizing the sugar moiety, others have been identified as salivary or bacterial enzymes and as immunoglobulins.

The carbohydrates of the matrix have received a great deal more attention, and at least some of the polysaccharides in the plaque matrix are well characterized. These are fructans (levans) and glucans. Fructans are synthesized in plaque from dietary sucrose and provide a storage of energy, which may be utilized by microorganisms in times

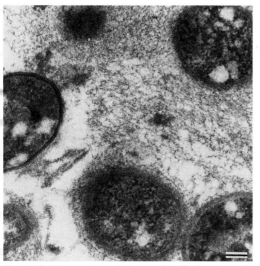

Fig. 3-20. Thin section of plaque with fibrillar intermicrobial matrix. Magnification X 47 500. Bar: 0.1 μm.

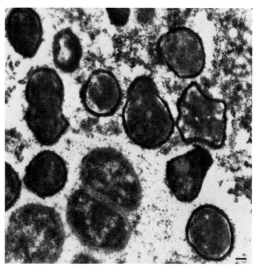

Fig. 3-21. Thin section of plaque with a granular or homogeneous intermicrobial matrix. Magnification X 19 000. Bar: 0.1 μm.

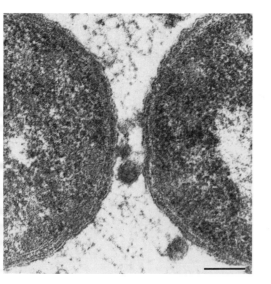

Fig. 3-22. Thin section of plaque with a region predominated by Gram negative bacteria. Between them vesicles surrounded by a trilaminar membrane (two thin electron dense layers with an electron lucent layer interposed between them). This substructure is also seen in the outermost endotoxin containing cell wall layer of the adjacent Gram negative bacteria. Magnification X 100 000. Bar: 0.1 μm.

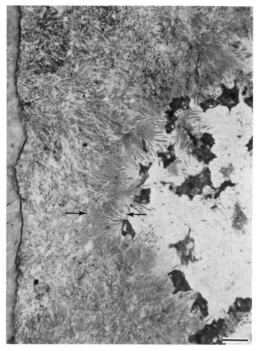

Fig. 3-23. Semithin section of subgingival plaque. To the left an electron dense cuticle bordering the enamel space. Filamentous bacteria are less predominating than in supragingival plaque. The surface toward the gingival tissue contains many spirochetes (between arrows). To the right in the illustration various host tissue cells. Magnification X 724. Bar: 10 μm. From Listgarten (1976).

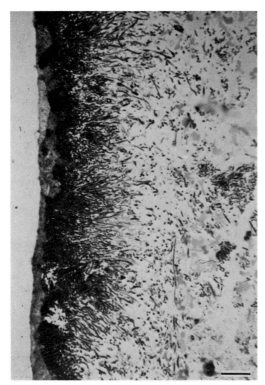

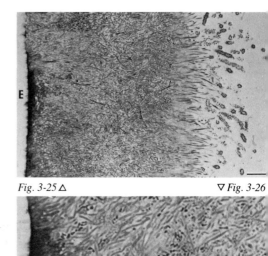

Fig. 3-25 △   ▽ *Fig. 3-26*

Fig. 3-24. Semithin section of supragingival plaque with a predominantly filamentous bacterial layer adherent to the enamel (to the left). Calcification of part of the plaque close to the tooth is evidenced by lighter staining. Magnification X 700. Bar: 10 μm. From Listgarten (1976).

Figs. 3-25. & 3-26. Semithin section of supragingival plaque on enamel (E), which has been dissolved prior to sectioning. Filamentous organisms predominate, and at the surface some of these are surrounded by cocci giving rise to corncob-like aggregations. Magnification X 708 and 1 300 X. Bars: 10 μm and 1 μm. From Listgarten (1976).

of low sugar supply. The glucans are also synthesized from sucrose. One type of glucan is dextran, which may also serve as energy storage. Another glucan is mutan and not readily degraded. It acts primarily, therefore, as a skeleton in the matrix in much the same way as collagen stabilizes the intercellular substance of connective tissue. It has been suggested that such carbohydrate polymers may be responsible for the change from a reversible to an irreversible adherence of plaque bacteria.

The small amount of lipids in the plaque matrix is as yet largely uncharacterized. Part of the lipid content is found in the small extracellular vesicles which may contain lipopolysaccharide endotoxins of Gram negative bacteria.

Subgingival plaque

The mechanisms involved in the formation of subgingival plaque are only partly elucidated. One reason is the difficulty in obtaining samples with subgingival plaque preserved in its original position between the soft tissues of the gingiva and the hard tissues of the tooth. Thus, there are only a limited number of studies on the detailed internal structure of human subgingival plaque (Schroeder 1970, Listgarten et al. 1975, Listgarten 1976, Westergaard et al. 1978). From these it is evident that in many respects sub-

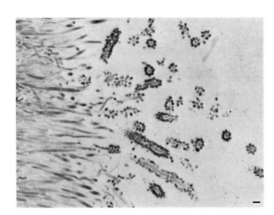

Fig. 3-27. The corncob formations seen at the plaque ▷ surface in Figs. 3-25 and 3-26. Magnification X 1 200. Bar: 1 µm. From Listgarten (1976).

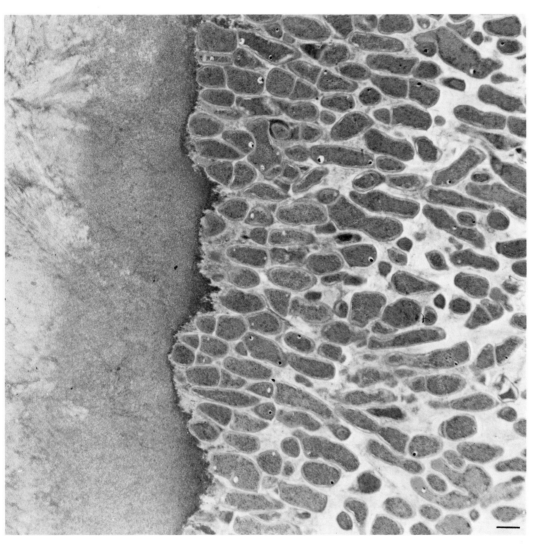

Fig. 3-28. Thin section of supragingival plaque on a root surface (to the left). The Gram positive bacteria are oriented in a palisading arrangement. Magnification X 6 000. Bar: 1 µm. From Listgarten (1976).

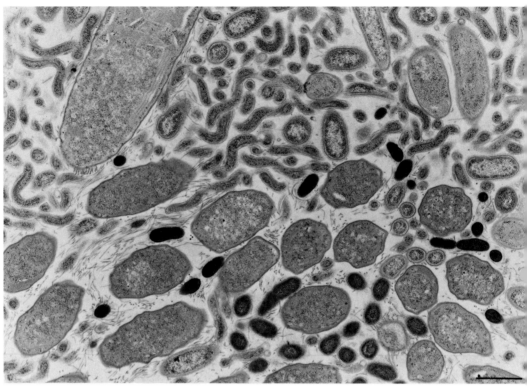

Fig. 3-29. Thin section of subgingival plaque from a deep periodontal pocket. Small microorganisms predominate, many of which are spirochetes. Magnification X 12 000. Bar: 1 µm. From Listgarten (1976).

gingival plaque resembles the supragingival variety, although the predominant types of microorganisms found vary considerably from those present coronally to the gingival margin.

Between subgingival plaque and the tooth an electron dense organic material is interposed, termed a cuticle (Fig. 3-23). This cuticle probably contains the remains of the epithelial attachment lamina originally connecting the junctional epithelium to the tooth with the addition of material deposited from the gingival exudate (Frank & Cimasoni 1970, Lie & Selvig 1975, Eide et al. 1983). It has also been suggested that the cuticle represents a secretory product of the adjacent epithelial cells (Schroeder & Listgarten 1977). Information is lacking concerning its chemical composition, but its location in the subgingival area makes it

unlikely that salivary constituents contribute to its formation.

The structure of subgingival plaque has some similarity to the supragingival variety, particularly when it concerns plaque associated with gingivitis without the formation of deep pockets. A densely packed accumulation of microorganisms is seen adjacent to the cuticular material covering the tooth surface (Fig. 3-24). The bacteria comprise Gram positive and Gram negative cocci, rods, and filamentous organisms. Spirochetes and various flagellated bacteria may also be encountered, especially at the apical extension of the plaque. The surface layer is often less densely packed and leukocytes are regularly interposed between the plaque and the epithelial lining of the gingival sulcus.

When periodontal disease has resulted in

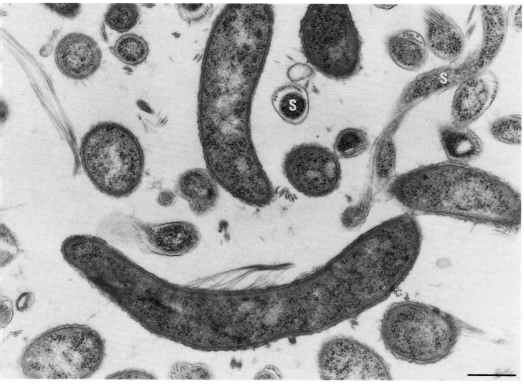

Fig. 3-30. Thin section of subgingival plaque from a deep periodontal pocket with many spirochetes (S) which are recognized by their axial filaments. In the lower part of the figure a curved organism with flagella at its concave surface. Magnification X 24 000. Bar: 0.5 μm. From Listgarten (1976).

a periodontal pocket, the appearance of the subgingival bacterial deposit becomes much more varied. The tooth surface may in this case either represent enamel or cementum from which the periodontal connective tissue is detached. Plaque accumulation on the portion of the tooth previously covered by periodontal tissues does not differ markedly from that observed in gingivitis (Fig. 3-25). In this layer filamentous microorganisms dominate (Figs. 3-26, 3-27, 3-28), but cocci and rods also occur. However, in the deeper parts of the periodontal pocket, the filamentous organisms become fewer in number, and in the apical portion they seem to be virtually absent. Instead, the dense, tooth facing part of the bacterial deposit is dominated by smaller organisms without particular orientation (Fig. 3-29).

The surface layers of microorganisms in the periodontal pocket facing the soft tissue are distinctly different from the adherent layer along the tooth surface, and no definite intermicrobial matrix is apparent (Figs. 3-29, 3-30). The microorganisms comprise a large number of spirochetes and flagellated bacteria. Gram negative cocci and rods are also present. The multitude of spirochetes and flagellated organisms are motile bacteria, and since there is no intermicrobial matrix between them, this outer part of the microbial accumulation in the periodontal pocket probably adheres very loosely, the soft tissue pocket wall probably being responsible for their retention. As plaque is, by definition, *bacteria that aggregate to the tooth*, it has been suggested that subgingival microorganisms should be redesignated subgingival flora rather than subgingival plaque, as the latter term may exclude the sig-

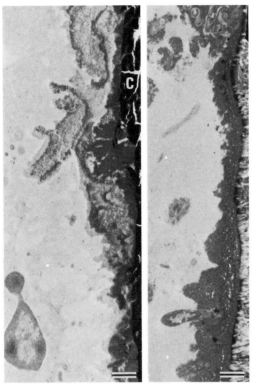

Fig. 3-31   *Fig. 3-32*

Fig. 3-31. Thin section of deposit in deep pocket o patient with juvenile periodontitis. The cementum (C is covered with cuticular material and cellular remnants. Magnification X 5 200. Bar: 1 μm. From Westergaard et al. (1978).

Fig. 3-32. Thin section of deposit in deep pocket o patient with juvenile periodontitis. A cuticle of uneven thickness is seen to the right on the cementum. A smal colony of degenerating bacteria adheres to the cuticle ir the upper part of the illustration, and below a single roc shaped microorganism is partly embedded in the cuti cle. Magnification X 5 400. Bar: 1 μm. From Wester gaard et al. (1978).

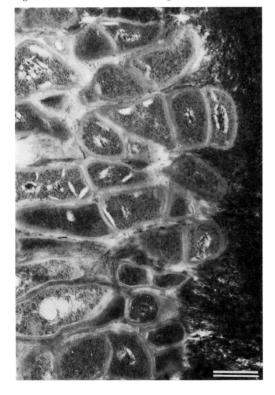

◁ *Fig. 3-33.* Thin section of plaque in deep pocket o patient with juvenile periodontitis. Densely packec Gram positive rods grow perpendicular to the cemen tum to the right in the illustration. Magnification X 21 500. Bar: 0.5 μm. From Westergaard et al. (1978).

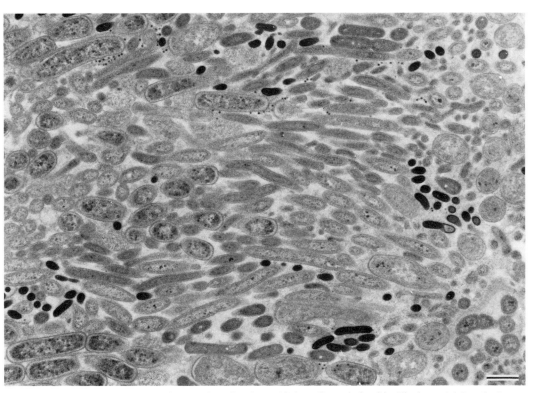

Fig. 3-34. Thin section of plaque in deep pocket of patient with juvenile periodontitis. The bacterial flora is characterized by cocci, rods or filamentous organisms, primarily of the Gram negative type. Magnification X 8 600. Bar: 1 µm. From Westergaard et al. (1978).

nificant motile portion of the bacterial population (Listgarten 1976).

Subgingival plaque has also been studied in cases of juvenile periodontitis (Listgarten 1976, Westergaard et al. 1978). It appears that the bacterial deposit in deep pockets from such patients is much thinner than found in adult forms of periodontal disease and that areas of the tooth surface in the periodontal pocket may be devoid of adherent microbial deposits. The cuticular material is characterized by an uneven thickness (Figs. 3-31, 3-32). The adherent layer of microorganisms, which also varies considerably in thickness, shows, equally, considerable variation in arrangement, and may exhibit a pallisaded organization of the bacteria (Fig. 3-33). The microorganisms in this layer are mainly cocci, rods or filamentous bacteria,

primarily of the Gram negative type (Fig. 3-34). A surface layer with some Gram positive cocci frequently associated with filamentous organisms in the typical corncob formation, may also be found with spirochetes in between.

The sequential events taking place during the development of subgingival plaque have not been studied in man. However, in dogs, subgingival plaque may develop in the gingival sulcus within a few days, if oral hygiene is discontinued (Matsson & Attström 1979, Ten Napel et al. 1983). From these studies it has been established that early dental plaque in the dog has many structural similarities with that occurring in man. This applies to the supragingival plaque (Fig. 3-35) as well as to the subgingival accumulations (Figs. 3-36, 3-37, 3-38, 3-39). These deposits may

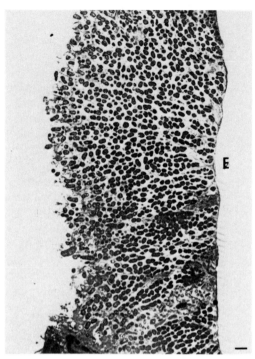

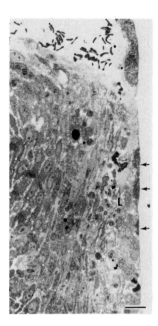

Fig. 3-37. Thin section of the gingival sulcus area in the Beagle dog. Plaque is seen at the orifice of the gingival sulcus in the upper part of the illustration. Subgingival plaque is deposited as discreet separate colonies on the tooth (arrows). Many leukocytes (L) migrate through the junctional epithelium to the subgingival portion of the tooth. Magnification X 700. Bar: 10 μm.

Fig. 3-35. Thin section of 14 day old supragingival plaque in the Beagle dog. Cocci or rods are present in a palisading arrangement perpendicular to the enamel (E). Magnification X 2 260. Bar: 1 μm.

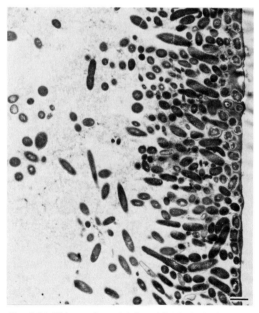

Fig. 3-36. Thin section of 4 day old subgingival plaque near the orifice of the gingival sulcus in the Beagle dog. Magnification X 5 000. Bar: 1 μm.

either appear as an apical continuation of the supragingival plaque, or as discrete aggregates at some distance from the supragingival deposit (Fig. 3-37). Old established subgingival plaque shows considerable variation of the bacterial composition between dogs: in some, a subgingival flora, dominated by spirochetes is seen, in others, colonies of Gram negative cocci and rods are found in the gingival crevice, whereas spirochetes are virtually absent (Soames & Davies, 1975, Theilade & Attström 1979). A characteristic feature of the subgingival plaque is the presence of a number of leukocytes interposed between the surface of the bacterial deposit and the gingival sulcular epithelium (Fig. 3-40). Some bacteria may be found between the epithelial cells, and evidence of phagocytosis (by polymorphonuclear leukocytes) is frequently encountered (Fig. 3-41).

Although subgingival plaque formation in the dog may not develop identically to that in man, the dog may still serve as a convenient model for investigating the basic phenomena governing the formation of subgingival plaque (Schroeder & Attström 1979).

Diet and plaque formation

Diet has frequently been considered to play a significant part in the development of dental plaque, yet for more than 50 years it has been known that dental plaque may form on human teeth in the absence of oral food intake (Howitt et al. 1928). Similar results have been obtained from studies in dogs (Egelberg 1965b) and monkeys (Bowen 1974).

On the other hand, it is similarly well established that diet may modify both the amount of plaque formed and its composition. Two different plaque forming modes of action may be operating. The diet may be such as to require vigorous chewing, thus activating the cleansing action of saliva, lips, cheeks and tongue, or it may be such as to favor plaque formation.

Consistency of diet
The plaque reducing effect of a hard, fibrous diet has been shown in dogs receiving raw bovine trachea (Egelberg 1965a). However, a similar marked effect of diets requiring vigorous chewing has not been demonstrated in man. The most likely explanation for this lack of effect, is that there are major differences in tooth anatomy. The tapered form of dog teeth and the diastemata between them probably makes the surfaces more accessible for cleansing action, while in man the dental plaque, located along the gingival margin of the teeth and interproximally, is not subject to friction from food during mastication (Wilcox & Everett 1963). It is therefore not surprising that several investigators have failed to demonstrate any effect on human plaque accumulation, even after excessive

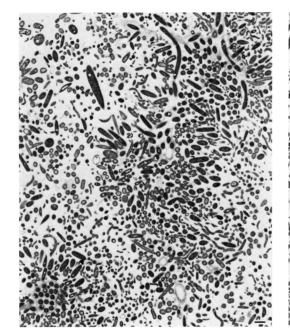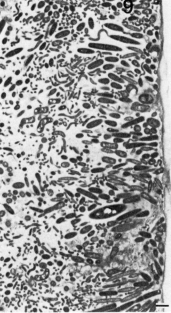

Figs. 3-38 & 3-39. Thin sections of 14 day old plaque in dog. The subgingival flora is characterized by a variety of different types of microorganisms including spirochetes with no apparent order of arrangement. Magnification X 2 750. Bar: 1 μm.

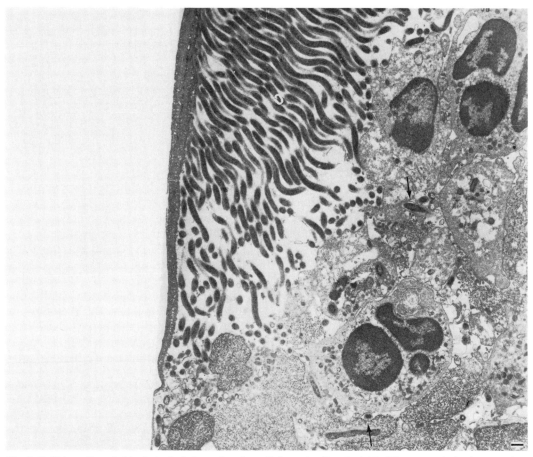

Fig. 3-40. Thin section of old subgingival plaque in a dog with long standing gingivitis. The most apical colony consists primarily of spirochetes attached to a dense cuticle and surrounded by migrated leukocytes. Single microorganisms are seen between them (arrows). Magnification X 2 650. Bar: 1 µm.

chewing of raw carrot, apple, etc. (Bergen-holtz et al. 1967, Lindhe & Wicén 1969, Wade 1971).

Composition of diet
The composition of diet has been considered to have a marked influence on plaque forma-tion, because diet together with saliva pro-vides nutrients for plaque microorganisms. Most studies of dietary effect on plaque per-tain to the carbohydrates. Fermentable sugars might be expected to increase plaque formation because of their action as addi-tional energy supply for the plaque micro-biota; they may also act as substrate for the

production of extracellular polysaccharides (Guggenheim 1970). However, the results from a number of studies regarding the effect of carbohydrates on plaque formation are contradictory, probably because of vary-ing trial design and limited subject availa-bility.

One study investigated 2 subjects over four 3 day periods of varying diets and with no oral hygiene (Carlsson & Egelberg 1965). Similar quantities of plaque were formed during periods when the participants used a carbohydrate free basic diet of protein and fat, and when this basic diet was sup-plemented at half-hourly intervals with either glucose or fructose. On the other hand, the basic diet plus a frequent intake of sucrose produced larger quantities of voluminous, turgid plaque, which had little tendency to spread coronally to the remaining surface areas. In a similar 7 day experiment with 10 subjects, essentially the same results were observed in 6 of the subjects (Carlsson & Egelberg 1965). In another 4 day experiment, 4 groups of students received either fructose, glucose, sucrose or sugar alcohol xylitol (Sheinin & Mäkinen 1971). Large individual variations in plaque formation were noted. The highest mean value in plaque index, as well as wet weight of plaque, was seen in the sucrose group and the lowest in the xylitol group. In a more recent, well controlled experiment, 24 subjects had a carbohydrate free diet for a 4 day period, and in comparable experiments, this diet was supplemented with sucrose-, xylitol- or sorbitol-containing sweets (Rateitschak-Plüss & Guggenheim 1982). This study also demon-

strated that more plaque formed during the diet period with sucrose supplements. On the other hand, in an experiment where the amount of plaque was assessed in subjects either on a low sucrose diet or a diet with hourly sucrose supplements, no difference could be found in the quantity of plaque measured by wet weight and by light absorbance of plaque suspensions (Folke et al. 1972). In a study of the effect of sucrose and glucose on early plaque formation, no increase could be demonstrated in plaque quantity as measured by microbial counts in sections of the deposits (Brecx et al. 1981). The possible explanation for the lack of effect may be that the few bacteria which were present in 4 h plaque had sufficient sugar available without supplements (Figs. 3-42, 3-43, 3-44, 3-45). These studies may indicate that the effect of dietary sugars on the amount of plaque forming in man is, generally, far less than theoretical expectation.

Some studies show no effect and others

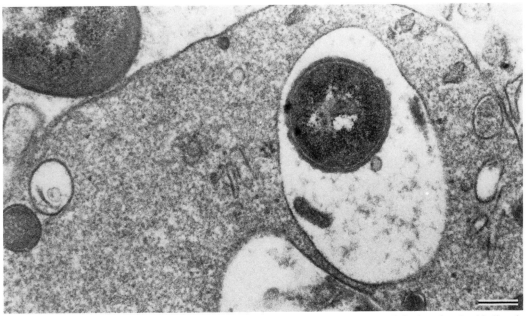

Fig. 3-41. Thin section of part of a leukocyte situated between subgingival plaque and the junctional epithelium in dog. The large membrane bound compartment of the leukocyte cytoplasm contains a phagocytized Gram negative microorganism. Another bacteria is in close apposition to the cytoplasmic membrane of the leukocyte. Magnification X 20 000. Bar: 0.5 μm.

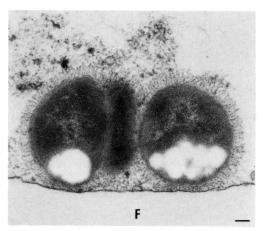

Fig. 3-42. Thin section of 4 h old supragingival plaque formed on plastic film (F) applied to the buccal surface of a premolar. During the period of development the person rinsed regularly with a 50% solution of sucrose. Two Gram negative organisms are seen with intracellular electron lucent areas in their cytoplasm. Magnification X 40 000. Bar: 0.1 μm.

ary sucrose is followed by lower proportions of *S. mutans* and higher proportions of *S. sanguis* in the plaque (de Stoppelaar et al. 1970). On the other hand, in short-term experiments with 1, 3 and 4 day old plaque, frequent supplements of glucose or sucrose to a low carbohydrate diet failed to influence the proportion of *S. mutans*, which was low in all groups (Carlsson 1967, Folke et al. 1972). In conclusion, plaque flora is apparently dependent to a much greater extent on the oral environment than on the transient presence of food (Bibby 1976). It is, nevertheless, evident that the quantitative proportions of some bacterial species may to some extent be modified by diet.

The assessment of the effect of diet on the chemical composition of plaque has dealt mainly with the carbohydrate metabolism. Plaque carbohydrates are primarily present

show statistically significant increases which, however, may be too small to have clinical significance, e.g. an increased extension of plaque coronally on the clinical crowns of the teeth may be inconsequential to the marginal periodontium.

Several studies have been performed to investigate whether dietary carbohydrates, and especially sucrose, have an influence on the bacterial composition of dental plaque. It has been known for many years that large numbers of lactobacilli in saliva are related to a high consumption of fermentable carbohydrates, and, that following restrictions of dietary sugar, the lactobacillus counts are reduced. However, lactobacilli constitute a very small proportion of the plaque flora (van Houte et al. 1972). Streptococci also might be expected to be influenced by dietary sugars. *S. mutans* and *S. sanguis* produce extracellular polysaccharides from sucrose, but not from other sugars. Sucrose seems to favor *S. mutans*, but not *S. sanguis* in plaque. Thus, in studies of long duration (weeks or months) frequent consumption of sucrose causes an increase in numbers of *S. mutans* (Gehring et al. 1974), and restriction of diet-

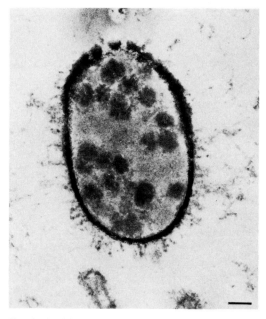

Fig. 3-43. Thin section of 4 h old supragingival plaque formed while the person performed regular rinses with water. The section is stained for the demonstration of carbohydrate. Although no dietary sugar was administered during the plaque formation period, intracellular polysaccharide granules are present in the microorganisms as well as in their cell walls. Magnification X 50 000. Bar: 0.1 μm.

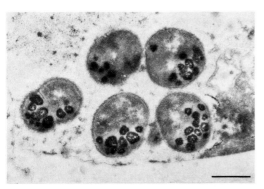

Fig. 3-44. Section comparable to that shown in Fig. 3-42, but specifically stained for the demonstration of polysaccharides. Thus the electron lucent areas in Fig. 3-42 represent intracellular polysaccharides. Magnification X 22 500. Bar: 0.5 µm.

as structural components of the microorganisms, as storage granules in the bacteria termed intracellular polysaccharides, and as extracellular polysaccharides in the matrix between the microorganisms (Wood 1969); carbohydrate constitutes about 20% of plaque dry weight (Hotz et al. 1972).

Intracellular polysaccharides of the glycogen-amylopectin type are synthesized by plaque bacteria from dietary sugars, such as sucrose, glucose and others, and in the absence of a sugar supply they are catabolized (Gibbons & Socransky 1962, Saxton 1969, Wood 1969). Thus, dietary restriction of carbohydrate seems to cause a marked reduction in the number of polysaccharide storing bacteria in plaque (van Houte 1964).

Extracellular polysaccharides in plaque comprise a variety of sugar polymers. Of these, fructans (levans) and glucans have received much attention in recent years. Fructans are synthesized in plaque from dietary sucrose, and, as with intracellular polysaccharides, they provide a storage component which is broken down when the sugar supply is insufficient. Thus, fructans constitute a variable, but always minor proportion of the extracellular polysaccharides in plaque (Critchley et al. 1967, Wood 1967, Higuchi et al. 1970, Leach et al. 1972, Gold et al. 1974). Glucans, which are also synthesized from sucrose, seem to be more important both quantitatively and functionally, and comprise a variety of different types of polymers. One of these is dextran which has predominance of α-1.6 linkages, and as some plaque bacteria possess the enzyme dextranase, the dextrans may also act as a storage carbohydrate. Another type of glucan characterized mainly by α-1.3 linkages is called mutan and does not seem to be broken down in plaque, so that its function is primarily that of structural stabilizer of the intermicrobial matrix (Guggenheim 1970, Hotz et al. 1972, Dewar & Walker 1975).

The carbohydrates, thus, play an important part in plaque development and maintenance. However, with the diversity of possible metabolic pathways dietary sugars can take in plaque, the lack of exact knowledge concerning the details of the clinical impact of variations in sugar consumption is not surprising.

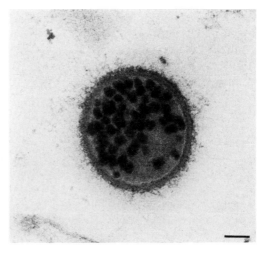

Fig. 3-45. Thin section of a bacteria from 4 hour old supragingival plaque formed while the person rinsed regularly with a 50% solution of glucose. Numerous granules containing intracellular polysaccharides have been demonstrated with a carbohydrate stain. Magnification X 50 000. Bar: 0.1 µm.

109

Dental calculus

The calcified deposits termed tartar or dental calculus have been recognized for centuries together with their detrimental effect on gingival tissue. In the middle of this century, renewed interest in dental calculus developed as a result of improved research methods, primarily the introduction of modern epidemiology applied to periodontal disease, and by the application of biochemical and biophysical techniques in the investigation of dental calculus.

Definition and classification of dental calculus

Dental calculus may be defined as calcified or calcifying deposits on the teeth and other solid structures in the oral cavity. It is classified as supragingival calculus when present on the visible clinical crowns of the teeth above the gingival margin. Calculus located apical to the gingival margin in the gingival sulcus or the periodontal pocket is termed subgingival calculus.

Clinical appearance and distribution of calculus

Supragingival calculus is yellow, white accretions usually located along the gingival margins of the teeth. However, the color may change to brown as a result of secondary staining from the use of tobacco or from food pigments. The distribution of supragingival calculus does not entirely follow that of supragingival plaque as the tendency for the latter to calcify into calculus varies within the oral cavity. The largest amounts of supragingival calculus are found opposite the openings of the major salivary ducts. Thus, copious amounts of supragingival calculus are often seen on the buccal aspects of the maxillary molars in the vicinity of the opening of the Stensen's duct of the parotid salivary gland, and on the lingual and even buccal surfaces of the mandibulary incisors opposite the orifice of the Warton's duct of the submandibular and the Bartholin's duct of the sublingual, salivary glands (Figs. 3-46, 3-47).

Subgingival calculus is brown to black in color and harder and often more tenaceously adherent to the tooth surface (Fig. 3-48). It is

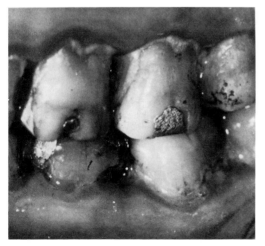

Fig. 3-46. Supragingival calculus along the gingival margin on the buccal surfaces of maxillary molars.

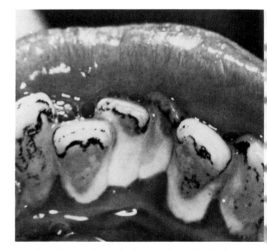

Fig. 3-47. Supragingival calculus along the gingival margin on the lingual surfaces of the mandibular cuspids and incisors.

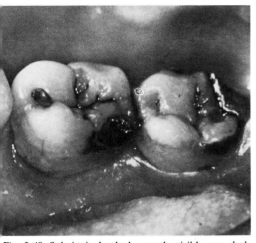

Fig. 3-48. Subgingival calculus partly visible as a dark concrement in the orifice of the gingival sulcus of the mandibular molars.

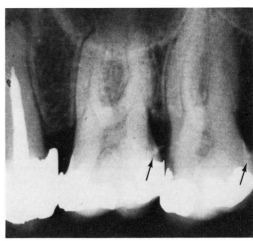

Fig. 3-49. Radiograph showing dental calculus (arrows) on the distal surfaces of two maxillary molars.

more evenly distributed on the various teeth, but on the individual tooth subgingival calculus is more prevalent on the approximal and lingual than on the buccal tooth surfaces.

Diagnosis of dental calculus

Supragingival calculus may be recognized by clinical inspection when present in sufficient amounts. Thin layers may, however, be overlooked if the tooth surface is moistened by saliva, which penetrates the porous surface of calculus. If the tooth surface is dried, a thin layer of calculus may have an appearance similar to that of a hypoplastic tooth surface, and its detection therefore requires probing or scraping with an instrument.

Subgingival calculus is often difficult to detect by clinical inspection, though its presence below the gingival margin may be indirectly diagnosed, if its dark color shines through the thin gingival margin, in the same way as a dark restoration or a dark endodontically treated root. Subgingival calculus may be seen by the detachment of the gingi-

val margin from the tooth by air blast or by appropriate instrument. Calculus in deeper periodontal pockets may be disclosed by probing, but this method of calculus detection is highly inefficient (Wærhaug 1978). Under certain circumstances calculus on the approximal surfaces of the teeth may be visible on radiographs (Fig. 3-49). This method of detection is also very uncertain, because the image of the calculus is dependent both on its density and on the radiographic technique. The correct diagnosis of subgingival calculus in deeper periodontal pockets, therefore, sometimes necessitates the reflection of the covering periodontal tissues during periodontal surgery.

Composition of dental calculus

Calculus consists of 70-80% inorganic salts, of which two-thirds are in crystalline form (Leung & Jensen 1958). Calcium and phosphorus constitute the major elements with a Ca/P ratio ranging from 1.66 to more than 2 (Leung & Jensen 1958, Little et al. 1963, Schroeder 1963, Little & Hazen 1964). Cal-

111

cium usually accounts for up to 40% of the inorganic weight, while the proportion of phosphorus approaches 20%. Small a-mounts of magnesium, sodium, carbonate and fluoride may be present as well, together with traces of other elements (for review see Theilade & Schroeder 1966, Schroeder 1969, Leach 1973).

The crystal forms in which inorganic constituents are present have been determined by various physical techniques of analysis, primarily X-ray and electron diffraction. The 4 principal crystal forms are hydroxy-apatite, $Ca_{10}(OH)_2(PO_4)_6$; magnesium whit-lockite, $Ca_3 (PO_4)_2$ in which the magnesium ion substitutes a small number of the calcium ions; octacalcium phosphate, $Ca_4 H(PO_4)_3$ $2H_2O$; and brushite $Ca HPO_4 2H_2O$ (Rowles 1964). Of these crystal types, the first 3 are variants of the hydroxyapatite lattice, which dominates many biological mineralized tissues such as bone, cementum, dentin and enamel. Brushite is the simple secondary calcium phosphate. The 4 crystal forms do not occur with the same frequency in all calculus samples, generally 2 or more are present in a sample. Their incidence varies with the age of the calculus sample (Schroeder & Baumbauer, 1966) as well as with its loca-

tion. Thus brushite is more common in sup-ragingival calculus, while magnesium whit-lockite is present particularly in the subgingi-val variety.

The organic portion of calculus has been analysed biochemically and histochemically in a number of studies (Mandel 1963, Little et al. 1964, 1966, Stanford 1966), from which it is evident that the bulk of the organic portion of calculus consists of proteins and carbohydrates, while lipids account for only a minor fraction; this composition is comparable to that of dental plaque (Silverman & Kleinberg 1967).

Structure of dental calculus

Study of the internal structure of dental calculus has been hampered by the high amount of inorganic constituents, which restricts sufficiently thin sectioning for subsequent examination. Calculus has been studied in a variety of ways including ground sections of undemineralized samples as well as regular sections of decalcified specimens with or without the presence of the adjacent tooth structure, and soft tissues. With the introduction of electron microscopy and the con-

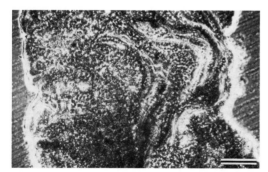

Fig. 3-50. Ground section of subgingival calculus. The tooth surface is represented to the left. A definite layering of the deposit is evident. Magnification X 90. Bar: 100 µm.

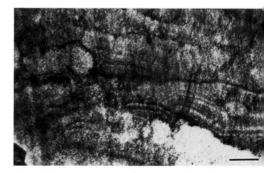

Fig. 3-51. Microradiograph of ground section of calculus. The tooth surface is at the bottom of the illustration. The degree of calcification varies from region to region. Unmineralized resting or incremental lines appear as radio lucent dark lines. Magnification X 77. Bar: 100 µm.

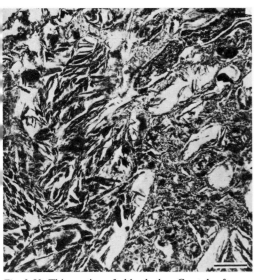

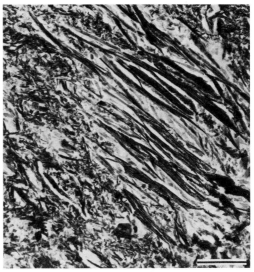

Fig. 3-52. Thin section of old calculus. Crystals of varying size are deposited in random orientation. The outlines of microorganisms are discernible; in the upper right corner a fully mineralized filamentous organism can be seen. Magnification X 17 000. Bar: 0.5 µm.

Fig. 3-53. Thin section of old calculus with a region of long ribbon shaped crystal with a preferred orientation. Magnification X 25 000. Bar: 0.5 µm.

comitant possibility of ultrathin sections, a clearer understanding of the nature of dental calculus has begun to emerge (Gonzales & Sognnaes 1960, Theilade 1960, Zander et al. 1960).

The examination of ground sections reveals that calculus is often a layered structure (Fig. 3-50) in which the degree of calcification varies in the different layers (Fig. 3-51) between which resting lines are frequently evident. In thin undecalcified sections, calculus is dominated by small needle shaped, inorganic crystals ranging in length from 5-100 nm, revealed by electron diffraction to consist of apatite. Other crystals appear as plates or long rods. Generally, the crystals are randomly oriented (Fig. 3-52), although in certain regions a particular orientation may prevail (Fig. 3-53). Within the mineralized material, it is possible to discern the outlines of calcified microorganisms (Fig. 3-54). A very significant feature of calculus (Fig. 3-55) is that its surface is covered by a layer of unmineralized plaque (Gonzales & Sognnaes 1960, Theilade 1960, Zander et al. 1960, Schroeder 1969).

Formation of calculus

Information on how calculus develops has to a large extent been obtained from studies in which Mylar® films were attached, for set

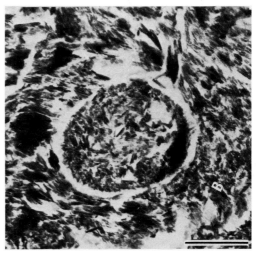

Fig. 3-54. Thin section of old calculus. The intermicrobial matrix and the microorganism are calcified to the same extent. Only the outline disguises the bacterium. Magnification X 31 000. Bar: 0.5 µm.

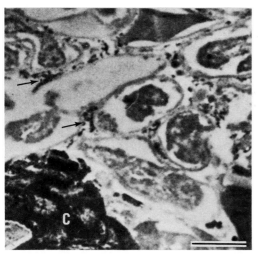

Fig. 3-55. Thin section of calculus (C). At its surface a layer of plaque with only small amounts of mineral precipitates (arrows) between the bacteria. Magnification X 28 000. Bar: 0.5 µm.

periods, to tooth surfaces known to form calculus. After removal the films were processed for either light or electron microscopy (Mandel et al. 1957, Voreadis & Zander,

1958, Mühlemann & Schneider 1959, Hazen 1960, Turesky et al. 1961, Schroeder et al. 1964, Theilade 1964, Schroeder 1965). From these studies it is evident that calculus formation is always preceded by plaque formation. The plaque accumulations serve as an organic matrix for the subsequent mineralization of the deposit.

Initially, small crystals are seen in the intermicrobial matrix (Fig. 3-56) frequently in close apposition to the external aspect of the bacteria. Gradually, the matrix between the microorganisms becomes entirely calcified, and eventually the bacteria also become mineralized (Fig. 3-57).

While the deposition of crystals within preformed plaque is the usual mode of calculus formation, minerals may also be deposited at the surface of supragingival plaque accumulations. In such foci the crystals are rod shaped. X-ray diffraction indicates that these crystals are calcium phosphate precipitated as brushite, $CaHPO_4,2H_2O$ (Schroeder 1964, Schroeder & Baumbauer 1966).

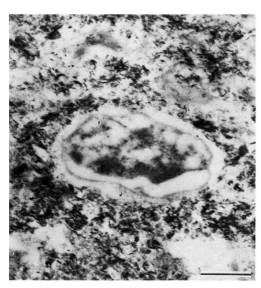

Fig. 3-56. Thin section of old plaque. A degenerating organism is surrounded by intermicrobial matrix in which initial mineralization has started by the deposition of small needle shaped electron dense apatite crystals. Magnification X 25 000. Bar: 0.5 µm. From Zander et al. (1960).

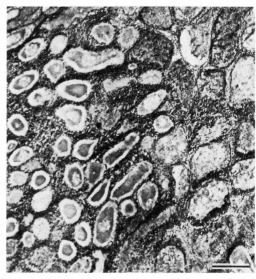

Fig. 3-57. Thin section of old mineralizing plaque. The intermicrobial matrix is totally calcified, and many microorganisms show intracellular crystal deposition. Magnification X 9 000. Bar: 1 µm.

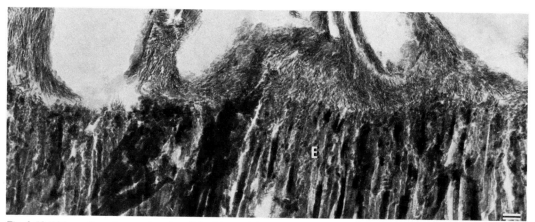

Fig. 3-58. Thin section of enamel surface (E) with overlying calculus. The enamel and calculus crystals are in intimate contact, and the latter extends into the minute irregularities of the enamel. Magnification X 35 000. Bar: 0.1 μm. From Selvig (1970).

The time required for the formation of supragingival calculus is, in some persons, less than 2 weeks, at which time the deposit may already contain about 80% of the inorganic material found in mature calculus (Mühlemann & Schroeder 1964). The first evidence of calcification may already occur after a few days (Theilade 1964). However, the development of a deposit with a crystal composition characteristic of old calculus requires months or years (Schroeder & Baumbauer 1966).

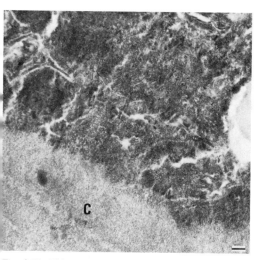

Fig. 3-59. Thin section of cementum surface (C) with overlying calculus. The calculus is closely adapted to the irregular cementum and is more electron dense and therefore harder than the adjacent cementum. To the right in the illustration part of an uncalcified microorganism. Magnification X 30 000. Bar: 0.1 μm. From Selvig (1970).

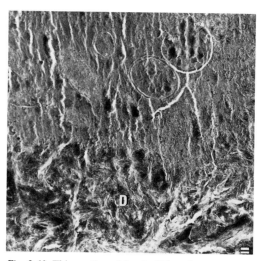

Fig. 3-60. Thin section of dentin (D) surface with overlying calculus. The interface between the calculus and dentin cannot be precisely determined as the calculus crystals fill in the irregularities of the dentin surface, which is devoid of cementum as a result of a previous scaling of the root surface. The circular profiles in the calculus surround completely calcified bacteria. Magnification X 18 000. Bar: 1 μm. From Selvig (1970).

Attachment of calculus to the teeth

Calculus often adheres tenaciously to the teeth, and hard, subgingival calculus may be especially difficult to remove. One reason for its firm attachment to the tooth surface may be that the pellicle beneath the plaque also calcifies, and thereby the calculus crystals come into intimate contact with the enamel, cementum or dentin crystals (Figs. 3-58, 3-59, 3-60) (Kopczyk & Conroy 1968, Selvig 1970, Canis et al. 1979). In addition, the surface irregularities are also penetrated by calculus crystals, so that the calculus is virtually locked to the tooth. This is particularly the case on exposed cementum where small pits occur at sites where the Sharpey's fibers previously inserted (Bercy & Frank 1980). Uneven root surfaces may be the result of carious lesions, small pieces of cementum may have been lost as a result of tear when the periodontal ligament was still attached (Moskow 1969), and, under such conditions, it becomes impossible to remove all calculus without the loss of some of the hard tissue of the teeth.

Mineralization theories

The question of why calcium phosphates precipitate as calculus has puzzled scientists for many years. Two aspects must be explained, first the nucleation of the crystallites, and secondly their growth. Saliva is a metastable solution for some calcium phosphates, namely apatite, octocalcium phosphate and whitlockite, and under certain conditions also with respect to brushite. This means that saliva is supersaturated with respect to the salts and thus able to support crystal growth, but that spontaneous precipitation does not occur unless the solution is seeded, e.g. by the presence of crystals on which new crystals can form. Crystals for this nucleation process are present in the tooth surface, but since they are covered by a pellicle, they are not readily available for this function. Several explanatory hypotheses have been offered for the initiation of the mineralization process, but the question remains unresolved; discussion of some of them follows: the carbon dioxide theory propounds that freshly secreted saliva leaving the openings of the salivary ducts has a CO_2 tension of about 60 mm Hg, while that prevailing in the oral cavity is considerably lower, somewhere between the CO_2 tension of the expired air (29 mm Hg) and that of the atmosphere (0.3 mm). This discrepancy will result in the escape of CO_2 from saliva, the pH of which will rise. When the pH of saliva increases, less calcium and phosphates can be accommodated in the ionized form, and consequently spontaneous precipitation may occur. Once crystallites are present, the physiological supersaturation accounts for this growth. This theory offers a plausible explanation for the occurrence of copious amounts of supragingival calculus near the orifice of the major salivary ducts. It cannot explain, however, the formation of subgingival calculus, which probably derives from the salts in the gingival exudate. Other mechanisms, however, might raise the pH in saliva or plaque, such as ammonia production. It has been observed that rapid calculus formers have an increased urea concentration of saliva (Mandel & Thompson 1967). Ammonia is a breakdown product from urea, and might result in a local pH increase in plaque.

When it was established that calculus forms by the calcification of plaque, and that certain changes could be demonstrated in plaque when the process of mineralization begins, it was proposed that the organic matrix could be acting as a seeding agent. When crystallization is nucleated by a compound of different chemical composition, the phenomenon is termed epitaxis. Although epitaxis has been claimed for the last 20 years to occur in biological mineralizations including calculus (Glimcher 1960), the compound(s) responsible has still not been identified. However, recently some progress has been made in characterizing fractions of the organic matrix that might be initiators. Thus, *in vitro* experiments with decalcified calculus have shown that extraction of the lipid component prevented remineralization of the calculus matrix, and later a proteolipid with nucleating property was partly characterized (Ennever et al. 1973, 1979). This does not preclude other organic compounds as nucleating factors. Furthermore, specific nucleators of apatite may not be essential, as it is possible for apatite crystals to transform from brushite and octocalcium phosphate (Barone et al. 1976).

The synthesis of the nucleating organic compounds is largely unknown, but it has been established that degenerating oral bacteria may calcify *in vitro* by deposition of calcium phosphate crystals of the same type as those found in calculus (Ennever 1960, Bowen & Gilmour 1961, Lie & Selvig 1974, Sidaway 1979). It is, therefore, reasonable to assign bacteria a key role in a possible epitactic mechanism for the mineralization process. This does not mean that they alone are responsible for producing nucleating compounds, since calculus formation, to a small extent, does occur in germ free rats by calcification of an organic matrix probably originating from saliva (Baer & Newton 1959, Fitzgerald & McDaniel 1960, Theilade et al. 1964).

Effect of calculus on periodontal tissues

The presence of calculus is invariably associated with periodontal disease (Wærhaug 1952, 1955, Lövdal et al. 1958). However, as calculus is always covered by an unmineralized plaque layer, it may be difficult to assess whether calculus *per se,* has a detrimental effect on the periodontal tissue. From epidemiologic data, however, it is evident that the correlation between plaque and gingivitis is much stronger than that between calculus and gingivitis (Silness & Löe 1964). It has been proposed that calculus may exert a detrimental effect on the soft tissues of the periodontium because of its rough surface. However, it has been clearly demonstrated that the roughness of a surface does not initiate gingivitis (Wærhaug 1956), and under certain circumstances a normal attachment may even be seen between the junctional epithelium and calculus (Listgarten & Ellegaard 1973). It has also been shown that autoclaved calculus may be encapsulated in connective tissue without causing marked inflammation (Allen & Kerr 1965).

The primary effect of calculus in periodontal disease, therefore, seems to be its retention site role for plaque. Large amounts of calculus may hamper the efficacy of daily oral hygiene and thereby accelerate plaque formation. In addition the calcified deposit may contain products toxic to soft tissue. Such products may either persist in the calculus from the period prior to its calcification, or they may enter its porous surface from the overlying plaque layer.

In conclusion, calculus is not the most significant etiological factor in periodontal disease. However, its presence makes sufficient plaque removal impossible for the therapist, and prevents patients from performing an efficient plaque control.

References

Allen, D. L. & Kerr, D. A. (1965) Tissue response in the guinea pig to sterile and non-sterile calculus. *Journal of Periodontology* **36**, 121-126.

Axelsson, P. & Lindhe, J. (1974) The effect of a preventive programme on dental plaque, gingivitis and caries in schoolchildren. Results after one and two years. *Journal of Clinical Periodontology* **1**, 126-138.

Axelsson, P. & Lindhe, J. (1981) Effect of controlled oral hygiene procedures on caries and periodontal disease in adults. Results after 6 years. *Journal of Clinical Periodontology* **8**, 239-248.

Baer, P. N. & Newton, W. L. (1959) The occurrence of periodontal disease in germ-free mice. *Journal of Dental Research* **38**, 1238.

Barone, J. P., Nancollas, G. H. & Tomson, M. (1976) The seeded growth of calcium phosphates. The kinetics of growth of dicalcium dihydrate on hydroxyapatite. *Calcified Tissue Research* **21**, 171-182.

Bercy, P. & Frank, R. M. (1980) Microscopie électronique à balayage de la surface du cément humain normal et carié. *Journal Biologie Buccale* **8**, 331-352.

Bergenholtz, A., Hugoson, A. & Sohlberg, F. (1967) Den plaqueavlägsnande förmåga hos någre mundhygieniske hjälpmedel. *Svensk Tandläkare Tidsskrift* **60**, 447-454.

Berthold, C.-H., Berthold, P. & Söder, P.-Ö. (1971) The growth of dental plaque on different materials. *Svensk Tandläkare Tidsskrift* **64**, 863-877.

Bibby, B. G. (1976) Influence of diet on the bacterial composition of plaques. In *Microbial Aspects of Dental Caries,* ed. Stiles, H. M., Loesche, W. J. & O'Brien, T. C., Special Supplement, Microbiology Abstracts, Vol. II, pp. 477-490. Washington D. C.: Information Retrieval Inc.

Black, G. V. (1911) Beginnings of pyorrhea alveolaris – treatment for prevention. *Dental Items of Interest* **33**, 420-455.

Bowen, W. H. (1974) Effect of restricting oral intake to invert sugar or casein on the microbiology of plaque in *Macaca fascicularis (irus).* *Archives of Oral Biology* **19**, 231-239.

Bowen, W. H. (1976) Nature of plaque. *Oral Sciences Reviews* **9**, 3-21.

Bowen, W. H. & Gilmour, M. N. (1961) The formation of calculus-like deposits by pure cultures of bacteria. *Archives of Oral Biology* **5**, 145-148.

Brecx, M. (1979) *Early Human Dental Plaque Formation. A Light and Electron Microscopic Study.* Thesis. Aarhus: Royal Dental College.

Brecx, M., Rönström, A., Theilade, J. & Attström, R. (1981) Early formation of dental plaque on plastic films. II. Electron microscopic observations. *Journal of Periodontal Research* **16**, 213-227.

Brecx, M., Theilade, J. & Attström, R. (1980) Influence of optimal and excluded oral hygiene on early formation of dental plaque on plastic films. A quantitative and descriptive light and electron microscopic study. *Journal of Clinical Periodontology* **7**, 361-373.

Brecx, M., Theilade, J. & Attström, R. (1981) Ultrastructural estimation of the effect of sucrose and glucose rinses on dental plaque formed on plastic films. *Scandinavian Journal of Dental Research* **89**, 157-164.

Brecx, M., Theilade, J. & Attström, R. (1983) An ultrastructural quantitative study of the significance of microbial multiplication during early dental plaque growth. *Journal of Periodontal Research* **18**, 177-186.

Burnett, G. W. & Schuster, G. S. (1978) In *Oral Microbiology and Infectious Disease.* Student Edition, pp. 158-160, 218-222. Baltimore: The Williams and Wilkins Company.

Canis, M. F., Kramer, G. M. & Pameijer, C. M. (1979) Calculus attachment. Review of the literature and new findings. *Journal of Periodontology* **50**, 406-415.

Carlsson, J. (1967) Presence of various types of non-haemolytic streptococci in dental plaque and in other sites of the oral cavity in man. *Odontologisk Revy* **18**, 55-74.

Carlsson, J. & Egelberg, J. (1965) Effect of diet on early plaque formation in man. *Odontologisk Revy* **16**, 112-125.

Crawford, A., Socransky, S. S. & Bratthall, D

(1975) Predominant cultivable microbiota of advanced periodontitis. *Journal of Dental Research* **54**, Special issue A, 97.

Critchley, P., Wood, J. M., Saxton, C. A. & Leach, S. A. (1967) The polymerisation of dietary sugars by dental plaque. *Caries Research* **1**, 112-129.

Dawes, C., Jenkins, G. N. & Tonge, C. H. (1963) The nomenclature of the integuments of the enamel surface of teeth. *British Dental Journal* **16**, 65-68.

De Stoppelaar, J. D., van Houte, J. & Dirks, D. B. (1970) The effect of carbohydrate restriction on the presence of *Streptococcus mutans, Streptococcus sanguis* and iodophilic polysaccharide-producing bacteria in human dental plaque. *Caries Research* **4**, 114-123.

Dewar, M. D. & Walker, G. J. (1975) Metabolism of the polysaccharides of human dental plaque. I. Dextranase activity of streptococci, and the extracellular polysaccharides synthesized from sucrose. *Caries Research* **9**, 21-35.

Eastcott, A. D. & Stallard, R. E. (1973) Sequential changes in developing human dental plaque as visualized by scanning electron microscopy. *Journal of Periodontology* **44**, 218-244.

Egelberg, J. (1965a) Local effect of diet on plaque formation and development of gingivitis in dogs. I. Effect of hard and soft diets. *Odontologisk Revy* **16**, 31-41.

Egelberg, J. (1965b) Local effect of diet on plaque formation and development of gingivitis in dogs. III. Effect or frequency of meals and tube feeding. *Odontologisk Revy* **16**, 50-60.

Egelberg, J. (1970) A review of the development of dental plaque. In *Dental Plaque*, ed. Mc Hugh, W. D., pp. 9-16. Edinburgh: Livingstone.

Eide, B., Lie, T. & Selvig, K. A. (1983) Surface coatings on dental cementum incident to periodontal disease. I. A scanning electron microscopic study. *Journal of Clinical Periodontology* **10**, 157-171.

Ennever, J. (1960) Intracellular calcification by oral filamentous organisms. *Journal of Periodontology* **31**, 304-307.

Ennever, J., Streckfuss, J. L. & Takazoe, I. (1973) Calcification of bacillary and streptococcal variants of *Bacterionema matruchotii. Journal of Dental Research* **52**, 305-308.

Ennever, J., Vogel, J. J., Boyan-Salyers, B. & Riggan, L. J. (1979) Characterization of calculus matrix calcification nucleator. *Journal of Dental Research* **58**, 619-623.

Fitzgerald, R. J. & McDaniel, E. G. (1960) Dental calculus in the germ-free rat. *Archives of Oral Biology* **2**, 239-240.

Folke, L. E. A., Gawronski, T. H., Staat, R. H. & Harris, R. S. (1972) Effect of dietary sucrose on quantity and quality of plaque. *Scandinavian Journal of Dental Research* **80**, 529-533.

Frank, R. M. & Brendel, A. (1966) Ultrastructure of the approximal dental plaque and the underlying normal and carious enamel. *Archives of Oral Biology* **11**, 883-912.

Frank, R. M. & Cimasoni, G. (1970) Ultrastructure de l'epithelium cliniquement normal du sillon et de jonction gingivo-dentaires. *Zeitschrift für Zellforschung und Mikroskopische Anatomie* **109**, 356-379.

Frank, R. M. & Houver, G. (1970) An ultrastructural study of human supragingival dental plaque formation. In *Dental Plaque*, ed. Mc Hugh, W. D., pp. 85-108. Edinburgh: Livingstone.

Gehring, F., Mäkinen, K. K., Larmas, M. & Scheinin, A. (1974) Turku sugar studies. IV. An intermediate report on the differentiation of polysaccharide-forming streptococci *(S. mutans). Acta Odontologica Scandinavica* **32**, 435-444.

Gibbons, R. J. & Socransky, S. S. (1962) Intracellular polysaccharide storage by organisms in dental plaques. *Archives of Oral Biology* **7**, 73-80.

Gibbons, R. J. & van Houte, J. (1975) Bacterial adherence in oral microbial ecology. *Annual Review of Microbiology* **29**, 19-44.

Glimcher, M. J. (1960) Specificity of the molecular structure of organic matrices in mineralization. In *Calcification in Biological Systems*, ed. Sognnaes, R.F., pp. 421-487. Washington, D.C.: AAAS Publication No. 64.

Gold, W., Preston, F. B., Lache, M. G. & Blechman, H. (1974) Production of levan and dextran in plaque *in vivo. Journal of Dental Research* **53**, 442-446.

Gonzales, F. & Sognnaes, R.F. (1960) Electron microscopy of dental calculus. *Science* **131**, 156-157.

Greene, J. C. (1960) Periodontal disease in India: report of an epidemiological study. *Journal of Dental Research* **39**, 302-312.

Greene, J. C. (1963) Oral hygiene and periodontal disease. *American Journal of Public Health* **53**, 913-922.

Greene, J. C. & Vermillion, J. R. (1960) The oral hygiene index: a method for classifying oral hygiene status. *Journal of the American Dental Association* **61**, 172-179.

Guggenheim, B. (1970) Extracellular polysaccharides and microbial plaque. *International Dental Journal* **20**, 657-678.

Hazen, S. P. (1960) *A Study of Four Week Old In Vivo Calculus Formation.* Thesis. Rochester, N.Y.: University of Rochester.

Hefferren, J. J., Cooley, R. O., Hall, J. B., Olsen, N. H. & Lyon, H. W. (1971) Use of ultraviolet illumination in oral diagnosis. *Journal of the American Dental Association* **82**, 1353-1360.

Higuchi, M., Iwami, Y., Yamada, T. & Araya, S. (1970) Levan synthesis and accumulation by human dental plaque. *Archives of Oral Biology* **15**, 563-567.

Hillam, D. G. & Hull, P. S. (1977) The influence of experimental gingivitis on plaque formation. *Journal of Clinical Periodontology* **4**, 56-61.

Hofstad, T., Kristoffersen, T. & Selvig, K. A. (1972) Electron microscopy of endotoxic lipopolysaccharide from *Bacteroides, Fusobacterium* and *Sphaerophorus*. *Acta Pathologica et Microbiologica Scandinavica,* Section B **80**, 413-419.

Hotz, P., Guggenheim, B. & Schmid, R. (1972) Carbohydrates in pooled dental plaque. *Caries Research* **6**, 103-121.

Howitt, B. F., Fleming, W. C. & Simonton, F. V. (1928) A study on the effects upon the hygiene and microbiology of the mouth of various diets without and with the use of the toothbrush. *Dental Cosmos* **70**, 575-588.

Kandarkar, S. V. (1973) Ultrastructure of dental plaque and acquired pellicle formed on the artificial tooth surface (araldite plate). *Journal of the Indian Dental Association* **45**, 122-129.

Kelstrup, J. & Theilade, E. (1974) Microbes in periodontal disease. *Journal of Clinical Periodontology* **1**, 15-35.

Kleinberg, I. (1970) Biochemistry of the dental plaque. *Advances in Oral Biology* **4**, 43-90.

Knowles, J. W., Burgett, F. G., Nissle, R. R., Schick, R. A., Morrison, E. C. & Ramfjord, S. P.(1979) Results of periodontal treatment related to pocket depth and attachment level. Eight years. *Journal of Periodontology* **50**, 225-233.

Kopczyk, R. A. & Conroy, C. W. (1968) The attachment of calculus to root planed surfaces. *Periodontics* **6**, 78-83.

Krembel, J., Frank, R. M. & Deluzarche, A. (1969) Fractionation of human dental plaque. *Archives of Oral Biology* **14**, 563-565.

Lang, N. P., Østergaard, E. & Löe, H. (1972) A fluorescent plaque disclosing agent. *Journal of Periodontal Research* **7**, 59-67.

Leach, S. A. (1973) Dental calculus. In: *Biological Mineralization,* ed. Zipkin, I., pp. 587-606. New York: John Wiley & Sons.

Leach, S. A., Appleton, J., Dada, O. A. & Hayes, M. L. (1972) Some factors affecting the metabolism of fructan by human oral flora. *Archives of Oral Biology* **17**, 137-145.

Leach, S. A. & Saxton, C. A. (1966) An electron microscopic study of the acquired pellicle and plaque formed on the enamel of human incisors. *Archives of Oral Biology* **11**, 1081-1094.

Leung, S. W. & Jensen, A. T. (1958) Factors controlling the deposition of calculus. *International Dental Journal* **8**, 613-626.

Lie, T. (1975) Growth of dental plaque on hydroxy-apatite splints. A method of studying early plaque morphology. *Journal of Periodontal Research* **9**, 135-146.

Lie, T. (1978) Ultrastructural study of early dental plaque formation. *Journal of Periodontal Research* **13**, 391-409.

Lie, T. & Selvig, K. (1974) Calcification of oral bacteria – an ultrastructural study of two stains of *Bacterionema matruchotii*. *Scandinavian Journal of Dental Research* **82**, 8-18.

Lie, T. & Selvig, K. A. (1975) Formation of an experimental dental cuticle. *Scandinavian Journal of Dental Research* **83**, 145-152.

Liljenberg, B. & Lindhe, J. (1980) Juvenile periodontitis. Some microbiological, histopathological and clinical characteristics. *Journal of Periodontology* **7**, 48-61.

Lindhe, J. & Axelsson, P. (1973) The effect of controlled oral hygiene and topical fluoride application on caries and gingivitis in Swedish schoolchildren. *Community Dentistry and Oral Epidemiology* **1**, 9-16.

Lindhe, J., Hamp, S.-E. & Löe, H. (1973) Experimental periodontitis in the Beagle dog. *Journal of Periodontal Research* **8**, 1-10.

Lindhe, J. & Wicén, P.-O. (1969) The effects on the gingivae of chewing fibrous foods. *Journal of Periodontal Research* **4**, 193-201.

Listgarten, M. A. (1976) Structure of the microbial flora associated with periodontal health and disease in man. A light and electron microscopic study. *Journal of Periodontology* **47**, 1-18.

Listgarten, M. A. & Ellegaard, B. (1973) Electron microscopic evidence of a cellular attachment between junctional epithelium and dental calculus. *Journal of Periodontal Research* **8**, 143-150.

Listgarten, M. A. & Helldén, L. (1978) Relative distribution of bacteria at clinically healthy and periodontally diseased sites in humans. *Journal of Clinical Periodontology* **5**, 115-132.

Listgarten, M. A., Mayo, H. & Amsterdam, M. (1973) Ultrastructure of the attachment device between coccal and filamentous microorganisms in "corn cob" formations in dental plaque. *Archives of Oral Biology* **8**, 651-656.

Listgarten, M. A., Mayo, H. & Tremblay, R. (1975) Development of dental plaque on epoxy resin crowns in man. A light and electron microscopic study. *Journal of Periodontology* **46**, 10-26.

Little, M. F., Bowman, L., Casciani, C. A. & Rowley, J. (1966) The composition of dental calculus. III. Supragingival calculus – the amino acid and saccharide component. *Archives of Oral Biology* **11**, 385-396.

Little, M. F., Bowman, L. M. & Dirksen, T. R. (1964) The lipids of supragingival calculus. *Journal of Dental Research* **43**, 836.

Little, M. F., Casciani, C. A. & Rowley, J. (1963) Dental calculus composition. I. Supragingival calculus: ash, calcium, phosphorus, sodium, and density. *Journal of Dental Research* **42**, 78-86.

Little, M. F. & Hazen, S. P. (1964) Dental calculus composition. II. Subgingival calculus: ash, calcium, phosphorus and sodium. *Journal of Dental Research* **43**, 645-651.

Löe, H. (1963) Epidemiology of periodontal disease, and evaluation of the relative significance of the aetiological factors in light of recent epidemiological research. *Odontologisk Tidskrift* **71**, 479-503.

Löe, H., Theilade, E. & Jensen, S. B. (1965) Experimental gingivitis in man. *Journal of Periodontology* **36**, 177-187.

Lövdal, A., Arno, A., Schei, O. & Wærhaug, J. (1961) Combined effect of subgingival scaling and controlled oral hygiene on the incidence of gingivitis. *Acta Odontologica Scandinavica* **19**, 537-555.

Lövdal, A., Arno, A. & Wærhaug, J. (1958) Incidence of clinical manifestations of periodontal disease in light of oral hygiene and calculus formation. *Journal of the American Dental Association* **56**, 21-33.

Mandel, I. D. (1963) Histochemical and biochemical aspects of calculus formation. *Periodontics* **1**, 43-52.

Mandel, I. D., Levy, B. M. & Wasserman, B. H. (1957) Histochemistry of calculus formation. *Journal of Periodontology* **28**, 132-137.

Mandel, I. D. & Thompson, R. H. (1967) The chemistry of parotid and submaxillary saliva in heavy calculus formers and non-formers. *Journal of Periodontology* **38**, 310-315.

Marshall, K. C., Stout, R. & Mitchell, R. (1971) Mechanism of the initial event in the sorption of marine bacteria to surfaces. *Journal of General Microbiology* **68**, 337-348.

Matsson, L. & Attström, R. (1979) Histologic characteristics of experimental gingivitis in the juvenile and adult beagle dog. *Journal of Clinical Periodontology* **6**, 334-350.

McDougall, W. A. (1963) Studies on dental plaque. II. The histology of the developing interproximal plaque. *Australian Dental Journal* **8**, 398-407.

Moskow, B. S. (1969) Calculus attachment in cemental separations. *Journal of Periodontology* **40**, 125-130.

Mühlemann, H. R. & Schneider, U. K. (1959) Early calculus formation. *Helvetica Odontologica Acta* **3**, 22-26.

Mühlemann, H. R. & Schroeder, H. E. (1964) Dynamics of supragingival calculus. In *Advances in Oral Biology,* ed. Staple, P. H., pp. 175-203. New York: Academic Press.

Nyvad, B., Fejerskov, O., Theilade, J., Melsen, B., Rölla, G. & Karring, T. (1982) The effect of sucrose or casein on early microbial colonization on Mylar and tooth surfaces in monkeys. *Journal of Dental Research,* **61**, 570.

Ørstavik, D. & Ruangsri, P. (1979) Effects of bactericidal treatments on bacterial adherence and dental plaque formation. *Scandinavian Journal of Dental Research* **87**, 296-301.

Öste, R., Rönström, A., Birkhed, D., Edwardsson, S. & Stenberg, M. (1981) Gas-liquid chromatographic analysis of amino acids in pellicle formed on tooth surface and plastic film *in vitro. Archives of Oral Biology* **26**, 635-641.

Ramfjord, S. P. (1961) The periodontal status of boys 11-17 years old in Bombay, India. *Journal of Periodontology* **32**, 237-248.

Ramfjord, S. P., Knowles, J. W., Nissle, R. R., Schick, R. A. & Burgett, F. G. (1973) Longitudinal study of periodontal therapy. *Journal of Periodontology* **46**, 66-77.

Rateitschak-Plüss, E. M. & Guggenheim, B. (1982) Effects of a carbohydrate-free diet and sugar substitutes on dental plaque accumulation. *Journal of Clinical Periodontology* **9**, 239-251.

Ritz, H. L. (1967) Microbial population shifts in developing human dental plaque. *Archives of Oral Biology* **12**, 1561-1568.

Ritz, H. L. (1969) Fluorescent antibody staining of Neisseria, Streptococcus and Veillonella in frozen sections of dental plaque. *Archives of Oral Biology* **14**, 1073-1084.

Rölla, G., Melsen, B. & Sönju, T. (1975) Sulphated macromolecules in dental plaque in the monkeys *Macaca irus. Archives of Oral Biology* **20**, 341-343.

Rönström, A. (1979) *Early Dental Plaque Formation on Plastic Film.* Thesis. Malmö: University of Lund.

Rönström, A., Attström, R. & Egelberg, J. (1975) Early formation of dental plaque on plastic films. 1. Light microscopic observations. *Journal of Periodontal Research* **10**, 28-35.

Rönström, A., Edwardsson, S. & Attström, R. (1977) *Streptococcus sanguis* and *Streptococcus salivarius* in early plaque formation on plastic films. *Journal of Periodontal Research* **12**, 331-339.

Rosling, B., Nyman, S. & Lindhe, J. (1976) The effect of systematic plaque control on bone regeneration in infrabony pockets. *Journal of Periodontology* **3**, 38-53.

Rowles, S. L. (1964) The inorganic composition of dental calculus. In *Bone and Tooth,* ed. Blackwood, H. J. J., pp. 175-183. Oxford: Pergamon Press.

Russell, A. L. (1963) International nutrition surveys: a summary of preliminary dental findings. *Journal of Dental Research* **42**, 233-244.

Saxe, S. R., Greene, J. C., Bohannan, H. M. & Vermillion, J. R. (1967) Oral debris, calculus and periodontal disease in the Beagle dog. *Periodontics* **5**, 217-225.

Saxton, C. A. (1969) An electron microscope investigation of bacterial polysaccharide synthesis in human dental plaque. *Archives of Oral Biology* **4**, 1275-1284.

Saxton, C. A. (1973) Scanning electron microscope study of the formation of dental plaque. *Caries Research* **7**, 102-119.

Schroeder, H. E. (1963) Inorganic content and histology of early calculus in man. *Helvetica Odontologica Acta* **7**, 17-30.

Schroeder, H. E. (1964) Two different types of mineralization in early dental calculus. *Helvetica Odontologica Acta* **7**, 117-127.

Schroeder, H. E. (1965) Crystal morphology and gross structures of mineralizing plaque and calculus. *Helvetica Odontologica Acta* **9**, 73-86.

Schroeder, H. E. (1969) *Formation and Inhibition of Dental Calculus.* Berne: Hans Huber Publishers.

Schroeder, H. E. (1970) The structure and relationship of plaque to the hard and soft tissues: electron microscopic interpretation. *International Dental Journal* **20**, 353-381.

Schroeder, H. E. & Attström, R. (1979) Effects of mechanical plaque control on development of subgingival plaque and initial gingivitis in neutropenic dogs. *Scandinavian Journal of Dental Research* **87**, 279-287.

Schroeder, H. E. & Baumbauer, H. U. (1966)

Stages of calcium phosphate crystallization during calculus formation. *Archives of Oral Biology* **11**, 1-14.

Schroeder, H. E. & De Boever, J. (1970) The structure of microbial dental plaque. In *Dental Plaque,* ed. McHugh, W. D., pp. 49-74. Edinburgh: Livingstone.

Schroeder, H. E., Lenz, H. & Mühlemann, H. R. (1964) Microstructures and mineralization of early dental calculus. *Helvetica Odontologica Acta* **8**, 1-16.

Schroeder, H. E. & Listgarten, M. A. (1977) *Fine Structure of the Developing Epithelial Attachment of Human Teeth.* Basel: S. Karger.

Selvig, K. A. (1970) Attachment of plaque and calculus to tooth surfaces. *Journal of Periodontal Research* **5**, 8-18.

Sheinin, A. & Mäkinen, K. K. (1971) The effect of various sugars on the formation and chemical composition of dental plaque. *International Dental Journal* **21**, 302-321.

Sidaway, D. A. (1979) A microbiological study of dental calculus. III. A comparison of the *in vitro* calcification of viable and non-viable microorganisms. *Journal of Periodontal Research* **14**, 167-172.

Silness, J. & Löe, H. (1964) Periodontal disease in pregnancy. II. Correlation between oral hygiene and periodontal condition. *Acta Odontologica Scandinavica* **22**, 121-135.

Silverman, G. & Kleinberg, I. (1967) Fractionation of human dental plaque and the characterization of its cellular and acellular components. *Archives of Oral Biology* **12**, 1387-1405.

Slots, J. (1976) The predominant cultivable flora in juvenile periodontitis. *Scandinavian Journal of Dental Research* **84**, 1-10.

Slots, J. (1977) The predominant cultivable microflora of advanced periodontitis. *Scandinavian Journal of Dental Research* **85**, 114-121.

Slots, J., Möenbo, D., Langebæk, J. & Frandsen, A. (1978) Microbiota of gingivitis in man. *Scandinavian Journal of Dental Research* **86**, 174-181.

Soames, J. V. & Davies, R. M. (1975) The structure of subgingival plaque in a beagle dog. *Journal of Periodontal Research* **9**, 333-341.

Socransky, S. S., Manganiello, A. D., Propas, D., Oram, V. & van Houte, J. (1977) Bacteriological studies of developing supra-gingival dental plaque. *Journal of Periodontal Research* **12**, 90-106.

Söderholm, G. (1979) *Effect of a Dental Care Program on Dental Health Conditions. A Study of Employees of a Swedish Shipyard.* Malmö: Department of Periodontology, Faculty of Odontology, University of Lund, Sweden.

Sönju, T. & Glantz, P.-O. (1975) Chemical composition of salivary integuments formed *in vivo* on solids with some established surface characteristics. *Archives of Oral Biology* **20**, 687-691.

Sönju, T. & Rölla, G. (1973) Chemical analysis of the acquired pellicle formed in two hours on cleaned human teeth. *Caries Research* **7**, 30-38.

Stanford, J. W. (1966) Analysis of the organic portion of dental calculus. *Journal of Dental Research* **45**, 128-135.

Suomi, J. D., Greene, J. C., Vermillion, J. R., Doyle, J., Chang, J. J. & Leatherwood, E. C. (1971) The effect of controlled hygiene procedures on the progression of periodontal disease in adults: results after third and final year. *Journal of Periodontology* **42**, 152-160.

Syed, S. A. & Loesche, W. J. (1978) Bacteriology of human experimental gingivitis: effect of plaque age. *Infection and Immunity* **21**, 821-829.

Ten Napel, J., Theilade, J., Matsson, L. & Attström, R. (1983) Ultrastructure of developing subgingival plaque in beagle dogs. *Journal of Dental Research* **62**, 495.

Theilade, E. & Theilade, J. (1970) Bacteriological and ultrastructural studies of developing dental plaque. In *Dental Plaque,* ed., McHugh, W. D., pp. 27-40. Edinburgh: Livingstone.

Theilade, E., Theilade, J. & Mikkelsen, L. (1982 a) Microbiological studies on early dentogingival plaque on teeth and Mylar strips in humans. *Journal of Periodontal Research* **17**, 12-25.

Theilade, E., Wright, W. H., Jensen, S. B. & Löe, H. (1966) Experimental gingivitis in man. II. A longitudinal clinical and bacteriological investigation. *Journal of Periodontal Research* **1**, 1-13.

Theilade, J. (1960) *The Microscopic Structure of Dental Calculus.* Thesis. Rochester, NY: University of Rochester.

Theilade, J. (1964) Electron microscopic study of

calculus attachment to smooth surfaces. *Acta Odontologica Scandinavica* **22**, 379-387.

Theilade, J. (1977) Development of bacterial plaque in the oral cavity. *Journal of Clinical Periodontology* **4**, extra issue No. 5, 1-12.

Theilade, J. & Attström, R. (1979) The distribution and ultrastructure of subgingival plaque in beagle dogs with gingival inflammation. *Journal of Periodontal Research* **14**, 254-255.

Theilade, J., Fejerskov, O., Karring, T., Rölla, G. & Melsen, B. (1982 b) TEM of the effect of sucrose on plaque formation on Mylar and tooth surfaces in monkeys. *Journal of Dental Research* **61**, 570.

Theilade, J., Fitzgerald, R. J., Scott, D. B. & Nylen, M. U. (1964) Electron microscopic observations of dental calculus in germfree and conventional rats. *Archives of Oral Biology* **9**, 97-100.

Theilade, J. & Mikkelsen, L. (1972) Ultrastructural study of dental plaque formation during the first 3-hour period. *Caries Research* **6**, 79.

Theilade, J. & Schroeder, H. E. (1966) Recent results in dental calculus research. *International Dental Journal* **16**, 205-221.

Tinanoff, N. & Gross, A. (1976) Epithelial cells associated with the development of dental plaque. *Journal of Dental Research* **55**, 580-583.

Turesky, S., Renstrup, G. & Glickman, I. (1961) Histologic and histochemical observations regarding early calculus formation in children and adults. *Journal of Periodontology* **32**, 7-14.

Van Houte, J. (1964) Relationship between carbohydrate intake and polysaccharide-storing organisms in dental plaque. *Archives of Oral Biology* **9**, 91-93.

Van Houte, J., Gibbons, R. J. & Pulkkinen, A. J. (1972) Ecology of human oral lactobacilli. *Infection and Immunity* **6**, 723-729.

Voreadis, E. G. & Zander, H. A. (1958) Cuticular calculus attachment. *Oral Surgery, Oral Medicine and Oral Pathology* **11**, 1120-1125.

Wade, A. B. (1971) Effect on dental plaque of chewing apples. *Dental Practitioner* **21**, 194-196.

Wærhaug, J. (1952) The gingival pocket. *Odontologisk Tidskrift* **60**, Supplement 1.

Wærhaug, J. (1955) Microscopic demonstration of tissue reaction incident to removal of dental calculus. *Journal of Periodontology* **26**, 26-29.

Wærhaug, J. (1956) Effect of rough surfaces upon gingival tissues. *Journal of Dental Research* **35**, 323-325.

Wærhaug, J. (1971) Epidemiology of periodontal disease. In *The Prevention of Periodontal Disease*, ed. Eastoe, J. E., Picton, D. C. & Alexander, A. G., pp. 1-19. London: Kimpton Publishers.

Wærhaug, J. (1978) Healing of dento-epithelial junction following subgingival plaque control. II. As observed on extracted teeth. *Journal of Periodontology* **49**, 119-134.

Westergaard, J., Frandsen, A. & Slots, J. (1978) Ultrastructure of the subgingival flora in juvenile periodontitis. *Scandinavian Journal of Dental Research* **86**, 421-429.

Wilcox, C. E. & Everett, F. G. (1963) Friction on the teeth and the gingiva during mastication. *Journal of the American Dental Association* **66**, 513-520.

Wood, J. M. (1967) The amount, distribution and metabolism of soluble polysaccharides in human dental plaque. *Archives of Oral Biology* **12**, 849-858.

Wood, J. M. (1969) The state of hexose sugar in human dental plaque and its metabolism by the plaque bacteria. *Archives of Oral Biology* **14**, 161-168.

World Health Organization (WHO) (1961) *Periodontal Disease*. Geneva: *WHO Technical Report Series* No. 207.

Zander, H. A., Hazen, S. P. & Scott, D. B. (1960) Mineralization of dental calculus. *Proceedings of the Society for Experimental Biology and Medicine, New York* **103**, 257-260.

Microbiology of Plaque Associated Periodontal Disease

A retrospective survey

The first described bacteria

In one of his letters to the Royal Society of London, Antony van Leeuwenhoek (1632-1723) wrote on September 17, 1683:

"Tis my wont of a morning to rub my teeth with salt, and then swill my mouth out with water: and often, after eating, to clean my back teeth with a toothpick, as well as rubbing them hard with a cloth: wherefore my teeth, back and front, remain as clean and white as falleth to the lot of few men of my years, and my gums (no matter how hard the salt be that I rub them with) never start bleeding. Yet notwithstanding, my teeth are not so clean thereby, but what there sticketh or groweth between some of my front ones and my grinders (whenever I inspected them with a magnifying mirror), a little white matter, which is as thick as if 'twere batter. On examining this, I judged (albeit I could discern nought a-moving in it) that there yet were living animalcules therein" (Dobell 1960).

Then follows the first description of bacteria from the human oral cavity. Antony van Leeuwenhoek further remarks:

"That all the people living in our United Netherlands are not as many as the living animals that I carry in my own mouth this very day."

He was obviously not far from the conclusion that bleeding of the gums was caused by the living animalcules he was studying. But it took over 200 years to realize that microorganisms cause disease.

The specificity of microbial action

The concept of the specific action of microbes was introduced by Louis Pasteur (1822-1895) in his studies on fermentation (Collard 1976). To prove his hypothesis that each type of fermentation was caused by specific microorganisms, Pasteur had to develop methods for the cultivation of each organism uncontaminated by any other species. He also had to develop methods for the sterilization of his media and glassware, as well as aseptic techniques for handling bacterial samples. The use of the naked flame, the hot-air oven and the autoclave all originated in his laboratory. By applying the concept of specificity of microbial action Pasteur was able to solve many of the problems arising in the production of wine and beer. Using the microscope, he was also able to show (1865), that a disease in silkworms was caused by a protozoan parasite.

Robert Koch (1843-1910) developed methods for staining bacteria in smears and he showed by the use of the microscope that a specific microorganism caused anthrax in cattle (1876). He was also the first to publish photomicrographs of bacteria (1877). The identity of microorganisms, however, can not usually be disclosed by microscopy. So when Koch in 1881 introduced the solid media technique, he initiated a veritable revolution in bacteriology. To obtain pure cultures of bacteria Pasteur had to use tedious liquid dilution methods, but with the solid media technique, mixed cultures could be isolated and pure single species cultures easily obtained. In the last two decades of the 19th century, the "Golden Era" of medical bacteriology, the causal organisms of the majority of the bacterial infections were isolated and characterized. Then studies on the mechanisms of pathogenicity, host response, and methods of prevention and treatment followed.

Koch's postulates

The criteria for distinguishing a pathogenic microorganism from an adventitious one are known as Koch's postulates:

1. the pathogenic organism is regularly found in the lesions of disease

2. it can be isolated in pure culture on artificial media
3. inoculation of this culture produces a similar disease in experimental animals
4. the organism can be recovered from the lesions in the animals.

Specific bacteria in periodontal disease

In Koch's laboratory worked a dentist, Willoughby Dayton Miller (1853-1907), who applied all the current bacteriological techniques to studies of the oral microbiota (Miller 1890). He was interested in many aspects of oral diseases and also in finding out whether any specific bacterium caused periodontal disease. From his studies in 1888-89 he drew the following conclusion:

"pyorrhaea alveolaris is not caused by any specific bacterium, which occurs in every case (like the tubercle-bacillus in tuberculosis), but various bacteria may participate in it, just as in suppurative processes not only one but generally various species have been found. Besides, as far as we know, there is no bacterium which, inoculated under the gums is able to provoke the disease in healthy persons."

but he also made the important remark:

"if there is a specific bacterium of pyorrhaea alveolaris it does not readily grow on gelatine ... At the same time the thought suggests itself that possibly the bacterium of pyorrhaea alveolaris, like so many mouth bacteria, is cultivable on none of the artificial nutrient media, which would of course render all experimenting useless."

It was not until quite recently that bacteriological techniques were developed which permit cultivation of the majority of the microorganisms of the oral cavity. The breakthrough came when careful dispersion of samples was combined with strict anaerobic techniques in which bacteria were protected from exposure to oxygen during various phases of the work in the laboratory. Now we have reached the point where the concept of specific bacteria in periodontal disease can again be tested.

The unique microbiota of the oral cavity

The oral cavity – an ecological system

The oral cavity with its microbiota is an ecological system of bewildering complexity (Bowden et al. 1979). It has been characterized as a river system (Appleton 1944), where sterile saliva arises from the salivary glands, washes all surfaces in the mouth, and passes many sites of prospering microbial life becoming, thus, strongly polluted before leaving the mouth. In running-water systems, life is proverbially rich and varied on solid surfaces, where the organisms achieve firm anchorage and a favorable nutritional environment. The mouth is the only site in the human body where such hard solid surfaces are found, i.e. the surfaces of the teeth.

From an ecological point of view the oral cavity is an open growth system. This means that nutrients and microbes are repeatedly introduced into and removed from the system (Lynch & Poole 1979). The flow rate of saliva is so high that the only organisms that are successful, are those which can *adhere* to the surfaces of the oral cavity, or are, in some other way, *retained*. Not only the *flow of saliva,* but also the *flow of the gingival fluid, chewing, oral hygiene procedures* and *desquamation of epithelial cells* from the mucous membranes serve to remove bacteria from the oral surfaces. Some bacteria may be retained simply by obtaining a refuge in pits and fissures, or in the protected areas in between the teeth. Other microorganisms have to rely on specific mechanisms of adherence in order to overcome the strong removal forces on the oral surfaces. The characteristics of the oral surfaces are unique and only specific bacteria have the ability to adhere. This means that the oral cavity harbors a unique microbiota and most of its members are not able to colonize any other site of the human body. The oral cavity consists of several distinct sites, each of which will support the growth of a charac-

teristic microbial community. Enormous differences, thus, exist in the composition of the microbiota on the mucous membranes, the tongue, the teeth and in the gingival sulcus area. It has even been demonstrated that the composition of the microbiota may vary from site to site on a single tooth surface.

Factors involved in the *adherence* of the microbes to the surfaces of the oral cavity are of primary ecological importance. An important ecological determinant of the oral cavity is also the *nutritional interrelation* between the host and the microbes. The composition of the microbiota is to a significant degree determined by the efficiency of various organisms to utilize the *available nutrients*.

For those organisms which become established the oral cavity will be like the "Garden of Eden". The humidity is high. The temperature, pH and carbon dioxide tension are optimal for growth. The oxygen tension varies in various sites and permits growth of aerobic as well as strictly anaerobic organisms. Saliva not only provides nutrients to the microbiota, but also buffers acidic fermentation products of the flora and removes inhibitory waste products.

In addition to the primary ecological determinants, bacterial adherence and nutrition, many other factors also influence the establishment of the organisms in the oral cavity, but before these factors are discussed, the primary determinants should be further considered.

Bacterial adherence

Bacterial adherence involves specific physicochemical mechanisms and is influenced not only by the interaction between surface structures of bacteria and colonizable surfaces, but also by the activity of saliva as a suspending fluid.

Characteristics of oral surfaces
The surfaces of lips, cheeks, palate, tongue,

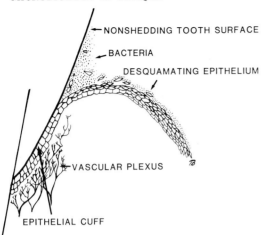

Fig. 4-1. The dentogingival area with bacterial aggregations on the solid tooth surface and bacteria colonizing the surface of the desquamating epithelium. In the gingival crevice area the epithelial cuff and the dense vascular plexus play an important part in the host defence against microbial invasion.

the epithelial turnover is higher in the dentogingival area than anywhere else in the mouth, this defence mechanism does not work very efficiently at this particular site. The reason is that the bacteria in contact with the epithelium are in addition firmly anchored to the solid nonshedding tooth surface. This is one of the reasons why this area presents so many unique features of host-parasite interactions.

Characteristics of bacterial surfaces
Most bacteria in nature are surrounded by highly hydrated matrices called glycocalyces (Costerton et al. 1981). These structures have only recently been recognized. The reason why they have been overlooked is that bacteria rapidly lose these structures when cultured in the laboratory and the glycocalyces are not visualized by conventional light or electron microscopy. In some bacteria the glycocalyx consists of a regular array of rod like glycoprotein appendages, but more often bacteria are surrounded by a glycocalyx composed of a matrix of polysaccharide fibers. The glycocalyx may be a coherent capsule or a more loosely, cell associated, extracellular polysaccharide. Many bacteria bear long nonflagellar appendages at their surfaces, which extend beyond the surface of the glycocalyx. These appendages can vary in length between 0.2 and 20 µm and the width of these structures ranges between 30 and 140 Å. They have many names, but are usually called *pili* or *fimbriae* (Ottow 1975).

The glycocalyces are often made up of heteropolysaccharides which bacteria can produce from any carbohydrate source. Some bacteria have in addition the capacity to form extracellular homopolysaccharides from sucrose (Guggenheim 1970, Walker 1978). These polysaccharides are synthesized from sucrose by enzymes, glycosyl transferases, excreted by *Streptococcus sanguis*, *Streptococcus salivarius* and *Streptococcus mutans*. There are different types of glycosyl transferases. Some cleave sucrose, release fructose and obtain energy for the extracellular conversion of the glucose

gums and teeth all provide different characteristics for bacterial colonization. All these surfaces are covered, however, by a highly hydrophilic confluent film of salivary mucins. These mucins have the form of a complex hydrated gel composed of a variety of high molecular weight glycoproteins. This surface film may be of importance in lubrication of the mucosa, in waterproofing and in protection against sudden changes in osmotic pressure, but it will also interfere with the bacterial adherence (McNabb & Tomasi 1981).

The most important difference among the oral surfaces, is the one between the mucosa, with its desquamating epithelium, and the solid tooth surface (Gibbons & van Houte 1975). On the tooth surface the salivary mucins are denatured (Pruitt 1977) and form a highly structured organic film called *pellicle* which serves as a solid ground for long lasting microbial life. On the desquamating epithelial surface, the bacteria must continually colonize 'virgin soil' (Fig. 4-1). The shedding surface of the oral mucosa is an important part of the host defence against bacterial invasion. Although

moieties of sucrose into highly branched glucans (Fig. 4-2). These glucans can be both 1.3-α- and 1.6-α-polymers. Those glucans which have a high percentage of 1.3-α-linkages are highly insoluble and are called *mutan,* while those with predominantly 1.6-α-linkages are soluble and are called *dextran.* The insoluble glucans are considered to play an important part as a matrix in the microbial aggregations on the teeth. Other glycosyl transferases cleave sucrose, release glucose and convert the fructose moieties of sucrose into *fructan.* This fructan is usually highly soluble and can be used as a source of carbohydrate by some of the bacteria of the oral microbiota (McGhee & Michalek 1981).

Physicochemical characteristics of bacterial adherence

An important characteristic of living cells is that they carry a net negative electric charge and thus tend to repel each other *electrostatically.* The tooth surface is also negatively charged and repels the cells (Marsh 1980). The cells are further influenced, however, by *electrodynamic* or *van der Waal's force.* These forces are attractive and of longer range than the repulsive electrostatic force. The attractive and repulsive forces will favor a separation of the bacteria at specific distances from the tooth surface (Fig. 4-3a). This separation gap is influenced by the presence of ions. An acid pH or an increased concentration of cations will decrease the gap (Fig. 4-3b). The importance of the glycocalyx for bacterial adherence is that the glycocalyx constitutes a hydrophilic extension beyond the highly charged surface of the bacterial cell and can thus bridge the separation gap between the bacteria and the tooth surface (Fig. 4-3c). When the glycocalyx comes into contact with the tooth surface other attractive forces such as hydrogen bonding, ion pair formation and dipole-dipole interaction can be established. The bacterial pili or fimbriae are usually long enough to protrude beyond the glycocalyx

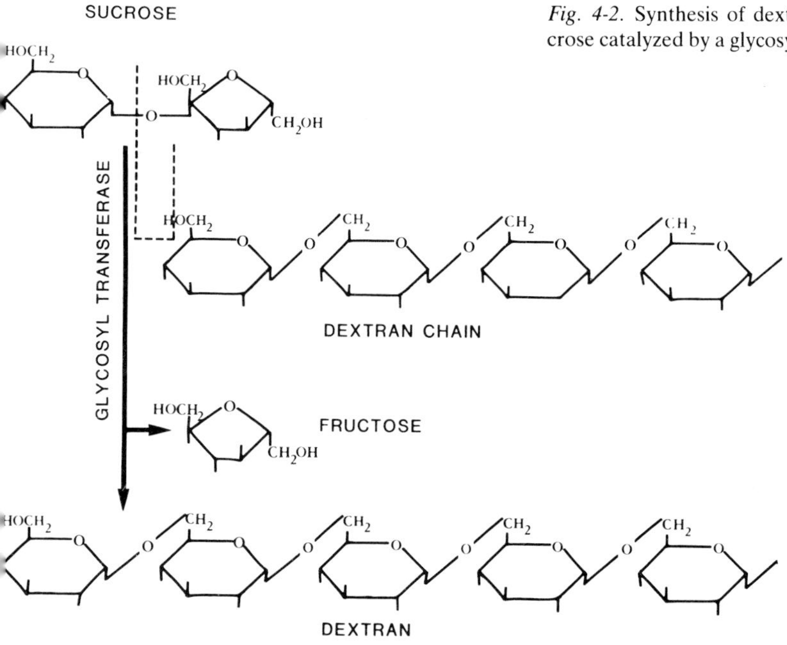

Fig. 4-2. Synthesis of dextran (1,6-α-glucan) from sucrose catalyzed by a glycosyl transferase.

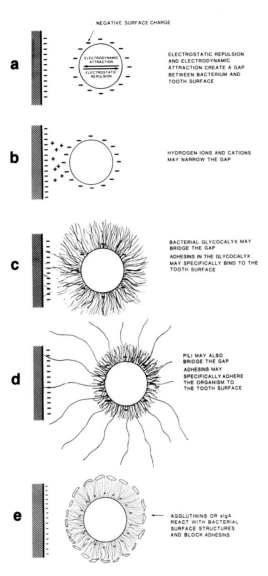

Fig. 4-3. Some factors which influence the adherence of a bacterial cell to a tooth surface.

and may therefore assist in bridging the separation gap and establishing the contact between the bacteria and the tooth surface (Fig. 4-3d).

The adhesion of bacteria to the tooth surface is probably in most cases determined by highly specific, yet unknown, mechanisms. Molecules called *adhesins* on the bacteria recognize specific receptor molecules on the tooth surface (Figs. 4-3c, d). These adhesins are often located on the pili or fimbriae (Beachey 1981). Adhesins which are proteins and recognize carbohydrate structures are called *lectins*. The carbohydrate groups of the glycoproteins of the pellicle may serve as receptors for such bacterial adhesins. Adhesins could also be enzymes which bind to their substrates. In some streptococci, the adhesins have been shown to be lipoteichoic acids which bind to albumin like proteins and to oral epithelial cells (Simpson et al. 1980). Lipoteichoic acids have also been implicated in the binding of Gram positive bacteria to the tooth surface. This conclusion is based on the observation that lipoteichoic acids will bind readily to hydroxylapatite, presumably through ionized phosphate groups and divalent cation bridging. The significance of this observation is, however, an open question, as all *in vitro* studies on adsorption of bacteria to hydroxylapatite, due to the fact that the hydroxylapatite of the tooth *in vivo* is always covered by an organic film, the pellicle (Wicken & Knox 1980). Another important problem with adherence studies *in vitro* is that most bacteria only develop their true glycocalyces when living in their natural environments (Costerton et al. 1981).

While the mucinous denatured film covering the solid tooth surface, pellicle, seems to facilitate the bacterial adherence, the mucinous film covering the oral mucosa may prevent bacteria from reaching receptor sites on the epithelial surfaces. Some of the salivary mucins *(agglutinins)* as well as *secretory immunoglobulin A* (sIgA) may react with bacterial surface structures (Fig. 4-3e) and in that way prevent the bacteria from adhering to the oral surfaces (Gibbons & van Houte 1975).

Enteric Gram negative bacilli are usually not found in the oral cavity, but may appear in the mouth of seriously ill patients. An interesting recent observation is that there is swift increase in protease activity of saliva and alterations in epithelial cell surfaces as reflected by loss of epithelial cell surface fibronectin in patients after major illnesses

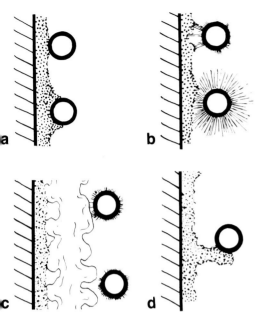

the pellicle there are laminated granular patterns (Lie 1979).

Structure of the microbial community on the tooth surface

In microscopic studies on the initial colonization of the tooth surface, single bacteria are usually seen to adhere to small irregularities in the surface of the pellicle (Figs. 4-4a, d). Some bacteria are attached to the pellicle by pili or fimbriae (Fig. 4-4b). Sometimes epithelial cells colonized by bacteria are seen on the tooth surface (Fig. 4-4c). The attached bacteria start to grow and multiply, and microorganisms in pits and grooves especially increase rapidly in number (Fig. 4-5a). From these initial areas of colonization, single layers of cells spread over the surface (Fig. 4-5b) and coalesce with neighboring areas of bacterial accumulation (Lie 1979). At this stage of bacterial accumulation, the mean bacterial generation time has been

These changes precede the colonization of the oral cavity by enteric Gram negative bacilli. Alterations in cell surface proteins may clear the way for the bacilli and expose binding sites normally present on the epithelial cell surfaces. Fibronectin is highly sensitive to proteolytic enzymes, but in addition many cell surface constituents may be altered in patients with severe illness or stress, and fibronectin is only one marker of a more generalized process (Woods et al. 1981).

Structure of the pellicle

The appearance of the pellicle may vary considerably. The mean thickness of 2 h pellicle is about 100 nm and increases to about 400 nm in 24-48 h. The structure of the pellicle is heterogeneous. Initially there are small globules or aggregations of amorphous material adsorbed to the tooth surface. Later globules of varying size and 3 and 7 nm wide fiber can be distinguished in the internal structure of the pellicle. In other areas of

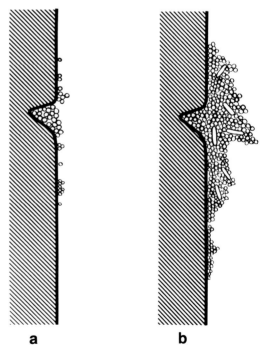

a   b

Fig. 4-5. Early bacterial aggregations in pits and grooves of the tooth surface (a). These bacteria increase rapidly in number and spread over the tooth surface (b) (Lie 1979).

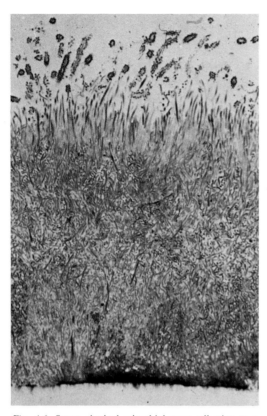

Fig. 4-6. Supra-gingival microbial mass adhering to a tooth with advanced periodontal disease. There are dense masses of filamentous organisms and "corncob" formations are seen on the surface of the microbial mass (Listgarten 1976). The tooth surface is located at the bottom of the illustration.

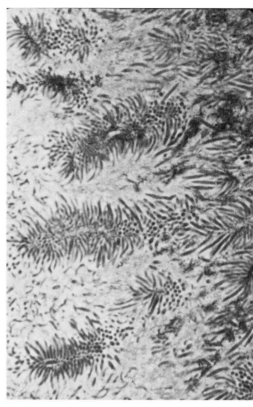

Fig. 4-7. "Test-tube brush" formations among the microbial masses in a gingival pocket. These structures are composed of filamentous bacteria to which the "bristles" (Gram negative rods) of the "brush" attach (Listgarten 1976).

estimated to be 3-4 h (Socransky et al. 1977). When germ free rats were infected with *Actinomyces viscosus,* the generation time on the tooth surface was 2.9 h. The generation time of *Streptococcus mutans* was 1.1 h (Beckers & van der Hoeven 1982).

The replicating bacteria will be unable to accumulate on the tooth surface unless there are retention mechanisms in operation. Mechanisms involved in bacterial adhesion to the tooth surface are also in effect when bacteria adhere to each other. Bacterial glycocalyces and salivary glycoproteins constitute a matrix which retains the microbial mass to the tooth surface. The cohesion of the mass is dependent on both unspecific and specific binding mechanisms. The "corncob" formations (Fig. 4-6) in which streptococci adhere to filaments of *Bacterionema matruchotii* (Mouton et al. 1980) or of *Actinomyces* (Cisar 1982), are very spectacular. Another example of intermicrobial cohesion is the "bristle brush" or "test-tube brush" formation commonly observed in the superficial layers of microbial masses in gingival pockets (Fig. 4-7). A characteristic of the microbial aggregations on the tooth is that the organisms are organized in a pattern perpendicular to the tooth surface (Figs. 4-8, 4-9). Filamentous organisms could thus play an important role in keeping the microbial mass together (Fig. 4-6; Listgarten 1976).

132

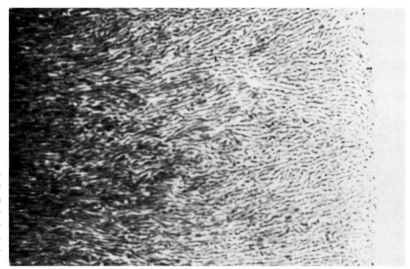

Fig. 4-8. A dense microbial mass adhering to the enamel of a tooth with healthy gingiva (Listgarten 1976). The tooth surface is located on the left-hand side of the illustration.

When gingival pockets develop, surfaces with new characteristics for bacterial colonization become exposed. The cemental root surface will be covered by an organic film composed of gingival fluid proteins instead of the salivary proteins which cover those parts of the teeth exposed to saliva. Although there is a flow of cells and fluid out of the gingival pocket, this is a rather stagnant environment compared to most other areas of the mouth. This means that the adherence capacity of the bacteria is not as decisive for their colonization in this area as in most other parts of the oral cavity. Along the gingival sulcus and in the gingival pocket there are usually many motile bacteria. It is likely that these bacteria have become established in the periodontal pocket because of their motility, although they may not be able to adhere either to the sulcular epithelial cells or to the root surface (Gibbons & van Houte 1975).

Microbial aggregations on the teeth often become mineralized by calcium phosphates. *Dental calculus* is formed. This calcified structure provides excellent sites for microbial retention on the teeth and in the deepened gingival pockets.

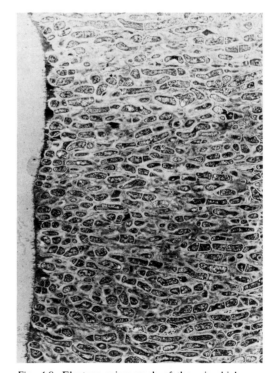

Fig. 4-9. Electron micrograph of the microbial mass (Fig. 4-8) close to the enamel surface. The bacteria are arranged perpendicular to the tooth surface and are embedded in an amorphous matrix (Listgarten 1976). The tooth surface is on the left-hand side of the illustration.

133

Nutritional interrelations between bacteria and the host

Bacterial nutritional requirements

In order to grow, the bacterial cell must be supplied with *sources of carbon* and *of energy* in addition to *nitrogen* and *essential inorganic ions*. Of the bacteria that adhere to specific sites of the oral cavity, only those will become established which are able to utilize efficiently the nutrients normally available. They must also have the capacity to respond rapidly to environmental change. Bacteria with simple nutritional requirements are able to grow and multiply if the environment supplies sugar, ammonium and other essential inorganic ions (Fig. 4-10). From these molecules the bacterial cell synthesizes its own cell constituents. In order to accomplish this, the bacterial cell has to have a complete set of enzymes to catalyze all the required chemical reactions. If some of these enzymes are lacking, essential molecules will not be formed and the organism will not be able to grow or multiply unless these molecules are provided by the environment. Many oral bacteria have incomplete cellular machineries and, therefore, require a number of amino acids, vitamins, purines and pyrimidines from the environment in order to grow and multiply (Mandelstam et al. 1982).

Nutrients provided by the host

The nutritional environment on the tooth surface is completely different from that in the periodontal pocket. On the tooth surface, the nutrients are provided by the *saliva*. The concentration of nutrients in saliva is, however, very low and our knowledge about the nutritional value of saliva is far from complete (Carlsson 1980). The concentration of glucose in parotid saliva has been reported to be 4-40 µM, pyruvate 17-70 µM and lactate 200-480 µM. The concentration of urea in parotid saliva is 2 mM, and of ammonia in whole saliva 2-6 mM. In whole saliva the concentration of individual amino acids varies between 5 and 150 µM. Most

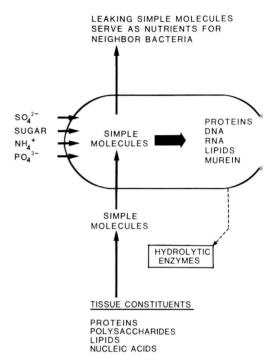

LEAKING SIMPLE MOLECULES SERVE AS NUTRIENTS FOR NEIGHBOR BACTERIA

SO_4^{2-}
SUGAR
NH_4^+
PO_4^{3-}

SIMPLE MOLECULES

PROTEINS
DNA
RNA
LIPIDS
MUREIN

SIMPLE MOLECULES

HYDROLYTIC ENZYMES

TISSUE CONSTITUENTS

PROTEINS
POLYSACCHARIDES
LIPIDS
NUCLEIC ACIDS

Fig. 4-10. Outline of bacterial nutrition. The nutritional requirements may be satisfied by ammonium, sugar and inorganic ions. Some bacteria will not grow and multiply unless some simple molecules such as amino acids vitamins, purines or pyrimidines are also provided by the environment. Some bacteria may release enzymes which hydrolyze macromolecules of the environment into these simple molecules.

water soluble vitamins have been detected in whole saliva. In order to grow and multiply on the tooth surface where saliva is the main source of nutrients, the bacteria must obviously have a high capacity to utilize nutrients available at low concentrations.

In the gingival pocket all the nutrients of the *tissue fluid* are available and the growth of very fastidious organisms will be supported. When epithelial and connective tissue cells disintegrate, valuable nutrients may also be available. The value of the diet as a source of nutrients for the oral microbiota is very limited (Carlsson 1980). One reason is that the dietary components remain in the mouth for only a short time. Another reason is that in order to grow, an organism has to be supplied with all the essential nutrients more or less simultaneously and the diet may lack some specific nutrients.

Bacteria, as mammalian cells, cannot utilize macromolecules, but only simple molecules such as sugars, amino acids, peptides and vitamins. In the digestive tract, proteins, lipids and polysaccharides are hydrolyzed by various enzymes into such simple molecules. The only digestive enzyme present in salivary secretions is amylase and it is relatively inefficient in converting starch. Many bacteria which colonize the gingival pocket, produce, however, very potent hydrolytic enzymes which can break down macromolecules. But such hydrolytic enzymes break down not only macromolecules of saliva and gingival fluid, but also attack the host tissue with deleterious results (Fig. 4-10).

Food webs

The bacterial cellular machinery is subjected to an elaborate system of control mechanisms in order to modulate all the different enzymatic processes (Mandelstam et al. 1982). It may happen, however, that in a given bacterial cell, some amino acids, vitamins, purines or pyrimidines are produced in higher quantities than can be assimilated. These products may then leak from the cell and be used as nutrients by neighbor cells in the microbial community. In the microbial communities established on the teeth and in the gingival pockets it is likely that such exchange of nutrients plays an important nutritional role. In Fig. 4-11 some possible nutritional interrelations are illustrated. The majority of the bacteria colonizing the mucous membranes and the teeth, such as

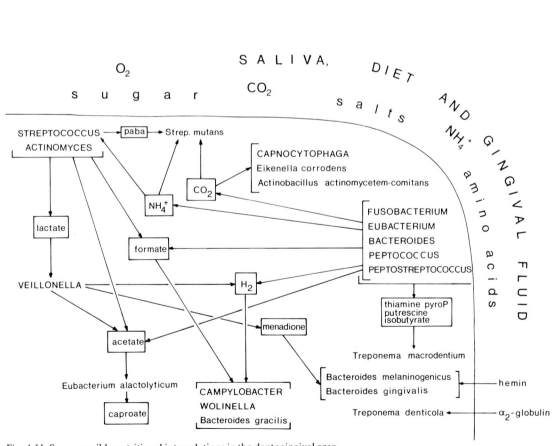

Fig. 4-11. Some possible nutritional interrelations in the dentogingival area.

streptococci and actinomyces, utilize saliva as the main nutrient source and sugars as the main energy source, while microorganisms colonizing the gingival pockets often utilize amino acids and simple peptides as energy sources (Loesche 1968). When amino acids are used as an energy source, carboxylic acid, ammonia and hydrogen sulfide are produced. The concentration of these substances may reach toxic levels in the gingival pockets. Butyrate and propionate formed by many of the bacteria colonizing the gingival pockets have recently been shown to be highly cytotoxic even in moderate concentration (Singer & Bruckner 1981). Although some of these substances may be toxic to the host, they may also be significant as nutrients for other bacteria. Ammonia is toxic at high concentration, but is also a very important source of nitrogen for many bacteria, even for streptococci. Ammonia is available in saliva as a result of bacterial hydrolysis of salivary urea and bacterial catabolism of amino acids. Carbon dioxide is an essential nutrient for many bacteria especially those colonizing gingival pockets. Some so-called "capnophilic" bacteria will not grow unless carbon dioxide is available.

Lactate, formate and hydrogen are excreted by many bacteria as a result of their energy metabolism. These products are subsequently used by other bacteria as an energy source. Fig. 4-11 shows that streptococci and *Actinomyces* produce lactate from sugars and that lactate is used by *Veillonella* as an energy source. In the catabolism of lactate by *Veillonella* hydrogen gas is formed which can be used by a number of organisms in the gingival pockets such as *Campylobacter, Wolinella* and *Bacteroides gracilis* (Tanner et al. 1981). Another organism colonizing the gingival pockets, *Eubacterium alactolyticum,* has the interesting ability to form caproic acid from acetic and butyric acids (Moore et al. 1982), and in this way the acidity of the environment is lowered.

Some bacteria have very specific nutritional requirements (Fig. 4-11). *Streptococcus mutans* requires p-amino benzoate and

this compound is produced by *Streptococcus sanguis* (Carlsson 1971). Black pigmented *Bacteroides* species may require vitamin K and hemin (Gibbons & MacDonald 1960). Vitamin K can be produced by many bacteria (Gibbons & Engle 1964) and hemin is made available when hemoglobin is broken down in the gingival pockets. Some bacteria also produce hemins. The requirement of vitamin K by *Bacteroides melaninogenicus* subspecies *intermedius* and *Bacteroides melaninogenicus* subspecies *melaninogenicus* could be substituted with the steroids, estradiol or progesterone (Kornman & Loesche 1982). *Treponema denticola* has a specific requirement for α_2-globulin and this globulin is only available in the gingival pockets (Socransky & Hubersak 1967). The requirement of *Treponema macrodentium* for thiamine pyrophosphate, putrescine and isobutyrate is satisfied by the concerted action of a number of organisms living in the gingival pockets (Socransky et al. 1964).

Oxygen and oxygen products as ecological determinants

Oxygen and oxygen products are very important ecological determinants because there are great variations in the ability of bacteria to grow and multiply at various levels of oxygen. Some bacteria are killed at extremely low oxygen levels, while others will grow only in the presence of oxygen. In relation to this spectrum of oxygen tolerance, the separation of bacteria into anaerobic and aerobic organisms is quite arbitrary. Microorganisms are identified as being *anaerobic* if they do not grow on the surface of blood agar in the presence of air, while bacteria that only grow in the presence of air are called *aerobic. Facultatively anaerobic* are microorganisms which grow under anaerobic as well as aerobic conditions.

Most bacteria, even oral streptococci, consume large quantities of oxygen and develop a low redox potential in their environment. This low redox potential may favor

$$O_2 \xrightarrow{H^+,e} H^+ + O_2^- \xrightarrow{H^+,e} H_2O_2 \xrightarrow{H^+,e} OH \cdot \xrightarrow{H^+,e} H_2O$$

OXYGEN   SUPEROXIDE   HYDROGEN   HYDROXYL   WATER
         ANION   PEROXIDE   RADICAL

$$H_2O$$
WATER

$$O_2^- + O_2^- + 2H^+ \xrightarrow{\text{SUPEROXIDE DISMUTASE}} H_2O_2 + O_2$$

$$H_2O_2 + H_2O_2 \xrightarrow{\text{CATALASE}} 2H_2O + O_2$$

$$H_2O_2 + RH_2 \xrightarrow{\text{PEROXIDASE}} 2H_2O + R$$

Fig. 4-12. Reduction of oxygen into water in 4 one-electron steps and the detoxification of the oxygen intermediates by the concerted action of superoxide dismutase, catalase and peroxidase.

the growth of some anaerobic bacteria, but the actual redox potential is usually of less importance for the survival and growth of the bacteria than the level of oxygen (Walden & Hentges 1975).

Intracellularly or in any site characterized by low redox potential, oxygen is converted into highly reactive, potentially destructive products. Oxygen is reduced in one-electron steps, and *superoxide anions* (O_2^-), *hydrogen peroxide* (H_2O_2), and *hydroxyl radicals* $(OH \cdot)$ are formed (Fig. 4-12). Of these products hydrogen peroxide and superoxide anions are not very toxic *per se*, but they can generate the more devastating hydroxyl radicals (Morris 1979, Halliwell 1981). Hydroxyl radicals are so very reactive that they fail to diffuse away from their site of formation. Hydrogen peroxide and superoxide anions become dangerous because they can reach the lethal target sites of the cell and generate *in situ* the highly reactive hydroxyl radicals. The oxygen products may damage cell membranes and inactivate enzymes, but one of the primary sites of damage in bacteria, as well as in mammalian cells exposed to hydrogen peroxide, is chromosomal

DNA. The DNA molecule may be randomly split into pieces.

In order to survive in an aerobic environment, bacterial as well as mammalian cells have to be equipped with an elaborate system of enzymes which disarms the harmful oxygen products. The concerted action of *superoxide dismutase, catalase* and *peroxidases* converts superoxide anions and hydrogen peroxide into water and thereby prevents the formation of hydroxyl radicals (Fig. 4-12). The cells are also equipped with enzyme systems which repair DNA and other cellular sites damaged by oxygen products. Organisms lacking some of these enzymes, may not be able to survive in an aerobic environment and are, *de facto*, anaerobic.

Bacterial growth within the mouth creates sites with various oxygen levels. The oxygen level and the redox potential are especially low in sites characterized by heavy accumulations of bacteria, e.g. in the gingival pockets where growth of even the extremely oxygen sensitive obligate anaerobes is supported (Globerman & Kleinberg 1979). In sites with high oxygen levels such as the mu-

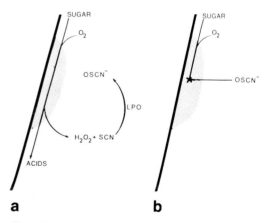

Fig. 4-13. A microbial mass taking up sugar and oxygen and excreting acids and hydrogen peroxide. Salivary lactoperoxidase (LPO) converts the hydrogen peroxide and salivary thiocyanate (SCN⁻) into the less toxic hypothiocyanite (OSCN⁻) (a). Hypothiocyanite diffuses into the microbial mass and inhibits the formation of acids and hydrogen peroxide (b).

cous membranes, the bacterial oxygen uptake, especially by the oral streptococci, may result in excretion of high amounts of hydrogen peroxide. This hydrogen peroxide is potentially dangerous for the epithelial cells of the mucous membrane, but saliva contains *lactoperoxidase* which converts hydrogen peroxide in the presence of salivary thiocyanate into water and hypothiocyanite (Hoogendoorn et al. 1977). Hypothiocyanite is much less toxic to the cells than hydrogen peroxide (Adamson & Carlsson 1982) and is in addition a potent inhibitor of glycolysis and hydrogen peroxide production by oral streptococci (Fig. 4-13). So lactoperoxidase-thiocyanate of saliva has a dual function. It detoxifies hydrogen peroxide and the product of this reaction, hypothiocyanite, serves as feed-back inhibitor of hydrogen peroxide production by the oral streptococci (Carlsson et al. 1983).

Other factors of ecological importance

Lactoferrin

Lactoferrin is an iron binding protein in saliva, milk and other exocrine secretions such as bile, pancreatic juice, and small intestinal secretions. Lactoferrin is also found in polymorphonuclear leukocytes. Several biological functions have been proposed for lactoferrin. Iron saturated lactoferrin may be involved in the transport of iron across the intestinal brush border and it may play a part in regulation of myelopoiesis (Pelus et al. 1981). It has also been shown to potentiate the hydroxyl radical formation from polymorphonuclear leukocytes (Ambruso et al. 1981). The unsaturated form of lactoferrin is bacteriostatic because it may deplete the environment of iron to a concentration which fails to support bacterial growth. Lactoferrin has also been reported to have a bactericidal effect *in vitro* (Arnold et al. 1980), but it is an open question whether the bacteriostatic or the bactericidal effects are of any ecological significance in the oral cavity.

Lysozyme

Lysozyme like lactoferrin is found in polymorphonuclear leukocytes and in secretions like saliva and tears. It is an enzyme which splits the bond between N-acetyl glucosamine and N-acetyl muramic acid in the murein of the bacterial cell wall. Lysozyme may have bacteriostatic or bactericidal effects *in vitro,* but the efficiency of the enzyme is strongly dependent on pH, ionic strength and various cell surface structures and it is not clear what role this enzyme has in the microbial ecology of the oral cavity (Iacono et al. 1982).

Bacteriocins

A bacteriocin is a protein, produced by a microorganism, which has the capacity to inhibit the growth of a limited number of other strains. The formation of a given bacteriocin is dependent on the presence of a corresponding plasmid. Bacteriocins are much more potent than antibiotics and have a more narrow antimicrobial spectrum. One molecule only may kill a microorganism. Some bacteriocins are nucleases and attack DNA. Others act on the cytoplasmic membrane, increasing its permeability to ions or inhibiting active transport. Although bacteriocins produced by oral bacteria have not yet been fully characterized, it is possible that bacteriocins may influence the microbial ecology of the oral cavity.

Composition of the microbiota in the dento-gingival area

Oral bacteria

Classification

More than 200 morphologically and biochemically distinct bacterial groups or species of bacteria are today recognized as normal inhabitants of the human oral cavity (Table 4-1; Moore et al. 1982). Many bacte rial strains isolated from the human oral cavity yet remain to be classified.

The object of classification is to group together bacteria with similar properties and to separate those with dissimilar properties. It is important to remember, however, that this is *an arbitrary process* and the form it takes is decided by the interest and knowledge of the persons making the classification. This means that new species will usually be created when the interest in a particular group of organisms increases. In recent years many new species from the human oral cavity have been described and it is important that this work on classification is continued, as the association of specific bacteria with particular diseases cannot be disclosed unless the bacteria have been identified. It will take many years before the oral microbiota has been properly described and classified. Until then our descriptions of the microbiota colonizing the dentogingival area will be incomplete. Demonstrated differences in composition of the microbiota at various pathological conditions of gingiva and periodontium will not necessarily be of pathogenic significance.

Cultivation

By using current bacteriological techniques about 70% of the bacteria disclosed by microscopy in a sample from the gingival margin may be cultivated in the laboratory. There are several reasons why not all bacteria are detected (Moore et al. 1982). Some of the bacteria do not find the conditions in the laboratory suitable for growth. Others may be killed by the methods we use in dispersing the bacterial masses we have sampled. On the other hand, if the bacterial sample is not properly dispersed the number and types of bacteria in the sample will be underestimated.

Gingivally accumulating bacteria

Clinically healthy gingiva

If the teeth are kept clean with proper oral hygiene measures, the gingiva remains healthy and only few bacteria are found along the gingival margin. If a person with such a healthy gingiva abstains from oral hygiene measures, bacteria accumulate on the teeth. After the first 8 h of abstention there are 10^3-10^4 bacteria per mm^2 tooth surface (Socransky et al. 1977). Streptococci and *Actinomyces viscosus* predominate, but also Gram negative facultatively anaerobic rods such as *Haemophilus, Eikenella* and *Actinobacillus actinomycetemcomitans* are found (Kilian et al. 1979). Within a day the number of bacteria increase 100- to 1000-fold. This rapid increase is above all dependent on the growth of *Streptococcus sanguis* on the tooth surface (Socransky et al. 1977).

In Fig. 4-14 the relative proportion of various bacterial groups in clinically healthy gingiva is presented. Most of the bacteria are facultatively anaerobic and the anaerobic bacteria only make up a minor portion of the flora (Slots 1977a). Among the facultatively anaerobic cocci *Streptococcus sanguis* is of particular interest since it adheres to the pellicle of the tooth surface and produces extracellular homopolysaccharides from sucrose. These polysaccharides play an important part in the accumulation of bacteria on the teeth. Among the facultatively anaerobic rods, *Actinomyces viscosus* seems to have specific affinity to the root surface (Ellen 1982). When hamsters or rats are infected with *Actinomyces viscosus* these bacteria adhere to the root surfaces and there is a rapid breakdown of the alveolar bone (Keyes & Jordan 1964).

Gingivitis

Accumulation of bacteria along the gingival margin for 3-4 days results in gingivitis. This inflammatory condition creates new opportunities for the growth of bacteria and a continuous change in the composition of the microbial community is initiated. Microscopic studies uncover 3 phases in the changes of the microbiota in a 2 week period (Theilade et al. 1966). During the first phase, the microbiota is dominated by Gram positive cocci, Gram positive rods and Gram negative cocci. During the second phase

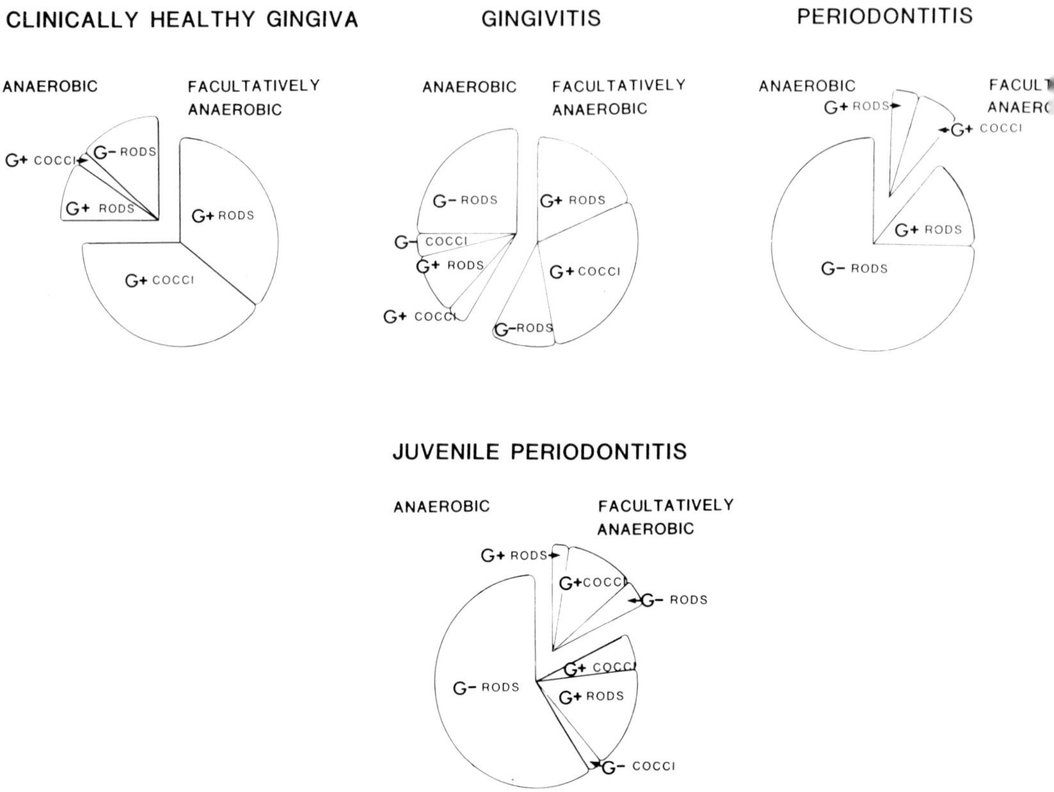

CLINICALLY HEALTHY GINGIVA

GINGIVITIS

PERIODONTITIS

JUVENILE PERIODONTITIS

Fig. 4-14. Relative proportions of various bacterial groups in clinically healthy gingiva and in microbial masses associated with gingivitis, periodontitis and juvenile periodontitis. (Adapted from Slots et al. 1976-1978).

filamentous organisms appear and during the third phase spirills and spirochetes (Theilade et al. 1966). When gingivitis has become established cultivation of the bacteria from the infected sites discloses an increase in number of anaerobic bacteria in relation to the facultatively anaerobic (Fig. 4-14; Slots et al. 1978). Among the anaerobic bacteria *Fusobacterium nucleatum* and *Bacteroides melaninogenicus* subspecies *intermedius* are often found (Socransky et al. 1982).

In acute necrotizing ulcerative gingivitis the microbiota is characterized by the presence of *Bacteroides melaninogenicus* subspecies *intermedius* as well as of *Treponema*, *Selenomonas* and *Fusobacterium* species (Loesche et al. 1982).

Advanced periodontal disease

In the early stages of periodontitis, the bacterial flora of the gingival pocket is similar to that of gingivitis (Williams et al. 1976, Darwish et al. 1978). Cultivation of samples from advanced cases of periodontal disease demonstrates a predominance of Gram negative anaerobic rods (Fig. 4-14; Slots 1977b, Darwish et al. 1978). Among these bacteria *Bacteroides gingivalis* seems to be of specific importance (Slots 1982). In the microscope it can also be observed that samples from advanced cases of periodontal disease usually contain high numbers of spirochetes (Listgarten & Helldén 1978, Loesche & Laughon 1982). In juvenile periodontitis special attention has been paid to the presence of *Actinobacillus actinomycetemcomi-*

ans and *Capnocytophaga* (Tanner et al. 1979, Slots et al. 1980, Hammond & Stevens 1982). It should be remembered, however, that the composition of the microbiota varies not only between various stages of periodontal disease, but also between individuals with similar symptoms. In addition the microbiota of the pockets may be different in various parts of the mouth and in various parts of a particular gingival pocket.

The criteria used by Koch for distinguishing a pathogenic microorganism from an adventitious one are not easily applicable to the pathogens in periodontal disease. Many potentially pathogenic organisms are, thus, regularly found both in healthy and in diseased sites. Some of them cannot be implanted in the oral cavity of experimental animals and from those organisms which can be implanted, it is not always clear whether the disease induced is the same disease as in humans.

In evaluating the etiologic role of a given microorganism in periodontal disease a number of characteristics of the organism have to be considered (Socransky 1979). A potential pathogen should be present in higher numbers at sites of pathology than in healthy sites or sites with different forms of disease. Elimination of this organism from the diseased sites should stop the progress of the active lesion. An increased or decreased cellular or humoral immune response to that organism in the presence of a consistent response to other organisms, might also be suggestive of a special role of that organism in the disease process. Animal pathogenicity testing could also give important information if the specific organism can actually be implanted in animals. The most important criterion, however, which could contribute to the understanding of its role as an oral pathogen is the possession of unique characteristics which could contribute to the pathogenesis of the disease. Some such characteristics of oral microorganisms will be discussed in the following parts of this chapter.

Host defence in the dentogingival area

Host-parasite interrelations

The microorganisms colonizing the oral cavity constitute a constant threat to the host tissues. In the healthy mouth, the host defence mechanisms match the attacks of the microorganisms, but as soon as the microorganisms at any site overcome this defence, an infection with tissue damage will develop.

The host defence works at various levels. An efficient defence against the microorganisms is provided by the intact surface of the mucous membranes, the desquamation of the epithelial cells, the salivary flow and various components of the salivary secretions. When the intact mucosal surface is broken, further protection is offered by various components of the body fluids and by the phagocytic cells.

In the dentogingival area the epithelial layer of the gingiva is penetrated by a solid body, the tooth. This creates a unique morphological situation, which the host defence mechanisms have to deal with. The contact area between the tooth and the soft tissues (i.e. the junctional epithelium) is a very weak structure in the host defence even if the capacity of defence in this region is reinforced by the epithelial cuff and the vascular plexus surrounding the tooth (Fig. 4-1) (Egelberg 1967). The unique feature to be handled by the host defence is that the bacteria may obtain a firm anchorage on the nonshedding tooth surface and will thereby remain in close contact, for a long time, with the soft tissues surrounding the tooth. This contact relationship triggers the defence mechanisms of tissues. The high efficiency of this gingival host defence is convincingly demonstrated, however, by the fact that periodontal disease in most situations progresses at a slow pace.

Defence by saliva

An important part of the defence is constituted by factors which interfere with bacterial adherence and prevent microorganisms from colonizing the dentogingival area. The salivary flow, the flow of gingival fluid, chewing, and oral hygiene procedures have previously been considered as important ecological determinants, but may equally be conceived as an important part of the host defence. Most of the bacteria entering the oral cavity are rapidly washed away by the salivary flow and swallowed. Only organisms which have the capacity to adhere to the surfaces of the oral cavity have a potential to remain in the oral cavity. But the salivary secretions also contain substances that can interfere with the bacterial adherence: agglutinins and secretory immunoglobulin A (sIgA). In addition the salivary component lysozyme may kill bacteria by lysing their cell wall, and the salivary lactoferrin may deprive the bacteria of essential iron.

Microbial perturbation of the salivary defence

The actual pathogens in periodontal disease have to be sought among those organisms, which, having survived defence by saliva, have found an adequate environment for their growth and multiplication in the dentogingival area. Of ultimate importance for these bacteria are *the surface characteristics* which contribute to their capacity for adherence or retention. They may also release products which interact with the humoral defence factors of saliva. Many strains of *Streptococcus sanguis* and *Streptococcus mitis* produce an *IgA protease* which breaks down the sIgA, thus removing this obstacle to their colonization of the oral surfaces (Kilian & Holmgren 1981, Plaut et al. 1982). Another way oral bacteria perturb the salivary immune defence is by *"antigenic shift and drift"*. The bacteria change their surface characteristics so they escape being recognized by the salivary immune systems (Gibbons & Qureshi 1980).

Little is known about the significance of the salivary lactoferrin and lysozyme in the host defence and how bacteria may evade these defence factors.

Humoral factors in the local defence

One of the first signs that the defence mechanisms against the bacteria colonizing the teeth are put into action, is a swelling of the vessels of the gingival margin (Egelberg 1967). This is followed by an increased vascular permeability, exudation of gingival fluid and migration of polymorphonuclear leukocytes into the gingival sulcus. This means that already, at this early phase, the gingival tissues have mobilized very potent parts of their defence forces.

The gingival fluid contains both *complement* factors and *specific antibodies*. Many members of the gingival microbiota induce an immune response in the host (Taubman et al. 1982, Tolo & Brandtzaeg 1982). The classical pathway of *complement activation* will be initiated when specific antibodies of IgG or IgM classes react with the bacteria. The alternative pathway of complement activation will be initiated by various bacterial cell constituents such as lipopolysaccharides, lipoteichoic acids and polysaccharides. The tissue consequences of this activation will be described elsewhere, and we will here consider only what the activation of the complement cascade means as far as protection of the tissues against bacterial invasion is concerned.

Among the fragments formed in the activation of the complement cascade, C3a and C5a play an important part in releasing histamine in the tissue. This leads to *increased vascular permeability* and to extensive transudation of serum components including complement and antibodies. C5a also has a strong *chemotactic effect* on polymorphonuclear leukocytes and will, thus, help in mobilizing these important defence forces. C3b is fixed to the bacterial cell surfaces and *facilitates phagocytosis* of the bacteria by the polymorphonuclear leukocytes and macrophages. An activation of the entire complement system leads to membrane damage and can cause lysis of Gram negative bacteria in the presence of lysozyme.

In addition to the part played by specific IgG and IgM antibodies in the activation of the complement system, IgG antibodies facilitate phagocytosis by binding to the bacterial cell surface. Antibodies of IgA, IgG and IgM classes prevent tissue damage by *neutralizing exotoxins* released by the bacteria. In addition to their role in preventing bacterial adherence and neutralizing bacterial exotoxins, IgA antibodies also have an important function in *preventing penetration of antigens* across the epithelial surface layer of the mucosa (McNabb & Tomasi 1981).

Microbial perturbation of the local humoral defence

An interesting recent finding is that some of the bacteria colonizing the gingival pockets produce *proteases which may degrade not only IgA but also IgG*. Strains of *Bacteroides gingivalis*, *Bacteroides asaccharolyticus*, *Bacteroides melaninogenicus* and *Capnocytophaga* possess this ability (Kilian 1981). This means that the *humoral immune defence mechanisms can actually be paralyzed* in infected gingival pockets. The degradation of IgA may facilitate the penetration and spread of potentially toxic substances, lytic enzymes and antigens released by the entire subgingival microbiota. Due to the importance of IgG antibodies in the defence mediated by phagocytes, the efficiency of this cellular defence may be impaired. The significance of the immune defence against chronic infections was recently demonstrated in experimental root canal infections in monkeys (Dahlen et al. 1982). In animals immunized against bacteria in the root canals, the periapical lesions were encapsulated and not so diffusely spread in the tissue as in non-immunized animals. An important point here is that although the immune defence mechanisms may lead to inflammation and tissue damage, as described in Chapter 5, they are in most cases beneficial for the host by preventing the spread of an infection into the tissue.

The subgingival microbiota may also *interfere with the function of the complement system*. It is known that bacterial proteases may degrade complement components (Densen & Mandell 1980). Cell surface constituents such as lipopolysaccharides released from the bacteria into the surrounding fluids may activate and degrade complement in these fluids. By causing this complement consumption at remote distances, bacteria may avoid fixation of C3b to their surfaces and thereby avoid phagocytosis (Horwitz 1982). It is not known, however, whether proteases or cell surface constituents released by members of the subgingival microbiota have the ability to paralyze the complement system of the gingival fluid. Ammonia generated by the normal metabolic activity of the kidney inhibits the function of the complement system (Braude 1981). This may mean that ammonia released by members of the subgingival microbiota in their catabolism of amino acids and peptides might equally menace the function of the complement system in the gingival pocket.

Microorganisms can also contrive sophisticated mechanisms capable of interfering with the host immune system and, thus, with the productions of humoral antibodies and cell mediated immune responses (Falcone & Campa 1981, Page 1982). There may be *inhibition of lymphoid tissue maturation* as well as *quantitative and qualitative modulations of the immune response*. The immunocompetence of the host is maintained by a delicate balance between stimulatory and suppressor cells, and bacterial constituents such as peptidoglycans, lipopolysaccharides, and lipoteichoic acids can interfere with the function of these cells. Thus, any bacterial constituent with mitogenic properties for B-lymphocytes may depress the host immune response by the activation of suppressor cells or by functioning as a polyclonal activator of B-lymphocytes. Although many members of the subgingival microbiota have mitogenic constituents their role in perturbing the host defence has not yet been elucidated.

Defence by phagocytes

Both polymorphonuclear and mononuclear leukocytes take part in the phagocytic defence of the dentogingival area and this defence is dependent on the presence of complement and often specific antibodies. In order to be effective, the phagocytes have to recognize the site of microbial invasion. They have to leave the blood vessels and migrate through the tissue to the site of invasion, where they have to ingest and kill the microorganisms (Densen & Mandell 1980). An activation of the complement cascade has an important function in this process. The binding of the complement fragment C5a to the surface of polymorphonuclear leukocytes determines the *adherence of the leukocytes to the vascular endothelium* close to the site of the microbial invasion (Wilton 1981). The migration of the leukocytes through the tissue to the site of infection *(chemotaxis)* may be determined by C5a and by substances released by metabolizing bacteria. Chemotactic substances are also produced by lymphocytes stimulated by specific antigens or mitogens, and by mast cells and basophils interacting with specific antigens or with the complement fragments C3a or C5a. The initial metabolites of the lipoxygenation of arachidonic acid are also chemotactic (Snyderman & Goetzl 1981).

During chemotaxis, the leukocytes release some of the contents of their lysosomes. The next step in the process of phagocytosis is the *attachment of the organism to the surface of the leukocyte*. To achieve this attachment C3b and/or specific antibodies, must often attach to the surface of the microorganism. After the attachment *the organism is ingested* and enclosed into a phagosome. This process triggers the leukocyte to *release oxygen products and lysosomal granule contents* into the phagosome and the extracellular milieu. The oxygen products include both singlet oxygen and superoxide anions as well as hydrogen peroxide and hydroxyl radicals. These oxygen products are in themselves *microbicidal,* but the most potent microbicidal mechanism

of the leukocyte is a reaction catalyzed by the lysosomal enzyme, myeloperoxidase, in the presence of hydrogen peroxide and chloride ions. The leukocytes also have microbicidal systems that work under anaerobic conditions (Root & Cohen 1981). The products released by the leukocytes not only kill invading microorganisms, but the oxygen products and the lysosomal proteases may cause *extensive tissue injuries* (Fantone & Ward 1982).

Microbial perturbation of the phagocytic defence

Microorganisms can elude the phagocytic defence in many ways (Densen & Mandell 1980). They can *fail to induce chemotaxis* and will, thus, not be detected by the phagocytes. The reason may be that their metabolism does not result in the production of a chemotactic substance or, that the microorganisms are not able to activate the chemotactic complement fragment C5a. Bacteria may also influence chemotaxis by producing substances which inhibit the motility of the leukocytes. *Capnocytophaga,* a member of the subgingival microbiota, has this capacity and it has been demonstrated that patients with their gingival pockets infected with this organism have a systemic defect in leukocyte function (Shurin et al. 1979). The normal functions of the leukocytes may also be impaired by subtoxic levels of some leukotoxins (Arbuthnott 1981).

Bacteria may also perturb the phagocytic defence by *avoiding attachment to the leukocytes*. Bacterial surface structures may prevent the attachment. Often such structures are capsules composed of polysaccharides but may also be proteins. Such bacteria can normally not be phagocytosed until the host has produced specific antibodies against the surface structures. These antibodies have to react with the surface, initiate the complement cascade, and thereby fragment C3b is fixed to the bacterial surface. As the leukocytes have receptors for C3b as well as for the Fc portion of IgG, the attachment to the bacteria can now be accomplished. The organisms may avoid this by the aforementioned "antigenic shift and drift" (Gibbons & Qureshi 1980) or by shedding substantial quantities of their surface antigens into the site of infection (Griffin 1982). These antigens react with the antibodies, and the immune complexes block the Fc and C3b receptors of the phagocytic cells and impair their ability to ingest the Fc- and C3b-coated organisms. Among the members of the subgingival microbiota, black pigmented *Bacteroides* have surface structures that may help in eluding the attachment to the leukocytes (Slots 1982).

After the microorganism has become attached to the leukocyte, it is usually ingested and killed. Some pathogenic bacteria such as gonococci may, however, *prevent the ingestion* after the attachment by increasing, in an unknown way, the rigidity of the leukocyte membrane (Densen & Mandell, 1980). It is presently unknown whether members of the subgingival microbiota can exert such effects on the leukocytes.

The attachment and ingestion of an organism induce a burst of metabolic oxidative activity in the leukocyte. This is essential for the normal bactericidal activity of this particular phagocyte. Some pathogenic bacteria can *inhibit this metabolic oxygen burst,* but it is not known if any of the members of the subgingival microbiota have this ability.

After the microorganism has been enclosed in a phagosome, it becomes exposed to toxic oxygen products, the myeloperoxidase system, lytic lysosomal enzymes and cationic proteins (Root & Cohen 1981). Usually only few of the pathogens can *resist these very potent microbicidal activities* for any significant length of time. Such pathogens, the intracellular parasites, have not yet been described from gingival pockets or the oral cavity.

An efficient way for the organism to elude all the phagocytic defence is to *kill the phagocytes.* Many pathogens possess leukotoxins and these toxins often play a key role in the pathogenicity of these organisms (Arbuthnott 1981). One predominant member of the subgingival microbiota, *Actinoba-*

cillus actinomycetemcomitans, possesses such a leukotoxin (Baeni et al. 1979). The presence of this toxin in the gingival pocket will paralyze the phagocytic defence against all the subgingival microbiota. Even subtoxic levels of the toxin may impair normal function of the leukocytes such as motility and phagocytic activity. The host defence in the form of specific antibodies may, however, have the capacity of neutralizing these effects of the leukotoxins.

The important part played by polymorphonuclear leukocytes in the defence of the periodontal tissues, was nicely demonstrated in dogs with low numbers of polymorphonuclear leukocytes after treatment with antileukocyte serum (Attström & Schroeder 1979). In the serum treated dogs bacteria advanced much more rapidly along the epithelial junction of the gingival crevice than in controls.

Microbial invasion of the periodontal tissue

The combined humoral and phagocytic defence of the dentogingival area efficiently protects the periodontal tissues from bacterial invasion. This protection is actually so efficient that it has been claimed that the members of the subgingival microbiota should be unable to invade tissues. A *bacterial invasion* of the junctional epithelium of the gingival pocket has been demonstrated, however, in acute ulcerative gingivitis (Fig. 4-15, Listgarten 1965) and in advanced cases of periodontal disease (Frank 1980, Saglie et al. 1982). Recently there was an interesting demonstration of invasion of subepithelial periodontal tissues by *Bacteroides melaninogenicus* subspecies *intermedius* in gnotobiotic rats (Allenspach-Petrzilka & Guggenheim 1982). Microbial invasion of the periodontal tissues may be more common than has been appreciated.

Bacteria growing in the tissue may damage the tissue by releasing *toxins, enzymes* and *metabolic waste products.* No exotoxins

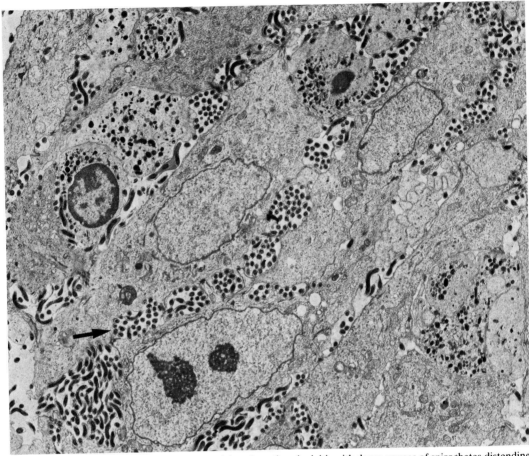

Fig. 4-15. Junctional epithelium in acute necrotizing ulcerative gingivitis with dense masses of spirochetes distending the space between the epithelial cells. (Listgarten 1965).

other than the leukotoxin produced by *Actinobacillus actinomycetemcomitans* have been shown to be produced by members of the subgingival microbiota. Various enzymes are produced, however, which may degrade intercellular tissue components. Phosphatases, aminopeptidases, proteases, phosphoamidases and glycosidases have been demonstrated (Slots 1981) as well as hyaluronidase, chondroitin sulfatase and fibrinolysin (Nitzan et al. 1978, Steffen & Hentges 1981). Black pigmented *Bacteroides* may produce proteases which degrade a number of proteins. Some of these proteins may play important parts in the host defense against bacterial infections. Not only the immunoglobulins IgG, IgA and IgM may be degraded, but also fibrinogen, transferrin, haptoglobin, ceruloplasmin and albumin (Werner & Müller 1971). Of particular interest is that the protease inhibitor α_1-antitrypsin has been reported to be annihilated by a strain of black pigmented *Bacteroides* (Werner & Müller 1971). Also phospholipase A is formed by members of the subgingival microbiota (Bulkacz et al. 1979), an enzyme which may contribute to the formation of prostaglandins in the tissue (Lewis & Austen 1981). Bacteria in the gingival pockets may also release waste products from their metabolism in cytotoxic levels. This may be ammonia, hydrogen sulfide, indol and carboxylic acids such as butyrate and propionate. To what extent these products may contribute to the periodontal tissue destruction remains unknown.

Much has been learned in the past few years about the microbiology of plaque associated periodontal disease. This growth in our understanding has given us a solid basis for formulating new questions concerning the microbiology and pathophysiology of this disease. The answers to these questions will not only increase our knowledge, but also influence our way of treating the various phases of periodontal disease.

Table 4-1. Some recognized microbial genera and species in the oral cavity

	Gram positive bacteria		Gram negative bacteria	
	Aerobic and facultatively anaerobic	Anaerobic	Aerobic and facultatively anaerobic	Anaerobic
Cocci	**Streptococcus** S. milleri S. mitis S. mutans S. salivarius S. sanguis **Staphylococcus** S. epidermidis **Micrococcus**	**Streptococcus** S. constellatus S. intermedius S. morbillorum **Peptostreptococcus** P. anaerobius P. micros **Peptococcus** P. magnus P. prevotii	**Neisseria** N. flavescens N. mucosa N. sicca N. subflava **Branhamella** B. catarrhalis	**Veillonella** V. alcalescens V. parvula **Acidaminococcus** A. fermentans
Rods	**Actinomyces** A. naeslundii A. viscosus **Bacterionema** B. matruchotii **Rothia** R. dentocariosa **Lactobacillus** L. acidophilus L. brevis L. buchneri L. casei L. cellobiosus L. delbrueckii L. fermentum L. plantarum L. salivarius	**Actinomyces** A. israelii A. meyeri A. odontolyticus **Arachnia** A. propionica **Eubacterium** E. alactolyticum E. brachy E. lentum E. nodatum E. saburreum E. timidum **Lactobacillus** L. catenaforme L. crispatus **Bifidobacterium** B. dentium B. eriksonii **Propionibacterium** P. acnes P. freudenreichii P. jensenii **Clostridium**	**Haemophilus** H. aphrophilus H. influenzae H. parainfluenzae H. paraphrophilus H. segnis **Actinobacillus** A. actinomycetem- comitans **Capnocytophaga** C. gingivalis C. ochracea C. sputigena **Eikenella** E. corrodens **Campylobacter** C. sputorum	**Bacteroides** B. asaccharolyticus B. buccae B. buccalis B. capillus B. denticola B. gingivalis B. gracilis B. loescheii B. melaninogenicus ss. intermedius B. melaninogenicus ss. melaninogenicus B. oris B. oralis B. pentosaceus **Fusobacterium** F. naviforme F. nucleatum **Leptotrichia** L. buccalis **Campylobacter** C. concisus **Selenomonas** S. sputigena **Wolinella** W. recta

Other organisms				
Mycoplasma M. orale M. salivarium M. homini	**Treponema** T. denticola T. macrodentium T. oralis T. vincentii	**Candida** C. albicans	**Entamoeba** E. gingivalis	**Trichomonas** T. tenax

References

Adamson, M. & Carlsson, J. (1982) Lactoperoxidase and thiocyanate protect bacteria from hydrogen peroxide. *Infection and Immunity* **35**, 20-24.

Allenspach-Petrzilka, G. E. & Guggenheim, B. (1982) *Bacteroides melaninogenicus* subsp. *intermedius* invades rat gingival tissue. *Journal of Dental Research* **61**, IADR Abstract 728.

Ambruso, D. R., & Johnston Jr., R. B. (1981) Lactoferrin enhances hydroxyl radical production by human neutrophils, neutrophil particulate fractions, and an enzymatic generating system. *Journal of Clinical Investigation* **67**, 352-360.

Appleton, J. L. T. (1944) In: *Bacterial Infection with Special Reference to Dental Practice.* 3rd ed., pp. 301-316. Philadelphia: Lea & Febiger.

Arbuthnott, J. P. (1981) Membrane-damaging toxins in relation to interference with host defence mechanisms. In *Microbial Perturbation of Host Defences,* ed. Grady, F. O. & Smith, H., pp. 97-120. London: Academic Press.

Arnold, R. R., Brewer, M., & Gauthier, J. J. (1980) Bactericidal activity of human lactoferrin: Sensitivity of a variety of microorganisms. *Infection and Immunity* **28**, 893-898.

Attström, R. & Schroeder, H. E. (1979) Effect of experimental neutropenia on initial gingivitis in dogs. *Scandinavian Journal of Dental Research* **87**, 7-23.

Baehni, P., Tsai, C.-C., McArthur, W. P., Hammond, B. F. & Taichman, N. S. (1979) Interaction of inflammatory cells and oral microorganisms. VIII. Detection of leukotoxic activity of a plaque-derived Gram-negative microorganism. *Infection and Immunity* **24**, 233-243.

Beachey, E. H. (1981) Bacterial adherence: Adhesin-receptor interactions mediating the attachment of bacteria to mucosal surfaces. *Journal of Infections Diseases* **143**, 325-345.

Beckers, H. J. A. & van der Hoeven, J. S. (1982) Growth rates of *Actinomyces viscosus* and *Streptococcus mutans* during early colonization of tooth surfaces in gnotobiotic rats. *Infection and Immunity* **35**, 583-587.

Bowden, G. H. W., Ellwood, D. C. & Hamilton, I. R. (1979) Microbial ecology of the oral cavity. *Advances in Microbial Ecology* **3**, 135-217.

Braude, A. I. (1981) Bacterial interference with nonspecific nonphagocytic defences. In *Microbial Perturbation of Host Defences,* ed. Grady, F. O. & Smith, H., pp. 31-47. London: Academic Press.

Bulkacz, J., Newman, M. G., Sokransky, S. S., Newbrun, E. & Scott, D. F. (1979) Phospholipase A activity of microorganisms from dental plaque. *Microbios Letters* **10**, 79-88.

Carlsson, J. (1971) Growth of *Streptococcus mutans* and *Streptocóccus sanguis* in mixed culture. *Archives of Oral Biology* **16**, 963-965.

Carlsson, J. (1980) Symbiosis between host and micro-organisms in the oral cavity. *Scandinavian Journal of Infectious Diseases,* Supplement **24**, 74-78.

Carlsson, J., Iwami, Y. & Yamada, T. (1983) Hydrogen peroxide excretion by oral streptococci and the effect of lactoperoxidase and thiocyanate. *Infection and Immunity* **40**, 70-80.

Cisar, J. O. (1982) Coaggregation reactions between oral bacteria: Studies of specific cell-to-cell adherence mediated by microbial lectins. In *Host-Parasite Interactions in Periodontal Diseases,* ed. Genco, R. J. & Mergenhagen, S. E., pp. 121-131. Washington, D. C.: American Society for Microbiology.

Collard, P. (1976) *The Development of Microbiology.* Cambridge: Cambridge University Press.

Costerton, J. W., Irvin, R. T. & Cheng, K.-J. (1981) The bacterial glycocalyx in nature and disease. *Annual Review of Microbiology* **35**, 299-324.

Dahlen, G., Fabricius, L., Heyden, G., Holm, S. E. & Möller, Å. J. R. (1982) Apical periodontitis induced by selected bacterial strains in root canals of immunized and non-immunized monkeys. *Scandinavian Journal of Dental Research* **90**, 207-216.

Darwish, S., Hyppa, T. & Socransky, S. S. (1978) Studies of the predominant cultivable microbiota of early periodontitis. *Journal of Periodontal Research* **13**, 1-16.

Densen, P. & Mandell, G. L. (1980) Phagocyte strategy vs. microbial tactics. *Reviews of Infectious Diseases* **2**, 817-838.

Dobell, C. (1960) *Antony van Leeuwenhoek and*

His "Little Animals". New York: Dover Publications.

Egelberg, J. (1967) The topography and permeability of the vessels at the dento-gingival junction in dogs. *Journal of Periodontal Research,* Supplement Nr. 1.

Ellen, R. (1982) Oral colonization by Gram-positive bacteria significant to periodontal disease. In *Host-Parasite Interactions in Periodontal Diseases,* ed. Genco, R. J. & Mergenhagen, S. E., pp. 98-111. Washington, D.C.: American Society for Microbiology.

Falcone, G. & Campa, M. (1981) Bacterial interference with the immune response. In *Microbial Perturbation of Host Defences,* ed. Grady, F. O. & Smith, H., pp. 185-210. London: Academic Press.

Fantone, J. C. & Ward, P. A. (1982) Role of oxygen-derived free radicals and metabolites in leukocyte-dependent inflammatory reactions. *American Journal of Pathology* 107, 397-418.

Frank, R. M. (1980) Bacterial penetration in the apical pocket wall of advanced human periodontitis. *Journal of Periodontal Research* 15, 563-573.

Gibbons, R. J. & Engle, L. P. (1964) Vitamin K compounds in bacteria that are obligate anaerobes. *Science* 146, 1307-1309.

Gibbons, R. J. & MacDonald, J. B. (1960) Hemin and vitamin K compounds as required factors for the cultivation of certain strains of *Bacteroides melaninogenicus. Journal of Bacteriology* 80, 164-170.

Gibbons, R. J. & Qureshi, J. V. (1980) Virulence-related physiological changes and antigenic variation in populations of *Streptococcus mutans* colonizing gnotobiotic rats. *Infection and Immunity* 29, 1082-1091.

Gibbons, R. J., & van Houte, J. (1975) Bacterial adherence in oral microbial ecology. *Annual Review of Microbiology* 29, 19-44.

Globerman, D. Y. & Kleinberg, I. (1979) Intraoral PO_2 and its relation to bacterial accumulation on the oral tissues. In *Saliva and Dental Caries,* ed. Kleinberg, I., Ellison, S. A. & Mandel, I. D., pp. 275-291. Washington, D. C.: Information Retrieval.

Griffin, Jr., F. M. (1982) Mononuclear cell phagocytic mechanisms and host defence. In *Advances in Host Defense Mechanisms,* ed.

Gallin, J. I. & Fauci, A. S., Vol. 1, pp. 31-55. New York: Raven Press.

Guggenheim, B. (1970) Extracellular polysaccharides and microbial plaque. *International Dental Journal* 20, 657-678.

Halliwell, B. (1981) Free radicals, oxygen toxicity and aging. In *Age Pigments,* ed. Sohal R. S., pp. 1-62. Amsterdam: Elsevier/North-Holland Biomedical Press.

Hammond, B. F. & Stevens, R. H. (1982) *Capnocytophaga* and *Actinobacillus actinomycetemcomitans:* Occurrence and pathogenic potential in juvenile periodontitis. In *Host-Parasite Interactions in Periodontal Diseases,* ed. Genco, R. J. & Mergenhagen, S. E., pp. 46-61. Washington, D.C.: American Society for Microbiology.

Hoogendoorn, H., Piessens, J. P., Scholtes, W. & Stoddard, L. A. (1977) Hypothiocyanite ion; the inhibitor formed by the system lactoperoxidase-thiocyanate-hydrogen peroxide. I. Identification of the inhibiting compound. *Caries Research* 11, 77-84.

Horwitz, M. A. (1982) Phagocytosis of microorganisms. *Reviews of Infectious Diseases* 4, 104-123.

Iacono., V. J., MacKay, B. J., Pollock, J. J., Boldt, P. R., Ladenheim, S., Grossbard, B. L. & Rochon, M. L. (1982) Roles of lysozyme in the host response to periodontopathic microorganisms. In *Host-Parasite Interactions in Periodontal Diseases,* ed. Genco, R. J. & Mergenhagen, S. E., pp. 318-342. Washington, D.C.: *American Society for Microbiology.*

Keyes, P. H. & Jordan, H. V. (1964) Periodontal lesions in the syrian hamster. III. Findings related to an infectious and transmissible component. *Archives of Oral Biology* 9, 377-400.

Kilian, M. (1981) Degradation of immunoglobulins A1, A2, and G by suspected principal periodontal pathogens. *Infection and Immunity* 34, 757-765.

Kilian, M. & Holmgren, K. (1981) Ecology and nature of immunoglobulin A1 protease-producing streptococci in the human oral cavity and pharynx. *Infection and Immunity* 31, 868-873.

Kilian, M., Larsen, J., Fejerskov, O. & Thylstrup, A. (1979) Effects of fluoride on the initial colonization of teeth *in vivo. Caries*

Research **13**, 319-329.

Kornman, K. S. & Loesche, W. J. (1982) Effects of estradiol and progesterone on *Bacteroides melaninogenicus* and *Bacteroides gingivalis*. *Infection and Immunity* **35**, 256-263.

Lewis, R. A. & Austen, K. F. (1981) Mediation of local homeostasis and inflammation by leukotrienes and other mast cell-dependent compounds. *Nature* **293**, 103-108.

Lie, T. (1979) Morphologic studies on dental plaque formation. *Acta Odontologica Scandinavica* **37**, 73-85.

Listgarten, M. A. (1965) Electron microscopic observations on the bacterial flora of acute necrotizing ulcerative gingivitis. *Journal of Periodontology* **36**, 328-339.

Listgarten, M. A. (1976) Structure of the microbial flora associated with periodontal health and disease in man. *Journal of Periodontology* **47**, 1-18.

Listgarten, M. A. & Helldén, L. (1978) Relative distribution of bacteria at clinically healthy and periodontally diseased sites in humans. *Journal of Clinical Periodontology* **5**, 115-132.

Loesche, W. J. (1968) Importance of nutrition in gingival crevice microbial ecology. *Periodontics* **6**, 245-249.

Loesche, W. J. & Laughon, B. E. (1982) Role of spirochetes in periodontal disease. In *Host-Parasite Interactions in Periodontal Diseases*, ed. Genco, R. J. & Mergenhagen, S. E., pp. 62-75. Washington, D.C.: American Society for Microbiology.

Loesche, W. J., Syed, S. A., Laughon, B. E. & Stoll, J. (1982) The bacteriology of acute necrotizing ulcerative gingivitis. *Journal of Periodontology* **53**, 223-230.

Lynch, J. M. & Poole, N. J. (ed.) (1979) *Microbial Ecology: A Conceptual Approach*. Oxford: Blackwell Scientific Publications.

Mandelstam, J., McQuillen, K., & Dawes, I. (ed.) (1982) *Biochemistry of Bacterial Growth*. Oxford: Blackwell Scientific Publications.

Marsh, P. (1980) *Oral Microbiology*. Walton-on-Thames: Thomas Nelson & Sons.

McGhee, J. R. & Michalek, S. M. (1981) Immunobiology of dental caries: Microbial aspects and local immunity. *Annual Review of Microbiology* **35**, 595-638.

McNabb, P. C. & Tomasi, T. B. (1981) Host defense mechanisms at mucosal surfaces. *Annual Review of Microbiology* **35**, 477-496.

Miller, W. D. (1890) *The Micro-Organisms of the Human Mouth*. Reprint 1973. Basel: S. Karger.

Moore, W. E. C., Ranney, R. R. & Holdeman, L. V. (1982) Subgingival microflora in periodontal disease: Cultural studies. In *Host-Parasite Interactions in Periodontal Diseases*, ed. Genco, R. J. & Mergenhagen, S. E., pp. 13-26. Washington, D.C.: American Society for Microbiology.

Morris, J. G. (1979) Nature of oxygen toxicity in anaerobic microorganisms. In *Strategies of Microbial Life in Extreme Environments*, ed. Shilo, M., pp. 149-162. Weinheim: Verlag Chemie.

Mouton, C., Reynolds, H. S. & Genco, R. J. (1980) Characterization of tufted streptococci isolated from the "corn cob" configuration of human dental plaque. *Infection and Immunity* **27**, 235-245.

Nitzan, D., Sperry, J. F. & Wilkins, T. D. (1978) Fibrinolytic activity of oral anaerobic bacteria. *Archives of Oral Biology* **23**, 465-470.

Ottow, J. C. G. (1975) Ecology, physiology, and genetics of fimbriae and pili. *Annual Review of Microbiology* **29**, 79-108.

Page, R. C. (1982) Lymphoid cell responsiveness and human periodontitis. In: *Host-Parasite Interactions in Periodontal Diseases*, ed. Genco, R. J. & Mergenhagen, S. E., pp. 217-224. Washington, D.C.: American Society for Microbiology.

Pelus, L. M., Broxmeyer, H. E. & Moore, M. A. S. (1981) Regulation of human myelopoiesis by prostaglandin E and lactoferrin. *Cell and Tissue Kinetics* **14**, 515-526.

Plaut, A. G., Gilbert, J. V. & Burton, J. (1982) Bacterial immunoglobulin A proteases and mucosal diseases: Use of synthetic peptide analogs to modify the activity of these proteases. In *Host-Parasite Interactions in Periodontal Diseases*, ed. Genco, R. J. & Mergenhagen, S. E., pp. 193-201. Washington, D.C.: American Society for Microbiology.

Pruitt, K. M. (1977) Macromolecular components of oral fluids at tooth surfaces. *Swedish Dental Journal* **1**, 225-240.

Root, R. K. & Cohen, M. S. (1981) The microbicidal mechanisms of human neutrophils and eosinophils. *Reviews of Infectious Diseases* **3**, 565-598.

Saglie, R., Newman, M. G., Carranza Jr., F. A. & Pattison, G. L. (1982) Bacterial invasion of gingiva in advanced periodontitis in humans. *Journal of Periodontology* **53**, 217-222.

Shurin, S. B., Socransky, S. S., Sweeney, E. & Stossel, T. P. (1979) A neutrophil disorder induced by *Capnocytophaga*, a dental microorganism. *New England Journal of Medicine* **301**, 849-854.

Simpson, W. A., Ofek, I., Sarasohn, C., Morrison, J. C. & Beachey, E. H. (1980) Characteristics of the binding of streptococcal lipoteichoic acid to human oral epithelial cells. *Journal of Infectious Diseases* **141**, 457-462.

Singer, R. E. & Buckner, B. A. (1981) Butyrate and propionate: Important components of toxic dental plaque extracts. *Infection and Immunity* **32**, 458-463.

Slots, J. (1976) The predominant cultivable organisms in juvenile periodontitis. *Scandinavian Journal of Dental Research* **84**, 1-10.

Slots, J. (1977a) Microflora in the healthy gingival sulcus in man. *Scandinavian Journal of Dental Research* **85**, 247-254.

Slots, J. (1977b) The predominant cultivable microflora of advanced periodontitis. *Scandinavian Journal of Dental Research* **85**, 114-121.

Slots, J. (1981) Enzymatic characterization of some oral and nonoral Gram-negative bacteria with the API ZYM system. *Journal of Clinical Microbiology* **14**, 288-294.

Slots, J. (1982) Importance of black-pigmented *Bacteroides* in human periodontal disease. In *Host-Parasite Interactions in Periodontal Diseases*, ed. Genco, R. J. & Mergenhagen, S. E., pp. 27-45. Washington, D.C.: American Society for Microbiology.

Slots, J., Möenbo, D., Langebaek, J. & Frandsen, A. (1978) Microbiota of gingivitis in man. *Scandinavian Journal of Dental Research* **86**, 174-181.

Slots, J., Reynolds, H. S. & Genco, R. J. (1980) *Actinobacillus actinomycetemcomitans* in human periodontal disease: A cross-sectional microbiological investigation. *Infection and Immunity* **29**, 1013-1020.

Snyderman, R. & Goetzl, E. J. (1981) Molecular and cellular mechanisms of leukocyte chemotaxis. *Science* **213**, 830-837.

Socransky, S. S. (1979) Criteria for the infectious agents in dental caries and periodontal disease. *Näringsforskning* **23**, Supplement 17, 16-21.

Socransky, S. S. & Hubersak, C. (1967) Replacement of ascitic fluid or rabbit serum requirement of *Treponema dentium* by α-globulin. *Journal of Bacteriology* **94**, 1795-1796.

Socransky, S. S., Loesche, W. J., Hubersak, C & MacDonald, J. B. (1964) Dependency o *Treponema microdentium* on other oral organisms for isobutyrate, polyamines, and a controlled oxidation-reduction potential. *Journal of Bacteriology* **88**, 200-209.

Socransky, S. S., Manganiello, A. D., Propas, D., Oram. V. & van Houte, J. (1977) Bacteriological studies of developing supra-gingival dental plaque. *Journal of Periodontal Research* **12**, 90-106.

Socransky, S. S., Tanner, A. C. R., Haffajee, A D., Hillman, J. D. & Goodson, J. M. (1982 Present status of studies on the microbial etiology of periodontal diseases. In *Host-Parasite Interactions in Periodontal Diseases,* ed. Genco, R. J. & Mergenhagen, S. E., pp. 1-12 Washington, D.C.: American Society for Microbiology.

Steffen, E. K. & Hentges, D. J. (1981) Hydrolytic enzymes of anaerobic bacteria isolated from human infections. *Journal of Clinical Microbiology* **14**, 153-156.

Tanner, A. C. R., Badger, S., Lai, C.-H., Listgarten, M. A., Visconti, R. A. & Socransky, S. S. (1981) *Wolinella* gen. nov., *Wolinella succinogenes* (*Vibrio succinogenes* Wolin et al.) comb. nov., and description of *Bacteroides gracilis* sp. nov., *Wolinella recta* sp. nov., *Campylobacter concisus* sp. nov., and *Eikenella corrodens* from humans with periodontal disease *International Journal of Systematic Bacteriology* **31**, 432-445.

Tanner, A. C. R., Haffer, C., Bratthall, G. T., Visconti, R. A. & Socransky, S. S. (1979) A study of the bacteria associated with advancing periodontitis in man. *Journal Clinical Periodontology* **6**, 278-307.

Taubman, M. A., Ebersole, J. L. & Smith, D. J. (1982) Association between systemic and local antibody and periodontal diseases. In *Host-Parasite Interactions in Periodontal Diseases,* ed. Genco, R. J. & Mergenhagen, S. A., pp. 283-298. Washington, D. C.: American Society for Microbiology.

Theilade, E., Wright, W. H., Jensen, S. B. & Löe, H. (1966) Experimental gingivitis in man. II. A longitudinal clinical and bacteriological investigation. *Journal of Periodontal Research* **1**, 1-13.

Tolo, K. & Brandtzaeg, P. (1982) Relation between periodontal disease activity and serum antibody titers to oral bacteria. In *Host-Parasite Interactions in Periodontal Diseases*, ed. Genco, R. J. & Mergenhagen, S. E., pp. 270-282. Washington, D. C.: American Society for Microbiology.

Walden, W. C. & Hentges, D. C. (1975) Differential effects of oxygen and oxidation-reduction potential on the multiplication of three species of anaerobic intestinal bacteria. *Applied Microbiology* **30**, 781-785.

Walker, G. J. (1978) Dextrans. In *Biochemistry of Carbohydrates II,* ed. Manners, D. J., Vol. 16, pp. 75-126. Baltimore: University Park Press.

Werner, H. & Müller, H. E. (1971) Immunoelektrophoretische Untersuchungen über die Einwirkung von *Bacteroides-, Fusobacterium-, Leptotrichia-* und *Sphaerophorus-* Arten auf menschliche Plasmaproteine. Zentralblatt fuer Bakteriologie, Parasitenkunde, Infektionskrankheiten und Hygiene, Abteilung 1: Originale, **216,** 96-113.

Wicken, A. J. & Knox, K. W. (1980) Bacterial cell surface amphiphiles. *Biochimica et Biophysica Acta* **604**, 1-26.

Williams, B. L., Pantalone, R. M. & Sherris, J. C. (1976) Subgingival microflora and periodontitis. *Journal of Periodontal Research* **11**, 1-18.

Wilton, J. M. A. (1981) Microbial interference with inflammation and phagocyte function. In *Microbial Perturbation of Host Defences,* ed. Grady, F. O. & Smith. H., pp. 67-96. London: Academic Press.

Woods, D. E., Straus, D. C., Johanson, Jr., W. G. & Bass, J. A. (1981) Role of salivary protease activity in adherence of Gram-negative bacilli to mammalian buccal epithelial cells *in vivo. Journal of Clinical Investigation* **68**, 1435-1440.

CHAPTER 5

Pathogenesis of Plaque Associated Periodontal Disease

Introduction

Periodontal disease probably comprises a group of different disorders all of which affect the supporting structures of the teeth and which may result in loss of teeth.

Clinically, periodontal disease is characterized by inflammatory alterations of the gingiva, such as swelling and redness of the gingival margin and bleeding on gentle prob-ing in the gingival sulcus/pocket area. Other important clinical symptoms of periodontal disease include (1) reduced resistance of the periodontal tissues to probing – increased probing depth or pocket depth – and (2) gingival recession. In most patients the severity of various clinical symptoms of periodontal disease varies not only from tooth to tooth but also from one tooth surface to another. In subjects with advanced periodontal disease (3) migration of teeth and the development of spaces between teeth are often seen as well as (4) tilting of premolars and molar with a resulting reduction of the height of the bite.

Radiographically, periodontal disease is evidenced by loss of alveolar bone. Bone loss which occurs at different rates around different teeth and tooth surfaces in the dentition results in an even ("horizontal") or an angular ("vertical") outline of the alveolar bone crest. While many teeth in a given patient may suffer from advanced loss of bone, some teeth or tooth surfaces may be almost unaffected and surrounded by an alveolar bone of normal height. Hence, clinical and radiographic findings imply that periodontal disease develops in a characteristic (specific) way around each individual tooth (tooth surface) in the dentition.

In a histological section, periodontal disease is identified by the presence of inflammatory cell infiltrates in the connective tissue beneath the pocket epithelium adjacent to a tooth surface harboring microbial plaque. Within the infiltrated connective tissue, inflammatory cells, such as plasma cells, lymphocytes, blast cells, macrophages and neutrophils, accumulate in a tissue compartment which has a low density of fibroblasts, collagen and matrix components.

Current concepts regarding the etiology nd pathogenesis of periodontal disease are erived from the results of *epidemiological tudies, analyses of autopsy material, clinical -ials* and *animal experimentation.*

Findings from *epidemiological studies* ave consistently revealed a close relation-hip between the age of a population, the ral hygiene conditions and the frequency nd severity of periodontal disease. Hence, he parameters measuring dental plaque, alculus (oral hygiene) and periodontal dis-ase, increase in numerical value with ncreasing age of the subjects in a given opulation.

From *analyses of human autopsy material* t has been realized that a close topographi-al relationship exists between the location f the microbial deposit on the tooth surface nd the extension of the inflammatory lesion n the adjacent soft tissue. As long as the nicrobial deposit is only present on the rown of the tooth, the lesion is limited to he supraalveolar connective tissue. When, owever, microbial plaques are found on the oot cementum, the areas previously ccupied by periodontal ligament and alveo-ar bone are also the seat of lesions. In fact, neasurements made by Waerhaug (1952) uggest that the distance, from the periphery f the microbial deposit on the tooth surface o the lateral and apical extension of the nflammatory cell lesion in the soft tissue, eldom exceeds 1-2 mm. In addition, a nar-ow zone (1 mm) of normal connective tissue s frequently recognized between the infil-rate and the alveolar bone (Waerhaug 979). Since the periodontal ligament and he alveolar bone frequently contain no nflammatory cell infiltrates, many forms of laque associated periodontal disease may e classified as (i) gingivitis without, or (ii) ;ingivitis with, loss of connective tissue ttachment.

Clinical trials of short duration have evealed that a normal, noninflamed gingiva an be established in young individuals who ave a high standard of oral hygiene. If such ndividuals abstain from mechanical tooth leaning, microorganisms start to colonize

the tooth surfaces. Within a few days inflam-matory changes can be seen in the adjacent gingiva. These inflammatory alterations are resolved when correct tooth cleaning mea-sures are resumed (Löe et al. 1965). Further-more, the initiation of gingivitis was pre-vented in individuals with normal gingiva and clean teeth by the daily use, over several weeks, of chlorhexidine digluconate – an antimicrobial compound which prevents the colonization of bacteria on the tooth surface – as a substitute for mechanical tooth clean-ing (Löe & Rindom Schiött 1970). This demonstrates that microorganisms which form plaques on the teeth, contain or release components which induce or mediate inflammatory changes in the gingiva.

Results from *long-term clinical trials* have provided additional information regarding the relationship between plaque, calculus and periodontal disease in humans. Thus, research reports by Lövdal et al. (1961), Ramfjord et al. (1968, 1975), Suomi et al. (1971), Lindhe & Nyman (1975), Axelsson & Lindhe (1978, 1981), Knowles et al. (1979), Nyman & Lindhe (1979) and others, have revealed that in patients with advanced periodontal disease, gingival inflammation was resolved and further destruction of the attachment apparatus was prevented by scal-ing and root planing in conjunction with poc-ket elimination procedures, and the subse-quent adoption of a careful oral hygiene program. In subjects with untreated periodontal disease, on the other hand, a gradual loss of attachment and alveolar bone can be seen (Axelsson & Lindhe 1981). Findings from long-term clinical trials demonstrate, thus, that the progressive and destructive character of periodontal disease is maintained only in areas which harbor subgingival plaque.

Finally, *experiments in animals (dogs)* have revealed that chronic plaque associated gingivitis in the presence of a subgingival microbiota, may develop into progressive and destructive periodontal disease. Thus, in dogs which for a period of several years accumulated plaque and calculus, the overt gingivitis (without loss of connective tissue

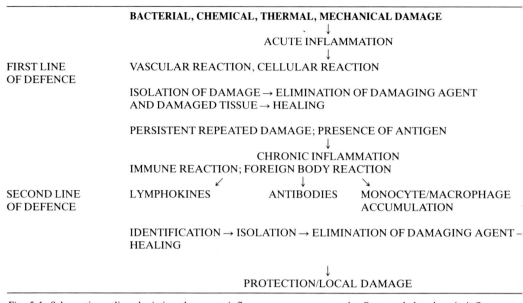

Fig. 5-1. Schematic outline depicting the acute inflammatory process as the first, and the chronic inflammator process as the second line of host defence.
Note that in both conditions there is a delicate balance between protection and local tissue damage. This means tha protection of the organism is achieved at the price of local damage.

attachment and bone) gradually shifted to periodontal disease including not only gingival inflammation but also loss of connective tissue attachment and alveolar bone (Saxe et al. 1967, Lindhe et al. 1975).

Taken together, the above described research data clearly indicate that most forms of periodontal disease are plaque associated disorders. Furthermore, there are reasons to assume that most, if not all, plaque associated periodontal disorders start as an overt inflammation in the gingiva. If left untreated, the lesion may spread in an apical direction and eventually result in loss of connective tissue attachment and supporting alveolar bone.

Basic phenomena in inflammation

Inflammatory lesions occurring in the gingiva are no different from similar lesions in other tissue compartments. The location extension and composition of gingiva inflammatory lesions are influenced, however, by the morphology and physiology of the tissues of the dentogingival region. In order to understand how inflammator lesions adapt to local conditions, some important fundamental mechanisms in both acute and chronic local inflammation will be described, as well as reactions which ma cause tissue damage.

The acute inflammatory reaction may be regarded as the *first line of defence* in the tissue following irritation or damage, while the so-called "chronic" inflammatory reaction may be looked upon as the *second line o defence* (Fig. 5-1). The characteristics o both lines of defence will be used to illustrate mechanisms which operate when the health gingiva turns into inflamed tissue and, subsequently, when an overt gingival lesion progresses to a lesion associated with loss of connective tissue attachment and alveolar bone i.e. destructive periodontal disease.

Acute inflammation

Acute inflammatory reaction is initiated in connective tissue following irritation or damage, e.g. of microbial, chemical, thermal or mechanical origin. The inflammatory reaction is comparatively "stereotyped", characterized by the occurrence of well defined, predictable vascular and cellular changes resulting in transient or permanent damage to normal tissue constituents (cells, fibers and matrix), with consequent impairment or loss of the normal function of the affected tissue (Ryan & Majno 1977).

Healing is an important feature of acute inflammatory reaction. Healing follows when the agent initiating the inflammatory response has been eliminated or partly inactivated.

The main objective of local inflammatory reaction is to protect exposed tissue against the penetration of noxious substances (or damage) as well as to establish conditions favorable to the regeneration or repair of tissue structures damaged in this combat. Local inflammatory reaction should, thus, be regarded as beneficial in the sense that it isolates damaging substances, thereby protecting more distant parts of the body (Mims 1977).

Even if an acute inflammatory reaction has a comparatively "stereotyped" course, variations in the intensity of the local response are often seen. Such variations may be related to differences between individuals or tissues in their ability to respond to the irritant. For example, under otherwise identical conditions, an inflammatory reaction in skin is not as intense as in oral mucosa. Factors, such as the vascularity of the tissue and the turnover of different, tissue components at the inflamed site, also influence the intensity of the acute inflammatory reaction. Furthermore, the nature of the damaging factor (microbial, chemical, thermal, mechanical) may influence the course and duration of the acute inflammatory reaction. Finally, the duration of exposure to irritation also influences the character of the tissue reaction (Ryan & Majno 1977).

An inflammatory lesion can be detected in a biopsy sampled from the gingiva and examined in the microscope long before pathological alterations can be seen clinically. The clinical characteristics of an inflamed tissue/organ should be regarded as the net effect of all the different alterations occurring in it. The clinical evaluation of a condition, therefore, should not be used, either as the only measure of disease, or to describe the intensity of the inflammatory reaction. However, the classical symptoms of inflammation, i.e. redness, heat, swelling, pain and impaired function, are valid for most local inflammatory conditions.

Vascular reactions

Vascular reactions rapidly develop following damage, their purpose being to provide the damaged area with the plasma proteins and fluid necessary for a rapid isolation of both the irritant and the damaged tissue. They also quickly bring both antibacterial substances and mediators of the inflammatory process, to the site of damage. Vascular reactions may be regarded as one part of the initial defence reaction (*first line of defence*) of the tissue and are characterized by *vascular dilatation* and a *decrease* of the *velocity* of the blood flow through the microvascular system of the affected part of the tissue.

Concomitantly with the dimensional alterations of the microvascular system, the *permeability* of the vessels is increased (Fig. 5-2). This change is first detected in the post-capillary venules of the microvascular system of the affected area. During normal function, there is "free" transport (pinocytosis; through a system of pinocytotic vesicles in the endothelial cells) of water, electrolytes and low molecular weight substances (e.g. albumin) between the vascular system and the surrounding connective tissues while the penetration of larger molecules is prevented. The increased vascular permeability in acute inflammation results partly from increased hydrostatic pressure in the microvascular system and partly from contraction of the endothelial cells located on the inner aspects of the walls

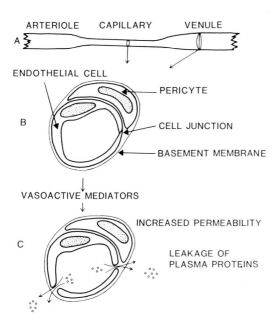

Fig. 5-2. Schematic illustration depicting the terminal vascular bed and the mechanisms of increased vascular permeability. Under normal conditions the terminal vessels are freely permeable to small molecules, salt and water. The intercellular junctions between the endothelial cells are closed. Via the influence of vasoactive mediators the endothelial cells become separated and increased vascular permeability occurs. Large molecules and plasmaproteins leak into the surrounding tissue. A number of inflammatory mediators present in plasma are activated when they enter the perivascular tissue.

of the post-capillary venules. In the latter process the junctions between the endothelial cells are opened and macromolecules can leave the vascular system and enter the surrounding tissue (Fig. 5-6).

The altered vascular permeability is often mediated by biochemically active substances (mediators). Vasoactive amines, *histamine* and *serotonin,* are primarily responsible for the increased vascular permeability during the first or "rapid" phase of the acute inflammatory reaction. Inactive precursors to such mediators are present in the matrix of connective tissue and in the granules of mast cells. Following exposure of tissue to an irrit-

ant, vasoactive amines are released from the mast cells. Other substances which can increase vascular permeability in acute inflammation are *prostaglandins* and *kinins* (kallikreinogen-Kallikrein). These substances are present in plasma but can also be produced by connective tissue cells. Mediators of increased permeability are also released during the process of coagulation (the Hageman factor which can activate the clotting cascade) and from the complement systems. In addition, the inflammatory cells, the leukocytes, contain and produce substances which, when released from the cells, can induce alterations in vascular permeability (Table 5-1).

The different mediators involved in the process of increasing vascular permeability cooperate, and in a given phase one or more can be active. Increased vascular permeability can occur without such mediators, i.e. following mechanically or thermally induced severe tissue trauma with direct damage to the vascular system. It should be understood that the mechanisms responsible for increased vascular permeability in acute inflammation are related to the nature and intensity of the irritant.

An immediate increase in vascular permeability can be detected within sec or min following the exposure of tissue to irritation/trauma and is found to continue for about 15-30 min. This type of vascular reaction mainly affects postcapillary venules which have a diameter of less than 100 microns. The mediators (e.g. histamine) responsible for this so-called "rapid phase" of the acute inflammatory reaction are often released from mast cells or from the injured tissue matrix (Table 5-1).

Table 5-1. Some important mediators of increased vascular permeability

Plasma	Tissues and cells
Bradykinin	Histamine
Kallikrein	Serotonin
Plasminogen activator	Prostaglandins
C3 fragment	Lysosomal material
C5 fragment	Lymphokines
Fibrin products	

An immediate but prolonged increase in permeability will develop after direct damage to the vascular system. This permeability change may persist for several days, and will not disappear until the injured vessel has been blocked, e.g. by coagulation. This kind of vascular damage frequently occurs when the tissue is exposed to intense heat (burn).

A monophasic increase in permeability often occurs after minor tissue damage while following moderate damage, a biphasic response develops. In cases of severe damage, the 2 phases of increased permeability can coincide to establish a prolonged monophasic increase in vascular permeability (Fig. 5-3).

Cellular reactions

Acute inflammatory reaction causes leukocytes, neutrophilic granulocytes (neutrophils) and monocytes, to leave the vascular system and enter the adjacent connective tissue. In the process of emigration the leukocytes first adhere to the walls of the venules of the microvascular system and after adhesion is established, they migrate through the endothelial cell junctions. It is important to understand that this migration is neither the result of, nor results in, increased vascular permeability.

The emigration of leukocytes is initiated and maintained by the presence of cell attractive, so-called *chemotactic factors* believed to be deposited in the intercellular junctions of the endothelial cells as well as in the extravascular compartments (Table 5-2). Leukocytes adhering to the vessel wall are stimulated to move through the endothelial cell junctions by chemotactic stimulation.

When tissue is exposed to a relatively mild irritant, migration of neutrophilic granulocytes will reach a maximum at approximately 4-6 h after injury and subsequently decline. Mononuclear leukocytes (monocytes) start to migrate from the vessels at approximately 4 h after injury and this migration reaches a peak at 18-24 h (Fig. 5-4).

As stated above, migration of both neutrophilic granulocytes and mononuclear cells is the result of chemotactic stimulation.

In the early phase of inflammatory reaction neutrophilic granulocytes are responsible for phagocytosis of foreign particles, noxious material, microorganisms. Neutrophilic granulocytes contain in their cytoplasm numerous granules (lysosomes) which harbor enzymes and antibacterial substances as well as mediators of inflammation. Neutrophilic granulocytes also contain large amounts of glycogen which means that through glycolysis the cells can also function in environments of low oxygen tension.

The phagocytosis of microorganisms by neutrophilic granulocytes is phasic. First the microorganism becomes attached to the cell membrane. Through an invagination of the cell surface, accomplished by the fusion of pseudoarms, a membrane bound *phago-*

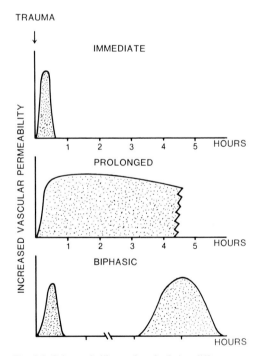

Fig. 5-3. Schematic illustration depicting different types of alterations in vascular permeability. *Immediately increased* vascular permeability occurs following minor tissue damage. A *prolonged increase* develops following more severe damage while a *biphasic response* arises following moderate tissue damage.

Table 5-2. Some important factors chemotactic to neutrophilic granulocytes

	Plasma	**Tissues and cells**	**Others**
Neutrophils:	Complement fragments, C5, C567 Kallikrein fibrin fragments Plasminogen activator	Prostaglandins Lysosomal material from neutrophils Lymphokines Collagen fragments	Bacterial products
Monocytes:	Complement fragments: C3, C5 Kallikrein Plasminogen activator	Lysosomal material from neutrophils Lymphokines	Bacterial products

some incorporating the microorganism is produced. In the phagosome the microorganism is transported into contact with *lysosomes.* The membrane of the phagosome and the membranes of one or several lysosomes merge. The lysosomal enzymes are emptied into the phagosome and a *phagolysosome* is formed. After phagocytosis and exposure to the lysosomal enzymes, most microorganisms are inactivated and subsequently disintegrated (Fig. 5-5, Table 5-3).

A deficiency in the number or function of neutrophilic granulocytes decreases the ability to combat infection and potentially lethal situations may develop. Examples of such conditions are neutropenia, agranulocytosis and/or certain forms of leukemia (Mims 1977).

The presence in the tissue of humoral antibodies against invading microorganisms stimulates and enhances the process of phagocytosis. The surface of the neutrophilic granulocyte harbors specific receptors (Fc-receptors) for antibody molecules. Via such Fc-receptors the microorganism becomes firmly adherent to the leukocyte, thereby facilitating phagocytosis.

During and following the process of phagocytosis, part of the lysosomal material of the leukocyte is disposed into the host tissue. Lysosomal enzymes released from phagocytosing neutrophils can cause pronounced breakdown of host tissue. Thus, phagocytosis not only counteracts the irritant (e.g. the infection) in the host tissue but

lysosomal material may cause additional tissue damage. Studies within different fields of medicine have clearly documented that tissue damage resulting from acute inflammation is, to a large extent, caused not by the microorganisms and their products *per se* but by the lysosomal material released from neutrophilic granulocytes which accumulate in affected connective tissue. For example tissue damage in the form of abscesses is considered to be the result of lysosomal enzymes

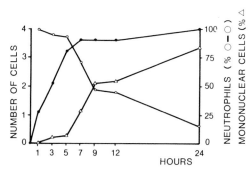

Fig. 5-4. Schematic illustration depicting alterations in the number of leukocytes and composition of the cellular exudate with time in a skin window lesion. Observe that the number of leukocytes rapidly increases up to 7 h following damage. Thereafter there is no obvious change in their number. In early inflammatory processes, the neutrophilic granulocytes dominate the cellular exudate, while after 9-12 h the majority of leukocytes are mononuclear cells, mainly monocytes/macrophages.

released from neutrophilic granulocytes participating in the defence of the host against infection (Ryan & Majno 1977).

The monocytes and their transmuted form, the macrophages (which develop when the monocytes are stimulated during the local inflammatory reaction), are cells which generally have functions similar to those of neutrophilic granulocytes. Thus, macrophages contain large numbers of lysosomes and participate in the phagocytosis of micro-organisms and noxious material. The macrophages are also engaged in the first phase of a process which leads to an immune reaction (Page & Schroeder 1981). Macrophages contain organelles with synthetic potential in their cytoplasm. Antigens which are phagocytosed by macrophages are altered through active processes in the cell and changed to a molecular form which can

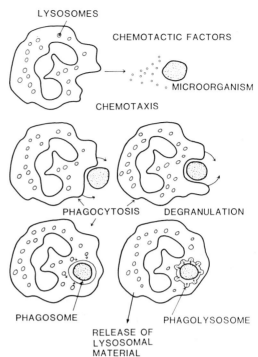

Fig. 5-5. Schematic illustration depicting phagocytosis. Leukocytes are attracted to bacteria as the result of chemotaxis. Following contact between the microorganism and the leukocyte, the cell extends pseudoarms and engulfs the microorganisms. The bacterium is trapped in a phagosome in the cytoplasm of the cell. The lysosomal membranes merge with the membrane of the phagosome and the lysosomal material is emptied into the phagosome which is now termed *phagolysosome* (degranulation). The lysosomal substances are activated and the microorganism disintegrates. The process of degranulation also leads to release of lysosomal material into the extracellular tissue compartments. When such a release occurs from a large number of accumulated neutrophilic granulocytes, tissue damage may result.

Table 5-3. Some enzymes and antibacterial components present in phagocytosing leukocytes

Enzymes
Acid hydrolases
β-glycerophosphatase
β-glucuronidase
N-acetyl-β-glucosaminidas
Mannosidase
Arylsulphatase
β-galactonidase
Proteases (cathepsins)

Neutral proteases
Cathepsin G
Elastase
Collagenase
Cationic proteins
Myeloperoxidase
Lysozyme
Lactoferrin
Acid phosphatase
Alkaline phosphatase
Antibacterial components
Acid pH
Cationic proteins
Lysozyme
Lactoferrin
Superoxid anion
H_2O_2

be recognized by the cells of the immune system, the lymphocytes.

Where exudation and phagocytosis, i.e. acute inflammation, are effective in eliminating the irritant, healing is soon initiated. During healing of connective tissue lesions, substances are released which mediate an increased proliferation and metabolic activity of fibroblasts.

161

Chronic inflammation/immune reaction

Where the local inflammatory reaction is insufficient to eliminate infectious material (antigens), an immune response may be elicited. The main purpose of the immune response is to identify and bind the noxious agent (the antigen) and to activate the phagocytes (neutrophilic granulocytes, macrophages). Through these functions, *the second line of defence*, the antigen is neutralized and decomposed and the host is protected (Fig. 5-1). Monocytes/macrophages, lymphocytes and plasma cells accumulate locally in tissue at the site of antigen deposition. A substance with nonantigenic properties will cause a foreign body reaction characterized by the accumulation of macrophages at the reaction site. The immune reactions as well as the acute inflammatory reaction should be regarded as defence mechanisms which limit the possibility for noxious substances or bacteria to penetrate further into the tissue. Immune reactions have 2 major parts and include:

1. production of antibodies – the humoral reaction
2. participation of certain lymphocytes – the cell mediated reaction.

In most situations both reactions occur simultaneously but one or the other may predominate depending on the character of the antigen to which the tissue is exposed (Fig. 5-6).

Antigen/antibody mediated reaction

Antibodies. Antibodies are produced by *plasma cells* which develop from lymphocytes belonging to the B-lymphocyte series. B stands for the bursa dependent system. The bursa is an organ still present in birds (Bursa of Fabricius). Through the influence of this structure lymphocytes are differentiated which have the capacity to react with an antigen by antibody production. The development of B-lymphocytes via a blast stadium into mature plasma cells occurs in different steps. Recently it was demonstrated that B-lymphocytes may also produce

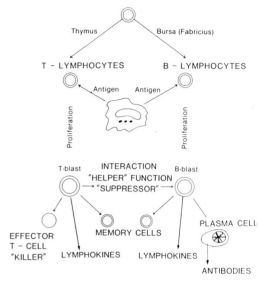

Fig. 5-6. Simplified schematic illustration of the main functions of the immune system. Note the interaction between the macrophages and the immune system as well as the interaction between the T- and B-cells. Both reactions lead to the release of factors that defend the tissue but which at the same time directly or indirectly may cause local tissue damage.

certain lymphokines (see: cell mediated immune reaction) (Page & Schroeder 1981).

Antibodies are produced by plasma cells present either at the site of reaction and/or in the lymphoid tissue (lymph nodes, tonsils, spleen, Payer's patches in the gut). Antibodies to some antigens can be synthetized by plasma cells without the participation of T-cells (see: cell mediated immune reaction). In many cases, however, the plasma cell requires assistance from the T-cell. Antibodies are released from plasma cells and deposited either in the tissues of the reaction site or in the lymph node from which they enter the circulation. The plasma cells produce antibodies, immunoglobulins (IG) with a single specificity and most of the cells produce immunoglobulins of the IgG or IgM class. Comparatively fewer plasma cells contain IgD and IgE. Some plasma cells located close to mucous membranes produce IgA-antibodies. Immunoglobulins of the IgA ype are of importance for the protection of he mucosal lining.

Antibody and antigen molecules combine n to an immune complex. The antigen is lereby bound and its biological effect is, in many cases, neutralized.

Complement. Immune complexes (anti-gen/antibody complexes) play an important part in development and maintenance of local inflammatory reaction (Page & Schroeder 1981). Activation of the *comple-ment system* is a very important result of the formation of immune complexes. The com-plement system is a series of at least 9 diffe-ent proteins present in plasma. During the early phase of acute inflammatory reaction, plasma proteins, including the components of the complement system, accumulate out-side the vessels. Proteins of the complement system after contact with most antigen/anti-body complexes are altered to biologically active substances (the classical way of com-plement alteration).

The components of the complement sys-em can be best described as enzymes acti-vated in a predetermined sequence. The activation of complement results in the for-mation of mediators for the local inflammat-ory reaction. Factors released by the activa-ion of the third component of complement, C3, induce increased vascular permeability and enhance phagocytosis by neutrophilic granulocytes and macrophages. A factor with similar properties is produced by the activation of C5. Furthermore, a combina-ion of components C5, C6 and C7 is also chemotactic for neutrophils. Additionally, products similar to kinins are released which nduce increased vascular permeability (Fig. 5-7).

Apart from the induction of local inflam-matory reaction, the activated complement, although an effective defence against bac-eria may also induce damage to cell mem-branes when the activation occurs in fibro-blast membranes of the host tissue.

Thus, by the production of antibodies, the antigenic substance is identified and neut-alized, and the complement system is acti-vated by the antigen antibody complex. The

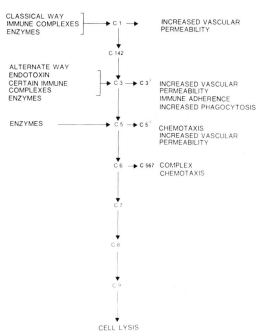

COMPLEMENT ACTIVATION VIA

Fig. 5-7. Schematic illustration of the complement sys-tem and its activation by various processes. Note that following activation of complement, fragments are released which increase vascular permeability, are chemotactic to leukocytes and may induce cell lysis, e.g. cause local inflammation and tissue damage.

immune complex is subsequently eliminated by the acute inflammatory reaction (exuda-tion and phagocytosis) initiated and main-tained by the activated components of com-plement.

Enzymes from bacteria, and lysosomal enzymes from neutrophilic granulocytes can, without the participation of immune complexes, also activate the complement system as well as endotoxin from Gram negative bacteria. Factors chemotactic for leukocytes and vasoactive substances are hereby generated via the so-called *"alterna-tive pathway"* of complement activation. The complement system may also be acti-

Table 5-4. Some important lymphokines released from stimulated lymphocytes

Factor		Effect
MIF	Migration inhibition factor	Inhibits the migration of macrophages
LIF	Leukocyte inhibition factor	Inhibits the migration of leukocytes
LMF	Lymphocyte mitogenic factor	Stimulates proliferation of lymphocytes
SRF	Skin reaction factor	Causes inflammation when injected intradermally
LT	Lymphotoxin	Cytotoxic to other cells (fibroblasts etc.)
MAF	Macrophage activating factor	Activates macrophages
OAF	Osteoclast activating factor	Activates osteoclasts

Factors chemotactic to neutrophilic granulocytes, monocytes and lymphocytes.

vated by factors involved in the process of coagulation. It is important to realize that by the activation of the complement system, either via immune complexes or non-specific reactions, mediators are released which are important for the 2 fundamental processes of the acute inflammatory reaction: increased vascular permeability, and activation and migration of neutrophils and macrophages (Ryan & Majno 1977).

Cell mediated immune reaction

Cell mediated immune reaction is managed by cells belonging to the T-lymphocyte series. These cells are differentiated in the thymus. Cellular immune reaction does not involve antibody production in the traditional sense. Instead substances, *lymphokines,* are synthesized and released from T-lymphocytes when they come into contact with an antigen they are programmed to react to (sensitized). Lymphokines are involved in defence of the host against bacteria and foreign cells and have the potential to mediate different phases of local inflammatory reaction (Page & Schroeder 1981).

Some lymphokines prevent macrophages from migrating from the reaction site (MIF) and stimulate the synthetic and phagocytic activity of the macrophages (MAF). Substances chemotactic to neutrophilic granulocytes, monocytes/macrophages and lymphocytes, have also been demonstrated among

lymphokines. Lymphotoxin (LT) is a lymphokine which has a nonspecific cytotoxic effect on other cells, and it can also cause damage to host tissue cells. Other lymphokines (LMF) stimulate proliferation of nonsensitized lymphocytes and activate osteoclasts (OAF) to produce bone resorption (Table 5-4).

It should be noted that many immune processes involve a combination of B-cell and T cell reactions, though some antigens elicit only one or the other immune reaction, some giving rise primarily to B-cell, other to. T-cell reactions. Furthermore, as stated above, a B-cell reaction is dependent on the presence of T-cells (T-helper and T-suppressor). This dependency may be one reason for the relative absence of pure B- or T-cell reactions.

Comments

This brief review of the more important mechanisms involved in acute and chronic inflammatory reactions emphasizes that both should be regarded as primarily protective. Thus, in most instances the organism is successfully defended against the antigen e.g. the infection. It is important to note that cellular and vascular reactions may be initiated by different mechanisms. The final response, increased vascular permeability and migration of inflammatory cells from the vascular system into the reaction site is, however, similar. It is also obvious that even if the immune reactions are longstanding, the tissue changes seen in chronic inflammation have some features in common with those in acute inflammation. However, while acute inflammation is of transient character, chronic inflammation is not resolved until the irritating agent/agents, as well as damaged components of the host tissue, have been neutralized and/or removed. Healing can not progress to functional reconstitution until the irritating agent or substance has been neutralized or removed.

One further difference between chronic and acute inflammation, is the proliferation in the chronic condition of the vessels in the affected tissue. The reason for this proliferation is not known, but it may be assumed, however, that the proliferation of the vasculature is an expression of a greater demand for nutrition and drainage.

Plaque associated periodontal disease

Normal gingiva

In order to fully understand and evaluate different symptoms of gingival inflammatory disease, a thorough and detailed knowledge of the structural composition and function of the healthy periodontium is a fundamental prerequisite. The anatomy of the gingiva and the attachment apparatus were described in Chapter 1; summarized below are some important features:

Clinically, the *normal gingiva* is characterized by its pink color, firm consistency and by the scalloped outline of the gingival margin. The interdental papillae are firm, do not bleed on gentle probing and occupy the space below the contact area of neighboring teeth.

In a histological section, the *normal gingiva* is characterized by a keratinized oral epithelium which fuses with a junctional

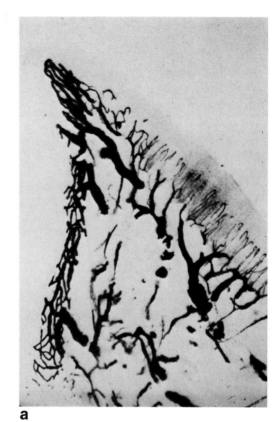

a

Fig. 5-8a. Buccolingual section of healthy gingiva in a dog. The gingival vessels were, prior to death of the animal, filled with a carbon suspension. Note the presence of a thin vascular network beneath the junctional epithelium to the left in the photomicrograph. This vascular network is present in the connective tissue below the entire surface of the junctional epithelium.

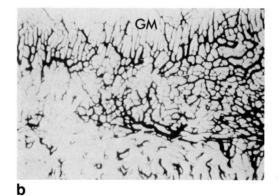

b

Fig. 5-8b. The vascular plexus is shown in a mesio-distal section. The thin vessels are anastomosing with each other to a vascular system of uniform density below the entire junctional epithelium. (From Egelberg 1967).

165

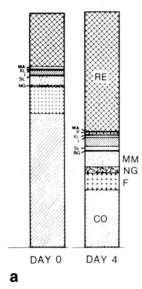

DAY 0   DAY 4

a

Fig. 5-9a. Alterations in gingival connective tissue during the first 4 days of gingivitis development in beagles. Note the reduction of the collagen content and the enhanced leukocyte infiltration; in particular neutrophilic granulocytes and monocytes/macrophages (RE: residual tissue, MA: mast cells, P: plasma cells, XL: blast lymphocytes, I: immunoblasts, SL: small lymphocytes, BG: basophilic granulocytes, MM: monocytes/macrophages, NG: neutrophilic granulocytes, F: fibroblasts, CO: collagen). (From Schroeder et al. 1975).

epithelium, which via hemidesmosomes establishes a firm attachment to the tooth surface. The area between the 2 epithelia is occupied by collagenous structures, most of which are organized in densely packed, distinctly outlined fiber bundles. Immediately below the junctional epithelium there is a vascular plexus, a dentogingival plexus, which contains numerous venules (Fig. 5-8). No infiltrates of inflammatory cells can be distinguished but the marginal portion of the junctional epithelium harbors a few neutrophilic granulocytes and mononuclear cells. A gingival sulcus is seldom seen. A careful analysis of the composition of *normal gingiva* reveals that almost 40% of the volume is occupied by epithelial structures (oral epithelium 30%, junctional epithelium 10%) and 60% by connective tissue components such as collagen fibers, matrix, cells, vessels and nerves (Fig. 5-9). Isolated inflammatory cells are present either in the connective tissue immediately below the junctional epithelium and/or around vessels

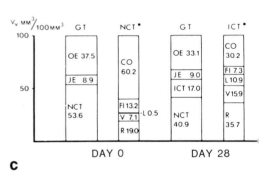

DAY 0   DAY 28

c

Fig. 5-9c. Composition of the gingiva (GT), noninfiltrated (NCT) and infiltrated (ICT) gingival connective tissue on day 0 (normal gingiva) and on day 28 of gingivitis in beagles. Note that the infiltrated connective tissue portion amounts to 17% of the free gingival margin on day 28 and that the collagen content is reduced from approximately 60% on day 0 to 30% on day 28 in the area were the inflammatory infiltrate has become established. Note also that in this area (on day 28) a reduction in fibroblast proportion has occurred, as well as an increase of vessels and residual tissue. OE: oral epithelium, JE: junctional epithelium, NCT: noninfiltrated connective tissue, ICT: infiltrated connective tissue, CO: collagen fibers, FI: fibroblasts, V: vascular structures, L: leukocytes, R: residual tissue. (From Lindhe & Rylander 1975).

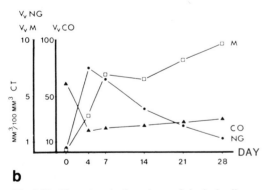

b

Fig. 5-9b. Alterations in the volume of gingival collagen (CO), neutrophilic granulocytes (NG) and mononuclear leukocytes (M) from day 0 to day 28 during the development of gingivitis in beagles. Observe the marked reduction of collagen content between day 0 and day 4, but also that collagen volume remains on this low level throughout the 28 days of experiment. (From Lindhe & Rylander 1975).

in areas more distant to the junctional epithelium (Attström et al. 1975, Lindhe & Rylander 1975).

Such *normal gingivae* can be established under experimental conditions in humans who, daily over several weeks, exercise meticulous plaque control measures, but should be distinguished from *clinically healthy gingivae*.

In *clinically healthy gingivae* a small infiltrate of inflammatory cells is always present in the coronal portion of the connective tissue (Page & Schroeder 1976). This infiltrate which occupies around 3-5% of the connective tissue volume and which is always in contact with the junctional epithelium, harbours lymphocytes, neutrophils and monocytes/macrophages in a compartment of the tissue rich in vascular structures but poor in collagen. A gingival sulcus, 0.1-0.5 mm deep, is always found between the coronal portion of the junctional epithelium and the tooth surface. The sulcus develops as a result of continuous bacterial and mechanical irritation, disappears after debridement and the initiation of chemical plaque control measures and should be distinguished from the

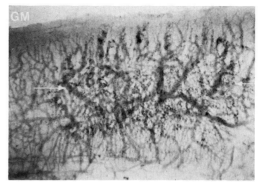

Fig. 5-10. Mesiodistal section of a gingiva showing the vascular network below the junctional epithelium. In the area between the arrows a filter paper-strip has been introduced into the junctional epithelium whereby an increased permeability of the gingival vessels has been induced. The increased vascular permeability is in this case identified by the presence of carbon particles which prior to biopsy were injected intravenously. The carbon particles have become trapped in the open endothelial junctions, and so-called vascular labelling has occurred. GM: gingival margin. (From Egelberg 1967).

pathologically deepened pocket (see below) (Schroeder 1973, 1977, Page & Schroeder 1982).

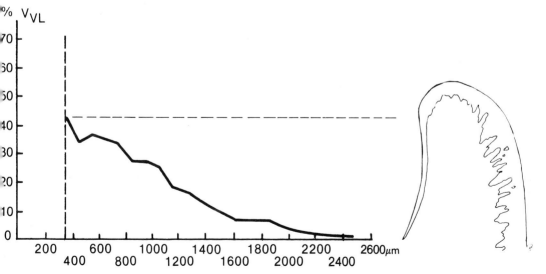

Fig. 5-11. Volume of leukocytes in the junctional epithelium expressed as the percentage of the total volume of the junctional epithelium. Observe that the volume of leukocytes decreases in apical direction and approaches 0 in the most apical portion. Within the junctional epithelium, the mononuclear leukocytes are located in more basal layers, while the neutrophilic granulocytes are present primarily in the superficial portions of the junctional epithelium. (From Schroeder 1973).

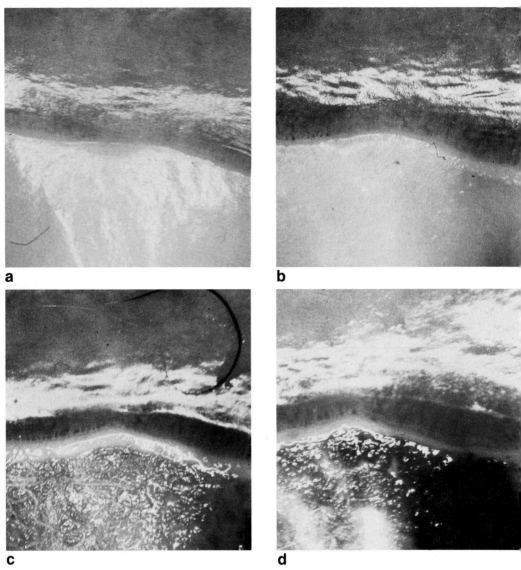

Fig. 5-12a-d. Gingival alterations which have occurred during a period of gingivitis development in beagles. a: day 0, b: day 4, c: day 14, d: day 28. Note the gradually developing inflammatory changes in the gingiva. Note the vascular reaction which is illustrated by a gradually increased number of vessels in the gingival margin. Plaque is present on the tooth surfaces.

The vascular plexus (dentogingival plexus) containing a large number of venules is the source from which the gingival fluid is derived (Fig. 5-10). Mechanical and/or chemical irritation of the tissue of the gingival margin results in an increased permeability of the vessels of the dentogingival plexus.

Fluid and plasma proteins leak out into the gingival sulcus via the connective tissue and the junctional epithelium (Egelberg 1967, Cimasoni 1974).

In the junctional epithelium of *normal* gingivae as well as in *clinically healthy* gingivae, neutrophilic granulocytes and mono-

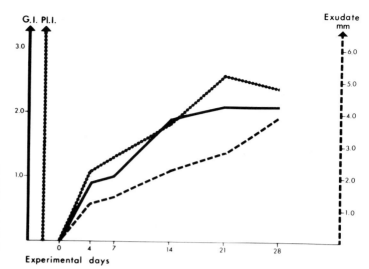

Fig. 5-12e. Alterations in Gingival Index, Plaque index and the amount of gingival fluid during a period of developing gingivitis in beagles. Note the gradual increase of all parameters during an experimental period of 28 days. (From Lindhe & Rylander 1975).

nuclear leukocytes are present (Fig. 5-11). The leukocytes, which more or less continuously migrate from the dentogingival vessels via the junctional epithelium to the gingival sulcus, indicate the presence in the gingival sulcus region of factors *chemotactic* for these cells. Saliva contains, and plaque forming bacteria release, such chemotactic factors. Leukocyte migration is minute in *normal* and *clinically healthy* gingivae but is markedly enhanced when bacteria accumulate and grow on the tooth surface (Attström 1971).

The ability of the *normal* and *clinically healthy* gingiva to defend the periodontium against irritating substances is excellent. Single microorganisms and other foreign substances placed in the dentogingival region are rapidly eliminated or removed. This is accomplished by (i) gingival fluid flow, (ii) migrating and phagocytosing leukocytes, (iii) shedding of surface cells from oral and junctional epithelia (Schroeder 1977, Page & Schroeder 1982).

As long as large amounts of microorganisms are prevented from colonizing the gingival third of the tooth surface the defence mechanisms of the gingiva are capable of preserving the integrity of the tissue.

Gingival inflammation

Inflammatory changes in the gingiva develop when microorganisms colonize the marginal portion of a tooth surface. The inflammation is only clinically observable after approximately 1 week of undisturbed bacterial growth. After 10-20 days of continuous plaque growth, clinically manifest gingivitis is established in most individuals. Clinically, the alterations are characterized

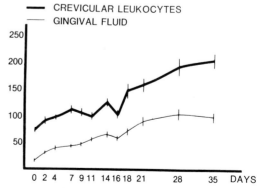

Fig. 5-13. Alterations in number of crevicular leukocytes and in gingival fluid during a period of developing gingivitis in beagles. Note the gradual increase of leukocytes and fluid flow during the experimental period. (From Attström & Egelberg 1971).

169

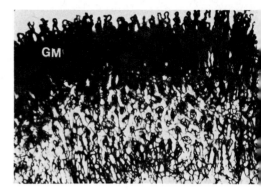

Fig. 5-14a.

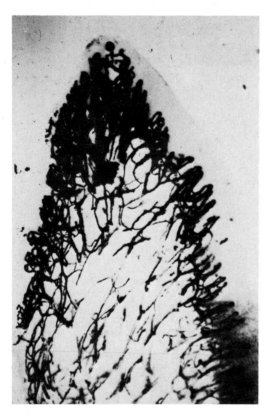

Fig. 5-14b.

Fig. 5-14a. Buccolingual section of chronically inflamed gingiva in a dog. The vessels have been filled with a contrasting carbon suspension. Note the wide and tortuous vessels below the junctional epithelium to the left in the illustration. Compare with the vasculature in healthy gingiva in Fig. 5-8. The pronounced vascular reaction in this area is a result of plaque accumulation.

Fig. 5-14b. Mesiodistal section of a gingiva illustrating the vessels below the junctional epithelium of chronically inflamed gingiva. Note vascular dilation and proliferation at the level of the gingival margin (GM). Note also that vascular proliferation has occurred in the apical part of the vascular plexus. (From Egelberg 1967).

by gingival redness and swelling and increased tendency of the soft tissue to bleed on gentle probing (Fig. 5-12). If the microbial plaque is removed at this stage and proper plaque control measures instituted the inflammatory alterations soon disappear (Löe et al. 1965, Lindhe & Rylander 1975).

The clinically detectable signs of disease constitute the net effect of a number of different events which can only be identified by microscopic examination of the affected tissue.

The tissue alterations which occur during the development of gingivitis will be described below with respect to vascular, cellular and immunologic changes.

Vascular reactions

Alterations of the vasculature of the dentogingival plexus can already be noted 1 day after the onset of plaque formation. The vasculature exhibits an increased permeability which is clinically detectable by an increased gingival fluid flow (Fig. 5-13). This alteration is the result of bacterial influence and/or the ensuing inflammatory reaction on the vessels of the dentogingival plexus (Attström & Egelberg 1971, Lindhe & Rylander 1975, Schroeder et al. 1975). Between 4-7 days after microbial colonization, some of the vessels of the dentogingival plexus increase in size. With time, the course of the vessels is also changed and the number of functioning vascular units increases both as a result of proliferation and of opening of previously inactive vascular units (Fig. 5-14). It is possible to detect clinically the alterations in number and course of the dentogingival vasculature after about 10 days of plaque growth (Söderholm & Egelberg 1973).

170

Cellular reactions

Increased migration and accumulation of neutrophilic granulocytes and monocytes/-macrophages into the junctional epithelium and gingival sulcus region can be observed after 2-4 days from the onset of plaque accumulation. The enhanced cellular migration is mainly the result of increased concentration of chemotactic factors of bacterial origin in the sulcus region (Lindhe & Rylander 1975, Payne et al. 1975, Schroeder et al. 1975). This migration to the dentogingival region gradually increases during the development of gingivitis. Even if the increased gingival fluid flow and the enhanced migration of leukocytes occur simultaneously, it should be remembered that *vascular changes* and *cellular migration* are phenomena which are probably mediated by *different factors* (Attström 1971).

The rate of migration of leukocytes is not stabilized until 1 month after the onset of plaque accumulation. The steady state of leukocyte migration and gingival fluid flow illustrates that a balance has now been achieved between the irritation produced by the dental plaque and the response of the tissue (Attström & Egelberg 1971).

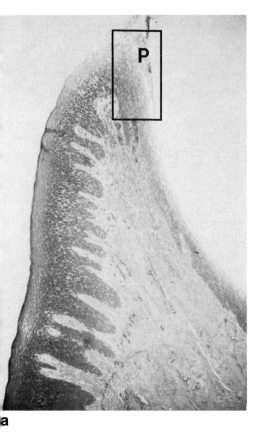
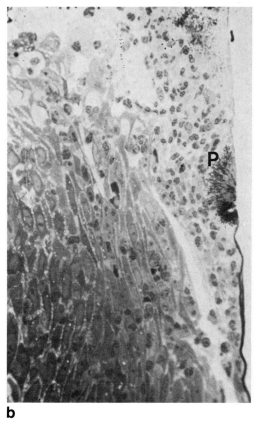

a   b

Fig. 5-15a, b. Buccolingual section of the gingiva on day 4 of developing gingivitis in a beagle. Note plaque (P) in the sulcus region and increased cellularity in the coronal part of the connective tissue below the junctional epithelium. Observe that the vessels appear dilated and note also the presence of leukocytes in the coronal part of the junctional epithelium and at the surfaces of the subgingival plaque.

171

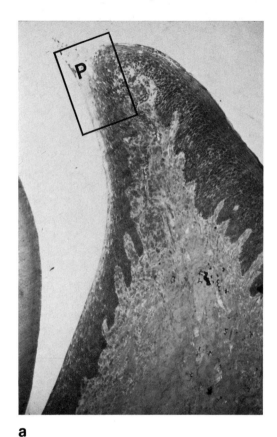
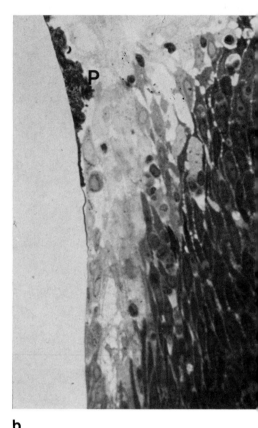

a   b

Fig. 5-16a, b. Buccolingual section of the gingiva on day 7 of developing gingivitis in a beagle. Note the subgingival extension of plaque (P), as well as the increased cellularity in the connective tissue below the junctional epithelium.

Histopathology of the gingival/periodontal lesions

The initial lesion

Within the first 2-4 days of initial plaque accumulation, marked changes occur in the junctional epithelium and connective tissue of the coronal part of the free gingival margin. Neutrophilic granulocytes and monocytes/macrophages migrate in large numbers from the vessels into the connective tissue immediately below the junctional epithelium and further into this epithelium (Fig. 5-15; Page & Schroeder 1976).

The inflammatory reaction at this stage of development is, thus, characterized by cell migration and cell accumulation combined with exudation of serum proteins from the dentogingival vessels into the surrounding connective tissue. Perivascular collagen as well as collagen supporting the coronal portion of the junctional epithelium is removed. Depositions of fibrin and degenerated inflammatory cells can frequently be observed within the infiltrate. In the coronal part of the junctional epithelium leukocytes accumulate in large numbers and a gingival sulcus is often formed. The inflamed area in the connective tissue is small and comprises only about 5-10% of the total connective tissue volume. However, the tissue alterations at this site are pronounced. The collagen content of the infiltrated portion of the connective tissue is reduced by 60-70%. The small cellular infiltrate is dominated by neutrophilic granulocytes and monocytes/ma-

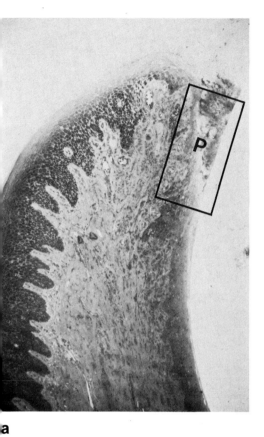
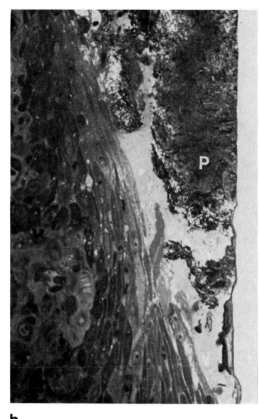

a   b

Fig. 5-17a, b. Buccolingual section of the gingiva on day 21 of developing gingivitis in a beagle. Note the extension of the subgingival plaque (P) as well as the increased cellularity and vascularity of the connective tissue.

crophages although lymphoid cells are also present. The participation of lymphocytes in this initial reaction points to the initiation of an immune response which will characterize the next phase of disease development (defence) (Fig. 5-9).

The early lesion

The character of the inflammatory reaction in the connective tissue alters within 7-14 days of undisturbed plaque accumulation. Vascular changes as well as the accumulation of leukocytes are now more pronounced than in the initial lesion. The cell infiltrate which is still localized immediately below the junctional epithelium contains mainly small and medium sized lymphocytes. Some of these lymphocytes (B-cells) will probably

develop into antibody producing plasma cells while others (T-cells) will change into cells responsible for cell mediated immune reactions. Some fibroblasts residing in the infiltrate, exhibit pronounced signs of degeneration (cellular vacuolization; Fig. 5-16; Schroeder & Page 1972).

Towards the end of the second week the size of the infiltrate will have increased and the reaction site will now occupy approximately 10-15% of the connective tissue volume of the free gingiva. Furthermore, the basal cells of the junctional epithelium have proliferated and rete peg formations can be seen piercing the coronal part of the infiltrate of the early lesion.

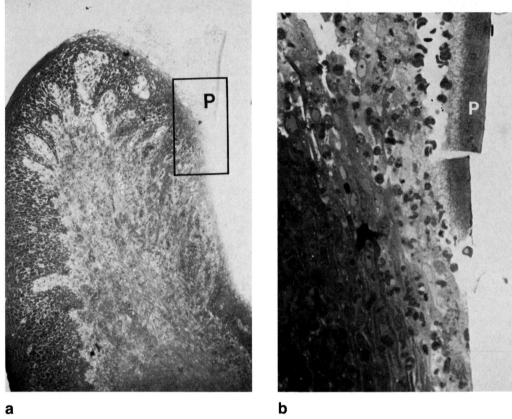

a   **b**

Fig. 5-18a, b. Buccolingual section of the gingiva on day 28 of gingivitis development in a beagle. Note the extension of the subgingival plaque (P) and the increased vascularity and cellularity of the connective tissue below the junctional epithelium. Note rete pegs in the junctional epithelium. The area between the subgingival plaque and the superficial cells of the junctional epithelium is occupied primarily by neutrophilic granulocytes.

INFILTRATED CONNECTIVE TISSUE

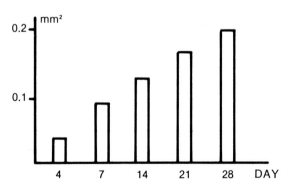

Fig. 5-19. Diagram showing the increase in size of the infiltrated connective tissue during the development of gingivitis in beagles. (From Matsson & Attström 1979).

The established lesion

With further exposure to plaque, the infiltrate will change in both size and quality. The cell infiltrate, which in the early lesion was dominated by lymphocytes, at this later stage is characterized by the large number of mature plasma cells. The infiltrated, collagen poor, connective tissue area extends in both lateral and apical directions deeper into the tissue (Figs. 5-17, 5-18, 5-19). Inflammatory cells can now, frequently, also be detected around vessels in more distant parts of the gingival connective tissue. The dentogingival epithelium now proliferates, extends into the connective tissue infiltrate by rete peg formations, and is converted into a pocket epithelium. This pocket epithelium

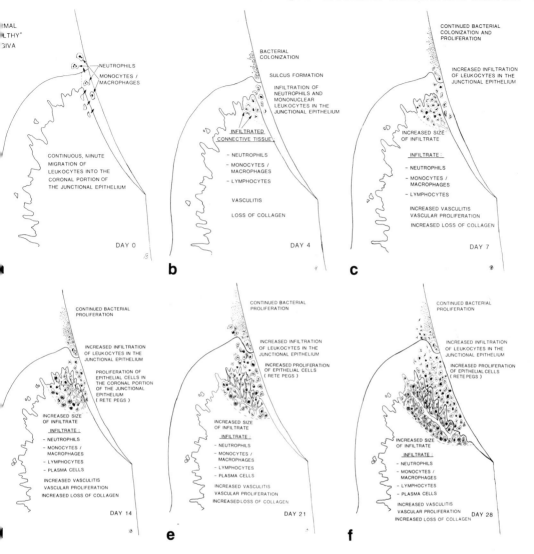

Fig. 5-20a-f. Schematic illustration depicting some alterations of the gingival tissues during the development of gingivitis. Note the continuous increase in the size of the infiltrated area in the connective tissue. Also observe the gradual development of an infiltration of leukocytes in the junctional epithelium.

1) does not attach to the tooth surface, (2) is often thin and in part ulcerated and (3) is *infiltrated* by lymphocytes and plasma cells, and is *transmigrated* by neutrophilic granulocytes. Vascular loops from the dentogingival plexus are often seen immediately below the thin epithelial structures.

Alterations which occur in epithelium and connective tissue during development of gingivitis result in changes of morphology and function of gingival tissue (Fig. 5-20; Table 5-5). In the early phases of gingivitis development, accumulation of leukocytes, primarily neutrophilic granulocytes, in the coronal part of the junctional epithelium causes it to lose contact with the tooth surface. A *deepened gingival sulcus* is formed and the tooth surface thereby becomes accessible for

Table 5-5. Summary of some important histopathological alterations during the gradual development of gingivitis

	Day 4	Day 7	Day 14	Day 21	Day 28
Neutrophils and mononuclear leuko-cytes in the junctional epithelium	————————————————————————				
Increased vascular permeability	————————————————————————				
Vascular proliferation			————————————————		
Neutrophils and monocytes/macro-phages in the connective tissue	————————————————————————				
Lymphocytes	————————————————————————				
Plasma cells				————————————	
Infiltrate size	————————————————————————				
Collagen destruction	————————————————————————				

Solid line indicates when the change can be noted and the gradual increase to day 28. From day 28 the changes take place more slowly, probably as a result of the fact that a balance has been established between the bacteria in the gingival sulcus and the defence response in the tissue.

subgingival bacterial colonization. Deposits of sub-gingival plaque can already be observed from 1-2 weeks after the start of experimental gingivitis. Subgingivally located bacteria release chemotactic factors for leukocytes. These cells migrate through the dentogingival epithelium and form a layer of phagocytic cells between the surface of the microbial plaque and the surface of the pocket epithelium described above (Fig. 5-15).

The advanced lesion
The progressive alterations of the dentogingival epithelium by which this epithelium is deprived of its contact with the tooth surface and converted into pocket epithelium allows the further apical downgrowth of subgingival plaque. Concomitantly with apical propagation of microorganisms, pathological, ulcerated pockets of varying depths develop, *pathologically deepened pockets* (Müller-Glanser & Schroeder 1982). Apical propagation of subgingival plaque is accompanied by apical and lateral propagation of inflammatory cell infiltrate in connective tissue.

Plasma cells, most of which produce IgG antibodies, dominate the lesion, but lymphocytes and macrophages are also present. The area of collagen destruction is increased and, sooner or later, the principal fiber investing in the root surface can become included in the infiltrate and degraded. The dentogingival epithelium is, thus, enabled to proliferate over the root surface, alveolar bone resorption is induced, and, in most cases of advanced disease, the infiltrated portion of the gingiva is separated from the resorbed alveolar bone by a band of intact collagen fiber bundles.

Pathogenic mechanisms in gingival inflammation

Since most, if not all, forms of human periodontal disease are associated with the presence of a subgingival microbiota, it conceivable that inflammatory lesions are caused, directly or indirectly, by factor dependent on such subgingival microbiota.

Cytotoxic reaction

The microbiota of the tooth surface contains and releases *enzymes* such as proteases, hyaluronidases, collagenases, etc. (Slots 1979). Such enzymes could be the direct cause of epithelial and connective tissue damage, and be, at least partly, responsible for tissue destruction in gingival lesions. It has been demonstrated that soluble substances from human dental plaque applied to normal dog or monkey gingiva, rapidly penetrate junctional epithelium and induce both enhanced migration of inflammatory cells from the dentogingival vessels and increased vascular permeability (Helldén & Lindhe 1973, Kahnberg et al. 1976).

A lipopolysaccharide, *endotoxin* from Gram negative bacteria, may activate the complement system (induce acute inflammation) and is, in addition, cytotoxic to host cells. Endotoxin could, therefore, contribute some of the tissue changes observed in gingival lesions. It has been suggested that teichoic acid from Gram positive bacteria has a similar effect (Wilton & de Almeida 1980).

It was recently demonstrated that a *leukotoxin* produced by a Gram negative rod, *Actinobacillus actinomycetemcomitans,* has the capacity to interfere with the vitality and function of phagocytosing leukocytes (Baehni et al. 1979).

Proteins or polysaccharides produced and released from the subgingival microbiota could mediate accumulation of inflammatory cells and cause exudation of plasma proteins from dentogingival vasculature and endogenous mediators of inflammatory reaction could be subsequently released and activated. Thus, once an inflammatory reaction is initiated, mediators, released from the host, could, to a certain extent, maintain conditions favoring migration of neutrophilic granulocytes and macrophages and vascular exudation.

Immune reaction

Most of the substances produced by plaque microbiota are antigenic, therefore elicit a general and a local immune reaction (Fig. 5-

21). Immune reactions protect gingival tissue against antigens produced by plaque microbiota. It has been demonstrated that immunizing dogs with plaque antigens may give the animals a better ability to combat infectious substances produced by plaque formed during experimental gingivitis (Rylander et al. 1976). However, even if immune reactions are protective in character, the inflammatory reactions by which foreign substances are identified and removed may also cause damage to gingiva and periodontium.

Antibody mediated reaction

The inflammatory cell infiltrate of established and advanced gingival lesions is characterized by the presence of large numbers of plasma cells (Page & Schroeder 1981). Most plasma cells produce immunoglobulins of the IgG class. A small number of plasma cells produces IgA and some also IgM. As previously discussed, antibodies may participate in the defence of gingival tissue by neutralizing toxins and enzymes from plaque. Furthermore, antibodies may decrease penetration of tissue by bacterial products (antigens) from the gingival sulcus/-pocket. In experimental animals immunized against a protein, the penetration via the

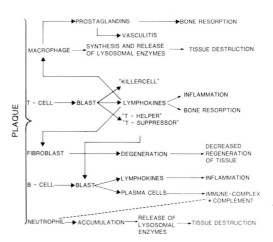

Fig. 5-21. Schematic illustration depicting the interaction between dental plaque and the immune system and the effects of this interaction on tissue.

junctional epithelium of a topically applied antigen was decreased as compared with nonimmunized animals.

Antibodies, both within the plasma cells and extracellularly, are present in the connective tissue and the extracellular space of the junctional epithelium. When an antigen and an antibody combine to protein aggregates (immune complexes) in the tissue, complement is activated and factors chemotactic to neutrophilic granulocytes are formed. In particular, activation of the fifth component of complement, C5, releases such chemotactic factors. Activation of complement also releases factors which cause increased vascular permeability. Immune complexes deposited in gingival tissue may thereby cause increased migration and accumulation of neutrophilic granulocytes and increased exudation of plasma proteins from the adjacent vasculature. Neutrophils have the capacity to phagocytose the antigen/antibody complex. In the process of phagocytosis, however, neutrophilic granulocytes will release some of their lysosomal enzymes into the surrounding tissue. These lysosomal enzymes can in turn cause tissue damage and increase the intensity of inflammatory reaction. Thus, in an attempt to defend the tissue against antigenic material a reaction is elicited which may cause tissue damage (Fig. 5-22).

Gingival lesions are characterized by the presence of a large number of neutrophilic granulocytes within and immediately below the dentogingival epithelium. There are reasons to assume that these leukocytes are in part responsible for tissue destruction in periodontal disease. This assumption is supported by the fact that connective tissue damage is decreased in animals which, during a phase of initial plaque accumulation, have been depleted of their circulating neutrophils (Attström & Schroeder 1979). In animals with chronic gingival inflammation, experimental reduction of the neutrophilic granulocytes also resulted in decreased lysosomal enzymes in the junctional epithelium and decreased gingival fluid flow (Fig. 5-23; Attström et al. 1971, Rylander et

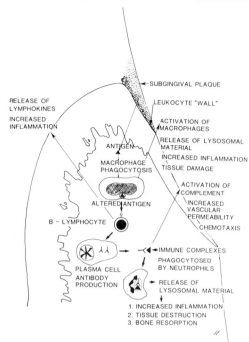

Fig. 5-22. Schematic illustration of possible effects of antigen/antibody reactions on gingival tissue. Antigen from dentogingival plaque enter the connective tissue through the junctional epithelium. In the connective tissue, the antigen is phagocytosed by macrophages which alter the antigens into a form recognizable by the B-lymphocytes (Recognition). The B-lymphocytes are stimulated to proliferate and develop into plasma cells which produce antibodies directed against the penetrating antigen. Antigen/antibody complexes are formed (Binding) and these immune aggregates activate complement which in turn induces increased vascular permeability and chemotaxis of leukocytes. The neutrophilic granulocytes phagocytose the immune complexes (Elimination). In this process the neutrophils release lysosomal material in the surrounding tissue. Increased inflammation, tissue destruction and bone resorption can result. Activated B-lymphocytes also release lymphokines which can cause enhanced inflammation. The activated macrophages release lysosomal material which may induce increased inflammation and tissue damage.

al. 1975). These observations could imply that lysosomal material, released from neutrophilic granulocytes during phagocytosis might mediate tissue damage in periodontal disease.

As previously described, complement often in activated form, is present in the dentogingival region. Thus, the third (C3) the fifth (C5) as well as the fourth (C4), components of complement have been demonstrated both within gingival tissue and in samples from the gingival sulcus region (Attström et al. 1975). Experimental reduction of complement in animals with induced hypersensitivity to certain plaque antigens, decreased the intensity of gingival cellular and vascular reactions to this particular plaque material (Kahnberg et al. 1977).

Activation of the complement system can also stimulate neutrophilic granulocytes (and macrophages) to produce and release prostaglandins. Prostaglandins are proteins which not only can enhance vascular permeability but also activate osteoclasts (Page & Schroeder 1981). The immune system, therefore, through complement activation can (1) mediate vascular and cellular reactions and (2) cause or induce bone resorption. The complement system may also be activated by enzymes and endotoxin from subgingival microbiota. Complement activated in this manner has a similar effect on neutrophils as described above. The relative importance of these mechanisms in gingival inflammation is presently not understood. However, it is likely that they all participate in gingivitis and contribute to tissue destruction.

In an experiment in the monkey Ranney & Zander (1970) demonstrated that topical application of an antigen to the gingival sulcus resulted in a gingival immune reaction. If the animals were immunized to the antigen and the applications were performed frequently enough, an intense inflammatory reaction developed. This reaction was associated with resorption of alveolar bone and apical proliferation of junctional epithelium. This experiment demonstrates that immune reactions mediated through antibodies and complement activation may generate destruction of the entire periodontium.

Immediate hypersensitivity reactions are elicited by antibodies of the IgE type (cytophilic antibodies) attached to the surface of mast cells. When such IgE antibodies are combined with their antigen, the mast cells degranulate and release lysosomal material which includes histamine and serotonin, substances which increase permeability of the adjacent vasculature. The presence of IgE antibodies specifically directed against oral microorganisms has been demonstrated in gingival tissue (Nisengard 1974). It has also been demonstrated that the concentration of histamine is higher in inflamed gingiva than in normal gingiva, and that mast cells are degranulated to a larger extent in inflamed than in normal tissues. Furthermore, some patients with advanced periodontal disease reacted with an immediate hypersensitivity reaction in the skin following topical application of antigens from certain plaque forming bacteria.

Cell mediated immune reaction

The presence of lymphocytes in gingival lesions indicates that cell mediated immune reactions can occur in the periodontium

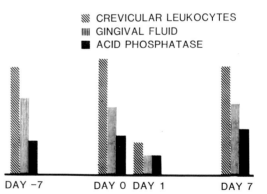

Fig. 5-23. Alterations in crevicular (sulcus) leukocytes, gingival fluid and acid phosphatase in samples from the dentogingival region during experimental neutropenia in dogs with chronically inflamed gingiva. On day 0 the dogs were injected with antineutrophil serum. This resulted in a pronounced reduction of neutrophils in the blood but also in the gingival sulcus on day 1. In combination with the reduction of (crevicular) sulcus leukocytes, a decreased concentration of acid phosphatase and a decrease in the flow of the gingival fluid were observed. All parameters returned to preexperimental levels when the animals on day 7 of the experiment had regained a normal number of neutrophils in the blood. (From Attström et al. 1971).

(Fig. 5-24). In such reactions lymphocytes, upon exposure to antigens to which they are sensitized, produce lymphokines. Such lymphokines can cause migration of inflammatory cells from the vascular system and induce increased vascular permeability. Other lymphokines are cytotoxic and can cause damage to connective tissue cells. Thus, if the cell mediated immune reaction takes place close to fibroblasts, these cells may degenerate (Schroeder & Page 1972). Degenerated fibroblasts have a decreased capacity to produce collagen and matrix substance. Of particular significance is the ability of some lymphokines to mediate accumu-

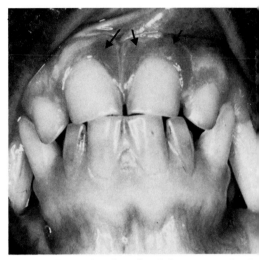

Fig. 5-25. Delayed, cell mediated, immune reaction in the gingiva of a sensitized monkey. Multiple applications of the antigen on the gingiva were performed during a 21 day period. During the experimental period the gingiva gradually developed signs of gingivitis (arrows).

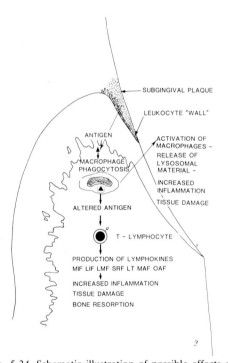

Fig. 5-24. Schematic illustration of possible effects of cellmediated immunity on the gingival tissue. Antigens from subgingival plaque penetrate into the connective tissue through the junctional epithelium. Macrophages phagocytose the antigen and alter it to a form recognizable by the immune system *(Recognition)*. The T-lymphocytes are stimulated to proliferate and release lymphokines. Such lymphokines may cause increased inflammation, tissue damage and bone resorption. In these activities the antigen is bound *(Binding)* and eliminated *(Elimination)*. The activation of the macrophages leads to release of lysosomal material which may cause increased inflammation and tissue damage (compare Fig. 5-22).

lation of monocytes/macrophages and stimulate these phagocytosing cells to an increased synthetic activity. By this stimulation the capacity of macrophages to produce and release lysosomal enzymes and prostaglandins into surrounding tissue is enhanced. The resultant tissue destruction may be similar to that produced by the release of lysosomal material from neutrophilic granulocytes. Lymphokines are also released from sensitized lymphocytes, possibly activating osteoclasts and initiating bone resorption (Figs. 5-25, 5-26; Page & Schroeder 1981).

As opposed to normal gingiva, gingivitis and advanced periodontal disease induce circulating lymphocytes with an increased ability to react to antigens from certain plaque forming microorganisms. Some experiments have shown an apparent correlation between the severity of periodontal disease and the number of sensitized lymphocytes; other studies, however, have failed to confirm this. In recent years the specificity of cell mediated immune reaction in gingiva has been questioned. It has been assumed that the major part of the lymphocyte reaction is caused by nonspecific cell stimulation by mitogens released either by subgingival microbiota or by inflammatory reaction (Page & Schroeder 1981).

Conclusions

A number of factors which may induce gingival inflammation and cause tissue damage have been described. It has been suggested that substances released from plaque are only to a limited extent the cause of direct tissue damage; phagocytosing leukocytes and the immune system will neutralize the biological effect of these plaque substances. Major tissue damage in gingivitis is probably caused by endogenous mechanisms, in particular the release of lysosomal enzymes from neutrophilic granulocytes and macrophages seems to be of importance.

Pathogenesis of periodontal disease

Clinical considerations

Results from epidemiologic studies and long-term clinical trials have revealed that plaque associated periodontal disease *increases in severity* with age in any human population (see Chapter 2). The onset as well as the progression of periodontal disease may certainly vary from one population to another and from one tooth to another (Löe et al. 1978, Axelsson & Lindhe 1981) but, once initiated, the disease (in the populations examined) appears to maintain a progressive and destructive character. Based on such findings and interpretations periodontal disease has been recognized as a slowly progressive (chronic) disorder which

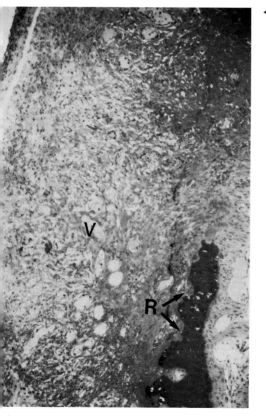

◁ *Fig. 5-26a.* Histopathology of a cell mediated immune reaction in the gingiva of a monkey (see Fig. 5-24). Observe the inflammatory reaction in the connective tissue and the resorption lacuna in the bone (arrows). The tissue reaction was intense. The infiltrate consisted primarily of mononuclear leukocytes. (V: vessels, R: resorption lacuna).

Fig. 5-26b. Numerous osteoclasts (OCL) are seen along the bone surface.
▽

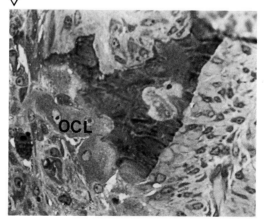

in an adult individual is likely to cause an average loss of attachment of around 0.1-0.2 mm per tooth surface per year (or 1-5 μm per day; Waerhaug 1977). This appreciation of a generalized, chronic, progressive and destructive periodontal disease, has had a profound influence on the development and utilization of diagnostic and therapeutic measures in periodontics.

Clinical observations, as well as results from epidemiological studies, have emphasized that chronic periodontal disease develops and progresses at different rates in different parts and surfaces of the dentition. Thus, while in an adult many sites may suffer from advanced periodontal tissue breakdown, other sites may be entirely devoid of or show only mild signs of disease. A diagram of the development and progress of a typical chronic, destructive disease in a given individual (e.g. Mr. Munksgaard) is presented in Fig. 5-28. Different dentitional sites are identified by letters (A-M). Certain sites (A, C, D, F, H, K and M) are depicted as not being exposed to periodontal disease, while others (B, E, G, I, J and L) develop destructive periodontal disease (vertical bars) – including loss of attachment and alveolar bone – at different times throughout life. In the affected sites periodontal disease, once initiated, progresses slowly until the tooth is lost. Mean values describing periodontal disease (e.g. probing depth, attachment level or height of the alveolar bone) in Mr. Munksgaard's dentition reveal an annual rate of progression of around 0.1-0.2 mm.

This *increase in severity* of periodontal disease with age may result from:
1) the introduction of new diseased sites
2) further breakdown of already diseased sites
3) slow, progressive breakdown of one diseased site (E) coupled with new outbreaks at new sites, e.g. J, B.

But is this appreciation of periodontal disease correct? Observations of humans with evidence of advanced periodontal disease who failed to show continued disease progress in the absence of therapy (Moskow

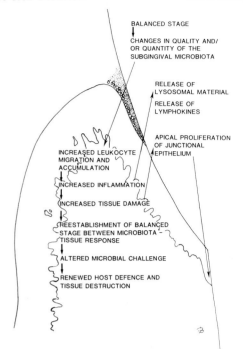

Fig. 5-27. Schematic illustration of a burst of progression in periodontal disease. The gingival tissue is in a balanced state with the microbiota in the plaque. A change in quantity and/or quality occurs in the sub-gingival microbiota. This results in an enhanced (acute) inflammatory response. The reaction counteracts the bacterial activity but also results in tissue damage. Destruction of the collagen fibers apical to the junctional epithelium enables it to further proliferate apically on the root surface.

1978, Axelsson & Lindhe 1981) are difficult to explain by the data outline in Fig. 5-27. Recently Socransky et al. (1983) calculated the progress of periodontal disease (attachment level changes) in a group of 65 adults who were monitored over 7 years during which they received no form of periodontal therapy. The annual loss of attachment per tooth surface/individual was found to be 0.18 mm; a figure similar to those reported from epidemiological studies and demonstrating *increase in severity* with age of periodontal disease. A closer analysis of the data, however, revealed that only 12% of all examined surfaces suffered additional attachment loss during the 7 years of observation. It was also interesting to observe that only 40% of the tooth surfaces, which in the first 3 years suffered attachment loss, showed further periodontal tissue breakdown in the next 4 years. These findings, therefore, fail to support the concept that once initiated, periodontal disease, if left untreated, will slowly but inevitably progress.

Haffajee et al. (1983) monitored the attachment levels in a group of 22 individuals with untreated periodontal disease. They examined 3,414 tooth surfaces once every 2 months and detected that only about 3% of these surfaces lost additional attachment during 1 year. The extent of the additional periodontal destruction (attachment loss) *where it occurred,* however, ranged between 2-5 mm. Rates of destruction of this magnitude are certainly not compatible with the concept of a slow progressive disease process, because if continued at these rates, the teeth involved would have been lost within a few years. The pattern of progress described above strongly indicates that human periodontal disease is not only a *site specific* but also a *cyclic* disorder, which progresses in "bursts" of comparatively short duration interrupted by longer (or shorter) periods of quiescence.

Fig. 5-29 depicts periodontal disease according to this cyclic disease concept. As in Fig. 5-28, certain sites (A, C, D, F, H, K and M) within the patient's dentition are free from signs of destructive periodontal disease throughout that individual's life. Other sites (G, I, J and L) demonstrate one active "burst" of destructive disease resulting in a minor (G and L) or pronounced (I and J) episode of attachment loss. These sites (G, I, and L) may never demonstrate destructive disease again. Other sites (B and E), however, may be exposed to several "bursts" of destructive disease at varying time intervals.

Recently published data thus suggests that periodontal disease progresses with acute episodes of inflammation ("bursts") of short duration interrupted by extended periods of quiescence during which there seems to be an equilibrium between the infectious com-

ponents of the subgingival microbiota and the local host response.

Histopathological observations

Microscopic examination of a *clinically healthy gingival unit* reveals the presence of a small infiltrate which occupies an area of the coronal portion of the connective tissue immediately lateral to the junctional epithelium. This infiltrate contains immune cells, mainly lymphocytes, and a small number of neutrophilic granulocytes (neutrophils) and macrophages. The presence of chemotactic factors, mainly originating from the sparse Gram positive microbiota of the gingival sulcus, promotes neutrophilic granulocytes and macrophages to leave the microvascular system of the infiltrated area, transmigrate the coronal portion of the junctional epithelium and enter the gingival sulcus. During the course of this migration, the leukocytes phagocytose the bacterial products which together with the neutrophilic granulocytes and macrophages are shed in the oral cavity (Page & Schroeder 1982).

As long as the number of bacteria present in the gingival sulcus region is small:
1) the integrity of the junctional epithelium and its attachment to the tooth surfaces is maintained

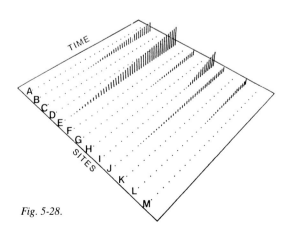

Fig. 5-28.

2) the number of migrating neutrophilic granulocytes and macrophages is minute
3) the size and composition of the connective tissue infiltrate remain unaltered.

In other words, a delicate equilibrium is maintained between the microbiota and the host; the gingiva appears healthy on clinical inspection. It is important to realize that this equilibrium – *clinically healthy gingiva* – may be maintained both for years, even decades, in many gingival sites, and in individuals who in other areas of the dentition develop advanced disease. If, in a particular gingival site, microorganisms are suddenly allowed to colonize the tooth surface in increasing numbers, this equilibrium may, however, be challenged. The microbiota undergoes not only quantitative but also qualitative changes. Gram positive and Gram negative rods and spirochetes are in increasing numbers included in the plaque (Listgarten & Helldén 1978, Slots 1979).

The *chemotactic stimulus* is thereby enhanced and the migration of neutrophilic granulocytes and macrophages is markedly increased as well as the flow of gingival fluid (Page & Schroeder 1982). Thus, the tissue responds to the microbial challenge by an acute inflammatory reaction (the first line of defence). More leukocytes are engaged in the process of phagocytosis and consequently more lysosomal material will be released which:

1) in the connective tissue participates in the destruction of collagen and increases the size of the lymphoid infiltrate; immune competent cells increase in numbers with both lymphocytes and plasma cells included in the infiltrate
2) in the coronal portion of the junctional epithelium causes injury to the host cells; the intercellular substance is degraded and the barrier function of this part of the epithelium becomes impaired as well as its attachment to the tooth. Thereby more apical parts of the tooth surface become accessible for bacterial colonization. *A subgingival microbiota may be established.*

But the bacterial products which enter the junctional epithelium and the connective tissue in increasing amounts are not only chemotactic to neutrophilic granulocytes and macrophages but also *antigens*. Consequently the local immune reaction is triggered and in this reaction both lymphocytes and plasma cells participate. In the early stages of developing gingivitis, lymphocytes dominate the inflammatory cell population while in later stages, in the established gingival lesion, plasma cells dominate the leukocyte population of the infiltrated area (Page & Schroeder 1976). The immune response (the *second line of defence*) evidently engages the humoral as well as the cell mediated limb of the host defence.

After a few days or weeks of exaggerated host defence, however, a new delicate equilibrium between the microbiota and the host tissue has been established at this particular site. Clinically this site is characterized by gingival redness, swelling and bleeding on probing, i.e. *chronic or established gingivitis*. This new equilibrium may remain unaltered for months, years or decades. In most individuals, also in those with advanced disease in many parts of the dentition, sites are recognized which show signs of established gingivitis but where no loss of connective tissue attachment has occurred.

But new microbial challenges, or new bursts of inflammation may sooner or later appear in a gingival site harboring subgingival microbiota and an established lesion

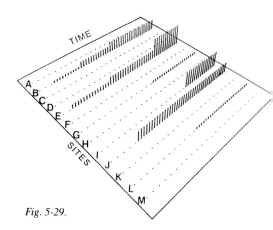

Fig. 5-29.

Such later occurring defence reactions may also engage more apical parts of the periodontium but are otherwise largely similar to those previously described, i.e. an acute inflammatory reaction (increased exudation and migration of neutrophilic granulocytes and macrophages) combating chemotactic and antigenic material released from the subgingival microbiota and an immune response which will identify and neutralize the microbial antigens and thereby protect more distant parts of the periodontium from exposure to microbial products (Fig. 5-29). The accumulation of neutrophilic granulocytes and macrophages in more apical parts of the dentogingival epithelium results in a destruction of this tissue and in the exposure of more apical portions of the tooth for microbial colonization. The enhanced immune response, including collagen breakdown, allows the infiltrate to propagate apically. Thus, the burst of inflammation will result in a further apical expansion of the area of host defence and in a further apical displacement of microbial plaque (Schroeder & Lindhe 1975, Schroeder & Attström 1980, Page & Schroeder 1982). But again after a few days or weeks of exaggerated host response an equilibrium is established which in turn may remain unchallenged for extended periods of time.

In many periodontal sites which harbor a subgingival microbiota, sooner or later, depending on the composition of the microbiota and the quality and duration of the host response, the repeated bursts of inflammation will result in a spread of the connective infiltrate to a position apical of the cementoenamel junction. The principal fibers investing in the root cementum are now degraded and a gingival lesion including loss of *connective tissue attachment* is established. Between the "bursts" of activity, which at different times may engage different sites in the dentition, however, there are longer or shorter periods of quiescence indicative of the presence of an equilibrium between challenging and defending factors in the dentogingival region. There are reasons to believe that the difference between a gingival site with no or only limited amounts of attachment loss and a site with advanced disease, rests mainly on the number of acute episodes of inflammation, (or bursts of activity, or challenges to the equilibrium) to which these two sites have been exposed. Finally, the possibility should be emphasized that, at least in advanced stages of disease, the bursts of acute inflammation may develop as a consequence of microbial invasion of the infiltrated portion of the connective tissue (Frank 1980, Saglie et al. 1982).

References

Attström, R. (1971) Studies on neutrophil polymorphonuclear leukocytes at the dento-gingival junction in gingival health and disease. *Journal of Periodontal Research,* Supplement 8.

Attström, R. & Egelberg, J. (1971) Presence of leukocytes within the gingival crevices during developing gingivitis in dogs. *Journal of Periodontal Research* **6**, 110-114.

Attström, R., Graf-de Beer, M. & Schroeder, H. E. (1975) Clinical and histological characterization of normal gingiva in dogs. *Journal of Periodontal Research* **10**, 115-127.

Attström, R., Laurell, A.-B., Larsson, U. & Sjöholm, A. (1975) Complement factors in

gingival crevice material from healthy and inflamed gingiva in humans. *Journal of Periodontal Research* **10**, 19-27.

Attström, R. & Schroeder, H. E. (1979) Effect of experimental neutropenia on initial gingivitis in dogs. *Scandinavian Journal of Dental Research* **87**, 7-23.

Attström, R., Tynelius-Bratthall, G. & Egelberg, J. (1971) Effects of experimental leukopenia on gingival inflammation in dogs. II. Induction of leukopenia by heterologous anti-neutrophil serum. *Journal of Periodontal Research* **7**, 200-210.

Axelsson, P. & Lindhe, J. (1978) Effect of controlled oral hygiene procedures on caries and periodontal disease in adults. *Journal of Clinical Periodontology* **5**, 133-151.

Axelsson, P. & Lindhe, J. (1981) The significance of maintenance care in the treatment of periodontal disease. *Journal of Clinical Periodontology* **8**, 281-295.

Baehni, P., Tsai, C.-C., McArthur, N. P., Hammond, B. & Taichman, N. S. (1979) Interaction of inflammatory cells and oral microorganisms VIII. Detection of leukotoxic activity of a plaque-derived Gram-negative microorganism. *Infection and Immunity* **24**, 233-243.

Cimasoni, G. (1974) The crevicular fluid. In *Monographs in Oral Science,* 3, ed. Mayers. H. M. Basel: Karger.

Egelberg, J. (1967) The topography and permeability of vessels at the dentogingival junction in dogs. *Journal of Periodontal Research* **2**, Supplement 1.

Frank, R. M. (1980) Bacterial penetration in the apical pocket wall of advanced human periodontitis. *Journal of Periodontal Research* **15**, 563-573.

Haffajee, A. D., Socransky, S. S. & Goodson, I. M. (1983) Comparison of different data analyses for detecting changes in attachment level. *Journal of Clinical Periodontology* **10**, in press.

Helldén, L. & Lindhe, J. (1973) Enhanced emigration of crevicular leucocytes mediated by factors in human dental plaque. *Scandinavian Journal of Dental Research* **8**, 123-129.

Kahnberg, K.-E., Lindhe, J. & Attström, R. (1977) The effect of decomplementation by carragheenan on experimental initial gingivitis in hyperimmune dogs. *Journal of Periodontal Research* **12**, 479-490.

Kahnberg, K.-E., Lindhe, J. & Helldén, L. (1976) Initial gingivitis induced by topical application of plaque extract. A histometric study in dogs with normal gingiva. *Journal of Periodontal Research* **11**, 218-225.

Knowles, J. W., Burgett, F. G., Nissle, R. R., Shick, R. A., Morrison, E. C. & Ramfjord, S. P. (1979) Results of periodontal treatment related to pocket depth and attachment level 8 years. *Journal of Periodontology* **50**, 225-233.

Lindhe, J., Hamp, S.-E. & Löe, H. (1975) Plaque induced periodontal disease in beagle dogs. A 4-year clinical, roentgenographical and histometric study. *Journal of Periodontal Research* **10**, 243-255.

Lindhe, J. & Nyman, S. (1975) The effect of plaque control and surgical pocket elimination on the establishment and maintenance of periodontal health. A longitudinal study of periodontal therapy in cases of advanced disease. *Journal of Clinical Periodontology* **2**, 67-79.

Lindhe, J. & Rylander, H. (1975) Experimental gingivitis in young dogs. *Scandinavian Journal of Dental Research* **83**, 314-326.

Listgarten, M. A. & Helldén, L. (1978) Relative distribution of bacteria at clinically healthy and periodontally diseased sites in humans. *Journal of Clinical Periodontology* **5**, 115-132.

Löe, H., Anerud, A., Boysen, H. & Smith, M. (1978) The natural history of periodontal disease in man. The rate of periodontal destruction before 40 years of age. *Journal of Periodontology* **49**, 607-620.

Löe, H. & Rindom Schiött, C. R. (1970) The effect of mouthrinses and topical application of chlorhexidine on the development of dental plaque and gingivitis in man. *Journal of Periodontal Research* **5**, 79-83.

Löe, H., Theilade, E. & Jensen, S. B. (1965) Experimental gingivitis in man. *Journal of Periodontology* **36**, 177-187.

Lövdal, A., Arno, A., Schei, O. & Waerhaug, J. (1961) Combined effect of subgingival scaling and controlled oral hygiene on the incidence of gingivitis. *Acta Odontologica Scandinavica* **19**, 537-555.

Matsson, L. & Attström, R. (1979) Histologic characteristics of experimental gingivitis in the juvenile and adult beagle dog. *Journal of Clinical Periodontology* **6**, 334-350.

Mims, C. A. (1977) *The Pathogenesis of Infectious Disease.* London, New York, San Francisco: Academic Press.

Moskow, B. S. (1978) Spontaneous arrest of advanced periodontal disease without treatment: an interesting case report. *Journal of Periodontology* **49**, 465-468.

Müller-Glanser, W. & Schroeder, H. E. (1982) The pocket epithelium: A light- and electron-microscopic study. *Journal of Periodontology* **53**, 133-144.

Nisengard, R. J. (1974) Immediate hypersensitivity and periodontal disease. *Journal of Periodontology* **45**, 344-350.

Nyman, S. & Lindhe, J. (1979) A longitudinal study of combined periodontal and prosthetic treatment of patients with advanced periodontal disease. *Journal of Periodontology* **50**, 163-169.

age, R. C. & Schroeder, H. E. (1976) Pathogenesis of inflammatory periodontal disease. A summary of current work. *Laboratory Investigations* **33**, 235-249.

age, R. C. & Schroeder, H. E. (1981) Current status of the host response in chronic marginal periodontitis. *J. Periodontol.* **52**, 477-491.

age, R. C. & Schroeder, H. E. (1982) *Periodontitis in Man and Animals. A comparative review.* Basel: Karger.

ayne, W. D., Page, R., Ogilvie, A. L. & Hall, W. B. (1975) Histopathologic features of the initial and early stages of experimental gingivitis in man. *Journal of Periodontal Research* **10**, 51-64.

Ramfjord, S. P., Knowles, J. W., Nissle, R. R., Burgett, F. G. & Shick, R. A. (1975) Results following three modalities of periodontal therapy. *Journal of Periodontology* **46**, 522-526.

Ramfjord, S. P., Nissle, R. R., Shick, R. A. & Cooper, Jr., H. (1968) Subgingival curettage versus surgical elimination of periodontal pockets. *Journal of Periodontology* **39**, 167-175.

Ranney, R. R. & Zander, H. A. (1970) Allergic periodontal disease in sensitized squirrel monkeys. *Journal of Periodontology* **41**, 12-21.

Ryan, G. B. & Majno, G. (1977) Acute inflammation. A review. *American Journal of Pathology* **86**, 185-276.

Rylander, H., Attström, R. & Lindhe, J. (1975) Influence of experimental neutropenia in dogs with chronic gingivitis. *Journal of Periodontal Research* **10**, 315-323.

Rylander, H., Lindhe, J. & Ahlstedt, S. (1976) Exerimental gingivitis in immunized dogs. *Journal of Periodontal Research* **11**, 339-348.

Saglie, R., Newman, M. G., Carranza, Jr., F. A. & Pattison, G. L. (1982) Bacterial invasion of gingiva in advanced periodontitis in humans. *Journal of Periodontology* **53**, 217-222.

Saxe, S. R., Greene, J. C., Bohannan, H. M. & Vermillion, J. R. (1967) Oral debris, calculus and periodontal disease in the beagle dog. *Periodontics* **5**, 217-224.

Schroeder, H. E. (1973) Transmigration and infiltration of leukocytes in human junctional epithelium. *Helvetica Odontologica Acta* **17**, 6-15.

Schroeder, H. E. (1977) Histopathology of the gingival sulcus. In *Borderland between Caries and Periodontal Disease,* ed. Lehner, T., pp. 43-78. New York: Academic Press.

Schroeder, H. E. & Lindhe, J. (1975). Conversion of established gingivitis in the dog into destructive periodontitis. *Archives oral Biology* **20**: 775-782.

Schroeder, H. E. & Attström, R. (1980) Pocket formation: a hypothesis. In *Borderland Between Caries and Periodontal disease,* Vol. II, ed. Lehner, T. & Cimasoni, G., pp. 99-123. London: Academic Press.

Schroeder, H. E., Graf-de Beer, M. & Attström, R. (1975) Initial gingivitis in dogs. *Journal of Periodontal Research* **10**, 128-142.

Schroeder, H. E. & Page, R. C. (1972) Lymphocyte-fibroblast interactions in the pathogenesis of inflammatory gingival disease. *Experientia* **28**, 1228-1230.

Slots, J. (1979) Subgingival microflora and periodontal disease. *Journal of Clinical Periodontology* **6**, 351-382.

Socransky, S. S., Haffajee, A. D., Goodson, J. M. & Lindhe, J. (1983) Changing concepts of destructive periodontal disease. *Journal of Clinical Periodontology* **10**. In press.

Söderholm, G. & Egelberg, J. (1973) Morphological changes in gingival blood vessels during developing gingivitis in dogs. *Journal of Periodontal Research* **8**, 16-20.

Waerhaug, J. (1952) The gingival pocket. Anatomy pathology deepening and elimination. *Odontologisk Tidsskrift* **60**, Supplement.

Waerhaug, J. (1977) Subgingival plaque and loss of attachment of periodontosis as evaluated on extracted teeth. *Journal of Periodontology* **48**, 125-130.

Waerhaug, J. (1979) The infrabony pocket and its relationship to trauma from occlusion and subgingival plaque. *Journal of Periodontology* **50**, 355-365.

Wilton, J. M. A. & de Almeida, O. P. (1980) The comparative inflammatory effect of dental plaque, Lipopolysaccharide, Lipoteichoic acid, dextran and levan on leukocytes in the mouse peritoneal cavity. In *Borderland between Caries and Periodontal Disease,* Vol. II, ed. Lehner, T. & Cimasoni, G., pp. 83-97. London: Academic Press.

187

CHAPTER 6

Juvenile Periodontitis (Periodontosis)

Definition

Periodontosis (Orban & Weinmann 1942) or *Juvenile Periodontitis* (Manson & Lehner 1974) is a disease of the periodontium occurring in an otherwise healthy young individual. Other terms that have been used to describe this or similar disorders are e.g. "Diffuse Bone Atrophy", "Deep Cementopathia" (Gottlieb 1923, 1928) or "Precocious Periodontitis" (Sugarman & Sugarman 1977).

Juvenile Periodontitis is characterized by a rapid loss of connective tissue attachment and alveolar bone at more than one tooth in the permanent dentition. According to current concepts two basic forms of juvenile periodontitis may exist. In one form, *localized juvenile periodontitis*, only the first molars and the incisors are involved in the disease process. In the second form, *generalized juvenile periodontitis*, most teeth in the dentition are affected.

In a review paper Baer (1971) described *juvenile periodontitis* (periodontosis) as a well defined, clinical entity different from adult periodontal disease. He suggested that

this particular form of periodontal disease (1) makes its debut when children are between the ages of 11-13 years, (2) that the disease affects more females than males and (3) that there is a familial tendency to the disease. Baer further stated that the gingiva around the diseased teeth may have a normal texture and color, but that deep periodontal pockets are present at one or more proximal surfaces of the affected teeth. It was also claimed that in the initial lesion gross deposits of subgingival calculus are uncommon and that the amount of periodontal destruction observed at the disease sites is not commensurate with the amount of local irritants present. He averred that *juvenile periodontitis* has a typical appearance in the radiographs. Thus, angular bone loss can be observed at first molar and incisors. In the molar regions bone loss is frequently seen bilaterally.

Baer concluded that *juvenile periodontitis* (periodontosis) is a disease which progresses rapidly, meaning that within a 4-5 year period between 50-75% of the attachment apparatus of the diseased teeth may be involved in an inflammatory lesion. Fig. 6-1 illustrates the rate of disease progression in a 13 year old girl. In Fig. 6-1a initial signs of bone loss can be detected on the mesial aspect of 43, 41 and 31. Three years later when the girl is 16 years of age, bone loss has progressed (Fig. 6-1b) and approximately 50% of the alveolar bone in these tooth regions has been lost.

Epidemiology

Results from epidemiological studies suggest that between 0.1 and 3.4% of the age group 10-19 years suffer from juvenile

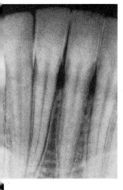
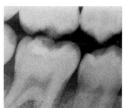
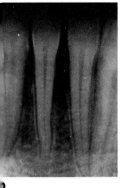
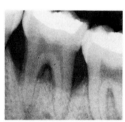

Fig. 6-1. Radiographs illustrating bone loss at the mesial spect of the lower first molar in a 13 year old girl (a), nd progression of disease 3 years later (b) when the girl ; 16 year old. Note also bone loss in the lower front ooth region (b).

eriodontitis. The disease seems to be more requent in Africa and the Middle East than n Europe or among the Caucasian popula- ions of North America. In a recent study by axén (1980) comprising more than 8,000 16 year old) children in Finland, only 0.1% f the examined subjects were found to suf- er from juvenile periodontitis. An heredit- ry tendency to the disease was also reported y Saxén.

Hörmand & Frandsen (1979) examined 56 individuals who had been referred to the)epartment of Periodontology, School of)entistry, in Copenhagen, Denmark, for pecialist treatment of advanced periodontal lisease. The patients were divided into 3 age ;roups: Group I, aged 12-18 years, Group I, aged 19-24 years, and Group III, aged 26-

32 years. In the youngest age group the female to male ratio was 5 to 1, while in the oldest age group the same relation was only 1.5 to 1. These findings tend to indicate that *juvenile periodontitis* initially affects more females than males but that this difference may be largely due to an earlier onset of the disease among females. The authors also assessed the number of teeth that were involved in periodontal disease lesions and reported that while only few teeth (4-6) were affected in younger individuals (12-15 years), with increasing age the number of affected teeth increased progressively. This could indicate that the generalized form of *juvenile periodontitis* has started as localized *juvenile periodontitis* which, left untreated, has spread. Consequently, Hörmand & Frandsen (1979) concluded that the typical pathogenesis of *juvenile periodontitis* com-

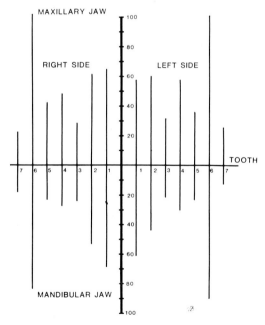

Fig. 6-2. The diagram illustrates the frequency of occurrence of juvenile periodontitis lesions in 1,314 teeth in 156 individuals. Note the high frequency of lesions among the first molars. (From Hörmand & Frandsen 1979).

189

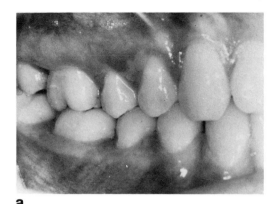

a

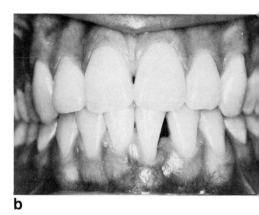

b

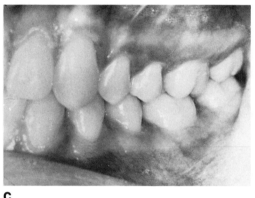

c

Figs. 6-3a, b, c. The clinical appearance of the periodontal tissues of a 15 year old girl suffering from juvenile periodontitis. Note the proper oral hygiene conditions and the scalloped outline of the gingival margin. In the lower front tooth region, the interdental papilla between teeth 31 and 32 is lost.

prises an initial involvement of first molar and/or incisors and a subsequent involvement of other teeth.

Fig. 6-2 depicts the distribution of attachment loss on 1,314 teeth in the 156 individuals examined by Hörmand & Frandsen. From this diagram it can be seen that the first molars are the teeth most frequently involved in the disease process followed by the central and lateral incisors in the upper and lower jaws. Thus, in most cases of *juvenile periodontitis* there seems to be a symmetrical involvement of first molars, incisors and a few additional teeth.

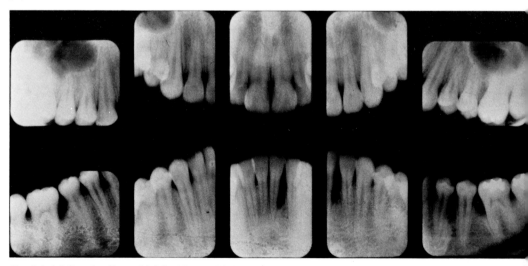

Fig. 6-4. A full oral radiograph of the 15 year old girl described in Fig. 6-3. Note the presence of angular bony defects at the mesial aspect of tooth 46, 36 and at the distal aspect of teeth 31.

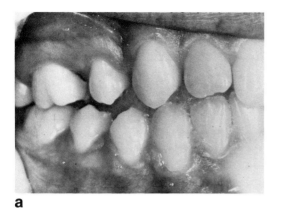

a

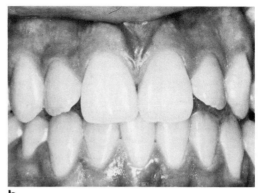

b

Clinical characteristics

Figs. 6-3a, b and c depict the clinical appearance of a 15 year old girl suffering from *juvenile periodontitis*. The interdental papilla between teeth 31 and 32 has lost some of its normal tissue volume, but the gingiva in the remaining part of the dentition is normal in texture and color. Fig. 6-4 presents the patient's full oral radiograph. Deep angular bony defects are seen on the mesial aspect of teeth 26, 36 and 46. In addition there is a deep angular bony defect at the distal surface of 31.

Figs. 6-5a, b and c present the clinical status of her 14 year old sister, whose gingiva in most parts of the dentition, also clinically, was normal, but bleeding was provoked by gentle probing in deep periodontal pockets at the mesial aspect of teeth 16, 26 and 46. Fig. 6-6a is her full oral radiograph. Angular bony defects can be seen at the mesial aspect of teeth 16, 26 and 46 (Fig. 6-6b).

Microbiology

Composition of the microbiota

Dark field microscopy. Liljenberg & Lindhe (1980) examined the microflora of the periodontal pockets of 8 patients with *localized juvenile periodontitis* and compared them with diseased sites in post-

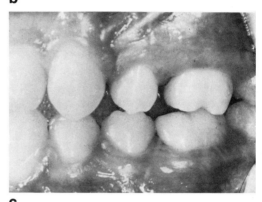

c

Figs. 6-5a, b, c. These figures illustrate the clinical appearance of a 14 year old girl. Note the excellent oral hygiene status. Bleeding on probing has been provoked in the gingivae at the mesial aspect of teeth 16 and 26.

juvenile periodontitis and advanced adult periodontitis. Only first molars and incisors were selected for examination. The sites examined fulfilled the following criteria: angular bony defects should be present, the probing depth should exceed 8 mm and bone loss should exceed 50% of the original height. The microbiota of the deep periodontal pockets was sampled with a curette and the sample subsequently examined by dark field microscopy. The following morphological forms were identified: coccoid cells, straight rods, filaments, fusiforms, curved and/or motile rods, and spirochetes. Fig. 6-7 depicts the composition of the subgingival plaque in the 3 categories of patients. It can be seen that

191

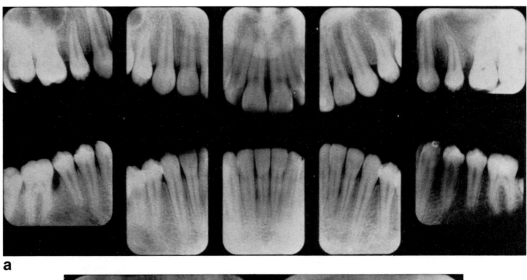

a

b

Figs. 6-6a, b. Full oral radiograph (a) of the dentition of the 14 year old girl described in Fig. 6-5. (b) A higher magnification of the first molar regions. Note the presence of angular bony defects at the mesial aspect of 16, 26 and 46.

while the postjuvenile periodontitis and adult periodontitis lesions were characterized by the presence of large numbers of spirochetes and motile and/or curved rods, the *juvenile periodontitis* lesions were dominated by coccoid cells and straight non-motile rods. In several *juvenile periodontitis* sites there were very few spirochetes present.

Ultrastructural studies have demonstrated a sparse but relatively characteristic microbial population in deep periodontal pockets

SUBGINGIVAL PLAQUE

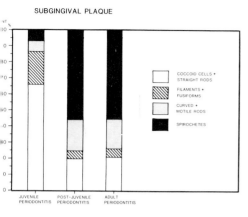

COCCOID CELLS +
STRAIGHT RODS

FILAMENTS +
FUSIFORMS

CURVED +
MOTILE RODS

SPIROCHETES

JUVENILE PERIODONTITIS | POST-JUVENILE PERIODONTITIS | ADULT PERIODONTITIS

6-7. The histogram describes the percentage rep-
entation of various microorganisms sampled in sub-
gival sites of juvenile periodontitis, postjuvenile
riodontitis and adult periodontitis lesions. Note that
juvenile periodontitis lesions there is a high portion
coccoid cells while in postjuvenile and adult
riodontitis lesions the microbiota is dominated by
rochetes. (From Liljenberg & Lindhe 1980).

of *localized juvenile periodontitis* (Listgarten 1976, Westergaard et al. 1978). A pellicle up to 20 μm in thickness is generally
present on the cementum surface (Fig. 6-8).
Masses of bacteria can be attached to this
pellicle but large root surface areas with
loosely attached or unattached bacteria regularly occur between islands of microbial
plaque. A zone free of pellicle and attached
bacteria is present in the most apical area of
the periodontal pocket.

The portion of the plaque which faces the
root cementum predominantly consists of
bacteria with a typical Gram positive cell
wall. More superficial plaque layers (Fig. 6-
9) are dominated by various Gram positive
rods, and the outermost layer contains
Gram negative rods, spirochetes and polymorphonuclear leukocytes. Listgarten
(1976) also examined the ultrastructure of

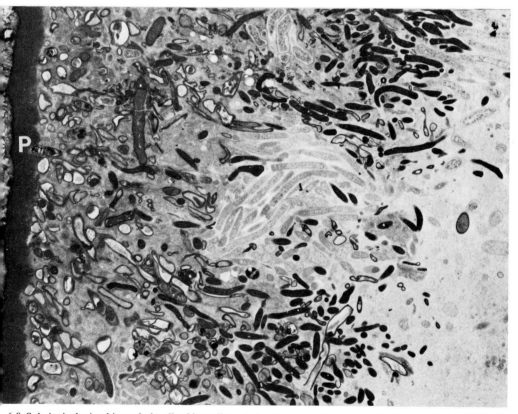

6-8. Subgingival microbiota of a localized juvenile periodontitis lesion. Cementum (C) is covered by a pellicle (P)
bacteria, many of which exhibit degeneration in the deep plaque layer. Note the high number of rod shaped
anisms. X 5,500 (courtesy of J. Westergaard).

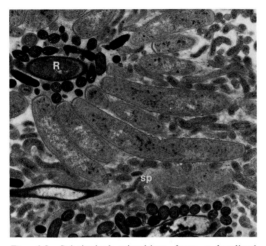

Fig. 6-9. Subgingival microbiota from a localized juvenile periodontitis lesion. Section of a rod shaped organism (R) surrounded by cocci and long Gram negative rods *(Capnocytophaga?). Numerous spirochetes (sp) occur peripherally to these bacteria. X 18,700 (courtesy of J. Westergaard).*

the microbiota in advanced incisor-molar lesions of individuals with postjuvenile periodontitis. The periodontal microflora of these patients resembled that of adult periodontitis.

The dominant cultivable microflora in localized juvenile periodontitis was studied by Slots (1976) and Newman & Socransky (1977) (Table 6-1). In both studies, Gram negative organisms comprised approximately ⅔ of the isolates from deep periodontal pockets. In contrast, these organisms averaged only about ⅓ of the isolates in control sites with normal gingiva. The dominant Gram negative bacteria in *juvenile periodontitis* included *Capnocytophaga* species, *Actinobacillus actinomycetemcomitans* and motile anaerobic rods mainly *Wolinella recta*. Species of *Streptococcus*, *Actinomyces* and *Peptostreptococcus* accounted for most of the Gram positive isolates.

Recent microscopic studies have revealed that microorganisms in *localized juvenile*

Table 6-1. Predominant cultivable microflora in patients with localized juvenile periodontitis[a]

	From Slots (1976)		From Newman & Socransky (1977)	
	Periodontitis lesions	"Normal" gingival sites	Periodontitis lesions	"Normal" gingival sites
Gram positive organisms	**34**	**60**	**38**	**75**
Facultative cocci	10	37	11	31
Anaerobic cocci	6	4	7	9
Facultative rods	3	12	8	8
Anaerobic rods	15	7	12	27
Gram negative organisms	**66**	**40**	**63**	**23**
Facultative cocci	0	1	2	2
Anaerobic cocci	2	3	9	12
Facultative, capnophilic or				
anaerobic rods	64	36	52	9
Capnocytophaga	many	?	many	?
Black pigmented *Bacteroides*	few	0	1	0
(Bacteroides gingivalis,				
saccharolytic species)				
Fusobacterium nucleatum	few	few	3	5
Actinobacillus actinomycetem-	13[b]	4[b]	4[c]	few[c]
comitans				

a) Data calculated as percentage of the total cultivable microflora
b) From Slots et al. (1980)
c) From Mandell & Socransky (1981)

Table 6-2. Virulence factors in bacteria associated with localized juvenile periodontitis (*A. actinomycetemcomitans*, *Capnocytophaga*) and generalized juvenile periodontitis (black-pigmented *Bacteroides* [*B. gingivalis*])

Virulence factors	Bacterial Species		
	A. actinomycetemcomitans	*Capnocytophaga*	Black pigmented *Bacteroides*
[1] Leukotoxin	variable	−	−
[2] Polymorphonuclear leukocyte chemo-taxis inhibition	+	+	+
[3] Endotoxin potency	strong	weak	weak
[4] Enzymes:			
Collagenase	variable	−	+
Trypsin like activity	−	variable	+, *B. gingivalis* −, saccharolytic species
Aminopeptidases	−	+	−
Immunoglobulin degradation	−	IgG-ase IgA1-ase	IgG-ase IgA1-ase variable, IgA2-ase
[5] Fibroblast inhibition	+	+	?
[6] Polyclonal B-cell activation	+	+	+

References:
1) Baehni et al. 1979, McArthur et al. 1981
2) Shurin et al. 1979, van Dyke et al. 1982
3) Hausmann et al. 1970, Hofstad 1970, Mansheim et al. 1978, Kiley & Holt 1980, Stevens et al. 1980b
4) Gibbons & MacDonald 1961, Kilian 1981, Slots 1981, Laughon et al. 1982, Rozanis & Slots 1982
5) Stevens et al. 1980a, Shenker et al. 1982
6) Bick et al. 1981.

periodontitis can invade the periodontal connective tissue (Gillett & Johnson 1982). Saglie et al. (1982) identified *A. actinomycetemcomitans* as being a prominent invading species. It is likely that these bacteria, which are capable of invading the gingiva and obtaining close proximity to the collagenous periodontal legament and the alveolar bone may play a particularly important part in the pathogenesis of the disease.

Data concerning the microbiota of lesions of *generalized juvenile periodontitis* are sparse. Baer & Socransky (1979) in 1 patient and Loesche et al. (1981) in 4 patients with *generalized juvenile periodontitis* showed that *Bacteroides gingivalis* comprised more than 30% of the cultivable subgingival microbiota.

Virulence factors

Several potentially tissue destructive mechanisms have been demonstrated in *juvenile periodontitis* microorganisms (Table 6-2):

1) Leukotoxin

Many *A. actinomycetemcomitans* strains produce a substance which can kill human polymorphonuclear leukocytes and monocytes. This leukotoxin may compromise the patient's ability to eliminate or control invading bacteria or bacterial products. On the other hand, more than 90% of patients with *localized juvenile periodontitis* develop neutralizing serum antibodies against the *A. actinomycetemcomitans* leukotoxin (Tsai et al. 1981). This antibody response may be of importance in controlling the effect of the leukotoxin and in modulating the progression of the disease.

2) Chemotaxis inhibition

Some of the Gram negative organisms found in juvenile periodontitis sites also produce nontoxic factors which inhibit the chemotaxis of human polymorphonuclear leukocytes. These inhibitors of chemotaxis may be important determinants of virulence because they may interfere with the ability of the leukocytes to reach the infectious agents.

3) Endotoxin

The lipopolysaccharide (endotoxin) from *A. actinomycetemcomitans* can elicit pathologic phenomena similar to those characterizing a periodontal lesion. Thus, the endotoxin can induce Schwartzman reactions, macrophage toxicity, platelet aggregation, complement activation and bone resorption. In contrast, the endotoxins from *Capnocytophaga* and black pigmented *Bacteroides* are only weakly toxic but may stimulate bone resorption in bone culture systems.

4) Enzymes

A. actinomycetemcomitans, Capnocytophaga and *Bacteroides* elaborate proteolytic enzymes which can degrade connective tissue constituents, activate the complement system or degrade immunoglobulins. Only a few other bacterial species from the oral cavity exhibit similarly high proteolytic activity.

5) Fibroblast cytotoxicity

A. actinomycetemcomitans and *Capnocytophaga* strains possess a fibroblast growth inhibitory factor. Inhibition of fibroblast proliferation may interfere with collagen synthesis and result in impaired gingival healing after challenge by oral bacteria.

6) Polyclonal B-lymphocyte activation

Several periodontal bacteria possess potent polyclonal B-lymphocyte activators. These bacterial factors may contribute to periodontal disease pathogenesis by inducing B-cells to produce antibodies with determinants unrelated to the activating agent. The polyclonal B-cell activators can also induce release of lymphokines, such as chemotactic factor(s) that mediate inflammatory reactions and osteoclast activating factor which may ultimately result in bone resorption.

Several potential mechanisms thus exist by which the *juvenile periodontitis* bacteria can cause periodontal destruction. Whether a multiplicity of pathogenic mechanisms or only a few are operative in the disease remains to be established.

Host response

Recent observations have indicated that the local as well as the general host response to the bacterial infection is interfered with in *juvenile periodontitis patients*.

Local host response

The local host response in the gingiva to the colonization of bacteria on the tooth surface involves (1) exudation of gingival fluid, (2) migration of neutrophils and macrophages with phagocytic capability into the junctional epithelium and gingival pocket area, and (3) the establishment of inflammatory cell infiltrates in the connective tissue beneath the dentogingival epithelium.

Findings reported by Murray & Patters (1980) have indicated that in patients with *juvenile periodontitis,* neutrophils in the gingival lesions have a reduced phagocytic capacity when compared with cells recovered from similar lesions of gingivitis and adult periodontitis. They also suggested that this dysfunction of the neutrophils was a localized phenomenon as only disease sites in patients with *juvenile periodontitis* showed this pathological alteration. These observations are consistent with findings by Baehni et al. (1979), Tsai et al. (1979) and McArthur et al. (1981) who demonstrated that *A. actinomycetemcomitans* has a capacity to interfere with the viability and function of neutrophils (see virulence factors).

The characteristic features of the inflammatory cell infiltrates of deep periodontal lesions in patients with *juvenile periodontitis,* postjuvenile periodontitis and adult periodontitis are illustrated in Fig. 6-10 (Liljenberg & Lindhe 1980). From the bars presented in Fig. 6-10 it can be seen that while the extracellular tissue (collagen and residual tissue) in lesions of postjuvenile periodontitis and adult periodontitis comprised between 50-60% of the tissue volume, in *juvenile periodontitis* sites, the extracellular tissue occupied only about 20% of the lesion. Since the majority of the cells in the *juvenile periodontitis* lesion were identified as plasma cells and blast cells, there are reasons to suggest that the *juvenile periodontitis* lesion is composed of a dense accumulation of plasma cells and blast cells.

General host response

Lehner et al. (1974) examined the role of humoral and cell mediated immunity in 34 patients with juvenile (14-21 years) and postjuvenile (22-29 years) periodontitis. They reported that the serum IgG, IgM and IgA were significantly *higher* in these patients than in healthy controls. In addition, patients in the *juvenile periodontitis* group showed an *impaired* lymphocyte blastogenic response to some selected Gram negative microorganisms but with the release of *positive* macrophage migration inhibition (MIF) activity. Recent studies by Ebersole et al. (1980) and Mouton et al. (1981) have confirmed the antibody data of Lehner et al. (1974) by showing that patients with *localized juvenile periodontitis* frequently have an increased antibody activity (serum IgG antibody) to *A. actinomycetemcomitans,* but a low titer of antibodies to *B. gingivalis.* Patients with adult periodontitis or generalized juvenile periodontitis on the other hand were found to have a high antibody titer to *B. gingivalis* but low titers to *A. actinomycetemcomitans.* These findings together with the available culture data imply that *localized juvenile periodontitis* on the one hand, and generalized forms of periodontitis on the other, are microbiologically different diseases.

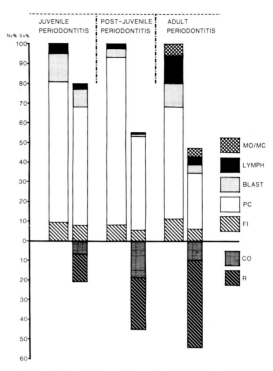

Fig. 6-10. Diagram illustrating the composition of the inflammatory cell infiltrate of periodontal lesions in patients with juvenile periodontitis, postjuvenile periodontitis and adult periodontitis. The wider bars illustrate the numerical density while the thin bars represent the volumetrical density of monocytes, macrophages, lymphocytes, blast cells, plasma cells, fibroblasts, collagen and residual tissues. (From Liljenberg & Lindhe 1980).

Results reported by Cianciola et al. (1977), Clark et al. (1977), Lavine et al. (1979) and van Dyke et al. (1980) have demonstrated that a majority of individuals with *juvenile periodontitis* have neutrophilic granulocytes in the circulating blood with an impaired capacity to react to chemotactic stimulus. Van Dyke et al. (1980) concluded that 26 out of 32 patients with *localized juvenile periodontitis,* but only 2 out of 23 with adult periodontitis, had neutrophils in the circulating blood with an improper ability to respond to chemotaxis. They suggested that the neutrophil dysfunction was caused by a cell associated defect of long duration. This observation indicates that examination of children and adolescents regarding neutrophil function may be a means of discriminating patients who run a risk of developing *juvenile periodontitis*.

Treatment

Data regarding the effect of treatment of *juvenile periodontitis* is sparse. Waerhaug (1977), from a retrospective study of 21 patients with juvenile periodontitis, who were monitored over a period of 8-32 years, reported that a treatment involving excision of the deepened pocket, root curettage and plaque control was effective in arresting the progression of the disorder. He stated: "the most important observation made in this material was that so-called periodontosis responds to total plaque control just as well as does ordinary advanced periodontitis". Baer & Socransky (1979) presented a long-term follow-up history of a patient with periodontosis and suggested that antibiotics such as tetracycline and penicillin can "be a helpful adjunct to patients' managements" including "full thickness flaps and curettage in affected areas".

Recently Lindhe (1982) studied the effect on *localized juvenile periodontitis* lesions of a treatment program which included tetracycline administration, surgical elimination of inflamed tissues, scaling and root planing and careful plaque control during healing. Treatment of *localized juvenile periodontitis* lesions was carried out on 16 individuals, aged 14-18 years. Lesions in first molars and incisors in individuals with adult periodontitis were treated in an identical manner and served as controls. A clinical examination was carried out first including assessments of oral hygiene, gingival conditions, probing depths and attachment levels. Periodic reproducible radiographs were taken from first molars and incisors to study alterations of the bony defects following treatment. After the clinical examination the patients were subjected to a treatment program involving: 1) administration of tetracycline (250 mg × 4/day for 2 weeks), 2) removal of granulation tissue after flap elevation, and 3)

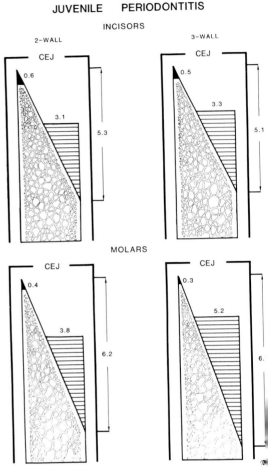

Fig. 6-11. Diagram describing the alterations of the morphology and height of angular bony defects in sites of juvenile periodontitis. In incisors as well as molars there was a slight posttherapeutic resorption of the bone crest (0.3-0.6 mm). Bone fill in the angular bony defects amounted to between 3.1 and 5.2 mm.

root curettage. After surgery the patients were instructed to rinse their mouths with a *0.2% chlorhexidine solution* for 2 min. twice a day during the first 2 postsurgical weeks. *Professional tooth cleaning* was carried out by a dental hygienist once every 3 months during a 2 year period. The patients were reexamined regarding their oral hygiene, gingival conditions, probing depth attachment levels and bone defect alterations 6, 12, 18 and 24 months following therapy.

It was observed that treatment of *localized*

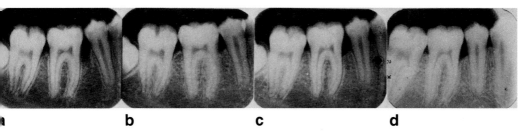

b   **c**   **d**

Fig. 6-12. A localized juvenile periodontitis lesion at the mesial surface of tooth 46 before therapy (a), 2 months (b), 12 months (c) and 24 months (d) following active therapy (administration of tetracycline, flap curettage and root surface instrumentation).

juvenile periodontitis in this way resulted in resolution of gingival inflammation, substantial gain of clinical attachment and refill of bone in the angular bony defects (Fig. 6-11). The clinical pattern of healing in the *juvenile periodontitis* sample was similar to that observed in patients with adult periodontitis. If anything, attachment gain and bone fill appeared to be somewhat faster in young patients with localized lesions than in older individuals (Fig. 6-12). Analysis of biopsy material obtained after therapy (Fig. 6-13) revealed that the previously diseased sites (juvenile as well as adult) had been

repopulated by a tissue, the composition of which was similar to that of normal gingiva.

This study, therefore, confirms the observations by Waerhaug (1977) that *juvenile periodontitis* lesions respond to treatment as well as do adult periodontitis lesions. It was, however, also observed that while no patient in the adult periodontitis group showed signs of recurrent disease during the 2 years of observation, 4 individuals and a total of 6 sites in the *juvenile periodontitis* group had to be retreated because of recurrence of inflammation, increasing probing depth and further loss of alveolar bone.

Fig. 6-13. Histogram of the composition of healthy gingival units and localized juvenile periodontitis lesions before and after therapy. The wide bars describe the numerical density and the thin bars the volumetrical density parameters. It can be seen that localized juvenile periodontitis lesions following therapy healed, i.e. tissue characteristics after treatment became similar to those of healthy gingiva. (From Lindhe 1982).

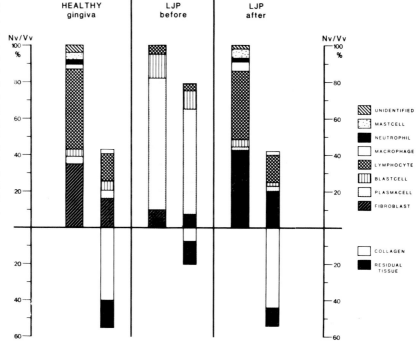

References

Baehni, P., Tsai, C-C., McArthur, W. P., Hammond, B. F. & Taichman, N. S. (1979) Interaction of inflammatory cells and oral microorganisms. VIII. Detection of leukotoxic activity of a plaque-derived gram-negative microorganism. *Infection and Immunity* **24**, 233-243.

Baer, P. N. (1971) The case for periodontosis as a clinical entity. *Journal of Periodontology* **42**, 516-520.

Baer, P. N. & Socransky, S. S. (1979) Periodontosis: Case report with long-term follow-up. *Periodontal Case Reports* **1**, 1-6.

Bick, P. H., Betts Carpenter, A., Holdeman, L. V., Miller, G. A., Ranney, R. R., Palcanis, K. G. & Tew, J. G. (1981) Polyclonal B-cell activation induced by extracts of gram-negative bacteria isolated from periodontally diseased sites. *Infection and Immunity* **34**, 43-49.

Cianciola, L. L., Genco, R. J., Paters, M. R., McKenna, I. & van Oss, C. J. (1977) Defective polymorphonuclear leukocyte function in a human periodontal disease. *Nature* **265**, 445-447.

Clark, R. A., Page, R. C. & Wilde, G. (1977) Defective neutrophil chemotaxis in juvenile periodontitis. *Infection and Immunity* **18**, 694-700.

Ebersole, J. L., Frey, D. E., Taubman, M. A., Smith, D. J. & Genco, R. J. (1980) Serum antibody response to A. actinomycetemcomitans (Y4) in periodontal diseases. *Journal of Dental Research* **59**, Special issue A, Abstract No. 249.

Gibbons, R. J. & MacDonald, J. B. (1961) Degradation of collagenous substrates by *Bacteroides melaninogenicus*. *Journal of Bacteriology* **81**, 614-621.

Gillett, R. & Johnson, N. W. (1982) Bacterial invasion of the periodontium in a case of juvenile periodontitis. *Journal of clinical Periodontology* **9**, 93-100.

Gottlieb, B. (1923) Die diffuse Atrophy des Alveolarknochens. *Zeitschrift für Stomatologie* **21**, 195.

Gottlieb, B. (1928) The formation of the pocket: diffuse atrophy of alveolar bone. *Journal of the American Dental Association* **15**, 462.

Hausmann, E., Raisz, L. G. & Miller, W. A. (1970) Endotoxin: stimulation of bone resorption in tissue culture. *Science* **168**, 862-864.

Hofstad, T. (1970) Biological activities of endoto-

xin from *Bacteroides melaninogenicus*. *Archives of Oral Biology* **15**, 343-348.

Hörmand, J. & Frandsen, A. (1979) Juvenile periodontitis. Localization of bone loss in relation to age, sex, and teeth. *Journal of Clinical Periodontology* **6**, 407-416.

Kiley, P. & Holt, S. C. (1980) Characterization of the lipopolysaccharide from *Actinobacillus actinomycetemcomitans* Y4 and N27. *Infection and Immunity* **30**, 862-873.

Kilian, M. (1981) Degradation of immunoglobulins A1, A2, and G by suspected principal periodontal pathogens. *Infection and Immunity* **34**, 757-765.

Laughon, B. E., Syed, S. A. & Loesche, W. (1982) API ZYM system for identification of *Bacteroides* spp., *Capnocytophaga* spp., and spirochetes of oral origin. *Journal of Clinical Microbiology* **15**, 97-102.

Lavine, W. S., Maderazo, E. G., Stolman, J., Ward, P. A., Cogen, R. B., Greenblatt, I. & Robertsson, P. B. (1979) Impaired neutrophil chemotaxis in patients with juvenile and rapidly progressing periodontitis. *Journal of Periodontal Research* **14**, 10-19.

Lehner, T., Wilton, M. A., Ivanyi, L. & Manson, I. D. (1974) Immunological aspects of juvenile periodontitis (periodontosis). *Journal of Periodontal Research* **9**, 261-272.

Liljenberg, B. & Lindhe, J. (1980) Juvenile periodontitis. Some microbiological, histopathological and clinical characteristics. *Journal of Clinical Periodontology* **7**, 48-61.

Lindhe, J. (1982) Treatment of localized juvenile periodontitis. In *Host-Parasite Interactions in Periodontal Disease*, ed. R. J. Genco & S. E. Mergenhagen. American Society for Microbiology. Washington, D.C:

Listgarten, M. A. (1976) Structure of the microbial flora associated with periodontal health and disease in man. A light and electron microscopic study. *Journal of Periodontology* **47**, 18.

Loesche, W. J., Syed, S. A., Morrison, E. C., Laughon, B. & Grossman, N. S. (1981) Treatment of periodontal infections due to anaerobic bacteria with short-term treatment with metronidazole. *Journal of Clinical Periodontology* **8**, 29-44.

Mandell, R. L. & Socransky, S. S. (1981) A selective medium for *Actinobacillus actinomycetemcomitans* and the incidence of the organ ism in juvenile periodontitis. *Journal of Periodontology* **52**, 593-598.

Mansheim, B. J., Orderdonk, A. B. & Kasper, D. L. (1978) Immunochemical and biologic studies of the lipopolysaccharide of *Bacteroides melaninogenicus* subspecies *asaccharolyticus*. *Journal of Immunology* **120**, 72-78.

Manson, J. D. & Lehner, T. (1974) Clinical feature of juvenile periodontitis (periodontosis). *Journal of Periodontology* **45**, 636-640.

McArthur, W. P., Tsai, C.-C., Baehni, P. C., Genco, R. J. & Taichman, N. S. (1981) Leukotoxic effects of *Actinobacillus actinomycetemcomitans*. *Journal of Periodontal Research* **16**, 159-170.

Mouton, C., Hammond, P. G., Slots, J. & Genco, R. J. (1981) Serum antibodies to oral *Bacteroides asaccharolyticus (Bacteroides gingivalis):* relationship to age and periodontal disease. *Infection and Immunity* **31**, 182-192.

Murray, P. & Patters, M. (1980) Gingival crevice neutrophil function in periodontal lesions. *Journal of Periodontal Research* **15**, 463-469.

Newman, M. G. & Socransky, S. S. (1977) Predominant cultivable microbiota in periodontosis. *Journal of Periodontal Research* **12**, 120-128.

Orban, B. & Weinmann, J. P. (1942) Diffuse atrophy of alveolar bone. *Journal of Periodontology* **13**, 31.

Rozanis, J. & Slots, J. (1982) Collagnolytic activity of *Actinobacillus actinomycetemcomitans* and black-pigmented *Bacteroides. Journal of Dental Research* **61**, Abstract No. 870, Annual meeting of the International Association of Dental Research.

Saglie, F. R., Carranza Jr., F. A., Newman, M. G., Cheng, L. & Lewin, K. J. (1982) Identification of tissue-invading bacteria in human periodontal disease. *Journal of Periodontal Research* **17**, 452-455.

Saxén, L. (1980) Juvenile periodontitis. *Journal of Clinical Periodontology* **7**, 1-19.

Shenker, B. J., Kushner, M. E. & Tsai, C.-C. (1982) Inhibition of fibroblast proliferation by *Actinobacillus actinomycetemcomitans. Infection and Immunity* **38**, 986-992.

Shurin, S. B., Socransky, S. S., Sweeney, E. & Stossel, T. P. (1979) A neutrophil disorder induced by capnocytophaga, a dental microorganism. *New England Journal of Medicine* **301**, 849-854.

Slots, J. (1976) The predominant cultivable organisms in juvenile periodontitis. *Scandinavian Journal of Dental Research* **84**, 1-10.

Slots J. (1981) Enzymatic characterization of some oral and nonoral gram negative bacteria with the API ZYM system. *Journal of Clinical Microbiology* **14**, 288-294.

Slots, J., Reynolds, H. S. & Genco, R. J. (1980) *Actinobacillus actinomycetemcomitans* in human periodontal disease: a cross-sectional microbiological investigation. *Infection and Immunity* **29**, 1013-1020.

Stevens, R. H., Sela, M. N., McArthur, W. P., Nowotny, A. & Hammond, B. F. (1980b) Biological and chemical characterization of endotoxin from *Capnocytophaga sputigena. Infection and Immunity* **27**, 246-254.

Stevens, R. H., Sela, M. N., Shapira, J. & Hammond, B. F. (1980a) Detection of a fibroblast proliferation inhibitory factor from *Capnocytophaga sputigena. Infection and Immunity* **27**, 271-275.

Sugarman, M. M. & Sugarman, E. F. (1977) Precocious periodontitis: A clinical entity and a treatment responsibility. *Journal of Periodontology* **48**, 397-409.

Tsai, C.-C., McArthur, W. P., Baehni, P. C., Evian, C., Genco, R. J. & Taichman, N. S. (1981) Serum neutralizing activity against *Actinobacillus actinomycetemcomitans* leukotoxin in juvenile periodontitis. *Journal of Clinical Periodontology* **8**, 338-348.

Tsai, C.-C., McArthur, W. P., Baehni, P. C., Hammond, B. F. & Taichman, N. S. (1979) Extraction and partial characterization of a leukotoxin from a plaque-derived gram-negative microorganism. *Infection and Immunity* **25**, 427-439.

van Dyke, T. E., Bartholomew, E., Genco, R. J., Slots, J. & Levine, M. J. (1982) Inhibition of neutrophil chemotaxis by soluble bacterial products. *Journal of Periodontology* **53**, 502-508.

van Dyke, T. E., Horoszewicz, H. U., Cianciola, L. J. & Genco, R. J. (1980) Neutrophil chemotaxis dysfunction in human periodontitis. *Infection and Immunity* **27**, 124-132.

Waerhaug, J. (1977) Plaque control in the treatment of juvenile periodontitis. *Journal of Clinical Periodontology* **4**, 29-40.

Westergaard, J., Frandsen, A. & Slots, J. (1978) Ultrastructure of the subgingival microflora in juvenile periodontitis. *Scandinavian Journal of Dental Research* **86**, 421-429.

Necrotizing Gingivitis

Necrotizing gingivitis (NG) is an inflammatory destructive gingival condition which exhibits characteristic clinical signs and symptoms, and which has been assumed to be at least partially due to etiological agents other than those producing common chronic marginal gingivitis. In its most typical acute form, it is characterized by interproximal necrotic ulcers. These ulcers are covered by a yellowish-white or greyish debris, they are painful to touch and bleeding is readily provoked.

NG has been known under several names. "Trench mouth", "ulceromembranous gingivitis", "acute necrotizing ulcerative gingivitis" (ANUG) and "Vincent's gingivitis" or "Vincent's gingivostomatitis" are some of the terms which have been used (Pickard 1973). The designation "ulcerative" or "ulcerating" is redundant, as necrotic lesions are always ulcerated. The association with the name Vincent is due to the fact that he first described the particular mixed *fusospirochetal* microbiota occurring in the so-called "Vincent's angina", where the necrotic areas are typically localized in the tonsils (Vincent 1898). The same mixed microbiota is found in NG lesions. Vincent's angina and NG usually occur independently of each other, however, and should therefore be regarded as separate disease entities. Vincent's angina occurs twice as frequently in females as in males (van Cauwenberge 1976), whereas *NG* has been reported to occur more frequently in males.

NG has features in common with the far more serious *cancrum oris* or "noma". This is a necrotizing and destructive, frequently mortal stomatitis in which the same mixed fusospirochetal flora dominates. It occurs almost exclusively in certain developing countries, mostly in children and in association with systemic diseases and malnutrition (Enwonwu 1972). Some researchers have suggested that *cancrum oris* always develops from preexisting *necrotizing gingivitis* (Emslie 1963) whereas others have been unable to confirm this observation (Pindborg et al. 1966, 1967, Sheiham 1966).

Unless properly treated, *NG* has a marked tendency for recurrence (Manson & Rand 1961). For such cases the designations "recurrent" or "chronic" have been used. If this condition is allowed to persist for some time, the disease may lead to considerable loss of periodontal support.

In this chapter the acute form will be termed *acute necrotizing gingivitis (ANG)*. The chronic or recurrent form will be termed *chronic necrotizing gingivitis (CNG)*. The collective term is *necrotizing gingivitis (NG)*.

Epidemiology

In industrialized countries ANG occurs particularly among young adults, 18-30 years of age. In a study conducted in the USA, Grupe & Wilder (1956) found ANG in 2.2% of 870 young military trainees. Giddon et al. 1964) found ANG in 2.5% of 326 students in their first college year. During the next year more students contracted the disease so that a total of 6.7% had encountered the disease during their first 2 college years. In a comprehensive study Pindborg (1951a) found NG in 6.0% of Danish military trainees.

ANG can be observed in all age groups, but in western countries it is practically never seen in children. In some developing countries, on the other hand, ANG is common even in early childhood, and is frequently associated with malnutrition or such systemic diseases as measles and malaria Pindborg et al. 1966, Sheiham 1966, Enwonwu 1972). Reports of epidemic-like ANG among soldiers were not uncommon some years ago. There is, however, no epidemiological or other scientific data to suggest that the disease is communicable, nor is there conclusive evidence to confirm a sex predilection in the occurrence of ANG.

Epidemiological investigations have identified 3 factors which seem to be related to increased frequency of ANG: *Poor oral hygiene, with preexisting simple chronic marginal gingivitis* is almost always seen in individuals who develop ANG. Thus, Pindborg 1951b) found that 87 out of 91 new cases of ANG had a preexisting chronic marginal gingivitis.

Smoking shows a clear association with ANG. Very few of those who develop ANG are nonsmokers. For instance, Pindborg 1951b) found only 1 nonsmoker among 57 ANG patients. The amount smoked also appears relevant. In a population examined by Goldhaber & Giddon (1964), 41% of subjects with ANG smoked more than 20 cigarettes daily. Only 5% of controls smoked as much as this and among the controls there were significantly more nonsmokers.

The third factor which seems to be related to the occurrence of ANG is *emotional stress.* Epidemiological investigations by Pindborg (1951a, b), Giddon et al. (1963), Goldhaber & Giddon (1964) and others, seem to indicate a more frequent occurrence of ANG in periods when the individuals are exposed to psychic or emotional stress. Such periods may be related *inter alia,* to problems in school, examinations, or with the beginning or the end of military service.

Clinical features

Acute necrotizing gingivitis (ANG)

Marginal necrosis
The most characteristic finding in ANG is necrotic lesions of the marginal gingiva. In the early stages, destruction is almost always localized to one or more interdental papillae. The first lesions are often seen interproximally in the lower anterior region, but they may occur in any interproximal space (Figs. 7-1, 7-3). In regions where lesions first appear there are usually also signs of preexisting chronic marginal gingivitis. The process commonly manifests itself with the occurrence of a necrotic ulcer on the tip of the papilla. The facial part tends to swell and becomes thickened with a rounded contour. The papillae do not always appear edematous at this stage; on the contrary, they may have a relatively firm consistency and gingival stippling is often maintained.

Necrosis develops rapidly. Within a few days the involved papillae are separated into one facial and one lingual portion with an interposed necrotic depression between them. In this central depressed portion, the necrosis produces considerable tissue destruction and a crater is formed. The necrosis may also extend laterally to the marginal gingiva along the oral or facial surfaces of the teeth. Necrotic zones originating from

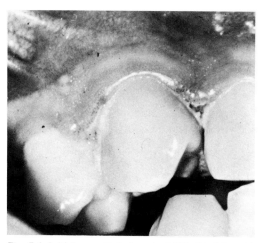

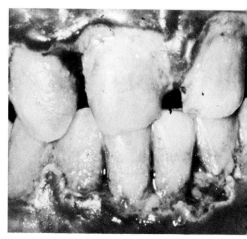

Fig. 7-1. Initial necrotic lesions in ANG. Mesial to 14 (13 is missing) initial crater formation is evident. The lesion near the tip of the interdental papilla distal to 14 is covered by a yellowish-white debris.

Fig. 7-2. Clinical photograph illustrating an advanc case of ANG. Confluent necrotic areas involving bo the papillae and the facial gingiva are seen. Lar amounts of yellowish-white soft debris cover both t necrotic zones and parts of the tooth surfaces.

neighboring interproximal spaces may merge and form a continuous necrotic area (Figs. 7-2, 7-4). These superficial necrotic lesions in ANG are primarily limited to the gingiva and only rarely do they cover the entire width of the attached gingiva. Usually only a relatively narrow zone of the marginal gingiva is afflicted.

The palatal and lingual marginal gingiva is less frequently involved than the corr sponding facial area. If other parts of th oral mucosa are involved in the process, t simultaneous occurrence of ANG ar another disease should be suspected. Th most likely systemic condition to be involve in such instances is herpetic gingivostoma tis (see under Differential diagnosis).

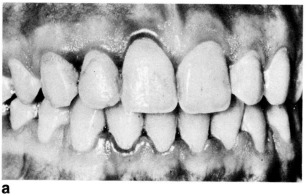

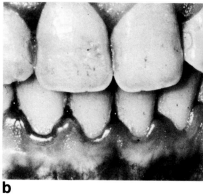

a   **b**

Fig. 7-3a. At this early stage of ANG, the first lesions can be seen in the lower anterior tooth region. The faci portions of the papillae are swollen and display a thickened, rounded margin. The necrotic areas are restricted to th interdental papillae and are still not very prominent.

Fig. 7-3b. Higher magnification of the incisor regions from the patient shown in Fig. 7-3a.

204

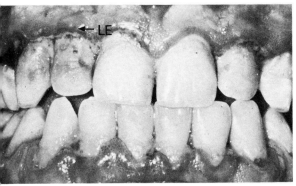
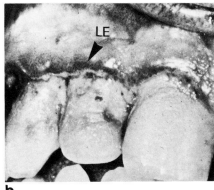

g. 7-4a. A typical case of ANG. In the lower anterior tooth region, necrotic areas are limited to the interproximal aces where they are mostly hidden by the swollen interdental papillae. In the upper anterior tooth region, necrotic eas can be seen both facially and approximally. At teeth 13, 12 and partially at 11, the necrotic areas form a ntinuous zone covered by large amounts of soft yellowish-white debris. The linear erythema (LE) is the relatively ell delineated red zone separating the marginal necrotic areas from the rest of the gingiva. In the upper anterior oth region white debris covers most of the free and attached gingiva.
g. 7-4b. Higher magnification of teeth 11, 12 and 13 shown in Fig. 7-4a. Note the linear erythema (LE).

ellowish-white debris

he soft yellowish-white or greyish material hich covers the necrotic zones has been rmed "pseudomembrane". This is not a ood term since the soft material bears little esemblance to a true membrane. It consists rimarily of leukocytes, erythrocytes, fibrin, ecrotic tissue remnants and masses of bacteria, and cannot be removed as a continuus membrane. Attempts to remove this aterial will cause it to break up, and the leeding, ulcerated connective tissue ecomes exposed. The soft deposits also over subgingival calculus which is frequently found in large amounts on approxiial surfaces of teeth next to the necrotic reas.

Personal oral hygiene in patients who conact ANG is usually poor. Moreover, brushag of teeth and contact with the acutely ıflamed gingiva is painful. There are therere frequently large amounts of plaque on ıe teeth especially along the gingival marin. A thin whitish film of bacteria and ebris may even cover the entire attached ingiva (Fig. 7-4). This film is composed of esquamated epithelial cells and some bacria in a meshwork of salivary proteins and,

possibly, fibrin deposits from the inflammatory exudate. It can be readily removed by a water spray.

Linear erythema

The zone between the marginal necrosis and the relatively unaffected gingiva usually exhibits a well demarcated narrow erythematous zone. This zone is called the linear erythema. It is caused by hyperemia of the vessels of the gingival connective tissue peripherally to the necrotic lesions (Fig. 7-4).

Bleeding

Acute inflammation and necrosis with exposure of the underlying connective tissue in ANG produces a marked tendency to bleeding. Bleeding may start spontaneously as well as in response to even gentle touch.

Pain

In the initial stages, when necrotic lesions in ANG are relatively few and small, pain is usually moderate. In more advanced cases the pain may be considerable and may be associated with a markedly increased salivary flow.

205

Foetor ex ore

A characteristic and pronounced foetor ex ore is often noticed in ANG, but it can vary in intensity and in some cases is not very noticeable. It should further be noted that strong foetor ex ore can also be found in such other pathological conditions of the oral cavity as chronic destructive periodontal disease. Strong foetor ex ore is, therefore, not pathognomonic for ANG.

Lymphadenitis

Swelling and tenderness of the regional lymph nodes may occur in ANG, particularly in advanced cases. Such lymphadenitis is usually confined to the submandibular lymph nodes, but the cervical lymph nodes may also be involved. In children with ANG, Jiménez & Baer (1975) found that lymphadenitis and increased bleeding tendency were the most pronounced clinical findings. Others, like Grupe & Wilder (1956), have not found lymphadenitis clearly characteristic of ANG.

Fever and malaise

There is no general agreement concerning the occurrence of fever and malaise in ANG. Investigations by Grupe & Wilder (1956), Goldhaber & Giddon (1964) and by Shields (1977) indicate that elevated body temperature is not common in ANG, and when present, the elevation of body temperature is usually moderate. Even a small decrease in body temperature in ANG has been described. The reason for disagreement on this point is thought to stem from a tendency to misdiagnose primary herpetic gingivostomatitis as ANG when it occurs in youth or young adults.

Chronic necrotizing gingivitis (CNG)

If inadequately treated or untreated, the acute phase of ANG will gradually subside. The condition becomes less unpleasant to the patient. The necrotic tissues do not,

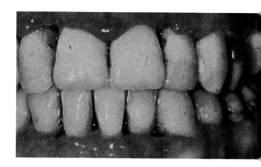

Fig. 7-5. In chronic necrotizing gingivitis (CNG) tenderness and pain may be relatively mild and the patient may therefore be able to maintain a better oral hygiene than in ANG. A thick, gingival margin exhibiting so called "reverse gingival architecture" is characteristic.

however, heal completely. The destruction of periodontal tissue continues, although at a slower rate and with less dramatic symptoms. This condition has been termed chronic necrotizing gingivitis (CNG) (Figs 7-5, 7-6). The necrotizing lesions persist as open craters, frequently filled by subgingival calculus and bacterial plaque. The characteristic yellowish-white, necrotic areas of the

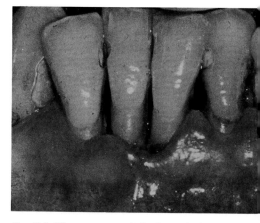

Fig. 7-6. The area around the lower incisors exhibits several findings typical of CNG: A thick rounded gingival margin, concave papillae, craters filled by subgingival calculus, and a relatively firm attached gingiva without obvious signs of acute lesions. The patient's oral hygiene is better than in most cases of ANG.

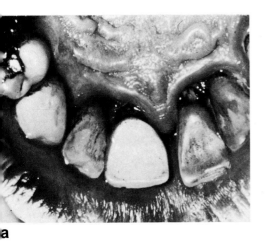

a

Fig. 7-7a. CNG with wide crater formation in the upper anterior tooth region. The patient's history and the clinical picture indicated that the formation of the defects had started several years earlier during an episode of ANG. The acute inflammation was not properly treated and later passed to a chronic stage with continuous tissue destruction in the interproximal craters.

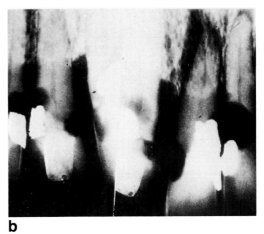

b

Fig. 7-7b. Radiographs of the interproximal areas of the upper anterior teeth of the patient shown in Fig. 7-7a. Note advanced interproximal osseous destruction and extensive caries lesions on root surfaces adjoining the interproximal craters.

acute phase usually disappear. Acute exacerbations with intervening quiescent periods may occur. In recurrent acute phases, subjective symptoms again become more noticeable and necrotic ulcers with masses of yellowish-white deposits reappear (Fig. 7-9). These masses are, however, frequently less conspicuous than in ANG, because they are located in preexisting interdental craters and are therefore not always readily detected.

A characteristic feature of CNG is a thickened and rounded gingival margin, which may give the impression of "reversed gingival architecture" (Figs. 7-5, 7-6, 7-8, 7-9). Adjoining interdental craters may fuse into one continuous trough like crater which contains large amounts of calculus and plaque. The facial and oral gingivae in such areas may be entirely separated and form two distinct flaps or "lips".

CNG may produce considerable destruction of supporting tissues. The most pronounced tissue loss usually occurs in association with the interproximal craters. Further-

more, carious lesions may be found on the exposed root surfaces (Fig. 7-7).

Diagnosis

The diagnosis of NG should be based on clinical signs and symptoms as described above. The patient's past history may also give valuable information. The patient has frequently noticed pain and bleeding from the gingiva, particularly upon touch. Fever and malaise may occur even though this is not characteristic for NG. Smoking and emotional or psychic stress predispose to the disease.

A bacterial smear which shows a dominance of fusobacteria and spirochetes may confirm the diagnosis, but in such smears a great variety of microorganisms may be found, and in some areas the fusospirochetal mixed flora may be less dominant. A biopsy will reveal superficial tissue necrosis with nonspecific inflammatory changes. The histopathological picture is not pathognomonic for NG, and biopsy is not usually indicated.

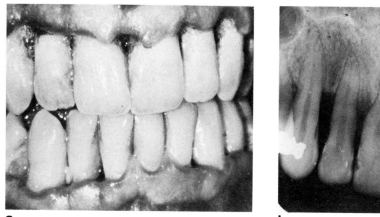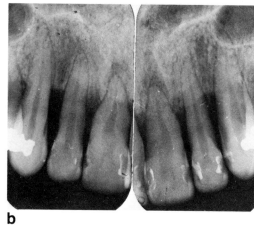

a   b

Fig. 7-8a. By local application of astringent medication a necrotizing gingivitis may be converted from acute to chronic form. This patient had been treated over a period of 14 months by repeated application of carbolfuchsin, without institution of proper cause related treatment. Note the characteristic "reverse gingival architecture".

Fig. 7-8b. Radiographs from the patient shown in Fig. 7-8 a exhibit advanced loss of alveolar bone. The tissue destruction has continued particularly in the interproximal areas. The "treatment" of the original condition only masked the tissue destruction by alleviating the acute symptoms.

Differential diagnosis

ANG may be confused with other diseases of the oral mucosa. Primary herpetic gingivostomatitis (PHG) is not infrequently mistaken for ANG (Fig. 7-10; Klotz 1973). The important differential diagnostic criteria for the two diseases have been listed in Table 7-1. It should be noted that in the USA and in northern Europe, ANG occurs very rarely in children, whereas PHG is most commonly found in children. If the body's temperature is markedly raised, to 38° C or more, PHG

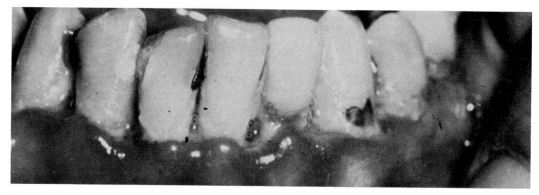

Fig. 7-9. CNG with recurrence or exacerbation of acute symptoms. This condition has sometimes been called recurrent necrotizing gingivitis. Necrosis, pain, increased bleeding tendency, etc. have recurred. The patient's history will assist the therapist to differentiate this condition from primary ANG. The necrotic lesions are localized to preexisting craters and the gingival contour is typical of CNG.

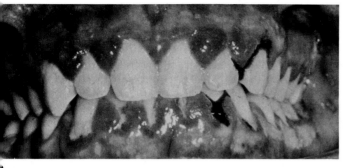
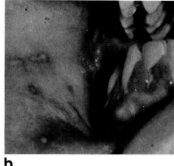

b

ig. 7-10a. Primary herpetic gingivostomatitis in an 18 year old male. The edematous swelling of the interproximal
apillae may produce an interdental morphology similar to approximal craters. These interdental areas may also be
overed by a moderate amount of yellowish-white debris. Marked color changes involving both oral mucosa and wide
reas of the attached gingiva can be seen as well as increased bleeding tendency. A small round ulcer is visible in the
uccal mucosa. The patient was a mouth breather.
ig. 7-10b. Buccal mucosa from the right side of the mouth of the patient shown in Fig. 7-10a. There are characteristic
erpetic lesions. They are flat, painful and covered by a greyish membranous debris, surrounded by an elevated
argin with a diffuse erythematous zone.

hould be suspected. ANG has a marked redilection for the interdental papillae, while PHG shows no such limitation and nay occur anywhere on the free or the ttached gingiva, or in the alveolar mucosa. n PHG the erythema is of a more diffuse character and may comprise the entire gingiva and parts of the alveolar mucosa. The vesicular lesions in PHG which disrupt and produce small ulcers surrounded by diffuse erythema, occur both on the lips and tongue as well as on the buccal mucosa. PHG and

able 7-1. Clinical criteria for the differential diagnosis between acute necrotizing gingivitis (ANG) and primary erpetic gingivostomatitis (PHG)

	ANG	PHG
Occurrence	Rare in children (in Europe, USA)	Most frequently seen in children
Fever, malaise	May occur, but is usually moderate	Temperature elevation, frequently marked, is characteristic
Sites of predilection	Preferentially occurs interdentally, penetrates deeply and spreads laterally. Rarely lesions outside the gingiva	No definite intraoral predilection sites. Diffusely spread over the entire gingiva. Lesions are frequently seen on lip and tongue, in the buccal and on other occasions in the oral mucosa
Lesion and erythema	Necrotic ulcers with yellowish-white debris and a narrow, linear erythema which sharply separates the lesions from the adjoining mucosa	Round, greyish small vesicles which disrupt and leave small ulcers without appreciable tissue destruction. Diffuse erythema
Foetor ex ore	Characteristic foetor has been reported as typical of the disease May not always be pronounced and is not pathognomonic	Foetor may be present, but is not regarded as being typical for this condition

ANG may occur simultaneously in the same patient, and in such cases there may be mucosal lesions outside the gingiva, and fever and general malaise tend to occur more frequently than with ANG alone.

Among oral mucosal diseases that have been confused with ANG, are desquamative gingivitis, benign mucous membrane pemphigoid, erythema multiforme exudativum, streptococcal gingivitis, gonococcal gingivitis, and others have been mentioned. All of these are described in Chapter 10 and are clinically quite distinct from ANG.

In some forms of leukemia, especially acute leukemia, necrotizing ulcers may occur in the oral mucosa and are not infrequently seen in association with the gingival margin, apparently as an exacerbation of an existing chronic inflammatory condition. The clinical appearance can resemble ANG lesions, and the symptoms they produce may be the ones that first make the patient seek professional consultation. In acute leukemia the gingiva often appears bluish-red and swollen with edema. Varying degrees of ulceration and necrosis occur, sometimes with formation of a "pseudomembrane". Generally, the patient has more marked systemic symptoms than with ordinary ANG, but can for a while feel relatively healthy. The dentist should be aware of the possibility that leukemias present such oral manifestations. Hematologic examination of the patient's blood may be indicated, whereas biopsy usually is not.

Treatment

In spite of the characteristic clinical and bacteriologic findings in NG, therapy should follow the same principal guidelines as for treatment of chronic gingivitis and periodontitis. Practical implementation of treatment may necessitate certain modifications, particularly because of the nature of the lesions, including pain and bleeding in the acute phase and great loss of interdental supporting tissues by crater formation.

Cause related treatment

Bleeding and sensitivity to touch may complicate both debridement and personal oral hygiene. Nevertheless, scaling should be attempted, as thoroughly as conditions will allow, even during the first consultation. Ultrasonic scaling may be preferable to the use of hand instruments. With minimal pressure against the soft tissues, ultrasonic cleaning may accomplish the removal of soft and mineralized deposits. The continuous water spray combined with adequate suction will allow good visibility. How far it is possible to proceed with debridement during the first visit will usually depend on the intensity of pain and the patient's tolerance of instrumentation.

Patients with ANG are not easily motivated to carry out a proper program of oral hygiene. They frequently have poor oral hygiene habits and possibly a negative attitude to dental treatment in general. As a result, some patients discontinue treatment as soon as pain and other acute symptoms are alleviated. Motivation and instruction should be planned to prevent this happening, and should be reinforced during later visits.

Instruction in tooth brushing and approximal cleaning should largely follow the recommendations of ordinary periodontal therapy. Some clinicians have emphasized the importance of gentle and light brushing during initial phases of ANG treatment. However, patients themselves generally apply oral hygiene measures with sufficient leniency because of bleeding and pain. If the dentist overemphasizes the importance of gentle brushing and interdental cleaning, it can result in unnecessarily inefficient oral hygiene. Clinical experience does, however, indicate that soft toothbrushes are preferable.

To support the patient's oral hygiene during the initial phase of treatment, frequent rinsing with a mixture of equal parts 3% H_2O_2 and lukewarm water is regarded by

ome as a useful aid. Twice daily rinses with
0.2% Hibitane (Chlorhexidine) is a very
effective adjunct to self performed oral
hygiene during the first 2 weeks of treatment.

Further treatment in ANG must be
adapted to the individual case. The efficiency of the patient's oral hygiene efforts
and the reduction of pain and bleeding will
determine the progression of therapy. The
patient should be seen at least once a week as
long as the acute symptoms persist. Systematic subgingival scaling with curettes, correction of restoration margins and polishing of
restorations and root surfaces should be performed during these visits in addition to supplementary oral hygiene instruction and
patient motivation.

Cause related treatment in CNG does not
differ appreciably from treatment of ordinary chronic periodontitis. Symptoms do not
complicate scaling and self performed oral
hygiene measures to the same extent as in
ANG. On the other hand, there are often
large amounts of subgingival calculus present in CNG, and depuration may require
considerable effort.

Surgical treatment

When the cause related phase of treatment
has been completed, necrosis and other
acute symptoms in ANG will have disappeared. The formerly necrotic areas have
healed and the gingival craters are reduced
in size, although as a rule some defects persist. In such areas bacterial plaque readily
accumulates, and the craters, therefore, predispose to recurrence of NG or further destruction because of a persisting chronic
inflammatory process, or both; these sites
require surgical correction.

In CNG, the soft tissue defects are usually
pronounced. The surrounding tissues are
often firm and fibrous and a gradual change
towards a more favorable topography in
response to treatment is less likely to occur
than in ANG. Surgical treatment therefore
is almost always necessary in CNG.

Shallow craters can be removed by simple

gingivectomy, while the elimination of deep
defects may require flap surgery. Thinning
of thick flap margins and correction of form
to achieve optimal interproximal coverage
and contour are important and may be technically demanding. Treatment of necrotizing
gingivitis has not been completed until all
gingival defects have been eliminated and
optimal conditions for future plaque control
have been established.

Drugs in treatment of NG

Miller & Greene (1958) have reported that
more than 100 different drugs have been suggested for the treatment of NG; this illustrates the uncertainty and confusion associated with treatment of this periodontal
disease.

Escharotics such as chromic acid and silver
nitrate or substances with an *astringent* and
possibly some *antibacterial effect* such as
gentian violet and carbolfuchsin, have been
widely used in the treatment of ANG (Fig. 7-
8). The rationale for using such substances
was probably that they appeared to alleviate
acute symptoms such as bleeding and pain
when applied to the inflamed gingiva. The
effect of escharotics is, however, extremely
difficult to control. The etching may penetrate deep into the periodontium and contribute to permanent destruction of healthy or
potentially healthy periodontal tissues.
There is considerably less danger of such
undesired effects associated with the use of
astringent substances. On the other hand,
some of these are regarded as potentially
carcinogenic. The effects of escharotics and
astringents are purely symptomatic and they
should therefore be avoided in the treatment
of NG. Recurrences are frequently seen
(Manson & Rand 1961) since such "therapy"
will only mask the destructive inflammatory
process, permitting it to continue into the
deeper portions of the periodontium.

Hydrogen peroxide and other oxygen
releasing agents also have a long-standing
tradition in the treatment of ANG. Hydrogen peroxide has been used as a caustic or
etching substance (30%), for debridement
(3%), and as a mouthrinse (equal portions

3% H_2O_2 and warm water). For debridement in necrotic areas and as a mouthrinse hydrogen peroxide is still used. It has been thought that the apparently favorable effects of hydrogen peroxide may be due to mechanical cleaning, and the influence on anaerobic bacterial flora of the liberated oxygen (Wennström & Lindhe 1979, Mac-Phee & Cowley 1981).

Hibitane (Chlorhexidine) in 0.2% solution is marketed in several European countries as a mouthrinse. Its effect is discussed elsewhere in this textbook. Hibitane is useful as a supplement to the patient's personal oral hygiene measures during the acute phase of ANG (see above). For an optimal effect of this medicament, it should be used only in conjunction with and in addition to systematic scaling and root planing. The Hibitane solution does not penetrate well subgingivally and the preparation is readily inactivated by exudates, necrotic tissues and masses of bacteria (Gjermo 1974). The effectiveness of Hibitane mouthrinses therefore is dependent upon a simultaneous thorough mechanical debridement.

Antibiotics and chemotherapeutics are aimed directly at the bacteria which are the direct cause of the inflammatory process in ANG. Penicillins and other broad-spectrum antibiotics such as tetracyclines are most effective. However, the important role of such medication in the treatment of other, more serious infectious diseases, calls for a restrictive attitude towards their use in less serious conditions such as ANG. Only in rare cases of ANG is the patient's general health affected to such an extent that the use of antibiotics is indicated. *Topical application* of broad-spectrum antibiotics is strictly contraindicated in the treatment of ANG.

Metronidazole (e.g. Flagyl, Rhodia®) has been found effective against spirochetes and has been used both locally and systemically in the treatment of ANG (Proctor & Baker 1971, Shinn 1976).

In conclusion, drugs are of limited usefulness in the treatment of NG, and only those producing improved plaque control in the cause related therapy phase, should be used.

Histopathology

The histopathologic picture of characteristic NG lesions reveals a nonspecific, acute necrotizing inflammation. The necrosis involves both the epithelium and the superficial layers of the connective tissue (Fig. 7-11). Normal tissue has been replaced by a meshwork of fibrin with degenerated epithelial cells, leukocytes and erythrocytes, and by bacteria and cellular debris. This layer corresponds to the yellowish-white debris which can be observed clinically. The viable connective tissue exhibits dilated and proliferating vessels and dense infiltrates of neutrophilic polymorphonuclear leukocytes. In the deeper layers, at some distance from the necrotic areas, the tissue exhibits signs of chronic inflammation and contains many plasma cells and monocytes. The necrotic area and the zone between this and the viable tissue contain large amounts of bacteria particularly fusobacteria and spirochetes (Figs. 7-12, 7-13, 7-14). Spirochetes have been reported to penetrate the superficial layers of the viable connective tissue. Listgarten (1965) in an electron microscopic investigation found large and medium sized spirochetes located as much as 0.25 mm below the necrotic surface. No other microorganisms were found to penetrate as deeply as this. Listgarten (1965) and Heylings (1967) also demonstrated compact masses of spirochetes and short, fusiform rods intercellularly in a presumably vital epithelium.

According to Listgarten (1965) the electron microscopic picture of the necrotic lesions in ANG exhibits 4 zones starting from the surface:

1. The bacterial zone, which consists of bacteria of varying sizes and forms including small, medium sized and large spirochetes.
2. The neutrophil rich zone, which contains many leukocytes with a dominance of neutrophilic granulocytes. Between these cells bacteria are observed, including many spirochetes.

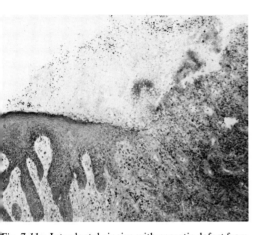

Fig. 7-11a. Interdental gingiva with necrotic defect from an ANG patient. The illustration shows the transition from the facial part of the gingival papilla to the interdental necrotic area. The lesion is covered by a thick layer of fibrin, leukocytes, erythrocytes and bacteria (X 48).

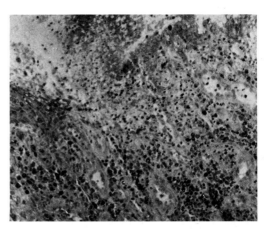

Fig. 7-11b. Section taken from the necrotic lesion near the intact epithelium. The sulcus and junctional epithelia are completely necrotized, only a small residue is visible to the left, and on top, bacterial masses with cellular debris. The necrotic part of the connective tissue and the region immediately subjacent to this area contains many polymorphonuclear leukocytes. In the deeper portion there is a dense infiltration of lymphocytes and particularly plasma cells, and the tissue contains many dilated vessels (X 128).

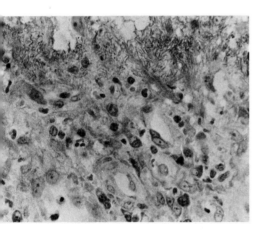

Fig. 7-11c. This section from the necrotic and spirochete infiltrated zones exhibits direct contact between bacteria and connective tissue. The tissue architecture is characterized by necrotic cells, disorganized collagen structures and accumulations of leukocytes. Several vessels are in close relation to the necrotic tissue. Among the bacteria, fusobacteria and spirochetes dominate, and close to the connective tissue practically only spirochetes are present (X 400).

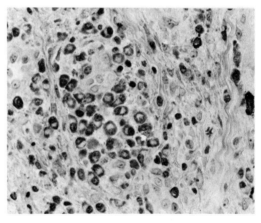

Fig. 7-11d. A viable connective tissue is seen peripherally to the necrotic lesion. This tissue is dominated by proliferating vessels, plasma cells and some monocytes forming a dense infiltrate. Intercellular collagen fibers can also be seen (X 400).

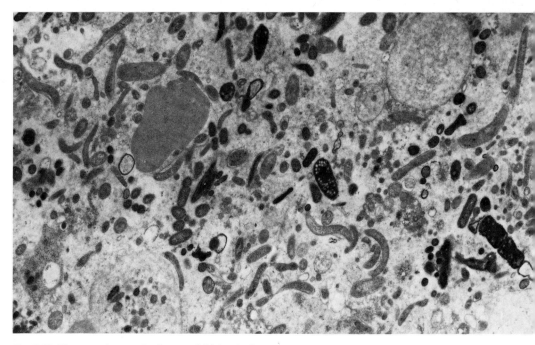

Fig. 7-12. Electron microscopic picture exhibiting the heterogeneous mixture of bacteria, cells and degenerated tissue components near the surface of the ulcerated connective tissue (X 8,000).

3. The necrotic zone, containing disintegrated cells, many large and medium sized spirochetes, and other bacteria which, judging from their size and shape, may be fusobacteria.
4. The spirochetal infiltration zone, where the tissue components appear intact, the tissue is infiltrated by large and medium sized spirochetes, but no other microorganisms can be seen.

Etiology

ANG is commonly regarded as an endogenous infection caused by a combined influence of several microorganisms. It has been suggested that ANG lesions may develop only if predisposing alterations in the resistance to infection of the host tissues have occurred. The most important predisposing conditions are *preexisting gingivitis, smoking* and *emotional/psychic stress*. Systemic diseases and malnutrition are of minor importance in industrialized countries, but may play an important role as ANG predispositional factors in developing countries.

The role of bacteria
Several observations support the concept that a particular microbiota plays a decisive role in the development of ANG. The condition shows a dramatic improvement when the patient is given such antibiotics as penicillin or tetracycline. A characteristic bacterial flora of fusobacteria and spirochetes is always present. Spirochetes and fusiform bacteria can invade the epithelium (Heylings 1967). The spirochetes can also invade the vital connective tissue (Listgarten 1965). Both fusobacteria and spirochetes can liberate endotoxins (Mergenhagen et al. 1961, Kristoffersen & Hofstad 1970). Experiments have shown

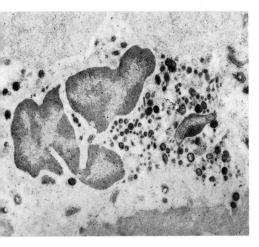

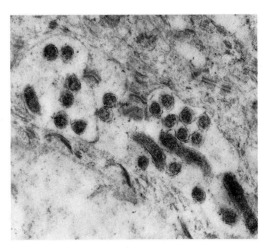

Fig. 7-13. Polymorphonuclear neutrophilic granulocyte from bacteria infiltrated area. Intracellularly, between the characteristic granulae, a phagocytosed spirochete is seen (X 9,000).

Fig. 7-14. Section from superficial layers of the epithelium near the periphery of the necrotic lesion. Spirochetes have invaded the widened intercellular spaces between the epithelial cells (X 16,000).

that these organisms possess biological activities which may contribute to the pathogenesis of ANG. Nevertheless, the exact role of the various microorganisms has not been clarified, and the fact that they are present in large numbers does not necessarily mean that they are of primary etiologic importance. Their presence could equally well result from secondary overgrowth.

Attempts to transmit the disease from one animal to another, or to produce necrotic lesions in experimental animals have failed to yield conclusive results (MacDonald et al. 1963). Several suspect microorganisms and several combinations of microorganisms can produce similar lesions in experimental animals. MacDonald et al. (1956) found that a combination of 4 different bacteria, none of them fusobacteria or spirochetes, had such properties. Further experiments gave indications that among the 4 bacterial species, *Bacteroides melaninogenicus* was the true pathogen (MacDonald et al. 1963). *B. melaninogenicus* may, under certain conditions, produce an enzyme which degrades native collagen (Gibbons & MacDonald 1961). It is still not clear, however, whether

this microorganism is of particular importance in the pathogenesis of ANG. The lesions produced in experimental animals may not be identical to those which occur in humans. It is also important to note that even if necrotic lesions can be transmitted by transmission of infectious material or bacterial cultures, this does not necessarily mean that the disease is truly contagious.

Our knowledge of the pathogenic mechanisms by which the bacterial flora produces the tissue changes characteristic of ANG is limited, particularly as it has been difficult to establish an acceptable animal experimental model. It seems reasonable to believe that several of the pathogenic mechanisms which have been associated with chronic gingivitis and periodontitis may also be of etiologic importance in ANG.

Several observations indicate that the effects of endotoxins are more prominent in ANG than in chronic gingivitis and periodontitis. The large masses of Gram negative bacteria liberate endotoxins in close contact with connective tissue. Endotoxins may produce tissue destruction both by direct toxic effects and indirectly, by

215

activating and modifying tissue responses of the host (Wilton & Lehner 1980). Through direct toxic effect, endotoxins may lead to damage of cells and vessels. Necrosis is a prominent feature in the so-called "Shwartzman-reaction" which is caused by endotoxins. Indirectly, endotoxins can contribute to tissue damage in several ways: they can function as antigens and elicit immune reactions, they can activate complement directly through the alternative pathway and thereby liberate chemotaxins, they can also activate macrophages and, acting as mitogens on B and T-lymphocytes, may influence the host's immune reactions. To what extent such reactions contribute to host defence or to tissue damage is not known. In addition, it has been shown, in *in vitro* experiments, that endotoxins can stimulate bone resorption.

Wilton et al. (1971) investigated the cellular and humoral immune responses in both necrotizing and chronic gingivitis. Titers of antibodies to *Actinomyces viscosus, Fusobacterium fusiforme* and *Veillonella alcalescens* were similar in patients with ANG and chronic gingivitis. This observation invalidates the theory that ANG is the result of a specific infection by one of these microorganisms. On the other hand, it supports the clinical finding that ANG always develops from a preexisting chronic gingivitis. Cellular immune responses were in accordance with these observations, but a stronger reaction to fusobacteria was taken as an indication that these microorganisms could be involved in the transition from chronic to acute gingivitis.

Preexisting gingivitis

Whether or not ANG may occur at all without preexisting gingivitis is uncertain. The mechanisms by which chronic gingivitis may predispose to the occurrence of ANG remain obscure. Several hypotheses have been advanced, among them changes in leukocyte function and changes in immune response. Wilton et al. (1971) found reduced

levels of IgG and increased levels of IgM in serum from ANG patients, and suggested that this might be an endotoxin effect, possibly also influencing the cellular immune response. Whether such changes predispose to development of ANG, or in fact reflect a response to ANG, remains to be determined.

Smoking

Smoking may predispose to ANG in several ways. Smokers in general have poorer oral hygiene and more frequently show signs of gingivitis than nonsmokers, and with increasing tobacco consumption the oral hygiene status tends to deteriorate further. Smoking may also influence tissue reaction to irritation. It is known that smoking leads to contraction of peripheral vessels and this phenomenon has been suggested as one mechanism by which smoking could predispose to ANG (Schwartz & Baumhammers 1972). Smoking also influences polymorphonuclear leukocytes. Kenney et al. (1977) found that oral leukocytes from smokers were less effective in phagocytosis than leukocytes from nonsmokers.

Emotional stress

The role of anxiety and psychic stress in the pathogenesis of ANG has been born out by both psychiatric and biochemical investigations (Moulton et al. 1952, Shannon et al. 1969, Maupin & Bell 1975). Goldhaber & Giddon (1964) and Manhold et al. (1971) have discussed various mechanisms through which stress may influence the gingival tissues. During periods of stress, actions and habits which are under the control of the patient may be influenced. Both the oral hygiene habits and the nutrition of the patient may suffer, and smoking habits may start or alter. In addition, host tissue resistance may be changed by mechanisms acting through the autonomic nervous system and endocrine glands, so that gingival circulation and salivary flow become affected.

References

Emslie, R. D. (1963) Cancrum oris. *Dental Practitioner* **13**, 481-485.

Enwonwu, C. O. (1972) Epidemiological and biochemical studies of necrotizing ulcerative gingivitis and noma (cancrum oris) in Nigerian children. *Archives of Oral Biology* **17**, 1357-1371.

Gibbons, R. J. & MacDonald, J. B. (1961) Degradation of collagenous substrates by *bacteroides melaninogenicus*. *Journal of Bacteriology* **81**, 614-621.

Giddon, D. B., Goldhaber, P. & Dunning, J. M. (1963) Prevalence of reported cases of acute necrotizing ulcerative gingivitis in a university population. *Journal of Periodontology* **34**, 366-371.

Giddon, D. B., Zackin, S. J. & Goldhaber, P. (1964) Acute necrotizing ulcerative gingivitis in college students. *Journal of the American Dental Association* **68**, 381-386.

Gjermo, P. (1974) Chlorhexidine in dental practice. *Journal of Clinical Periodontology* **1**, 143-152.

Goldhaber, P. & Giddon, D. B. (1964) Present concepts concerning the etiology and treatment of acute necrotizing ulcerative gingivitis. *International Dental Journal* **14**, 468-496.

Grupe, H. E. & Wilder, L. S. (1956) Observations of necrotizing gingivitis in 870 military trainees. *Journal of Periodontology* **27**, 255-261.

Heylings, R. T. (1967) Electron microscopy of acute ulcerative gingivitis (Vincent's type). *British Dental Journal* **122**, 51-56.

Jiménez, M. L. & Baer, P. N. (1975) Necrotizing ulcerative gingivitis in children: A 9 year clinical study. *Journal of Periodontology* **46**, 715-720.

Kenney, E. B., Kraal, J. H., Saxe, S. R. & Jones, J. (1977) The effect of cigarette smoke on human oral polymorphonuclear leukocytes. *Journal of Periodontal Research* **12**, 227-234.

Klotz, H. (1973) Differentiation between necrotic ulcerative gingivitis and primary herpetic gingivostomatitis. *New York State Dental Journal* **39**, 283-294.

Kristoffersen, T. & Hofstad, T. (1970) Chemical composition of lipopolysaccharide endotoxins from oral fusobacteria. *Archives of Oral Biology* **15**, 909-916.

Listgarten, M. A. (1965) Electron microscopic observations on the bacterial flora of acute necrotizing ulcerative gingivitis. *Journal of Periodontology* **36**, 328-339.

MacDonald, J. B., Sutton, R. M., Knoll, M. L., Medlener, E. M. & Grainger, R. M. (1956) The pathogenic components of an experimental fusospirochaetal infection. *Journal of Infectious Diseases* **98**, 15-20.

MacDonald, J. B., Socransky, S. S. & Gibbons, R. J. (1963) Aspects of the pathogenesis of mixed anaerobic infections of mucous membranes. *Journal of Dental Research* **42**, 529-544.

MacPhee, T. & Cowley, G. (1981) *Essentials of Periodontology*. 3rd ed., pp. 157-177. Oxford: Blackwell Scientific Publications.

Manhold, J. H., Doyle, J. C. & Weisinger, E. H. (1971) Effects of social stress on oral and other tissues. II. Results offering to a hypothesis for the mechanism of formation of periodontal pathology. *Journal of Periodontology* **42**, 109-111.

Manson, J. D. & Rand, H. (1961) Recurrent Vincent's disease. A survey of 61 cases. *British Dental Journal* **110**, 386-390.

Maupin, C. C. & Bell, W. B. (1975) The relationship of 17-hydroxycorticosteroid to acute necrotizing ulcerative gingivitis. *Journal of Periodontology* **46**, 721-722.

Mergenhagen, S. E., Hampp, E. G. & Scherp, H. W. (1961) Preparation and biological activities of endotoxin from oral bacteria. *Journal of Infectious Diseases* **108**, 304-310.

Miller, S. C. & Greene, H. I. (1958) A worldwide survey of acute necrotizing ulcerative gingivitis: A preliminary report. *Journal Dental Research* **13**, 66-81.

Moulton, R., Ewen, S. & Thieman, W. (1952) Emotional factors in periodontal disease. *Oral Surgery, Oral Medicine and Oral Pathology* **5**, 833-860.

Pickard, H. M. (1973) Historical aspects of Vincent's Disease. *Proceedings of the Royal Society of Medicine* **66**, 695-698.

Pindborg, J. J. (1951a) Gingivitis in military personnel with special reference to ulceromembranous gingivitis. *Odontologisk Revy* **59**, 407-499.

Pindborg, J. J. (1951b) Influence of service in armed forces on incidence of gingivitis. *Journal of the American Dental Association* **42**, 517-522.

Pindborg, J. J., Bhat, M., Devanath, K. R., Narayana, H. R. & Ramachandra, S. (1966) Occurrence of acute necrotizing gingivitis in South Indian children. *Journal of Periodontology* **37**, 14-19.

Pindborg, J. J., Bhat, M. & Roed-Petersen, B. (1967) Oral changes in South Indian children with severe protein deficiency. *Journal of Periodontology* **38**, 218-221.

Proctor, D. B. & Baker, C. G. (1971) Treatment of acute necrotizing ulcerative gingivitis with metronidazole. *Journal of the Canadian Dental Association* **37**, 376-380.

Schwartz, D. M. & Baumhammers, A. (1972) Smoking and periodontal disease. *Periodontal Abstracts* **20**, 103-106.

Shannon, I. L., Kilgore, W. G. & O'Leary, T. J. (1969) Stress as a predisposing factor in necrotizing gingivitis. *Journal of Periodontology* **40**, 240-242.

Sheiham, A. (1966) An epidemiological survey of acute ulcerative gingivitis in Nigerians. *Archives of Oral Biology* **11**, 937-942.

Shields, W. D. (1977) Acute necrotizing ulcera-tive gingivitis. A study of some of the contributing factors and their validity in an army population. *Journal of Periodontology* **48**, 346-349.

Shinn, D. L. (1976) Vincent's disease and its treatment. In *Metronidazole. Proceedings of the International Metronidazole Conference*, pp. 334-340. Montreal, Quebec, Canada, May 26-28.

Van Cauwenberge, P. (1976) De betekenis van de "fusospirillaire associatie" (Plaut-Vincent) *Acta Otorhinolaryngologica Belgica* **30**, 334-345.

Vincent, H. (1898) Sur une forme particulière d'engine differoide (engine à bacilles fusiformes). *Archives Internationales de Laryngologie* **11**, 44-48.

Wennström, J. & Lindhe, J. (1979) Effect of hydrogen peroxide on developing plaque and gingivitis in man. *Journal of Clinical Periodontology* **6**, 115-130.

Wilton, J. M. A., Ivanyi, L. & Lehner, T. (1971) Cell-mediated immunity and humoral antibodies in acute ulcerative gingivitis. *Journal of Periodontal Research* **6**, 9-16.

Wilton, J. M. A. & Lehner, T. (1980) Immunological and microbial aspects of periodontal disease. In *Recent Advances in Clinical Immunology*, No. 2, ed. Thompson, R. A., pp. 145-181. Edinburgh: Churchill Livingstone.

Trauma from Occlusion

Definition and terminology

Trauma from occlusion is a term used to describe pathological alterations or adaptive changes which develop in the periodontium as a result of undue force produced by the masticatory muscles. *Trauma from occlusion* is only one of many terms that have been used to describe such alterations in the periodontium. Other terms often used are: *traumatizing occlusion, occlusal trauma, traumatogenic occlusion, periodontal traumatism, overload*, etc. In addition to producing damage in the periodontal tissues, undue occlusal forces may also cause injurious effects to e.g. the temporomandibular joint, the masticatory muscles, and the pulp tissue. This chapter deals exclusively with the effects of trauma from occlusion on the periodontal tissues.

Trauma from occlusion was defined by Stillman (1917) as "a condition where injury results to the supporting structures of the teeth by the act of bringing the jaws into a closed position". WHO in 1978 defined *trauma from occlusion* as "damage in the periodontium caused by stress on the teeth produced directly or indirectly by teeth of the opposing jaw". Undue or traumatizing forces may act on an individual tooth or on groups of teeth in premature contact relationship; in conjunction with parafunctions such as clenching and bruxism; in conjunction with loss of premolar and molar teeth with an accompanying, gradually developing spread of the anterior teeth of the maxillary jaw, etc.

In the literature, the tissue injury associated with *trauma from occlusion* is often divided into *primary* and *secondary* varieties. The *primary* form includes a tissue reaction (damage), which is elicited around a tooth with normal height of the periodontium, while the *secondary* form is related to situations in which occlusal forces cause injury in a periodontium of reduced height. The distinction between a *primary* and *secondary* form of injury – primary and secondary occlusal trauma – serves no meaningful purpose, since the alterations which occur in the periodontium as a consequence of *trauma from occlusion* are similar and independent of the height of the target tissue, i.e. the periodontium. It is, however, important to understand that symptoms of *trauma from occlusion* may develop only when the magnitude of the load elicited by occlusion is so high that the periodontium around the exposed tooth cannot properly distribute the resulting forces whilst maintaining unaltered tooth position and stability as well as normal height and width of the ligament tissue. This means that in cases of severely reduced height of the periodontium even comparatively small forces may produce traumatic lesions or adaptive changes in the periodontium.

219

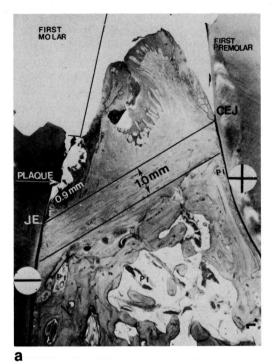
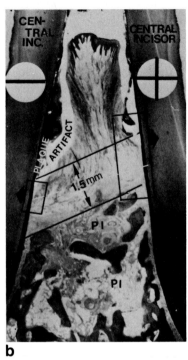

a   b

Figs. 8-1a, b. Microphotographs illustrating two interproximal areas with angular bony defects. ⊖ denotes a tooth no subjected and ⊕ denotes a tooth subjected to trauma from occlusion. In both categories ⊖ and ⊕, the distance between the apical cells of the junctional epithelium and the supporting alveolar bone is about 1-1.5 mm and the distance between the apical extension of plaque and the apical cells of the junctional epithelium about 1 mm. Since the apical cells of the junctional epithelium are located at different levels on the two adjacent teeth, the outline of the bone crest becomes oblique. A radiograph from such a site would disclose the presence of an angular bony defect at a nontraumatized ⊖ tooth.

Trauma from occlusion and plaque associated periodontal disease

Ever since Karolyi (1901) postulated that an interaction may exist between *trauma from occlusion* and *alveolar pyrrohea* different opinions have been presented in the literature regarding this possibility. Already in 1935 and 1938 Box and Stones reported findings from experiments in sheep and monkeys, the results of which seemed to indicate that "traumatogenic occlusion is an etiologic factor in the production of that variety of periodontal disease in which there is vertical pocket formation associated with one or a

varying number of teeth" (Stones 1938). The experiments by Box and Stones, however have been criticized because they lacked proper controls and the claim has been made that the experimental design did not justify the conclusions drawn.

The interaction between trauma from occlusion and plaque associated periodontal disease in humans has often been discussed in connection with *case reports* and with results from *analysis of human autopsy* material. In this chapter findings presented from case reports are not discussed. Results reported from examinations of autopsy material are difficult to appreciate properly and have also often been highly controversial. For example, Glickman (1965, 1967) claimed that the path along which plaque associated, inflammatory lesions spread can be changed if forces of an abnormal magnitude are acting on teeth harboring subgingival plaque. This would imply that the character of the progressive tissue destruction of the periodontium may alter. Instead of an even (horizontal) destruction of the periodontium and the alveolar bone, which occurs in conjunction with plaque associated lesions, areas which are also exposed to abnormal occlusal forces will develop angular bony defects and infrabony pockets. Waerhaug (1979), on the other hand, who examined similar autopsy preparations (Figs. 8-1a, b) concluded from his analysis that angular bony defects and infrabony pockets occur likewise in periodontal areas not affected by trauma from occlusion. The loss of connective tissue attachment and the resorption of bone around teeth are, according to Waerhaug, exclusively the result of an inflammatory lesion associated with subgingival plaque. According to this concept, angular bony defects in conjunction with infrabony pockets develop when the subgingival plaque on one tooth has reached a more apical level than the microbiota on the neighboring tooth, and when the volume of the alveolar bone surrounding the roots is comparatively large. Waerhaug's observations support findings presented by Prichard (1965) and Manson (1976) which imply that the pattern of loss of supporting structures is the result of an interplay between the form and volume of the alveolar bone and the apical extension of the microbial plaque on affected root surface. It may seem that the differences between the conclusions drawn by the two research groups concerning the reason for the development of angular bony defects are surprising. In this context it should be understood, however, that results from examinations of autopsy material must be interpreted with caution since it is impossible in retrospect to describe correctly the occlusion of the living individual.

Glickman's concept

Since the concept of Glickman regarding the effect of trauma from occlusion on the

spread of the plaque associated lesion is often cited, a short presentation of his theory seems pertinent.

The periodontal structures can be divided into 2 zones: (1) the *zone of irritation* and (2) the *zone of codestruction* (Fig. 8-2). The *zone of irritation* includes the marginal and interdental gingiva. The tissue in this zone is not affected by forces of occlusion. This means that gingival inflammation cannot be produced by trauma from occlusion but is the result of irritation from microbial plaque. The plaque associated lesion propagates in an apical direction by first involving the alveolar bone and only later the periodontal ligament area. The progression of this lesion often results in an even (horizontal) bone destruction. The *zone of codestruction* includes the periodontal ligament, the root cementum and the alveolar bone and is coronally demarcated by the transseptal (interdental) and the dentoalveolar collagen fiber bundles (Fig. 8-2). The tissue in this zone may become the seat of a lesion caused by "trauma from occlusion".

The fiber bundles which separate the *zone of codestruction* from the *zone of irritation* can be affected from 2 different directions: (1) from the inflammatory lesion maintained

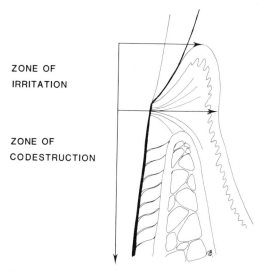

ZONE OF
IRRITATION

ZONE OF
CODESTRUCTION

Fig. 8-2. Schematic drawing of the zone of irritation and the zone of codestruction according to Glickman.

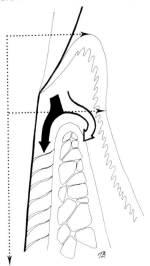

Fig. 8-3. The inflammatory lesion in the zone of irritation can, in teeth not subjected to trauma, propagate into the alveolar bone (open arrow), while in teeth also subjected to trauma from occlusion, the inflammatory infiltrate spreads directly into the periodontal ligament (filled arrow).

aggravating factor in periodontal disease (e.g. Macapanpan & Weinman 1954, Posselt & Emslie 1959, Glickman & Smulow 1962, 1965) while others have refused to accept the existence of a relationship between occlusal trauma and periodontal tissue breakdown (e.g. Lövdahl et al. 1959, Belting & Gupta 1961, Baer et al. 1963, Knowles 1967, Waerhaug 1979).

Much of what has been postulated concerning the effect of trauma from occlusion on the rate and pattern of progression of plaque associated periodontal disease is controversial and difficult to interpret properly. Because of this, it seems necessary to describe the contributions made by means of animal research to our present understanding of the effect of trauma from occlusion on the periodontal structures. Results from such experiments describing the reactions of the normal and, subsequently, the diseased periodontium to these forces are presented below.

by plaque in the *zone of irritation* and (2) from trauma induced changes in the *zone of codestruction.* Through this exposure from 2 different directions the fiber bundles may become dissolved and/or reoriented into a direction parallel to the root surface. The spreading of an inflammatory lesion from the *zone of irritation* directly down into the periodontal ligament (i.e. not via the interdental bone) may thereby be facilitated (Fig. 8-3). This alteration of the "normal" pathway of spread of the plaque associated inflammatory lesion results in the development of angular bony defects. Glickman (1967) in a review paper stated that "trauma from occlusion" is an etiological factor (codestructive factor) of importance in situations where angular bony defects combined with infrabony pockets are found around one or several teeth.

The validity of conclusions drawn from analysis of autopsy preparations has been questioned. Thus, a number of authors claim that trauma from occlusion may be an

The response of the periodontium to "trauma from occlusion"

Healthy periodontium with normal height

Orthodontic type trauma

The reaction of the periodontal tissues to traumatic forces initiated by occlusion has been studied principally in animal experiments. In early publications the reaction of the normal periodontium was studied following the application of forces which were inflicted on teeth in one direction only. Biopsies including tooth and periodontium were harvested after varying experimental time intervals and prepared for histologic examination. Analysis of the tissue sections (Häupl & Psansky 1938, Reitan 1951, Mühlemann & Herzog 1961, Ewen & Stahl 1962, Waerhaug & Hansen 1966, Karring et al. 1982) revealed the following: when a tooth is exposed to unilateral forces of a magnitude, frequency and duration that its periodontal tissues are unable to withstand and distribute while maintaining the stability of the tooth, certain well defined reactions develop in the periodontal ligament, eventually resulting in an adaptation of the periodontal structures to the altered functional demands. If the crown of a tooth is affected by such horizontally directed forces, the tooth tilts in the direction of the force (Fig. 8-4). This tilting results in the development of pressure and tension zones within the marginal and apical parts of the periodontium. The tissue reactions which develop in the *pressure zone* are characterized by increased vascularization, increased vascular permeability, vascular thrombosis, and disorganization of cells and collagen fiber bundles. If the magnitude of the forces is within certain limits allowing the maintenance of the vitality of the periodontal ligament cells, bone resorbing osteoclasts soon appear on the bone surface of the alveolus in the *pressure zone,* and a process of bone resorption is initiated. This phenomenon is called "direct bone resorption".

If the force applied is of higher magnitude, the result may be necrosis of the periodontal ligament tissue in the *pressure zone,* i.e. decomposition of cells, vessels, matrix and fibers (hyalinization). "Direct bone resorption" therefore cannot occur. Instead, osteoclasts appear in marrow spaces within the adjacent bone tissue where the stress concentration is lower than in the periodontal ligament and a process of undermining or "indirect bone resorption" is initiated. Through this reaction the surrounding bone is resorbed until there is a breakthrough to the hyalinized tissue within the *pressure zone*. This breakthrough results in a reduction of the stress in this area, and cells from the neighboring bone or adjacent areas of the periodontal ligament can proliferate into the *pressure zone* and replace the previously hyalinized tissue, thereby reestablishing prerequisites for "direct bone resorption". Irrespective of whether the bone resorption

TIPPING MOVEMENT

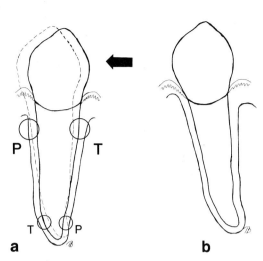

Figs. 8-4a, b. If the crown of a tooth is exposed to excessive, horizontally directed forces (arrow), pressure (P) and tension (T) zones will develop within the marginal and apical parts of the periodontium (a). Within the pressure and tension zones certain tissue alterations take place and the tooth starts to tilt in the direction of the force. When the tooth has escaped the trauma complete regeneration of the periodontal tissues takes place (b). There is no downgrowth of the dentogingival epithelium along the root surface.

is of a direct or an indirect nature the tooth tilts further in the direction of the force.

Concomitantly with tissue alterations in the *pressure zone,* including bone resorption, apposition of bone occurs in the *tension zone* in order to compensate for the increased width of the periodontal ligament in this area. The tooth thereby becomes temporarily hypermobile. When the tooth has tilted to a position where the effect of the forces is nullified, healing of the periodontal tissues takes place in both the *pressure* and the *tension zones* and the tooth becomes stable in its new position. In orthodontic tipping movements, gingival inflammation or loss of connective tissue attachment never occurs in a healthy periodontium, and there will be no apical migration of the dentogingival epithelium. In other words, the supraal-

BODILY MOVEMENT

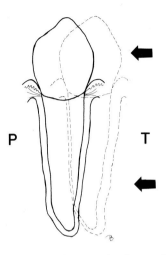

P   T

Fig. 8-5. When a tooth is exposed to forces which produce "bodily tooth movement", e.g. in orthodontic therapy, the pressure (P) and tension (T) zones, depending on the direction of the force, are extended in apical-coronal direction. Neither in conjunction with tipping nor in conjunction with bodily movements of teeth, is the supraalveolar connective tissue affected. Forces of this kind, therefore, will not induce inflammatory reactions in the gingiva. No apical down-growth of the dentogingival epithelium along the root surface occurs.

veolar connective tissue is not influenced by such tipping forces, since this structure is only (in the direction of the force) bordered by hard tissue (the tooth) on one side.

These tissue reactions do not differ fundamentally from those which occur as a consequence of *bodily tooth movement* in orthodontic therapy (Reitan 1951). The main difference is that the *pressure* and *tension* zones, depending on the direction of the force, are more extended in apical-coronal direction along the root surface than in conjunction with tipping movement (Fig. 8-5). Neither in conjunction with tipping nor in conjunction with bodily movements of the tooth, is the supraalveolar connective tissue affected by the force. Unilaterally directed forces, therefore, will not induce inflammat-

ory reactions in the gingiva or loss of connective tissue attachment.

Criticism has been made, however, of experiments in which only unilateral trauma is exerted on teeth (Wentz et al. 1958). It has been suggested that in humans, unlike in the animal experiments described here, the occlusal forces act alternately in one and then in the opposite direction. Such forces have been termed *jiggling forces*.

Jiggling type trauma

Experiments have also been reported in which traumatic forces were exerted on the crowns of the teeth alternately in buccal and lingual or mesial and distal directions and in which the teeth were not allowed orthodontically to move away from the force (e.g. Wentz et al. 1958, Glickman & Smulow 1968, Svanberg & Lindhe 1973, Meitner 1975, Ericsson & Lindhe 1982). In conjunction with so-called "*jiggling type trauma*" no clearcut *pressure* and *tension* zones can be identified but rather a combination of pressure and tension on both sides of the jiggled tooth (Fig. 8-6).

The tissue reactions in the periodontal ligament provoked by the combined *pressure* and *tension* were, however, found to be similar to those reported for the pressure zone in conjunction with orthodontically moved teeth, with the one difference that the periodontal ligament space gradually increased in width on both sides of the tooth. During the phase when the periodontal space gradually increased in width 1) inflammatory changes were present in the ligament tissue 2) active bone resorption occurred and 3) the tooth displayed signs of gradually increasing *(progressive)* mobility. When the effect of the forces applied had been compensated by the increased width of the periodontal space, the ligament tissue showed no signs of increased vascularity or exudation. The tooth was hypermobile but the mobility was no longer progressive in character. Distinction should thus be made between *progressive* on the one, and *increased* tooth mobility on the other hand.

In "*jiggling force*" experiments, per-

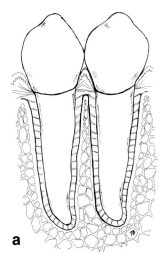

formed on animals with a normal periodontium, the supraalveolar connective tissue was not influenced by the occlusal forces, the reason again being that this tissue structure is bordered on one side only by hard tissue. This means that a gingiva which was noninflamed at the start of the experiment remained noninflamed, but also that an overt inflammatory lesion residing in the supraalveolar connective tissue was not aggravated by the jiggling forces.

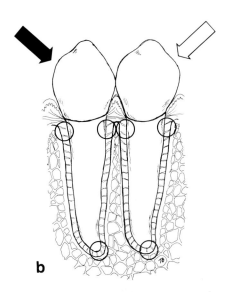

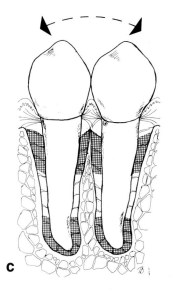

○ ACUTE INFLAMMATION
   COLLAGEN RESORPTION
   BONE RESORPTION
   CEMENTUM RESORPTION

⊞ WIDENED PERIODONTAL LIGAMENT SPACE
   NORMAL TISSUES
   INCREASED TOOTH MOBILITY
   NO LOSS OF CONNECTIVE TISSUE ATTACHMENT

Figs. 8-6a-c. Two mandibular premolars with normal periodontal tissues (a) are exposed to jiggling forces (b) as llustrated by the two arrows. The combined tension and pressure zones (encircled areas) are characterized by signs of cute inflammation including collagen resorption, bone resorption and cementum resorption. As a result of bone esorption the periodontal ligament space gradually increases in size on both sides of the teeth as well as in the eriapical region. When the effect of the force applied has been compensated for by the increased width of the eriodontal ligament space (c), the ligament tissue shows no sign of inflammation. The supraalveolar connective ssue is not affected by the jiggling forces and there is no apical downgrowth of the dentogingival epithelium.

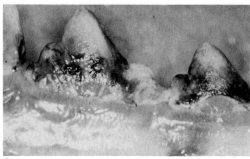

a

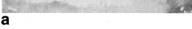

b

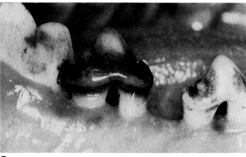

c

Figs. 8-7a-e. Dogs were allowed to accumulate plaque and calculus in the lower premolar regions (a). When around 50% of the periodontal tissue support had been lost (b) the animals were treated by scaling, root planing and pocket elimination. During surgery a notch was prepared in the root at the level of the bone crest. The dogs were subsequently placed on a plaque control program and 8 months later the teeth were surrounded by a healthy periodontium with reduced height (c). The lower fourth premolars in one side of the jaw were exposed to jiggling forces. As a consequence a widened periodontal ligament and increased tooth mobility resulted (d). This increase in tooth mobility and the development of widened periodontal ligament space did not, however, result in apical downgrowth of the dentogingival epithelium (e). The arrow indicates the apical extension of the junctional epithelium (JE) coinciding with the apical border of the notch (N), prepared in the root surface prior to jiggling.

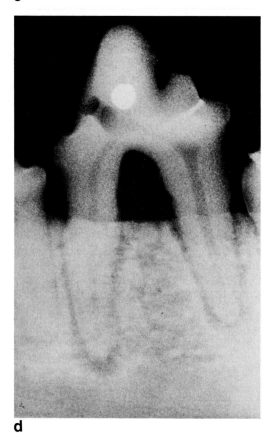

d

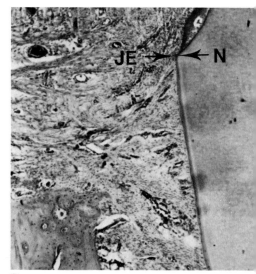

e

Healthy periodontium with reduced height

Progressive periodontal disease is characterized by gingival inflammation and a gradually developing loss of connective tissue attachment and alveolar bone. Treatment of periodontal disease, i.e. removal of plaque and calculus and elimination of pathologically deepened pockets, will result in the reestablishment of a healthy periodontium but with reduced height. The question is whether a healthy periodontium with reduced height has a capacity similar to that of the normal periodontium to adapt to traumatizing occlusal forces (secondary occlusal trauma).

This problem has also been examined in animal experiments (Ericsson & Lindhe 1977). Destructive periodontal disease was initiated in dogs by allowing the animals to accumulate plaque and calculus for a period of 6 months (Fig. 8-7). When around 50% of the periodontal tissue support had been lost (Figs. 8-7a, b), the progressive disease was subjected to treatment by scaling, root planing and pocket elimination. The animals were subsequently, during an 8 month period, enrolled in a careful plaque control program. During this period certain premolars were exposed to traumatizing jiggling forces. The periodontal tissues in the combined *pressure* and *tension* zones reacted to the forces by vascular proliferation, exudation and thrombosis, and bone resorption. In radiographs, widened periodontal ligaments (Fig. 8-7d) could be found around the traumatized teeth which also displayed progressive hypermobility. The gradual increase in the width of the periodontal ligament and the resulting progressive increase in tooth mobility took place during a period of several weeks but eventually terminated. The active bone resorption ceased and the markedly enlarged periodontal ligament tissue regained its normal composition in the histological section; healing had occurred (Fig. 8-7e). The teeth were extremely mobile but surrounded by periodontal structures which

had adapted to the altered functional demands.

During the entire experimental period the supraalveolar connective tissue remained unaffected by the jiggling forces. There was no further loss of connective tissue attachment and no further downgrowth of dentogingival epithelium (Fig. 8-7e). The results from this study clearly reveal that a healthy periodontium with reduced height has a capacity similar to that of a periodontium with normal height to adapt to altered functional demands (Fig. 8-8).

Plaque associated periodontal disease

Experiments carried out on humans and animals have demonstrated that *trauma from occlusion* cannot induce pathological alterations in the supraalveolar connective tissue, i.e. cannot produce inflammatory lesions in a normal gingiva or aggravate a gingival lesion associated with plaque and cannot induce loss of connective tissue attachment. The question remains if abnormal occlusal forces can influence the spread of the plaque associated lesion and enhance the rate of tissue destruction in periodontal disease. This has been studied in animal experiments (Lindhe & Svanberg 1974, Meitner 1975, Nyman et al. 1978, Ericsson & Lindhe 1982). In these experiments progressive and destructive periodontal disease was first initiated in dogs or monkeys by allowing the animals to accumulate plaque and calculus. Teeth thus involved in a progressive periodontal disease were also subjected to trauma from occlusion.

Jiggling forces were exerted on premolars and were found to induce certain tissue reactions in the combined *pressure/tension* zones. The periodontal ligament tissue in these zones, within a few days of the onset of the jiggling forces, displayed signs of inflammation: increased numbers of vessels, increased vascular permeability and exudation, thrombosis, retention of neutrophils and macrophages. On the adjacent bone sur-

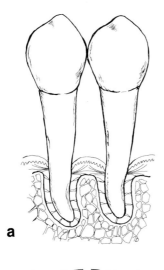

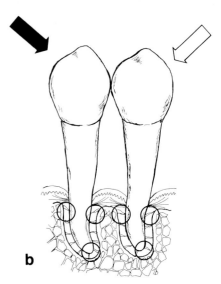

a

b

○ ACUTE INFLAMMATION
COLLAGEN RESORPTION
BONE RESORPTION
CEMENTUM RESORPTION

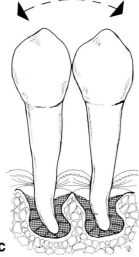

c

⊞ WIDENED PERIODONTAL LIGAMENT SPACE
NORMAL TISSUE COMPOSITION
INCREASED TOOTH MOBILITY
NO FURTHER LOSS OF CONNECTIVE
TISSUE ATTACHMENT

Figs. 8-8a-c. Two lower premolars are surrounded by a healthy periodontium with reduced height (a). If such premolars are subjected to traumatizing forces of the jiggling type (b) a series of alterations occurs in the periodontal ligament tissue (encircled areas). These alterations result in a widened periodontal ligament space (c) and in an increased tooth mobility but do not lead to further loss of connective tissue attachment.

faces there was a large number of osteoclasts. Since the teeth could not orthodontically move away from the jiggling forces, the periodontal ligament of both zones gradually increased in width, the teeth became hypermobile (progressive tooth mobility) and angular bony defects could be detected in the radiographs. The forces were nullified by the increased width of the periodontal ligament.

If the forces applied were of such magnitude that the periodontal structures could become adapted to the altered functional demands, the *progressive* increase of the tooth mobility terminated within a few weeks. The active bone resorption ceased out the angular bone destruction persisted as well as the *increased* tooth mobility. The periodontal ligament had an increased width but a normal tissue composition. Histological examination of biopsies revealed that this adaptation had occurred with no greater apical proliferation of the dento-gingival epithelium than was caused by the plaque associated lesion (Figs. 8-9a, b; Meitner 1975). This means that occlusal forces which allow adaptive alterations to develop in the *pressure/tension* zones of the periodontal ligament will not aggravate a plaque associated periodontal disease (Fig. 8-10).

If, however, the jiggling forces had such magnitude and direction that during the course of the study (6 months) the tissues in the *pressure/tension* zones could not become adapted, the injury in the *zones of codestruction* had a more permanent character. The periodontal ligament in the *pressure/tension* zones displayed for several months signs of inflammation (vascular proliferation, exudation, thrombosis, retention of neutrophils and macrophages, collagen destruction). Osteoclasts residing on the walls of the alveolus maintained the bone resorptive process which resulted in a gradual widening of the periodontal ligament in the *pressure/tension* zones (Fig. 8-11). As a consequence, the resulting angular bone destruction was continuous and the mobility of the teeth remained progressive. The plaque associated lesion in the "zone of irritation" and the inflammatory lesion in the "zone of codestruction" merged; the dentogingival

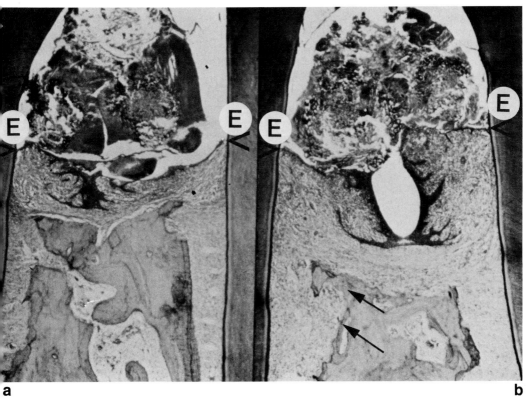

a   b

Figs. 8-9a, b. A composite photomicrograph illustrating the interdental space between two pairs (a and b) of teeth. The teeth have been subjected to experimental, ligature induced periodontitis and the teeth in (b) also to repetitive mechanical injury. In (b), there is considerable loss of alveolar bone and an angular widening of the periodontal ligament space (arrows). However, the apical downgrowth of the dentogingival epithelium in the two areas (a and b) is similar. E indicates the apical level of the dentogingival epithelium. (Courtesy of Dr. Meitner).

229

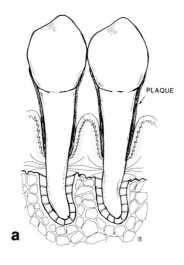

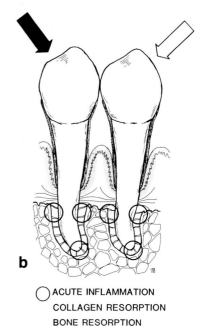

○ ACUTE INFLAMMATION
COLLAGEN RESORPTION
BONE RESORPTION
CEMENTUM RESORPTION

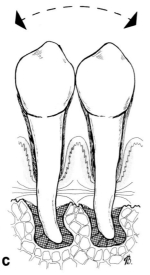

▦ WIDENED PERIODONTAL LIGAMENT SPACE
NORMAL TISSUE COMPOSITION
INCREASED TOOTH MOBILITY
NO FURTHER LOSS OF CONNECTIVE
TISSUE ATTACHMENT

Figs. 8-10 a-c. Two lower premolars with supra- and subgingival plaque, advanced bone loss and periodontal pockets of a suprabony character (a). Note the connective tissue infiltrate (shadowed areas) and the noninflamed connective tissue between the alveolar bone and the apical portion of the infiltrate. If these teeth are subjected to traumatizing forces of the jiggling type (b) pathological and adaptic alterations occur within the periodontal ligament space (encircled areas). These tissue alterations which include bone resorption result in a widened periodontal ligament space and increased tooth mobility but no further loss of connective tissue attachment (c).

epithelium proliferated in an apical direction and periodontal disease was aggravated (Figs. 8-12, 8-13; Lindhe & Svanberg 1974).

Recently a study was published from another experiment in the dog (Ericsson & Lindhe 1982) in which the effect was assessed of a prolonged period of jiggling force application on the rate of progression of plaque associated, marginal periodontitis. Thus, in dogs with continuing periodontal disease, certain teeth were exposed to jiggling forces during a period of 10 months.

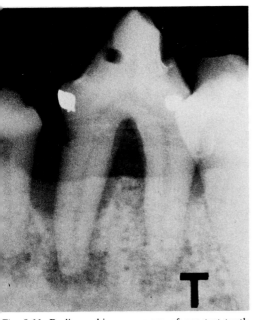

Fig. 8-11. Radiographic appearance of one test tooth (T) at the termination of an experiment in which periodontitis was induced by ligature placement and plaque accumulation and in which trauma of the jiggling type was induced. Note angular bone loss particularly around the mesial root of the lower premolar. (From Lindhe & Svanberg 1974).

in loss of connective tissue attachment. *Trauma from occlusion cannot induce periodontal tissue breakdown.* Trauma from occlusion does, however, result in resorption of alveolar bone leading to an increased tooth mobility which can be of transient or permanent character. This bone resorption with resulting increased tooth mobility should be regarded as a physiologic adaptation of the periodontal ligament and surrounding alveolar bone to the traumatizing forces, i.e. to altered functional demands.

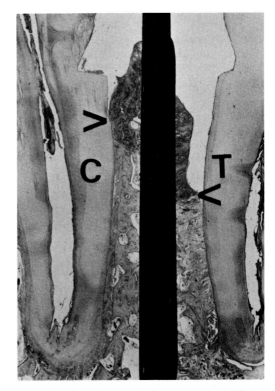

Fig. 8-12. Microphotographs from one control (C) and one test (T) tooth after 240 days of experimental periodontal tissue breakdown (C and T) and 180 days of trauma from occlusion of the jiggling type (T). The arrow heads denote the apical position of the dentogingival epithelium. The attachment loss is more pronounced in T than in C. (From Lindhe & Svanberg 1974).

Control teeth were not jiggled. Fig. 8-14a illustrates the marked periodontal tissue breakdown around a tooth which for several months was exposed to plaque infection combined with jiggling trauma and Fig. 8-14b illustrates a control tooth which was exposed to plaque infection only.

Conclusions

Experiments, carried out on humans as well as animals, have produced convincing evidence that neither unilateral forces nor jiggling forces, applied to teeth with a *healthy* periodontium, result in pocket formation or

231

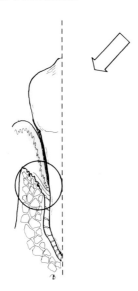

○ INCREASING PERIODONTAL LIGAMENT SPACE

INCREASING TOOTH MOBILITY

ENHANCED LOSS OF CONNECTIVE

TISSUE ATTACHMENT

Fig. 8-13. Illustration of a tooth where subgingival plaque has mediated the development of an infiltrated soft tissue (shadowed area) and an infrabony pocket. When trauma from occlusion of the jiggling type is inflicted (arrow) on the crown of this tooth, the associated pathological alterations occur within a zone of the periodontium (encircled area) which is also occupied by the inflammatory cell infiltrate (shadowed area). In this situation the increasing tooth mobility may also be associated with an enhanced loss of connective tissue attachment and further downgrowth of dentogingival epithelium.

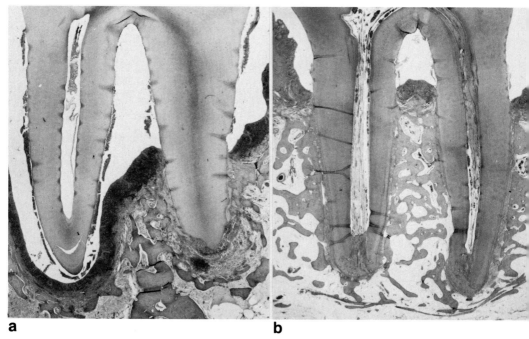

a
b

Figs. 8-14a-e. Fig. 8-14a illustrates the periodontal conditions around a tooth which has been exposed to trauma from occlusion (of the jiggling type) for 300 days in combination with plaque associated experimental periodontitis. Fig. 8-14b illustrates the condition of a control tooth from the same dog in which experimental periodontitis but no jiggling trauma had been in operation. Note the difference between (a) and (b) regarding the degree of bone destruction and proliferation of the dentogingival epithelium which in (a) has surrounded the apex of the tooth. Note also in (a) the location of the subgingival plaque at the apex of the root. (From Ericsson & Lindhe 1982).

In teeth with continuing plaque associated periodontal disease, trauma from occlusion may, however, under certain conditions enhance the rate of progression of the disease, i.e. act as a cofactor in the destructive process. From the clinical point of view, this knowledge strengthens the demand for proper treatment of plaque associated disease. This treatment will arrest the destruc- tion of the periodontal tissues even if the occlusal trauma persists. A treatment directed towards the trauma alone, i.e. occlusal adjustment or splinting, may reduce the mobility of the traumatized teeth but will not arrest the rate of further breakdown of the supporting apparatus. (For detailed discussion on treatment of teeth exhibiting increased mobility see Chapter l2).

References

Baer, P., Kakehashi, S., Littleton, N. W., White, C. L. & Lieberman, J. E. (1963) Alveolar bone loss and occlusal wear. *Periodontics* **1**, 91.

Belting, C. M. & Gupta, O. P. (1961) The influence of psychiatric disturbances on the severity of periodontal disease. *Journal of Periodontology* **32**, 219-226.

Box, H. K. (1935) Experimental traumatogenic occlusion in sheep. *Oral Health* **25**, 9-25.

Ericsson, I. & Lindhe, J. (1977) Lack of effect of trauma from occlusion on the recurrence of experimental periodontitis. *Journal of Clinical Periodontology* **4**, 115-127.

Ericsson, I. & Lindhe, J. (1982) The effect of longstanding jiggling on experimental marginal periodontitis in the beagle dog. *Journal of Clinical Periodontology* **9**, 497-503.

Ewen, S. J. & Stahl. S. S. (1962) The response of the periodontium to chronic gingival irritation and long-term tilting forces in adult dogs. *Oral Surgery, Oral Medicine and Oral Pathology* **15**, 1426-1433.

Glickman, I. (1965) Clinical significance of trauma from occlusion. *Journal of the American Dental Association* **70**, 607-618.

Glickman, I. (1967) Occlusion and periodontium. *Journal of Dental Research* **46**, Supplement 1, 53.

Glickman, I. & Smulow, J. B. (1962) Alterations in the pathway of gingival inflammation into the underlying tissues induced by excessive occlusal forces. *Journal of Periodontology* **33**, 7-13.

Glickman, I. & Smulow, J. B. (1965) Effect of excessive occlusal forces upon the pathway of gingival inflammation in humans. *Journal of Periodontology* **36**, 141-147.

Glickman, I. & Smulow, J. B. (1968) Adaptive alterations in the periodontium of the Rhesus monkey in chronic trauma from occlusion. *Journal of Periodontology* **39**, 101-105.

Häupl, K. & Psansky, R. (1938) Histologische Untersuchungen der Wirkungsweise der in der Funktions-Kiefer-Orthopedie verwendeten Apparate. *Deutsche Zahn-, Mund- und Kieferheilkunde* **5**, 214.

Karolyi, M. (1901) Beobachtungen über Pyorrhea alveolaris. *Österreichisch-Ungarische Viertejahresschrift für Zahnheilkunde* **17**, 279.

Karring, T., Nyman, S., Thilander, B. & Magnusson, I. (1982) Bone regeneration in orthodontically produced alveolar bone dehiscences. *Journal of Periodontal Research* **17**, 309-315.

Knowles, J. W. (1967) Occlusal interferences and loss of periodontal attachment. *IADR* Abstract No. 517.

Lindhe, J. & Svanberg, G. (1974) Influence of trauma from occlusion on progression of experimental periodontitis in the Beagle dog. *Journal of Clinical Periodontology* **1**, 3-14.

Lövdal, A., Schei, O., Waerhaug, J. & Arno, A. (1959) Tooth mobility and alveolar bone resorption as a function of occlusal stress and oral hygiene. *Acta Odontologica Scandinavica* **17**, 61-77.

Macapanpan, L. C. & Weinmann, J. P. (1954) The influence of injury to the periodontal membrane on the spread of gingival inflammation. *Journal of Dental Research* **33**, 263-272.

Manson, J. D. (1976) Bone morphology and bone loss in periodontal disease. *Journal of Clinical Periodontology* **3**, 14-22.

Meitner, S. W. (1975) *Co-destructive Factors of Marginal Periodontitis and Repetitive Mechanical Injury*. Thesis. Rochester, USA: Eastman Dental Center and The University of Rochester.

Mühlemann, H. R. & Herzog, H. (1961) Tooth mobility and microscopic tissue changes produced by experimental occlusal trauma. *Helvetica Odontologica Acta* **5**, 33-39.

Nyman, S., Lindhe, J. & Ericsson, I. (1978) The effect of progressive tooth mobility on destructive periodontitis in the dog. *Journal of Clinical Periodontology* **7**, 351-360.

Posselt, U. & Emslie, R. D. (1959) Occlusal disharmonies and their effect on periodontal diseases. *International Dental Journal* **9**, 367-381.

Prichard, J. F. (1965) *Advanced Periodontal Disease*. Philadelphia: W.B. Saunders.

Reitan, K. (1951) The initial tissue reaction incident to orthodontic tooth movement as related to the influence of function. *Acta Odontologica Scandinavica* **10**, Supplement 6.

Stillman, P. R. (1917) The management of pyorrhea. *Dental Cosmos* **59**, 405.

Stones, H. H. (1938) An experimental investigation into the association of traumatic occlusion with periodontal disease. *Proceedings of the Royal Society of Medicine* **31**, 479-495.

Svanberg, G. & Lindhe, J. (1973) Experimental tooth hypermobility in the dog. A methodological study. *Odontologisk Revy* **24**, 269-282.

Waerhaug, J. (1979) The infrabony pocket and its relationship to trauma from occlusion and subgingival plaque. *Journal of Periodontology* **50** 355-365.

Waerhaug, J. & Hansen, E. R. (1966) Periodontal changes incident to prolonged occlusal overload in monkeys. *Acta Odontologica Scandinavica* **24**, 91-105.

Wentz, F. M., Jarabak, J. & Orban, B. (1958) Experimental occlusal trauma imitating cuspal interferences. *Journal of Periodontology* **29** 117-127.

Interrelationships Between Periodontics and Endodontics

Introduction

Periodontal disease is but one of several diseases that present clinical and radiographic symptoms of inflammation of the supporting tissues. Hence, symptoms such as deep periodontal pockets, suppuration from such pockets, swelling of the marginal gingiva, fistulae, tenderness to percussion, increased mobility and angular bone destruction are not exclusively the result of plaque associated periodontal disease. These conditions may also be initiated and maintained by irritants in the root canal system of the affected tooth.

The differential diagnosis between an endodontic* and a marginal** lesion is seldom difficult, since endodontic lesions most often induce symptoms from the apical periodontium, while symptoms of the marginal lesions are usually confined to the coronal periodontium. However, the clinical symptoms may sometimes be confusing and their origin misinterpreted. What may appear as a marginal lesion may actually be a pulpal problem and *vice versa*. The establishment of a correct diagnosis may also be complicated by the fact that both marginal and endodontic lesions can simultaneously affect the same tooth. In such a situation, one of the lesions may either be the result of, or the cause of, the other, or the two lesions may constitute two separate processes which have developed independently.

Proper diagnosis of the various disorders affecting the pulpal and periodontal tissues is important in order to preclude unnecessary and even detrimental treatment. The clinician should, therefore, be well acquainted with the mechanisms involved in disease development as well as with available diagnostic measures.

The purpose of this chapter is to describe possible interrelationships between disease processes in the pulp and in the marginal periodontium. Emphasis will be placed upon

---

* In the following text the term *endodontic lesion* is used to denote an inflammatory process in the periodontal tissues resulting from noxious agents present in the root canal system of the tooth (usually a root canal infection).

** The term *marginal lesion* is used to denote an inflammatory process in the periodontal tissues resulting from plaque accumulation on the external tooth surfaces.

diagnosis and treatment. Since, in addition, endodontic treatment measures may induce alterations in the periodontium, and periodontal treatment measures may provoke alterations in the pulp, such complications will also be discussed.

Influence of pathologic conditions in the pulp on the periodontium

Vital pulp – pulpitis

Inflammatory alterations in the vital pulp seldom cause significant lesions in the periodontal tissues, i.e. rarely does the inflamed pulp produce sufficient amounts of irritants to induce severe lesions in the adja-

cent periodontium. Teeth with pulpitis, however, may occasionally demonstrate radiographic signs of inflammation in the apical periodontium, i.e. disruption of the lamina dura with widening of the periodontal ligament space or a minor periapical radiolucency. In such cases, clinical symptoms of spontaneous pain, thermal sensitivity or tenderness to percussion may or may not be present. Hence, it is important to point out that pulpitis does not cause pronounced destruction of the periodontal tissues.

Nonvital pulp – necrosis

Chronic periapical lesion

Involvement of the periodontal tissue is frequently a result of necrosis of the pulp. In the nonvital pulp microorganisms find condi-

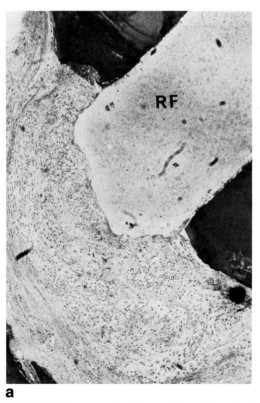

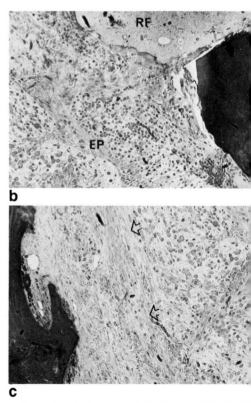

a   c

Fig. 9-1. Light microscopic demonstration of a small chronic inflammatory lesion associated with a rootfilled tooth (a). Close to the rootfilling (RF) numbers of plasma cells and lymphocytes have infiltrated the connective tissue. Epithelium (EP) has proliferated through the lesion (b). In peripheral parts only few inflammatory cells are seen and collagen rich connective tissue (arrows) adjacent to bone tissue circumscribes the lesion (c). (From Bergenholtz et al 1983).

ions which favor their growth. The bacteria will release various substances (enzymes, metabolites, antigens, etc.) which will emerge into the periodontium through canals and foramina that regularly connect the pulp chamber with the periodontal ligament. Once in the periodontium, the bacterial products may induce inflammatory alterations resulting in destruction of periodontal tissue fibers and resorption of adjacent alveolar bone. Resorption of tooth substance may also be observed. Most frequently, such inflammatory lesions develop around the apex of the tooth.

The extension of the periodontal tissue destruction is largely dependent on the virulence of the bacteria in the root canal and the capacity of the host to encapsulate and neutralize the bacterial products released into the periodontium. In most cases a balanced host-parasite stasis will develop and a chronic inflammatory process may remain unchanged in size for many years. However, cyst transformation may occasionally occur which, in turn, can result in extensive destruction of the alveolar bone.

Histopathologically, the chronic periapical inflammatory lesion is characterized by a richly vascularized, granulation tissue which, to a varying degree, is infiltrated by inflammatory cells (Fig. 9-1). The inflammatory cell composition of these lesions may vary, probably depending on the intensity and nature of the irritants affecting the periodontal tissues. In some lesions plasma cells and lymphocytes may predominate (Bergenholtz et al. 1983), as they do in advanced lesions of plaque associated periodontitis (Lindhe et al. 1980). In other lesions macrophages or neutrophilic granulocytes may be present in large numbers (Yanagisawa 1980, Stern et al. 1981, Weiner et al. 1982).

Lateral lesion
Inflammatory processes in the periodontium as a result of root canal infection may not only be localized at the tooth apex but may also appear along the lateral aspects of the root (Fig. 9-2) and in furcation areas of 2- and 3-rooted teeth (Fig. 9-3). In such cases the inflammatory process may be induced and maintained by bacterial products which reach the periodontium through accessory canals.

Accessory canals normally harbor vessels which connect the circulatory system of the pulp with that of the periodontal ligament. Such anastomoses are formed during the early phases of tooth development. During

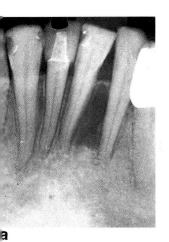 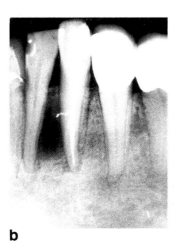 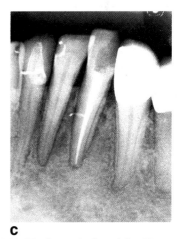

a   **b**   **c**

Fig. 9-2. Destruction of alveolar bone is observed between the roots of 31 and 32 (a). Vitality test indicated that 32 was nonvital. Endodontic treatment was performed (b). On condensing gutta percha into the canal, an accessory canal communicating with the bony defect was filled. Recall 2 years after treatment (c) demonstrated an obvious reduction of the bony lesion. (Courtesy of Dr. Conrad Jacobsson).

the completion of root formation several anastomoses become blocked and reduced in width by continuous deposition of dentin and root cementum. However, patent communications of varying size, number and location in the root, between the pulp and the periodontal ligament, may remain in adult individuals.

Accessory canals can be observed in all groups of teeth. The majority of the canals are found in the apical portion of the root. In the middle and cervical portions the incidence of accessory canals is small. In a study of 1140 extracted teeth from adult human subjects, DeDeus (1975) reported tha accessory root canals occurred in 313 teetl (27.4%). The canals were distributed on var ious levels in the roots as depicted in Fig. 9-4

In recent years considerable interest ha been devoted to the study of the occurrenc of accessory canals in the furcation area of 2 and 3-rooted teeth (Fig. 9-5). A variety o techniques has been used which may explai the divergent results obtained. Some studie report frequencies of furcation canals at bet ween 20% and 60% (Lowman et al. 1973 Vertucci & Williams 1974, Gutmann 1978) whereas others have failed to demonstrat the presence of such canals (Pineda & Kut tler 1972, Hession 1977).

Clinically it is seldom possible to identif accessory canals unless they have been fille with a radio-opaque material in conjunctio with endodontic therapy (Fig. 9-2b). A lateral position of a radiolucency associate with a pulpless tooth may also indicate th presence of an accessory canal (Fig. 9-2a).

The clinical significance of accessory ca nals in spreading infectious products from necrotic pulp to the periodontium is no clear, and no scientific documentation is ye available concerning· the incidence o endodontically derived lesions in the margi nal periodontium. Clinical observation demonstrate such lesions (Fig. 9-3) but th incidence is low.

No evidence has yet been presented indi cating that nonvital pulp can affect th periodontal tissues through normal walls o dentin and cementum. Even if the width o the dentinal tubules is large enough for th passage of both bacteria and bacterial prod ucts, an intact layer of cementum evidentl acts as an effective barrier for such penetra tion into the periodontal structures (Stallar 1968).

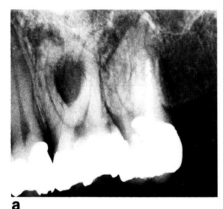

a

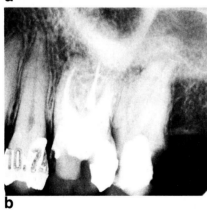

b

Fig. 9-3. Loss of interradicular bone of an upper molar simulating a marginal lesion (a). The process, however, had no marginal genesis as indicated by the following findings: (1) periodontal probing failed to identify a pocket, (2) the pulp was nonvital, (3) endodontic treatment resulted in complete resolution of the lesion (b). (Courtesy of Dr. Björn Ödesjö).

Acute periapical lesion

A chronic inflammatory lesion in th periodontal tissues, induced and maintaine by an infection in nonvital pulp, often has limited extension around the apex of th tooth or at the orifice of a lateral canal. How ever, following an acute exacerbation of chronic lesion, rapid and extensive destruction of the supporting tissues can occur. An acute periapical lesion can also develop as a direct extension of a pulpal abscess into the periapical tissues.

Abscesses derived from a periapical lesion drain off in different directions, of which drainage into the gingival sulcus/pocket is of particular interest with respect to the effect on the periodontal tissues. The process can be accompanied, albeit not always, by clinical signs of acute inflammation such as throbbing pain, tenderness to pressure and percussion, increased tooth mobility, and swelling of the marginal gingiva. Such symptoms are also typical of periodontal abscesses (see Fig. 9-20).

In general, drainage of periapical abscesses into the sulcus/pocket follows 1 of 2 routes (Fig. 9-6):
1) The suppurative lesion may produce a sinus tract along the periodontal ligament space (periodontal ligament fistulation; Fig. 9-6a). This usually results in only a narrow opening of the fistula into the gingival sulcus/pocket. *Such a fistula can readily be probed down to the apex of the tooth* (Fig. 9-

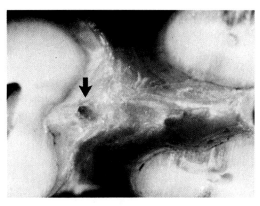

Fig. 9-5. Photograph of the furcation area of an extracted maxillary molar with cut roots demonstrating the opening of an accessory canal (arrow). Scanning electron microscopic observations indicate that the incidence of such furcation foramina is high (Burch & Hulen 1974, Koenigs et al. 1974), whereas the number of openings at the pulpal floor is small (Perlich et al. 1981). This suggests that furcation foramina at the external surface of the root do not necessarily represent patency to the pulpal chamber. (Courtesy of Dr. Robert C. Bowers).

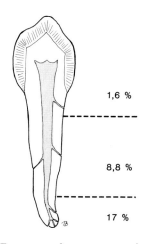

Fig. 9-4. Frequency of accessory canals at different levels of the root. The data are average values obtained from DeDeus (1975). Observations were made after the teeth had been rendered transparent and the root-canal system filled with China ink. The figures for the cervical portion of the root include those of the bi and trifurcations.

7b), *where no increased probing depth otherwise exists around the tooth.* In multi-rooted teeth a periodontal ligament fistulation can drain off in the furcation area. The resulting lesion often resembles a "through and through" furcation of a marginal lesion (Fig. 9-8).
2) A periapical abscess can also perforate the cortical bone close to the apex, elevating the soft tissue including the periosteum from the bone, to drain into the gingival sulcus/pocket (Fig. 9-6b). This type of drainage will result in a wide opening of the fistula into the sulcus/pocket (extraosseous fistulation), and is most often seen at the buccal aspect of the tooth. Since this type of fistula is not associated with loss of bone tissue at the inner walls of the alveolus, a periodontal probe cannot penetrate into the periodontal ligament space.

It is essential to be aware that both types of lesions described are strictly endodontic and are not marginally derived. Therefore, following proper endodontic treatment, both types of fistulae can be expected to heal rapidly without a persistent periodontal defect (Figs. 9-7, 9-8, 9-9); there is generally no need for adjunctive periodontal therapy. The endodontic treatment of the involved tooth should be performed without delay to prevent repeated exacerbations and the establishment of a permanent apical-marginal communication. If a periodontal ligament fistulation passes undetected or is left untreated, the potential exists that downgrowth of plaque and epithelium might occur along the affected root surface, which implies that in this situation endodontic treatment might have less chance of success, possibly having to be supplemented with adjunctive periodontal treatment.

Combined endodontic – marginal lesion

In cases of advanced loss of attachment resulting from plaque associated periodontal disease, an apical inflammatory lesion of endodontic origin may not have to expand far coronally to communicate with the marginal lesion. Apical-marginal communications of this type have been termed *"true combined endoperio lesions"* (Simon 1976,

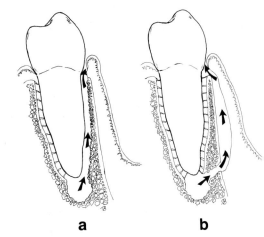

a　　　　　　　**b**

Fig. 9-6. Schematic illustration of drainage of a periapical abscess into the gingival sulcus/pocket a=periodontal ligament fistulation. b=extraosseou fistulation.

Harrington 1979). Such lesions are characterized by extensive loss of attachment resulting both from the root canal infection and the plaque accumulation on the external root surface. Treatment of such combined lesions does not differ from treatment given

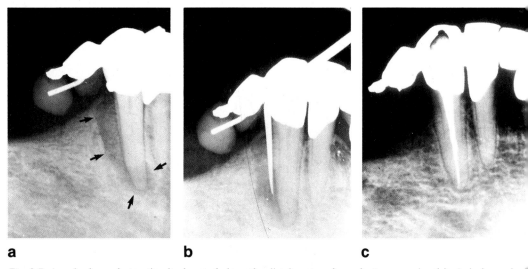

a　　　　　　　　　　**b**　　　　　　　　　　**c**

Fig. 9-7. Angular bone destruction is observed along the distal root surface of a lower canine (a). Apical-marginal communication was confirmed by periodontal probing (b). Endodontic treatment resulted in complete reestablishment of the periodontal structures demonstrating that the periodontal defect in this case was the result of endodontic infection only. (Courtesy of Dr. Ralph Milthon).

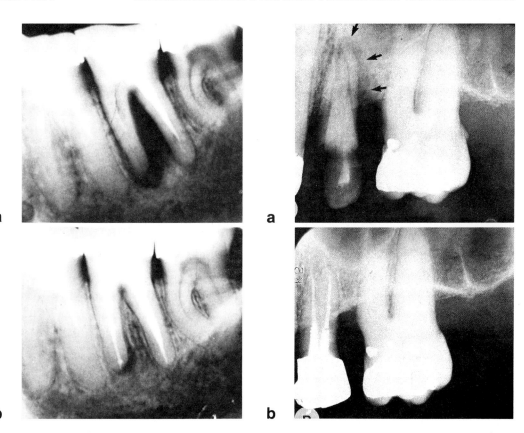

a

b

a

b

Fig. 9-8. Severe destruction of the bone tissue in the interradicular area and along the mesial root of a first mandibular molar following acute exacerbation of a periapical lesion (a). One year after endodontic treatment reformation of bone and reestablishment of a normal width of the periodontal ligament space occurred in the furcation area, while a small radiolucency persisted around the apex. (Courtesy of Dr. Sven-Erik Hamp).

Fig. 9-9. Radiolucent area along the distal root surface of tooth 25 combined with a horizontal marginal bone destruction (a). The tooth pulp was nonvital. Six months after endodontic treatment normal periodontal structures had been reformed in the previous area of angular bone destruction. (Courtesy of Dr. Conrad Jacobsson).

when the two disorders occur separately. The part of the lesion sustained by the root canal infection may usually be expected to resolve after proper endodontic treatment (Figs 9-9, 9-10). The part of the lesion caused by the plaque infection can also heal following periodontal therapy, although little or no regeneration of the attachment apparatus will occur (see Chapter 19). This suggests that the prognosis for regeneration of the attachment apparatus seems to be the more favorable, the larger the part of the lesion is, which is caused by pulpal disease. However, to what extent one or the other of the two

disorders (endodontic or marginal) has affected the periodontal tissues is clinically seldom possible to evaluate. This problem is illustrated by the case described in Fig. 9-10.

Conclusion: Where periodontal involvement, encompassing either the apical or the marginal periodontium or both, is associated with nonvital pulp, endodontic treatment is indicated. Debridement and disinfection of the root canal system should be performed prior to periodontal treatment. If an endodontic lesion is overlooked, periodontal treatment will not result in proper heal-

241

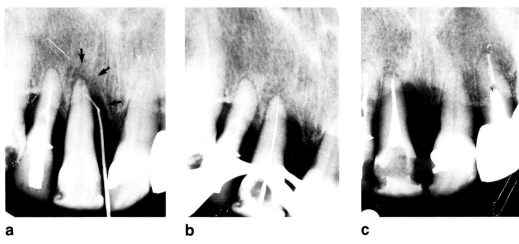

a   b   c

Fig. 9-10. At the mesial root surface of tooth 11 a deep, angular, bony defect extends to the apical level of the tooth. A gutta percha cone has been inserted into the gingival pocket as an indicator of its depth (a). The tooth exhibited markedly increased mobility in both horizontal and vertical direction. No other clinical symptoms of inflammation were present. Vitality tests indicated that the pulp was nonvital, suggesting the diagnosis of a combined lesion. A combined endodontic and periodontal treatment was attempted since extraction of the tooth would have resulted in extensive prosthetic treatment. Endodontic treatment (b) was instituted followed by scaling and root planing in conjunction with flap surgery. Treatment resulted in healing of the apical part of the destruction (c) and in the arrest of the progression of periodontal disease. However, the marginal part of the angular defect failed to heal with bone fill.

ing. It should be understood that a marginal lesion may be responsible for the entire loss of the supporting apparatus around a tooth and in addition, be the cause of the breakdown of the pulp tissue (see below). In such cases endodontic treatment alone will not contribute to healing.

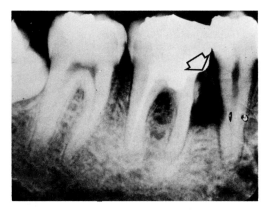

Fig. 9-11. Destruction of alveolar bone between tooth 45 and tooth 46 as a result of leakage of paraformaldehyde applied in order to devitalize the pulp of tooth 46. A bone sequestrum has formed (arrow).

Influence of endodontic treatment measures on the periodontium

When breakdown of the periodontal tissues is associated with a root filled tooth, endodontic etiology should be considered particularly if the root filling is defective. Infectious products may leak through apical or accessory canals to the periodontium from voids in the root filling. In addition, periodontal lesions may be caused by infectious products released from sites of root perforations or root fractures. Periodontal inflammatory lesions may also result from mechanical as well as chemical irritation initiated in conjunction with root canal preparation in endodontic therapy. Medication for canal irrigation and disinfection and materials for obturation used in modern endodontics, however, are comparatively well tolerated by the connective tissue of the periodontium, even if, during treatment they are forced into the periodontal ligament. On the other hand, strong antiseptic drugs used for root canal disinfection and pulp devitalization can cause damage to the periodontium. In particular, mortal pulp devitalization (mortal pulpotomy, mortal pulpectomy) utilizing paraformaldehyde is hazardous, since the agent may leak into the periodontal tissues, e.g. along the margins of temporary restorations or through accessory canals. Severe necrosis of the periodontal ligament and the alveolar bone may be the result of such leakage (Fig. 9-11).

Root perforation

During endodontic treatment, and in conjunction with preparation of root canals for insertion of posts, instrumentation can accidentally cause perforation of the root and wounding of the periodontal ligament. Perforations can be produced through the lateral walls of the root or through the pulpal floor in multirooted teeth. At the site of such perforations, an inflammatory reaction will develop in the periodontium. If the perforation is located close to the gingival margin, the resulting lesion can merge with the gingival sulcus/pocket. This may result in loss of attachment and downgrowth of dentogingival epithelium. Other complications in conjunction with root perforation can involve exacerbation of the periodontal inflammatory process and development of clinical symptoms, similar to those of a periodontal abscess: acute pain, swelling, drainage of pus into the pocket, increased mobility and further loss of fibrous attachment (Fig. 9-12).

Root perforations are identified by the occurrence of sudden pain and bleeding during preparation of root canals coronal to the working length. These symptoms, however, are hardly observable if the perforation is made in conjunction with pulpectomy performed under local anesthesia. In such cases the perforation may be detected during later treatment of the root canal by the presence of coagulated blood or granulation tissue

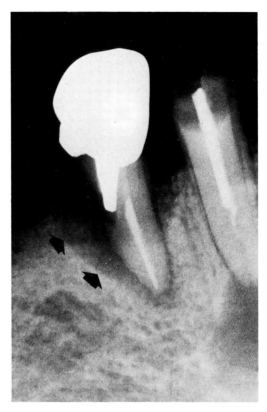

Fig. 9-12. Angular bone destruction at the distal root surface of a mandibular premolar (arrows). The root is perforated. Conceivably, this occurred in conjunction with preparation of the root canal for insertion of the dowel. Clinical symptoms involved drainage of pus from the pocket and increased tooth mobility. The tooth was extracted.

which has proliferated into the pulp from the site of perforation. Elimination of such granulation tissue can be accompanied by bleeding difficult to stop.

As soon as a root perforation has been detected, treatment should be initiated. Fig. 9-13 demonstrates the successful result of treatment of a perforation made in the furcation of a mandibular molar. Healing of lesions in the periodontium depends largely on whether bacterial infection can be excluded from the wound area by tight obturation of the perforation site. For various reasons this may be difficult to accomplish. If the perforation is made at an oblique angle

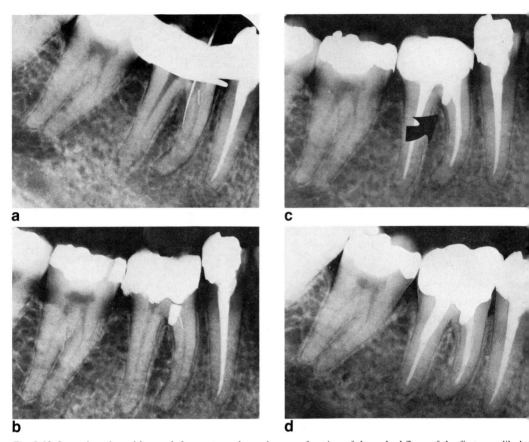

Fig. 9-13. In conjunction with search for root canal openings, perforation of the pulpal floor of the first mandibula molar occurred (a). The perforation was immediately obturated with gutta percha (b). One month after treatment slight radiolucency appeared at the perforation site in the periodontium (c). After an observation period of 2 year normal periodontal conditions had been reestablished both clinically and radiographically (d). (Courtesy of Dr Gunnar Heden).

in the lateral wall of the root and if it has been produced by a reamer or a root canal file, the artificial canal often has an oval shaped orifice into the periodontium. Obturation of such perforations with gutta percha can result in a defective seal and subsequent bacterial irritation of the periodontal tissues. Because of the internal sealing difficulties of lateral perforations, healing is unpredictable. Therefore, a questionable prognosis of such treatments should be anticipated.

The use of calcium hydroxide has been suggested for the treatment of root perforations, since this promotes healing of wounds in the dental pulp with the formation of hard tissue adjacent to the capping material (Fitz-gerald 1979). Recent experiments in monkeys (Beavers et al. 1982) have demonstrated that healing of perforations into the periodontium can also occur following sealing with a hard setting calcium hydroxide compound. However, healing was no characterized by the closure of the perforation with new hard tissue but with a layer of uninflamed connective tissue which formed adjacent to the medicament.

If the perforation is located in the cervical part of the root, obturation of the perforation with for example amalgam, can be attempted from the outer surface of the root and accomplished after the elevation of a flap.

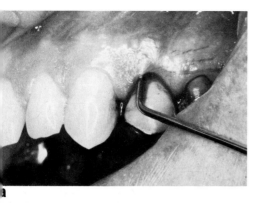

a

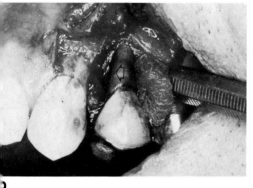

b

Fig. 9-14. Clinical photographs of a maxillary premolar with a longitudinal root fracture. A deep periodontal pocket was probed at the buccal aspect of the tooth (a). No other clinical symptoms were present. The elevation of a mucoperiosteal flap (b) revealed extensive loss of marginal bone at the buccal aspect of the root and a thin root fracture (arrow). (Courtesy of Dr. Claes Reit).

Root fracture

Root fractures can occasionally occur in endodontically treated teeth. Such fractures produce clinical and radiographic symptoms similar to those observed in endodontic and marginal lesions. A fracture can traverse the root in different directions either through the entire length of the root or at a more or less oblique angle towards the long axis of the tooth. A root fracture can involve the gingival sulcus/pocket area but may also be incomplete and confined to the alveolus area.

Root fractures can develop as a result of excessive forces used during lateral conden-sation of gutta percha in endodontic treatment or during cementing posts or inlays in endodontically treated teeth (Meister et al. 1980). It has also been suggested that root filled teeth, with time, will become more brittle and less resistant to bite forces and mechanical trauma. This hypothesis is supported by the observation that root fractures are often detected several years after the completion of endodontic treatment and restoration of the tooth. In a study comprising 32 root fractures, the average time between the completion of the endodontic treatment and the detection of root fracture was 3.25 years with a range varying between 3 days and 14 years (Meister et al. 1980).

It is often difficult to identify a root fracture. The clinical symptoms may vary in character. In certain cases, the symptoms are pronounced and include pain, tenderness and abscess formation – symptoms similar to those of a periodontal abscess or acute periapical lesion. In other instances, a narrow, local deepening of the periodontal pocket is the only symptom. Other symptoms occurring in conjunction with root fractures are tenderness to mastication, fistulous tract, mild pain and dull discomfort.

The fracture line is usually difficult to detect on clinical examination and only in exceptional cases it can be seen in the radiograph. Placement of iodine tincture on the root surface can be used to discover the fracture. Iodine entering the fracture space will show a dark line against the surrounding tooth substance. Indirect illumination of the tooth substance using fiber optics can also reveal fracture. Often the diagnosis of a fractured tooth can only be confirmed after exploratory surgery (Walton & Michelich 1982; Fig. 9-14).

As a result of bacterial growth in the fracture space, the adjacent periodontal ligament can soon become the seat of an inflammatory lesion causing the breakdown of connective tissue fibers and alveolar bone. This breakdown can be discovered radiographically (Fig. 9-15). The pattern of the bone destruction may be similar to that characterizing plaque associated marginal

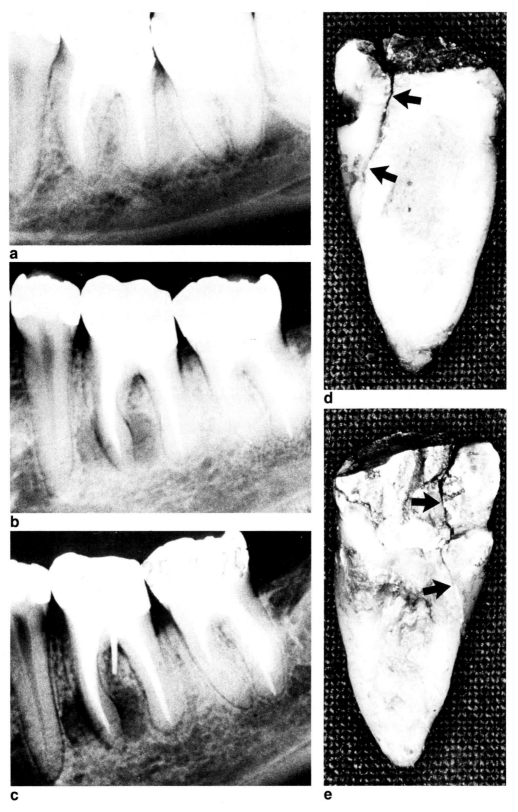

Fig. 9-15. A typical case of root fracture. The first mandibular molar had been asymptomatic for 15 years after completion of endodontic treatment. *Fig. 9-15a* shows normal periapical conditions in a radiograph taken 2 years after treatment. For a month the patient had slight pain and a tenderness on mastication that could not be relieved by occlusal adjustment. Radiographic examination (b) revealed an apical bone destruction adjacent to the mesial root. Within a narrow zone at the lingual aspect of the tooth, a deep periodontal pocket (10 mm) could be probed. A gutta percha point inserted into the pocket indicated marginal communication with the apical lesion (c). Clinical examination could not confirm the presence of a fracture. However, based on the findings that clinical and radiographic symptoms suddenly developed 15 years after therapy, and that a localized narrow pocket was found at a single tooth in a dentition otherwise free from periodontal disease, strongly suggested the presence of a root fracture. The tooth was extracted and the diagnosis confirmed. *Fig. 9-15d* shows the fracture line at the mesial aspect of the root and *Fig. 9-15e* at the distal aspect.

periodontitis or may resemble that of an endodontic lesion (Fig. 9-15). In addition, a diffuse widening of the periodontal ligament space along the lateral surfaces of the root may be indicative of a root fracture. Roots with fracture extending the entire length of the root should be extracted.

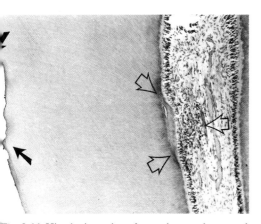

Fig. 9-16. Histologic section of a monkey tooth exposed to experimental periodontal tissue breakdown. Beneath resorptive defects in the external root surface a slight infiltrate of inflammatory cells and a small rim of irregular secondary dentin are observed in the pulp. (From Bergenholtz & Lindhe 1978).

Influence of periodontal disease on the condition of the pulp

The progressive breakdown of the attachment apparatus in periodontal disease and the formation of bacterial plaque on the detached root surfaces can occasionally induce pathologic changes in the pulp tissue. Bacterial products and substances released by the inflammatory process in the periodontium, may gain access to the pulp via exposed accessory canals, apical and furcal foramina, and dentinal tubules in a way similar to the spread of infectious products in the opposite direction from necrotic pulp to periodontal tissue.

Inflammatory alterations as well as localized necrosis of pulp tissue have been reported to occur adjacent to accessory canals exposed by periodontal disease (Seltzer et al. 1963, Rubach & Mitchell 1965). Severe breakdown of pulp, however, presumably does not occur until the periodontal disease process has reached a terminal stage, i.e. when bacterial plaque involves the main apical foramina (Langeland et al. 1974). This observation demonstrates that the pulp has a good capacity for defence against the injurious elements released by the lesion in the periodontium as long as the blood supply through the apical foramen is intact.

A clear-cut relationship between progressive periodontal disease and pulpal involvement does not invariably exist (Mazur & Massler 1965, Czarnecki & Schilder 1979). In an experiment in monkeys, Bergenholtz & Lindhe (1978) studied the nature and frequency of tissue changes in the pulp of teeth with moderate breakdown of the attachment apparatus. The majority of the roots examined (70%) exhibited no pathologic tissue changes in the pulp, despite the fact that approximately 30-40% of the periodontal attachment was lost. The remaining roots (30%) displayed small inflammatory cell infiltrates and/or formations of irregular secondary dentin in an area of the pulp subjacent to those root areas exposed by the destruction of the supporting apparatus. These tissue changes in pulp were frequently associated with root surface resorption (Fig. 9-16), suggesting that the irritation of the pulp had been transmitted through exposed dentinal tubules. This observation further suggests that the presence of an intact cementum layer may be important to the protection of pulp from injurious elements produced by lesions in the periodontium.

In the study by Bergenholtz & Lindhe (1978), destructive periodontal disease was produced experimentally during a comparatively short period (5-7 months), while in humans a similar degree of destruction of the periodontal tissues normally requires several years. It has been reported that the pulp of teeth with longstanding periodontal disease can develop changes such as fibrosis and dystrophic calcifications (Bender &

Seltzer 1972; Fig. 9-17). The number of blood vessels and nerve fibers can also be reduced. It may be speculated that tissue changes of this nature represent the accumulated response of pulp to relatively weak, but repeatedly occurring, insults to pulp tissue via accessory canals and dentinal tubules. The clinical significance of such tissue changes is not clear. Further research is needed to elucidate 1) to what extent inflammatory and degenerative tissue changes in the pulp result from periodontal disease and 2) if the pulp tissue in teeth with longstanding periodontitis is less resistant to additional injury, e.g. by scaling and root planing and restorative procedures.

Conclusion: Plaque associated periodontal disease rarely produces significant pathologic changes in pulp. In teeth with moderate breakdown of the attachment apparatus, the pulp is usually vital and in proper function. The vitality of the pulp is usually not lost until the periodontal lesion and bacterial plaques have reached the apical foramen.

Influence of periodontal treatment measures on the pulp

Scaling and root planing

Scaling and root planing not only remove bacterial deposits from the root surface but also cementum and superficial parts of dentin. Therefore, by this instrumentation, dentinal tubules may be exposed to microbial colonization. As a consequence, inflammatory reactions can be induced in the pulp by the penetration of bacterial products through the dentinal tubules (Bergenholtz & Lindhe 1975). It may be assumed that pathologic pulp reactions can also result from mechanical exposure of accessory canals by deep scaling.

The vitality of pulp, however, does not seem to be jeopardized by scaling proce-

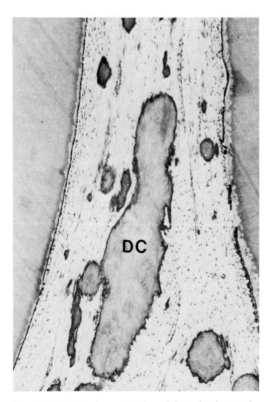

Fig. 9-17. Histologic preparation of the palatal root of a first maxillary molar exposed to extensive breakdown of the attachment apparatus, showing numerous dystrophic calcifications in the pulp (DC). The pulp tissue is noninflamed.

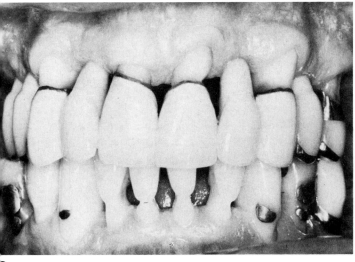
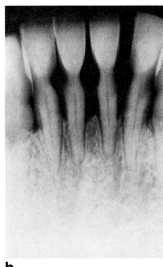

a   **b**

Fig. 9-18. Hourglass shaped teeth in the mandibular front region resulting from improper use of interdental tooth-brushes (a). The coronal portions of the pulp chamber are filled with hard tissue (b). One of the teeth (42) later had a crown fracture due to the weakening of tooth substance, but without clinical exposure of the pulp. (Courtesy of Dr. Sture Nyman).

dures, even though clinical symptoms of pulpitis may follow such measures (see below). In the experimental study in monkeys (Bergenholtz & Lindhe 1978), scaling of periodontally involved teeth did not enhance the severity and incidence of pathological tissue changes in pulp in comparison with untreated periodontally diseased teeth. In pulp tissue adjacent to scaled root surfaces, localized inflammatory alterations and secondary dentin formation were observed in some teeth while other teeth displayed normal pulp tissue morphology even though dental plaque had been allowed to accumulate on the root surfaces after scaling. The incidence of inflammatory alterations in the human dental pulp resulting from exposure of dentinal tubules by scaling is presently not known.

During the maintenance phase of periodontal therapy (see Chapter 13) scaling and planing of root dentin surfaces are frequently repeated procedures. At each recall session, the root surfaces are debrided and some dentin is removed. Irregular secondary dentin can form in the pulp following such treatment (Fig. 9-18).

Dentin hypersensitivity

Patients frequently complain of increased sensitivity of teeth to thermal, osmotic, and mechanical stimuli following periodontal treatment, including scaling and root planing. The symptoms usually peak during the first weeks after treatment and then gradually subside. The hypersensitivity can, however, persist and even become intense. Shorter or longer periods of tooth ache can also be provoked. In severe cases even minimal contact between a toothbrush and the root dentin may result in intense pain – a condition not only uncomfortable but one likely to diminish proper oral hygiene.

Considerable controversy exists regarding the etiology of root hypersensitivity and its underlying mechanisms. The problem has been debated in dental literature for many years (Peden 1977). It is conceivable that the symptoms are related to inflammatory alterations in the pulp, induced locally by bacterial products from the oral environment, which penetrate the exposed dentinal tubules. The inflammatory reaction, in turn, could reduce the pain threshold of the sen-

249

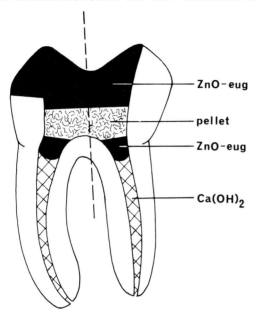

ZnO-eug

pellet

ZnO-eug

Ca(OH)$_2$

Fig. 9-19. Endodontic procedure prior to root resection. Root canals are filled with Ca(OH)$_2$ after canal preparation. The canal openings are sealed with zinc oxide-eugenol cement on top of which a cotton pellet and temporary cement are placed.

sory nerve receptors within the affected area of the pulp. The receptors may react faster and more intensely to external stimuli than normal teeth. Thus, the problem of hypersensitive root dentin seems to be dependent on the patency of the involved dentinal tubules. This assumption is supported by the fact that exposed dentin which is nonsensitive to touch and thermal changes, frequently shows deposition of mineralized material in the tubular openings in the surface layer (Hiatt & Johansen 1972). It is reasonable to assume that such an occlusion of the dentinal tubules would prevent transmission of both bacterial products and sensory nerve stimuli to the pulp.

In cases of severe dentin hypersensitivity, active treatment is urgent. Remedy is not always possible to obtain, however, with the methods presently available. A large number of different therapeutic methods have been recommended. These methods involve 1) topical application of chemical

substances to the dentin surface such as fluoride and formalin containing solutions, strontium chloride, corticosteroids, calcium hypophosphate, calcium hydroxide, etc., 2) electric deposition of chemical substances with the use of iontophoresis, 3) use of dentifrices containing "active substances" ($SrCl_2$, Na_2PO_3F, SnF_2), and 4) resin impregnation of the dentin. Unfortunately none of these methods has been proven to result in a predictable therapeutic effect.

Meticulous plaque control can lead to reduction of dentin hypersensitivity. It has been observed clinically that with time teeth in patients with proper oral hygiene habits develop hard, smooth and insensitive root surfaces. Electron microscopic examination of the dentin of such root surfaces has revealed that the tubular openings are obliterated by mineral deposits (Hiatt & Johansen 1972).

When severe symptoms of root sensitivity have emerged it is difficult to motivate the patient to maintain the degree of plaque control necessary to the natural occlusion of the dentinal tubules. In such situations an agent should be selected which has a reasonable capacity to block the tubular openings, at least temporarily, so that proper oral hygiene measures can be reinforced. Promising therapeutic effects have been reported following the treatment of hypersensitive root dentin with water-pastes of calcium hypophosphate (Hiatt & Johansen 1972) or calcium hydroxide (Levin et al. 1973, Green et al. 1977). These compounds are applied on the dentin surface for 1-5 min. in combination with burnishing the dentin surface with either tooth pick, rubber cup or dental tape. Immediate relief is often obtained by this treatment. The long-term result depends on whether proper oral hygiene can be established after treatment. The mode of action of this type of treatment is not clear. It has been assumed that the chemical agent denatures the organic contents of the tubules in the superficial part of the dentin, thus inducing the formation of a surface protein plug (Bergenholtz & Reit 1980). It is also possible that the compound during the burn-

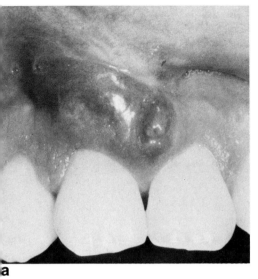

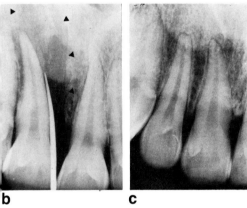

Fig. 9-20. Fig. 9-20a demonstrates a gingival swelling at the buccal aspect of tooth 11. Fig. 9-20b shows the radiographic appearance of the area. Note the advanced destruction of alveolar bone along the mesial aspect of the root (arrow heads). Fig. 9-20c shows healing of the area 7 months following periodontal treatment. (Courtesy of Dr. Harald Rylander).

ishing procedure is forced into the tubular opening and in this way creates a surface block. Further documentation is needed to demonstrate the efficacy and mode of action of this and other methods of treatment of dentin hypersensitivity. In desperate cases, where no remedy is achieved by topical treatment, pulpectomy of the vital pulp tissue and root filling may be the only therapeutic alternative.

Endodontic considerations in root resection of multirooted teeth in periodontal therapy

Treatment of periodontally diseased, multirooted teeth may involve separation and extraction of one or two roots (see Chapter 20). As a rule, endodontic treatment of the root to be retained should be performed prior to surgery. Information will, thus, be gained regarding the effect of the endodontic measures before alternative roots are extracted. This rule should be followed for both vital and nonvital teeth. The root canals of molars are sometimes difficult to prepare, in particular when the tooth has been exposed to long-standing periodontal disease. As mentioned above, such teeth can harbor both dystrophic calcifications and irregular secondary dentin formations that jeopardize proper endodontic treatment.

In multirooted teeth with advanced periodontal destruction it is not always possible to decide before surgery which root(s) can be preserved. As an alternative to permanent filling of all root canals in such teeth, pulpectomy can be performed and the canals temporarily filled with calcium hydroxide (see Fig. 9-19). Each of the canal openings is sealed with zinc oxide eugenol cement. Root separation can then be performed without bacterial contamination of the root canals. Permanent root filling of the root(s) retained is performed after surgery.

Instead of endodontic treatment, capping of the pulp exposed by the root separation has been advocated (Haskell et al. 1980). Sufficient documentation of the long-term result of such treatment, however, is lacking.

Differential diagnosis

In this chapter, several examples of lesions in the periodontium have been presented which are not associated with plaque accumulation on the root surfaces (see Figs. 9-7, 9-8, 9-9, 9-11, 9-12, 9-15). Two cases of plaque associated periodontitis are pre-

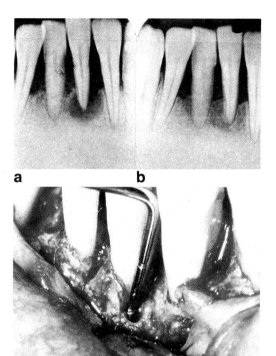

a   b

c

Fig. 9-21a. Demonstrates advanced destructions of alveolar bone including an angular bony defect simulating an endodontic periapical lesion around tooth 31. The pulp responded vital and the tooth was therefore periodontally treated with the use of a flap procedure (b). Fig. 9-21c (radiograph obtained 6 months after treatment) shows healing of the lesion. (Courtesy of Dr. Ingvar Magnusson).

sented below. These cases show clinical and radiographic symptoms similar to those of acute, periapical lesions, endodontic perforations or root fractures. The cases further demonstrate that diagnostic entities such as location, form and extension of radiolucencies, clinical symptoms of pain and swelling, increased probing depths, etc. are not always effective diagnostic tools for differentiating a marginal from an endodontic lesion.

The clinical photograph in Fig. 9-20a shows swelling of the marginal gingiva on the buccal aspect of tooth 11. This swelling had for a few days been preceded by severe throbbing pain. Radiographic examination (Fig. 9-20b) disclosed the presence of an

angular bone destruction that involved the apical regions of the tooth. In this case the pulp responded vital to testing (see below), indicating that the pathologic condition was not of endodontic etiology. Pocket debridement was combined with irrigation with 0.2% chlorhexidine digluconate solution and systemic administration of antibiotics. The lesion healed rapidly. Seven months following treatment new bone had formed around the apex and along the mesial root surface (c). This case demonstrates that the periodontal destruction observed was caused by plaque associated periodontal disease.

Fig. 9-21 illustrates another case of differential diagnostic interest. A radiograph taken of the front region of the mandibular jaw demonstrates bone destruction around the apex of tooth 31 in addition to a generalized horizontal loss of alveolar bone (a). The form and extension of the apical radiolucency around tooth 31 are similar to those resulting from an endodontic lesion. Clinically, a deep periodontal pocket could be probed along the distobuccal root surface. Vitality tests indicated that the tooth pulp was vital. Therefore, no endodontic treatment was performed. Following elevation of a mucoperiosteal flap, an angular bone destruction was found at the buccal aspect of the root without involving the apex. The wound area was debrided and the root surfaces were scaled. Rapid bone healing followed surgery (c) and the pulp of the tooth maintained its vitality.

The two cases described above (Figs. 9-20, 9-21) demonstrate that neither clinical symptoms nor radiographic findings always lead to the correct diagnosis. The only significant observation for the differential diagnosis was the pulp vitality.

Pulp vitality

Pulp vitality means that the pulp chamber is occupied by connective tissue supplied by nerves and blood vessels. Sensory nerve function is normally present. Vital pulp may be subjected to inflammatory and degenerative tissue changes.

Pulp vitality is easy to demonstrate when the pulp chamber is exposed and a bleeding sensitive tissue can be probed at the exposed site. In teeth where the pulp is surrounded by either hard tissue or restorative materials, pulp vitality must be determined by indirect means and is based on the assumption that vital pulp is able to respond to sensory stimuli such as mechanical, thermal and electric stimulation. This means that the *sensitivity* of the pulp is tested rather than the *vitality* of the pulpal tissue. There is, however, extensive documentation to support the concept that a tooth which responds to sensory stimuli is vital. Conversely, if a tooth does not respond to sensory stimuli, the pulp may be nonvital. It should be recognized, however, that false negative and false positive responses may occur with the testing methods commonly used.

Although it has been reported that necrotic teeth may respond to electric stimulation (Mumford 1967), this phenomenon cannot be an effect of sensory nerve function. Such a response is most likely the effect of a false positive recording due to transmission of electric current to the periodontal tissues. For example, electric current may leak to the gingiva from the tooth electrode along a moist tooth surface. Positive responses from necrotic pulp to electrical stimulation are exceptional provided that the testing procedure is performed carefully and according to proper principles.

Except for electrical stimulation, pulpal sensitivity can be examined by thermal stimulation with the use of ethyl chloride, carbon dioxide snow, ice, or heated gutta percha. Another testing method is mechanical stimulation by, for example, preparing a test cavity in dentin. Since false positive as well as false negative readings occur in conjunction with sensitivity testing, a combination of the various methods should always be used to ensure correct diagnosis.

Conclusion: The recognition of pulp vitality is important for differential diagnosis and for selection of primary measures for treatment of inflammatory lesions in the marginal and apical periodontium. Deep restorations, dental trauma, endodontic treatment, previous pulp capping, etc., are factors to consider when assessing the need for endodontic treatment as a part of the overall periodontal therapy. Location, form and extension of radiolucencies, as well as clinical symptoms of pain, tenderness, abscess formation, increased probing depth, etc., may not distinguish a marginal from an endodontic lesion.

References

Beavers, R., Bergenholtz, G., Cox, C. F., Fitzgerald, M., Syed, S. A., Baker, J. A. & Corcoran, J. F. (1982) Healing of furcal/lateral root lesions in Rhesus monkey teeth. *Journal of Dental Research* **61**, IADR Abstract No. 253.

Bender, I. B. & Seltzer, S. (1972) The effect of periodontal disease on the pulp. *Oral Surgery* **33**, 458-474.

Bergenholtz, G., Lekholm, U., Liljenberg, B. & Lindhe, J. (1983) Morphometric analysis of chronic inflammatory periapical lesions in root filled teeth. *Oral Surgery*. **55**, 295-301.

Bergenholtz, G. & Lindhe, J. (1975) Effect of soluble plaque factors on inflammatory reactions in the dental pulp. *Scandinavian Journal of Dental Research* **83**, 153-158.

Bergenholtz, G. & Lindhe, J. (1978) Effect of experimentally induced marginal periodontitis and periodontal scaling on the dental pulp. *Journal of Clinical Periodontology* **5**, 59-73.

Bergenholtz, G. & Reit, C. (1980) Reactions of the dental pulp to microbial provocation of calcium hydroxide treated dentin. *Scandinavian Journal of Dental Research* **88**, 187-192.

Burch, J. G. & Hulen, S. (1974) A study of the presence of accessory foramina and the topography of molar furcations. *Oral Surgery* **38**, 451-455.

Czarnecki, R. T. & Schilder, H. (1979) A histological evaluation of the human pulp in teeth with varying degrees of periodontal disease. *Journal of Endodontics* 5, 242-253.

DeDeus, Q. D. (1975) Frequency, location and direction of the lateral, secondary and accessory canals. *Journal of Endodontics* 1, 361-366.

Fitzgerald, M. (1979) Cellular mechanics of dentinal bridge repair using ^{3}H-thymidine. *Journal of Dental Research* 58, 2198-2206.

Green., B. W., Green, M. L. & McFall, W. T. (1977) Calcium hydroxide and potassium nitrate as desensitizing agents for hypersensitive root surfaces. *Journal of Periodontology* 48, 667-672.

Gutmann, J. L. (1978) Prevalence, location and patency of accessory canals in the furcation region of permanent molars. *Journal of Periodontology* 49, 21-26.

Harrington, G. W., (1979) The perio-endo question: Differential diagnosis. *Dental Clinics of North America* 23, 673-690.

Haskell, E. W., Stanley, H. & Goldman, S. (1980) A new approach to vital root resection. *Journal of Periodontology* 51, 217-224.

Hession, R. W. (1977) Endodontic morphology. A radiographic analysis. *Oral Surgery* 44, 610-620.

Hiatt, W. H., Johansen, E. (1972) Root preparation. I. Obturation of dentinal tubules in treatment of root hypersensitivity. *Journal of Periodontology* 43, 373-380.

Koenigs, J. F., Brilliant, J. D. & Foreman, D. W. (1974) Preliminary scanning electron microscope investigations of accessory foramina in furcation areas of human molar teeth. *Oral Surgery* 37, 773-782.

Langeland, K., Rodrigues, H. & Dowden, W. (1974) Periodontal disease, bacteria and pulpal histopathology. *Oral Surgery* 37, 257-270.

Levin, M. P., Yearwood, L. L. & Carpenter, W. N. (1973) The desensitizing effect of calcium hydroxide and magnesium hydroxide on hypersensitive dentin. *Oral Surgery* 35, 741-746.

Lindhe, J., Liljenberg, B. & Listgarten, M. (1980) Some microbiological and histopathological features of periodontal disease in man. *Journal of Periodontology* 51, 264-269.

Lowman, J. V., Burke, R. S. & Pelleu, G. B. (1973) Patent accessory canals: incidence of molar furcation region. *Oral Surgery* 36, 580-584.

Mazur, B. & Massler, M. (1964) Influence of periodontal disease on the dental pulp. *Oral Surgery* 17, 592-603.

Meister, F., Lommel, T. J. & Gerstein, H. (1980) Diagnosis and possible causes of vertical root fractures. *Oral Surgery* 49, 243-253.

Mumford, J. M. (1967) Pain perception threshold on stimulating human teeth and the histological condition of the pulp. *British Dental Journal* 123, 427-433.

Peden, J. W. (1977) Dental hypersensitivity. *Periodontal Abstracts* 25, 75-83.

Perlich, M. A., Reader, A. & Foreman, D. W. (1981) A scanning electron microscopic investigation of accessory foramens on the pulpal floor of human molars. *Journal of Endodontics* 7, 402-406.

Pineda, F. & Kuttler, Y. (1972) Mesiodistal and buccolingual roentgenographic investigation of 7,275 root canals. *Oral Surgery* 33, 101-110.

Rubach, W. C. & Mitchell, D. F. (1965) Periodontal disease, accessory canals and pulp pathosis. *Journal of Periodontology* 36, 34-38.

Seltzer, S., Bender, I. B. & Ziontz, M. (1963) The interrelationship of pulp and periodontal disease. *Oral Surgery* 16, 1474-1490.

Simon, J. H. S. (1976) Periodontal-endodontic treatment. In *Pathways of the Pulp*, ed. Cohen, S. & Burns, R. C., pp. 442-468. St. Louis: C. V. Mosby Co.

Stallard, R. E. (1968) Periodontal disease and its relationship to pulpal pathology. *Parodontologie and Academy Review* 2, 80-86.

Stern, M. H., Dreizen, S., Mackler, B. F., Selbst, A. G. & Levy, B. M. (1981) Quantitative analysis of cellular composition of human periapical granuloma. *Journal of Endodontics* 7, 117-122.

Walton, R. E. & Michelich, R. (1982) Pathogenesis of vertical root fracture. *Journal of Dental Research* 61, IADR Abstract No. 537.

Weiner, S., McKinney, R. V. & Walton, R. E. (1982) Characterization of the periapical surgical specimen. *Oral Surgery* 53, 293-302.

Vertucci, T. J. & Williams, R. G. (1974) Furcation canals in the human mandibular first molar. *Oral Surgery* 38, 308-314.

Yanagisawa, S. (1980) Pathologic study of periapical lesions. I. Periapical granulomas: clinical, histopathologic and immunohistopathologic studies. *Journal of Oral Pathology* 9, 288-300.

CHAPTER 10

Manifestation of Systemic Disorders in the Periodontium

<table>
<tr><td>

Infectious diseases
  Streptococcal gingivostomatitis
  Zoster
  Herpetic gingivostomatitis
  Vesicular stomatitis with exanthema
  Verruca vulgaris
  Secondary syphilis
  Reiter's syndrome
  Condyloma acuminatum
  Acute pseudomembranous candidiasis
  Chronic mucocutaneous candidiasis

Malignant systemic diseases
  Acute monocytic leukemia
  Acute erythremic myelosis

Endocrinopathies
  Diabetes mellitus
  Hypoadrenocorticism

Nutritional and metabolic disturbances
  Eosinophilic granuloma of bone

Blood diseases
  Thrombasthenia
  Thrombocytopenia
  Cyclic neutropenia

Diseases of the nervous system
  Melkersson-Rosenthal's syndrome

Diseases of the circulatory system
  Wegener's granulomatosis

Diseases of the digestive system
  Idiopathic gingival fibromatosis
  Recurrent aphthous ulcerations
  Homogeneous leukoplakia

</td><td>

  Nodular leukoplakia
  Crohn's disease

Diseases related to pregnancy, menstruation, and oral contraceptives
  Pregnancy gingivitis

Pregnancy granuloma
  Effect of menstruation
  Effect of oral contraceptives

Diseases of the skin
  Pemphigus vulgaris
  Benign mucous membrane pemphigoid
  Erythema multiforme exudativum
  Discoid lupus erythematosus
  Psoriasis
  Lichen planus

Diseases of the musculoskeletal system
  Dermatomyositis
  Osteitis deformans
  Scleroderma

Congenital anomalies
  Recklinghausen's neurofibromatosis
  Fallot's tetralogy
  White sponge nevus

Drug stomatitis
  Cytostatics
  Hydantoin derivatives

Industrial intoxications
  Lead
  Mercury

    References

</td></tr>
</table>

Infectious diseases

Streptococcal gingivostomatitis

Fig. 10-1 is from a 20 year old woman who had a sore throat and elevated temperature 2 days prior to the appearance of oral symptoms. Then gingivitis develops in the form of fiery red and swollen gingival mucosa. Furthermore there are small ulcerations asymmetrically along the gingival margin and on the top of the interdental papillae as can be seen from the illustration. These 2 changes, involvement of all areas of the gingiva and the asymmetric occurrence of lesions, indicate clearly that there is a systemic background. In this patient it is a streptococcal infection. Ulcerations are present in other areas of the oral mucosa. Formerly, *Streptococcus viridans* was considered to be the causative organism, but recent evidence associates the infection with β-hemolytic streptococci.

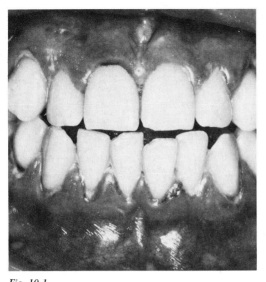

Fig. 10-1.

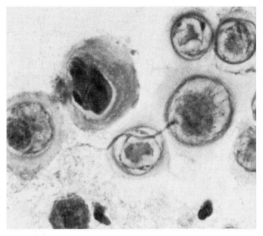

Fig. 10-3.

Zoster

Fig. 10-2 is from a 25 year old man who, some months before, had a kidney transplantation. There is now an affection of the right side of the oral cavity including the gingiva, consisting of vesicular elements of which a number have burst. Because of the

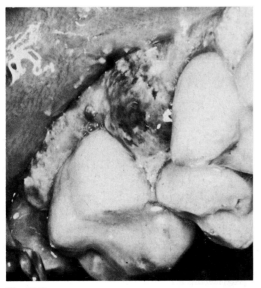

Fig. 10-2.

unilateral nature of the lesions and the result of a smear from a vesicle (Fig. 10-3) zoster is diagnosed. The most probable cause of zoster is a reactivation of varicella virus lying dormant in sensory ganglia of patients whose immunity to the virus has diminished. When the second or third divisions of the trigeminal nerve are affected, oral manifestations can occur in addition to the skin lesions. The most frequent locations for the lesions are the buccal mucosa, the tongue, the palate and the lips. It is rather rare to observe gingival changes as seen in Fig. 10-2. As a complication to immunosuppressive treatment, patients who have undergone transplantation, will often present with herpes simplex or zoster of the oral mucosa. Fig. 10-3 is a photomicrograph of a smear taken from one of the vesicles illustrated in Fig. 10-2. All the cells bear witness to a virus infection with abnormally large nuclei and scanty cytoplasm. Sometimes multinucleated cells are seen, but not here.

Herpetic gingivostomatitis

Fig. 10-4. When the herpes simplex virus affects the oral mucosa it results in a herpetic gingivostomatitis, usually seen in children

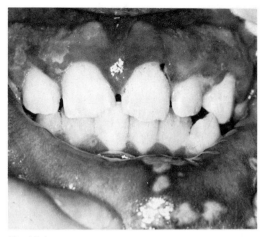

Fig. 10-4.

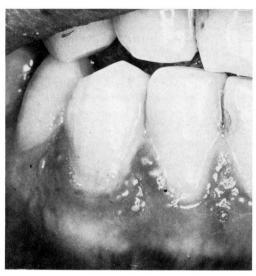

Fig. 10-5.

between the ages of 2 and 4, but in recent years, also diagnosed in a number of older age groups. After an incubation period of 1 week, the patients develop fever, swollen submandibular lymph nodes and a diffuse gingivitis. Fig. 10-4 is a typical example of herpetic gingivostomatitis in a 12 year old boy. There is marked edema of the marginal gingiva and occurrence of vesicles on the interdental papillae of 12,11 and 42,41. On the interdental papilla between 22,12 and on the labial mucosa there are burst vesicles covered by fibrin.

Vesicular stomatitis with exanthema

Fig. 10-5 illustrates vesicular elements corresponding to the marginal gingiva and the interdental papillae from a 26 year old man who experienced a burning sensation in the affected area. Vesicular stomatitis is better known by the name "hand-foot-and-mouth disease", and has been described as epidemic in certain countries. The disease is caused by Coxsackie virus Group A (5, 10 and 16) and more rarely by Group B (2 and 5). The disease, which should not be

confused with "foot-and-mouth disease" (stomatitis epizootica), usually lasts 1 week and is accompanied by only a slightly elevated temperature. Symptomless vesicles develop on hands, feet, and in the mouth, where the buccal mucosa is most frequently affected. Very often the symptoms are so mild that the patients seek neither dental nor medical advice.

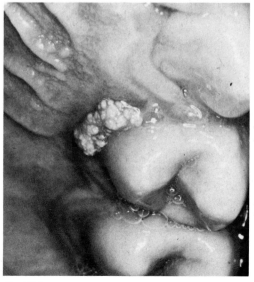

Fig. 10-6.

Verruca vulgaris

Fig. 10-6 shows, in a 12 year old boy, a gingival change in the form of a small, white, elevated lesion which was clinically diagnosed as a papilloma. It is easy to understand why confusion between a papilloma and a verruca may occur as they are very similar from a clinical point of view. In the verruca it is possible, by means of electron microscopy, to demonstrate virus particles in the epithelial cells. Virus is transferred to the mouth from verrucae (warts) on the hands when they are chewed. Oral verrucae are seen mainly in children, the favorite location being the mucosa of lip and tongue.

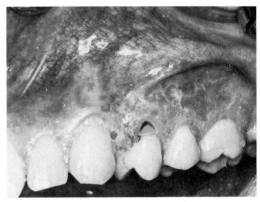

Fig. 10-8.

Secondary syphilis

Fig. 10-7 illustrates a comparative rarity: a gingival manifestation of syphilis in the secondary stage. Along the marginal gingiva of the extremely carious second molar there are 2 small, slightly elevated, white papules surrounded by a red halo. Indications of secondary syphilis are usually seen 6 weeks after the primary stage. The typical lesions of the oral mucosa are the so-called "syphilitic papules", plaques or mucous patches.

They are slightly elevated, whitish-grayish and, in most instances, surrounded by a red halo. Syphilitic papules, which may appear in any part of the oral mucosa, are either solitary or multiple and, most frequently, occur in areas exposed to trauma. Mucous patches are the most contagious lesions in acute syphilis because of their high content of spirochetes.

Reiter's syndrome

Fig. 10-8 shows peculiar, whitish, circinate, gingival changes with a central red area. The patient, a 34 year old man, suffers from arthritis, and the genital mucosa is also affected. These symptoms are characteristic of Reiter's syndrome, where other components are changes of the skin, eyes and oral cavity. The etiology of the syndrome is unknown but in 80-95% of patients the tissue type antigen HLA-B27 is present. The oral manifestations, observed in 20%, consist of erythematous areas surrounded by circinate, white lines as seen in Fig. 10-8.

Condyloma acuminatum

Fig. 10-9 illustrates, in a 44 year old man, a lesion which at first glance looks like an epulis of a papillomatous type. It is charac-

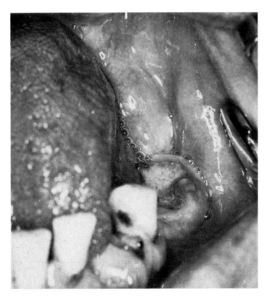

Fig. 10-7.

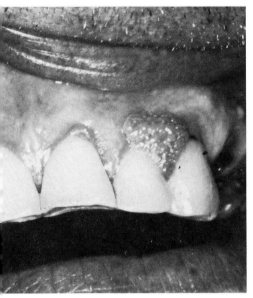

Fig. 10-9.

condylomas in the literature may be due to such lesions usually being diagnosed as papillomas, verrucae vulgares or fibro-epithelial hyperplasias. In most patients with oral condylomas an orogenital contact is revealed, together with genital condylomas of the partner.

Acute pseudomembranous candidiasis

Fig. 10-10 illustrates a rare phenomenon: an acute pseudomembranous candidiasis localized to the gingiva. It is surprising that *Candida albicans* infection so rarely affects the gingiva, and even more so, as oral Candida infections belong to the most frequent oral mucosal infectious diseases. The patient in Fig. 10-10 is a 55 year old man who suffers from Hodgkin's lymphogranulomatosis. He has been treated with cytostatics and antibiotics, predisposing the oral mucosa to development of both zoster and acute pseudomembranous candidiasis, the latter having the typical clinical appearance of creamy, pearly-white patches which can be scraped off. Because of the extensive patches it is difficult to identify the zoster lesions.

erized by its cauliflower-like appearance, typical of condyloma acuminatum. The patient has condylomas on the penis and the histologic examination of the removed "epulis" reveals structures characteristic of condyloma acuminatum. The rarity of oral

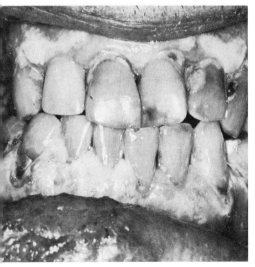

Fig. 10-10.

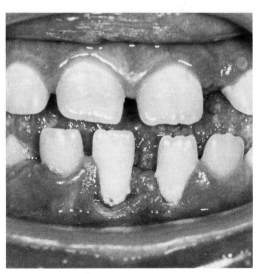

Fig. 10-11.

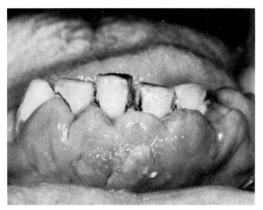

Fig. 10-12.

Chronic mucocutaneous candidiasis

Fig. 10-11 shows a gingival lesion in the form of a localized retraction of the gingiva of 31 and 41. The patient is a 10 year old boy who has suffered from affections involving nails, scalp and tongue since the age of 1. He has a rare form of a Candida infection, a mucocutaneous candidiasis, also called a candidal granuloma, usually starting early in life. The oral changes are very marked and the surface of the tongue has a lobulate appearance as a result of the longstanding infection. It is very rare that the disease affects the gingiva as seen in Fig. 10-11. The gingival lesions were surgically removed causing an improvement of the periodontal conditions.

Malignant systemic diseases

Acute monocytic leukemia

Fig. 10-12. Whereas chronic leukemia only rarely causes oral lesions, the acute forms are often associated with oral manifestations, which may be pronounced and quite disturbing. Fig. 10-12 demonstrates a very marked increase in gingival volume in a 32 year old woman who suddenly experienced

pain in the gingiva, enlarged lymph nodes of the neck and later an increase in temperature. The gingiva has lost its normal stippling and has a spongy appearance. There are very deep pseudopockets and the teeth are loose. The patient was referred to a department of internal medicine where the tentative diagnosis of leukemia was confirmed. Two weeks later the patient has died.

Acute erythremic myelosis

Fig. 10-13 is of a 28 year old woman suffering from an acute erythremic myelosis. There is a moderate enlargement of the gingiva, especially in the mandible. The disease is characterized by a generalized proliferation of the erythropoietic cells of the bone marrow, similar to the leukocytic proliferation in leukemia. The gingival changes, also comprising petechiae and ecchymoses, are to be distinguished from those seen in leukemia. The submucosal bleeding is due to a secondary thrombocytopenia.

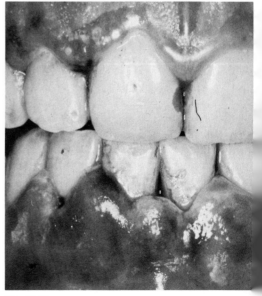

Fig. 10-13.

Endocrinopathies

Diabetes mellitus

Diabetes mellitus is a syndrome characterized by insufficient secretion of insulin, decreased glucose tolerance and a tendency for development of microangiopathy, neuropathy and arteriosclerosis.

The prevalence of diabetes varies in different countries, ranging from 0.5-2%. In children diabetes is usually insulin dependent, i.e. it requires exogenous insulin. More frequently diabetes affects the middle-aged and the old and can be controlled by dietary restrictions.

A hereditary background can be found in 5-40% of all newly diagnosed cases. Most often the etiology is unknown in diabetes patients. There are several diseases which either reduce the production of insulin (diseases of the pancreas, ageing and hemochromatosis) or cause a reduced effectiveness of insulin (acromegaly, Cushing's syndrome and obesity).

Insulin is secreted in the B-cells (β-cells), which make up for 75% of the pancreatic Langerhans' islands. Without insulin the transfer of glucose through certain cell membranes, especially muscle and fat cells, is insufficient, leading to an accumulation of glucose in the blood: hyperglycemia. Hyperglycemia changes the cell metabolism; hence the accumulation of ketones, which leads to further complications in the form of acidosis, coma, kidney lesions and retinopathy. Most changes can be explained through microangiopathy which involves a thickening of vessel walls and basement membranes with a PAS positive material. The clinical symptoms of diabetes mellitus are thirst, polyuria and loss of weight. The diagnosis is based on a glucose tolerance test, which reflects the blood level and utilization of glucose. It must, however, be emphasized that diagnosis of diabetes mellitus may be difficult.

The life of a diabetic is threatened by vascular diseases, especially of the coronary arteries. Blindness is also a severe complication. It has been discussed whether diabetics are more receptive to other than fungus infections, but no conclusions have been reached.

The oral manifestations of diabetes comprise, besides the periodontal: xerostomia, burning tongue, bad taste, and increased disposition to Candida infections.

Diabetically conditional periodontal changes have often been discussed in the literature, and it has been postulated that diabetes does not predispose to periodontal disease. Several studies in recent years have demonstrated, however, that there is a causal relationship.

It has recently been demonstrated that child diabetics with well controlled disease had more gingivitis than age matched controls without diabetes; both groups had the same plaque score (Faulconbridge et al. 1981)

In adults it has been shown, in a longitudinal study, that even patients with controlled diabetes, have more gingivitis and loss of epithelial attachment than nondiabetics (Cohen et al. 1970).

Recent data indicate that altered neutrophil function may be responsible for accelerated periodontal tissue breakdown in poorly controlled diabetics. An impaired

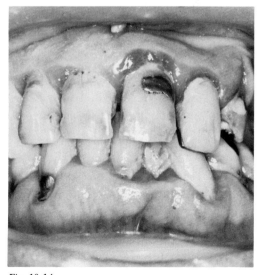

Fig. 10-14.

chemotactic and phagocytic activity of the polymorphonuclear leukocytes has been found in diabetics. Further, it has been demonstrated that there is a relationship between a positive family history of diabetes and depressed neutrophil chemotaxis (McCullen et al. 1981).

Fig. 10-14 demonstrates the periodontal conditions in a 56 year old man suffering from diabetes mellitus. Along the marginal gingiva are some limited granulomatous changes particularly at 21. The periodontal tissue around most of his teeth is the seat of advanced periodontal disease. The asymmetric location of the gingival changes should arouse suspicion of systemic disease.

Hypoadrenocorticism

Fig. 10-15 shows a dark staining of the gingiva involving all four regions. The patient is a 30 year old woman who suffers from hypoadrenocorticism, better known as Addison's disease. For several months the patient experienced dizziness, fatigue and observed an increased number of freckles in the face. The disease is caused by a hypofunction of the adrenal cortex. An early sign is a bronze-like pigmentation of the skin and a brownish, occasionally grayish-blackish, pigmentation of the oral mucosa. The pigmentation is due to an increased amount of melanin. Before a diagnosis of hypoadrenocorticism

is made on the basis of gingival pigmentation it should be remembered that the cause o gingival melanoplakia (apart from ethni background) may be intensive smoking; smoker's melanosis.

Nutritional and metabolic disturbances

Eosinophilic granuloma of bone

Fig. 10-16 shows a defect in the palatal gingival mucosa in a 15 year old male, who ha similar changes in the opposite side and o the gingiva corresponding to 17, 16, 26, 2 facially and 32, 33, 34 lingually. All lesion have a surface which is red, almos granulomatous, and below the adjacent nor mal mucosa. There is also a radiolucent are around the partially impacted 48 and 38 Biopsies taken from several of the lesions all show histologic changes typical of a eosinophilic granuloma of bone. Histiocy tosis X is a collective term for a group o reticuloendothelioses of unknown etiolog comprising eosinophilic granuloma of bone Hand-Schüller-Christian's disease, and Let terer-Siwe's disease. In all 3 forms

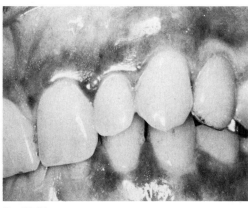

Fig. 10-15.

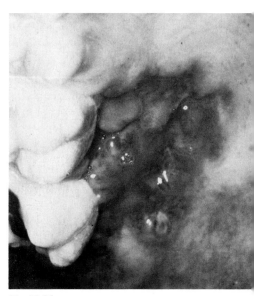

Fig. 10-16.

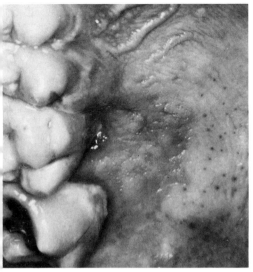

Fig. 10-17.

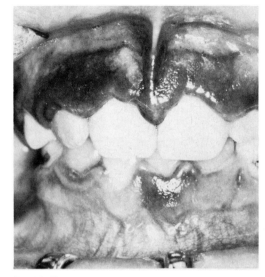

Fig. 10-18.

periodontal lesions can be observed. In the present patient corticosteroid was pre-scribed in the form of Prednisone tablets 5 mg 3 times daily. Fig. 10-17 is a picture taken 14 months later, demonstrating a marked improvement.

Blood diseases

Thrombasthenia

Fig. 10-18 illustrates an increase in volume, hyperemia and ecchymoses of the gingiva in an 8½ year old boy. At the age of 3 months the child was hospitalized for the first time, for epistaxis in connection with a cold. Marked ecchymoses and petechiae were found on both the body and face. The number of thrombocytes and other coagulation figures were normal and thrombas-thenia suspected. Laboratory investigations confirmed this. Hereditary thrombasthenia, also called Glanzmann's disease, is an auto-somal recessive inherited disorder charac-terized by a defective thrombocyte aggrega-tion. Before the child presented with the changes seen in Fig. 10-18, he had a herpetic gingivostomatitis. The gingival ecchymoses

can be seen as a parallel to the ecchymoses noted in the bleeding of the tonsils and nose, which were observed several times in the patient, shortly after infections of the upper respiratory tract. Fig. 10-19 illustrates his condition 10 days later, after treatment con-sisting of mouth rinsing 3 times daily with chlorhexidine (0.2%).

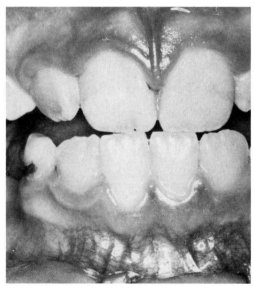

Fig. 10-19.

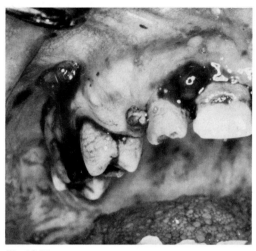

Fig. 10-20.

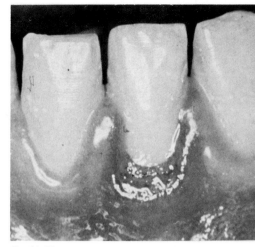

Fig. 10-21.

Thrombocytopenia

Fig. 10-20 shows very marked gingival bleeding in a 35 year old woman who, 8 days after a cesarean section, woke with a mouth full of blood, and ecchymoses of lips and cheeks. A thrombocytopenia was diagnosed but no decision was reached as to whether it was an essential idiopathic or a drug induced thrombocytopenia. Because of her condition, the patient could not be exposed to a provocation test. She received treatment with epsilon-amino-caproic acid (EACA) whereby the hemorrhagic diathesis disappeared and the number of thrombocytes increased. Drug induced thrombocytopenia is usually caused by cytostatics, barbiturates, and analgesics.

Cyclic neutropenia

In 1949 it was recognized that neutropenia, in some patients, had a cyclic course and the term cyclic neutropenia was introduced for a disease characterized by a dramatic fall in the number of circulating neutrophil leukocytes at 3 week periodic intervals. After 5-8 days the number of leukocytes increases, but it never reaches the normal level. The etiology of cyclic neutropenia is unknown. In the periods with a low number of leukocytes, the patient suffers from fever and general malaise. At the same time, changes occur on the skin and in the mouth. The oral lesions consist of a subacute gingivitis and/or aphthae-like ulcerations very often localized to the marginal gingiva, where recurrent aphthae are rarely seen. Furthermore, the neutropenic ulcerations have a punch-out appearance as can be seen in Fig. 10-21, which relares to an 8 year old boy whose cyclic neutropenia was identified through his gingival lesions. Fig. 10-22 shows severe periodontal changes in an 18 year old man

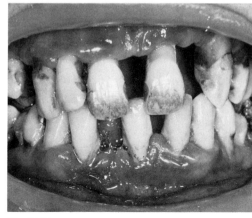

Fig. 10-22.

who since birth, with 3 week intervals, has suffered from malaise, skin eruptions and gingival symptoms. The result was a progressive marginal periodontitis with so much bone destruction that extraction was the only treatment possible. A very characteristic change, in both idiopathic and cyclic neutropenia, is sharply demarcated, hyperemic zones along the marginal gingiva. If such changes are found, the patient ought to receive a hematologic examination.

Diseases of the nervous system

Melkersson-Rosenthal's syndrome

Fig. 10-23 shows granulomatous changes of the mandibular gingiva in a 14 year old girl suffering from Melkersson-Rosenthal's syndrome (MRS). Usually the syndrome is described as a triad, consisting of recurrent edema of lips and/or buccal mucosa, recurrent facial paralysis, and fissured tongue. Related to the syndrome is Mischer's cheilitis. MRS, the etiology of which is unknown, is a rather rare disease, which usually affects younger individuals. There is no preference for sex and the syndrome is often seen in an incomplete form with edema as the constant symptom. In recent years it has been recognized that MRS can also affect

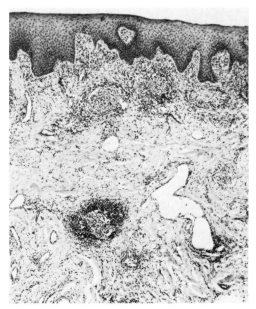

Fig. 10-24.

the palate, tongue and gingiva. Besides the gingival granulomas, the patient in Fig. 10-23 also has lesions of the upper lip and hard palate. Fig. 10-24 is a photomicrograph of a gingival biopsy from the patient in Fig. 10-23. Just below the epithelium there are 3 epitheloid cell granulomas, and deeper in the tissue 2 more granulomas can be observed; all are surrounded by an intense accumulation of lymphocytes and plasma cells. The histologic structure is very similar to that seen in sarcoidosis. Fig. 10-25 is from an 8 year old boy whose MRS began with gingival changes. The marginal gingiva in both maxilla and mandible exhibits with focal, granuloma-like, firm thickenings. The swellings, not symmetric, are slightly bluish-red and relatively well demarcated. In most cases the gingival changes are localized to the gingiva of the incisors and canines. In a Danish study comprising 30 patients with MRS, gingival changes were found in 5 of these patients. That gingival changes in MRS are reported so rarely, is possibly due to the fact that they are rather inconspicuous and consequently easy to overlook.

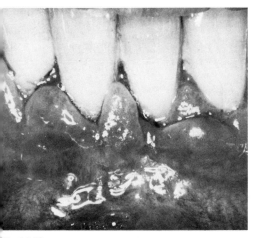

Fig. 10-23.

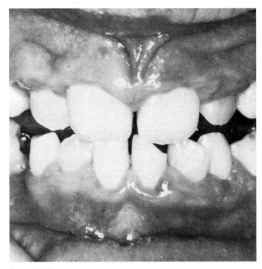

Fig. 10-25.

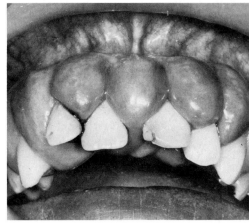

Fig. 10-28.

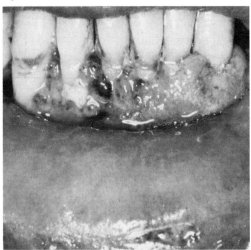

Fig. 10-26.

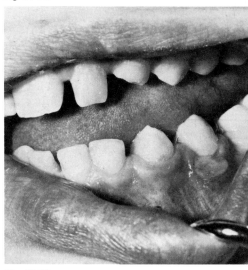

Fig. 10-29.

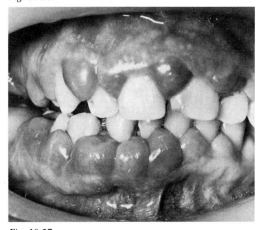

Fig. 10-27.

Diseases of the circulatory system

Wegener's granulomatosis

Fig. 10-26 shows gingival changes in a 4●
year old man with Wegener's granulomato
sis, a disease considered to be a disseminate●
form of malignant granuloma. Wegener'●
granulomatosis is a rapidly fatal disease
characterized by a necrotizing granulo

matosis of the respiratory tract, showing marked arteritis associated with granulomatous lesions of the kidneys and lungs. Like the malignant granuloma, Wegener's granulomatosis may begin with chronic nasal infection or oral changes. This happened to the patient in Fig. 10-26. Her disease began with a painful palatal ulceration and crust formation in the nose. On admission, the patient also had fungating masses of the mandibular gingiva. Within a few weeks the patient died from lesions in the kidneys.

Diseases of the digestive system

Idiopathic gingival fibromatosis

Fig. 10-27 illustrates a very pronounced swelling of the gingiva, mostly affecting the interdental papillae, in a 26 year old woman, who has for many years suffered from gingival enlargement. In the premolar and molar areas the enlargement is so marked that the teeth are covered to the occlusal surfaces. There is no history of phenytoin medication, so the lesion can only be classified as an idiopathic gingival fibromatosis. The molars were extracted because of extensive bone loss. Four years later the patient represents with gingival enlargement by now so severe (Fig. 10-28), that the interdental papillae can be lifted so that it can be observed that the roots of the teeth are denuded to 5 mm from the collum. The patient discloses that she suffers from hypertrichosis, a phenomenon reported to occur in a number of cases of idiopathic gingival fibromatosis.

Recurrent aphthous ulcerations

Fig. 10-29 shows aphthae located to the marginal and alveolar gingiva of 34 in a 10 year old boy who has had recurrent aphthous ulcerations (RAU) for the last 4 years. The aphthae heal spontaneously within 1 week. The gingiva is a most unusual location for RAU.

Clinically RAU are fibrin covered ulcerations of varying size and surrounded by a red halo. RAU is one of the most frequent oral mucosal diseases with reported prevalences ranging from 11-65%. The etiology is still unknown; stress and trauma may in some cases be eliciting factors. New investigations seem to indicate that RAU may be due to autoimmunity in oral mucosa, or to hypersensitivity to certain streptococci. When a gingival ulceration is recognized, and local factors can be excluded, neutropenia should be kept in mind as an etiologic factor. Fig. 10-30 is a photomicrograph of a biopsy from an early RAU. At the margins of the picture squamous epithelium of normal thickness can be observed, whereas the central part has only 1-2 layers of epithelial cells. The destruction of the other epithelial areas is due to a fibrinoid necrosis of the connective tissue. A mild inflammatory reaction is present.

Homogeneous leukoplakia

Fig. 10-31 shows a homogeneous leukoplakia limited to the areolar and alveolar gingivae and parts of the buccal groove. A mild gingival retraction points at energetic tooth brushing, which, however, is not enough to cause such an intense hyperkeratosis. Another etiologic factor is the 20 cigarettes the patient smokes daily. It is peculiar that the leukoplakia has spared the marginal gingiva of 16. Most oral leukoplakias are caused by heavy tobacco consumption, which can be cigarettes, cigars, cheroots, pipe, snuff and chewed tobacco. It is rather rare to observe leukoplakias on the gingiva, which may be explained by the fact that the marginal and alveolar gingivae are normally keratinized, apparently by a protective structure.

Nodular leukoplakia

Fig. 10-32 is an example, in a 50 year old man, of so-called "nodular" leukoplakia

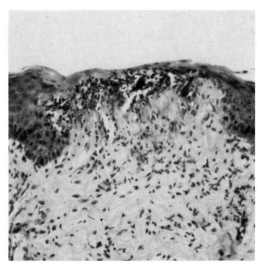

Fig. 10-30.

lial dysplasia which means an increased possibility for malignant transformation compared to homogeneous leukoplakia. Eigh years later the patient developed a squamous cell carcinoma in the affected area.

Crohn's disease

Fig. 10-33 is from the palate of a 27 year old man referred for necrotizing gingivitis of the incisor area. In the buccal groove there are linear, hyperplastic folds from which a biopsy is taken. As the histologic examination shows epitheloid cells, the patient was referred to a department of gastroenterology where Crohn's disease was diagnosed. Crohn's disease is a chronic inflammatory granulomatous disorder of unknown etiology. The patient in question also had gingival lesions as can be seen from Fig. 10-33. They are reddish and slightly elevated.

A biopsy from the area shows the typical features of Crohn's disease: epitheloid cell granuloma with some giant cells surrounded by a lymphocytic infiltration (Fig. 10-34).

located on the gingiva and part of the labial groove. In some parts of the leukoplakia a number of white nodules can be identified. The patient is a heavily addicted smoker. A biopsy from the nodular area shows epithe-

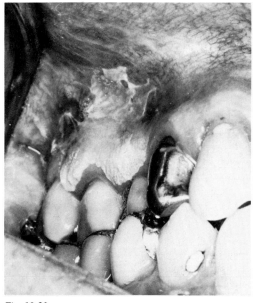

Fig. 10-31.

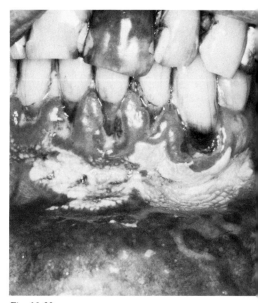

Fig. 10-32.

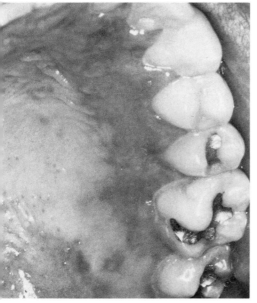

Fig. 10-33.

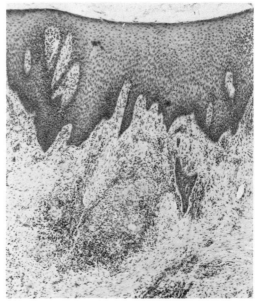

Fig. 10-34.

Diseases related to pregnancy, menstruation, and oral contraceptives

Pregnancy gingivitis

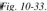It seems beyond any doubt that pregnancy may cause gingival changes. However, the reported frequency of so-called "pregnancy gingivitis" varies between 30-100%, reflecting the diversity of opinion which exists. According to studies using well defined indices, a gingival change is noticeable in pregnant women from the second month of gestation, reaching a maximum in the eighth month. During the last month of gestation a definite decrease occurs. Furthermore, it has been found that the state of the gingiva immediately after parturition is similar to that at the second month of pregnancy (Löe & Silness 1963). The same investigators also found that, although the gingiva of the molar teeth showed the highest scores throughout pregnancy, the greatest relative increase was observed around the anterior teeth. The interproximal areas are by far the most frequent sites of gingival inflammation both during pregnancy and after parturition.

Several studies have suggested that gingivitis during pregnancy is a result of the increased levels of progesterone and its effect on the microvasculature (Hugoson 1970). It has also been proposed that exaggeration of the gingival inflammatory response during pregnancy could be due to hormonal changes altering tissue metabolism (Löe & Silness, 1963).

The prevalence of gingivitis in pregnancy seems to be offset to some degree by a concomitant decrease in debris accumulation (Adams et al. 1974). During pregnancy both the gingival-periodontal index and horizontal tooth mobility are increased (Cohen et al. 1971).

Clinically, the gingival changes in pregnancy are characterized by a fiery red color of the marginal gingiva and interdental papillae. At the same time, the gingiva becomes enlarged, with the swelling mainly affecting the interdental papillae. The gingi-

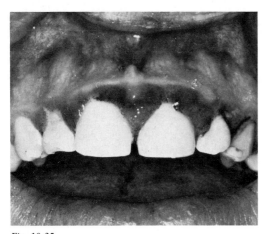

Fig. 10-35.

...va shows an increased tendency to bleed, and, in advanced cases, the patients sometimes even experience slight pain. Fig. 10-35 shows the increased volume of the marginal gingiva and the interdental papillae in a 20 year old woman in the fifth month of pregnancy. The gingival changes have been present from the third month.

Pregnancy granuloma

Apart from the generalized gingival changes, pregnancy may also give rise to the formation of tumor-like growths, epulides, along the gingival margin. A number of terms have been suggested, such as "pregnancy tumor", "epulis gravidarum", and "pregnancy granuloma". The last-mentioned term is to be preferred, because the histologic structure is similar to the structure in pyogenic (telangiectatic) granuloma. The reported frequency of pregnancy granuloma varies from 0-5% (Tiililä 1962). Occurring more frequently in the maxilla, favoring the vestibular aspect of the anterior region, it usually arises during the second trimester though occasionally earlier, and often shows rapid growth, although seldom becoming larger than 2 cm in diameter. After parturition, the granuloma begins to regress spontaneously and sometimes disappears entirely. Pregnancy granuloma is mostly a pedunculated soft growth of interdental origin with a fiery red color and often with small fibrin covered areas like those seen in Fig 10-36, from a 31 year old woman in the eighth month of pregnancy. Pregnancy granulomas will frequently bleed when touched, and have a tendency to recur rapidly.

Effect of menstruation

Some investigators have reported gingiva changes during the menstrual cycle, while others have denied the existence of such changes. Using gingival fluid measurements as an indicator of gingival inflammation, variations in the amount of fluid can be correlated to the different phases of the menstrual cycle (Lindhe & Attström 1967).

Effect of oral contraceptives

Several studies have shown that women taking hormonal contraceptives have an increased prevalence of gingivitis accompanied by a higher gingival fluid flow Recent studies have confirmed these observations and have demonstrated that there i a statistically significant increase in gingival inflammation related to the duration of drug therapy (Pankhurst et al. 1981).

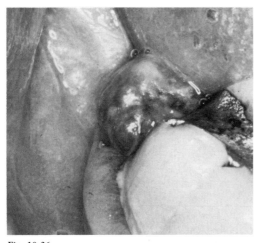

Fig. 10-36.

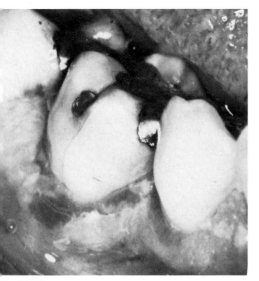

Fig. 10-37.

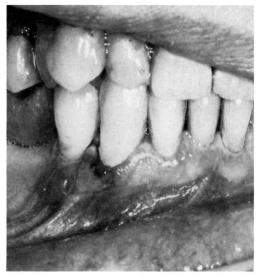

Fig. 10-39.

Diseases of the skin

Pemphigus vulgaris

Fig. 10-37 shows gingival change in a 43 year old woman who has had increasing oral mucosal trouble. The changes, consisting of blisters which burst during eating, began in the palate later spreading to the entire oral mucosa. The gingival change in Fig. 10-37 is

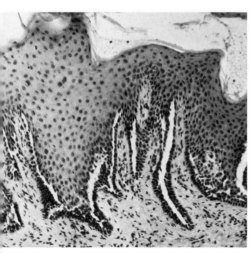

Fig. 10-38.

erythematous with focal spots of fibrin. In the periphery of the lesion there are flakes of epithelium. A biopsy from the palate shows an intraepithelial bulla in its early stage of development (Fig. 10-38). Pemphigus is a chronic bulla forming disease of skin and mucous membranes with a severe prognosis and autoimmune pathogenesis. All patients will show oral lesions in the course of the disease, and in approximately 60% the oral manifestations are its first indication. Because of the humid environment and trauma, the bullae of the oral mucosa will rupture shortly after formation, leaving a nonspecific ulceration, which sometimes makes it very difficult to arrive at a correct diagnosis. Pemphigus vegetans is another type of pemphigus having a milder course than the vulgaris type. It is characterized by fungus-like proliferations in areas where a bulla has developed. Like the vulgaris type, pemphigus vegetans often has its debut in the mouth.

Fig. 10-38 is a photomicrograph of a biopsy from the patient in Fig. 10-37. There is a split in the epithelium between the basal cells and the most profound cells of the spinal cell layers. In the split, fluid has accumu-

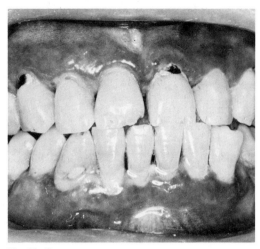

Fig. 10-40.

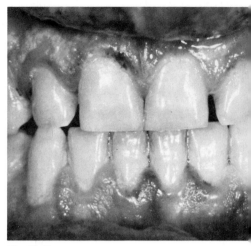

Fig. 10-42.

lated which in later stages leads to the formation of a bulla. The split in the epithelium is called acantholysis and it is pathognomonic for pemphigus. The acantholysis is due to loss of cohesion between the epithelial cells, a phenomenon caused by an immunologic reaction. Serum from patients with pemphigus contains an antibody with specificity directed against the cell surface in the epithelium from skin and mucous membranes.

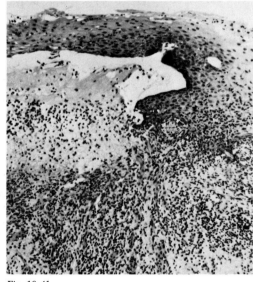

Fig. 10-41.

Benign mucous membrane pemphigoid

Fig. 10-39 shows a bulla on the alveolar gingiva of 44 and a burst bulla at 43. It is from 55 year old man who for 6 months had an itching, burning sensation of the gingiva and other areas of the mouth. Besides the changes mentioned above, the gingiva pervaded the seat of erythema and there was total loss of normal stippling. The fluid filled bulla was excised and studied histologically. The bulla proved to be subepithelial, thus compatible with the diagnosis of benign mucous membrane pemphigoid. Further confirmation of the diagnosis was found in the presence of bullae on the conjunctiva.

It is rare to find the disease in men, the patients are usually women over the age of 50. Fig. 10-40 shows a very diseased gingiva mucosa in a 57 year old woman, who for 1 years had suffered from disturbing gingival symptoms. It can be seen from the illustration that the gingiva has lost its stippling and is fiery red. In several areas, flakes of epithelium can be seen. Histologi examination of a biopsy from an area where the epithelium is intact, showed a subepithelial accumulation of fluid (Fig. 10-41) consistent with diagnosis of benign mucous membrane pemphigoid. There is no doubt that most of the cases of so-called "desquamative" gingivitis are benign mucous membrane pemphigoid. A smaller number can be identified as erosive lichen planus. Fig. 10-41 is a photomicrograph of a biopsy from the patient in Fig. 10-40. There is subepithelial fluid accumulation which has caused an atrophy of the overlying epithelium. There is marked chronic inflammation of both the fluid and the connective tissue. By means of immunofluorescence microscopy it can be demonstrated that the basement membrane area is the seat of an accumulation of immunoglobulins, which is the result of an antibody reaction against antigens in the basement membrane. Pemphigoid is classified into bullous pemphigoid and benign mucous membrane pemphigoid, both characterized by subepithelial bulla formation and identical oral lesions. However, the latter are more rare in bullous pemphigoid, which is dominated by skin changes.

Erythema multiforme exudativum

Fig. 10-42 illustrates gingival changes in the form of small ulcerated lesions in a 28 year old man with erythema multiforme exudativum. For some days the patient had influenza-like symptoms and oral discomfort. Such symptoms are typical of erythema multiforme exudativum, which is normally described eponymously. The disease is characterized by stomatitis, conjunctivitis, balanitis, and skin changes. It occurs especially in the young and more frequently in men. The course of the disease is acute and may sometimes be dramatic with a high temperature and general malaise. The patients are often disturbed by a pronounced crust formation on the lips. Not all patients have gingival changes. When present they are not diagnostic for the disease, as can be seen from Fig. 10-42. The picture, however, demonstrates an asymmetry of the gingival lesions which points towards a systemic background. Fig. 10-43 illustrates marked mucosal changes in a 23 year old man, who, shortly after angina, experienced blisters on

the labial mucosa. Within 6 days fever, red eyes and labial affections appeared. Although the disease is vesiculo-bullous, it is rare to see fluid filled blisters; they burst quickly and become covered by fibrin. Note also the gingival changes in Fig. 10-43; they are asymmetric and nonspecific. Further, the gingiva is the seat of accumulation of desquamated epithelial cells caused by lack of mastication and tooth brushing.

Discoid lupus erythematosus

Fig. 10-44 is from a 43 year old woman who for 4 years had an alteration of the right maxillary gingiva. The change consisted of erythema associated with an irregular white pattern with a number of pinpoint excrescences. These are the clinical expressions of horn pearls, which can be identified histologically. Corresponding to the marginal gingiva of 15 and the interdental papilla between 14 and 13 some constrictions or furrows can be seen. They are most probably due to a marked downgrowth of epithelial rete ridges. As the patient has a facial skin rash, the suspicion of discoid lupus erythematosus (DLE) was raised and a biopsy taken from the gingival lesion. The histologic examination confirms the tenta-

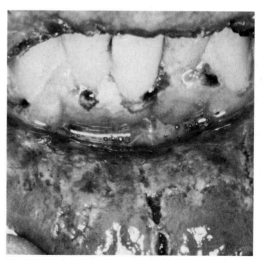

Fig. 10-43.

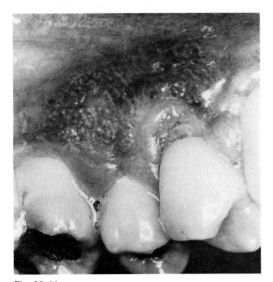

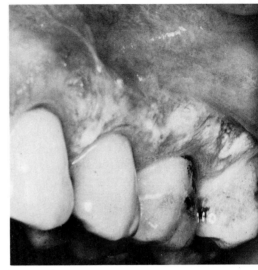

Fig. 10-44.

Fig. 10-45.

tive diagnosis. Lupus erythematosus is an autoimmune disorder which occurs in a chronic discoid and an acute disseminated form. Fig. 10-45 illustrates another type of gingival change in a patient with DLE. This change is more like lichen planus because of striae-like configurations which could simulate striae of Wickham. A more detailed

examination, however, reveals that diagnosis of lichen planus can be neither clinically nor histologically sustained. As the patient, a 33 year old woman, smokes 15 cigarettes daily it is possible to assume that tobacco has changed an originally typical DLE lesion to a more homogeneous white. It should, however, be admitted that in some

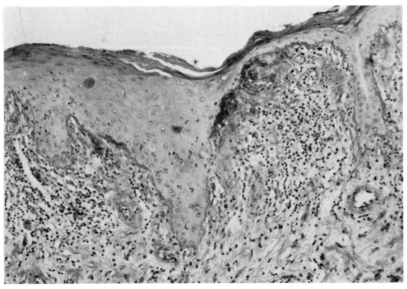

Fig. 10-46.

cases it is difficult, clinically as well as histologically, to make the differential diagnosis between oral changes of DLE and lichen planus. In such instances an immunologic study will be decisive. Fig. 10-46 is a photomicrograph of the biopsy of the lesion in Fig. 10-44. The histologic section is stained with PAS, which more clearly than hematoxylin-eosin shows the presence of immunoglobulins juxtaepithelially, particularly of IgM. The photomicrograph further illustrates the differences in the thickness of the epithelium, which explains that some areas (the atrophic) appear red clinically, whereas other (the hyperplastic) appear white.

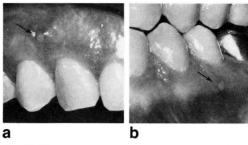

a   **b**

Fig. 10-47.

Psoriasis

Fig. 10-47 shows 2 very small, yellow excrescences in a 20 year old woman who for 7 years has suffered from psoriasis, a common, chronic, recurrent inflammatory skin disease. The skin lesions are round, well defined, erythematous affections often of a silver-white color. It is still debated whether psoriasis has oral manifestations. Some investigators feel they have demonstrated, in psoriatic patients, very small, greyish-white elements as illustrated in Fig. 10-47. Histologic examination of these elements has shown abscesses in the superficial part of the epithelium.

Lichen planus

Figs. 10-48-52. Lichen planus is a relatively common chronic, inflammatory skin disease of unknown etiology accompanied by small (flat), polygonal, red-brown papules, the surface of which is characterized by fine, small, and keratinized lines, the so-called "Wickham's striae". Lichen is often associated with oral manifestations. The prevalence of oral lichen planus is approximately 1%, and slightly higher in women. Among patients with oral lichen planus only 30% will show skin lesions. The oral manifestations present a rather varied picture. Usually the oral lesions are classified into reticular, papular, plaque, atrophic-ulcerative, and bullous types. It should not, however, be forgotten that 2 or more types can be found in the same patient. The gingival mucosa is often affected in patients with oral lichen planus. The appearance of the lesions is dependent upon the location in the mouth. Thus, physiologically keratinized mucosa, i.e. palate and gingiva, will not exhibit such well defined Wickham striae as non-keratinized mucosa. This fact is clearly illustrated in Fig. 10-48, a 45 year old women

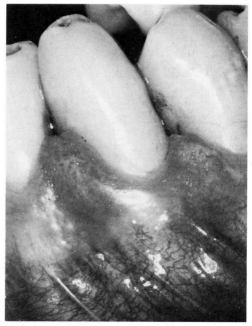

Fig. 10-48.

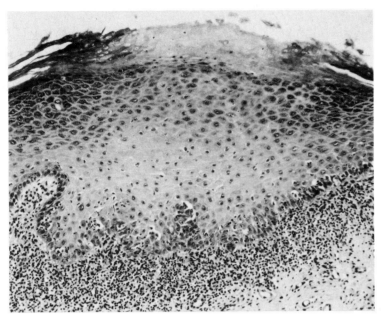

Fig. 10-49.

with lichen planus lesions on the interdental papillae. Although the Wickham's striae are wider and less well defined than usual, they can still be identified. A histologic examination will in most cases confirm a clinical suspicion of lichen planus. Fig. 10-49 is a photomicrograph of a biopsy which contained a stria of Wickham. All features characteristic of lichen planus can be seen in the picture. There is hyperorthokeratosis and hyperplasia of the epithelium corresponding to Wickham's striae. Furthermore, there is a "sawtooth" appearance of the rete ridges which are also marked by degenerativ changes in connection with the band-lik accumulation of lymphocytes in the juxtaepithelial connective tissue. A more diffuse type of gingival manifestation of lichen planus is seen in Fig. 10-50, a 46 year old woman who for 1 year had cutaneous lichen planus affections. The gingival lesion is quite similar to the gingival lesion caused by discoid lupus erythematosus as demonstrated in Fig. 10-45. In the patient of Fig. 10-50 both sides of the buccal mucosa showed typical reticular elements. On the picture both confluent striae of Wickham and a red atrophic area are visible. An accentuation of the atrophic element can be seen in Fig. 10-51, a 43 year old woman who for 1 month had itching sensations in the gingiva. Clinically the changes are characterized by alternating white and red (erythematous) areas all over the gingiva. The erythematous areas, caused by atrophic epithelium and subepithelia

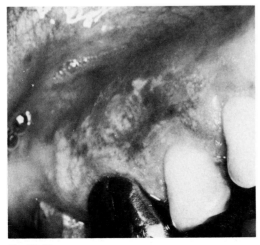

Fig. 10-50.

276

inflammation, appear dark on the illustration. Sometimes strong symptoms of disturbance were experienced after tooth brushing or eating of spicy food. The patient also reported aggravation in periods of psychic stress. In some patients, the epithelium becomes so atrophic that it bursts spontaneously or by a light trauma, giving rise to an ulcerative (erosive) type of oral lichen planus. This condition is illustrated in Fig. 10-52 from a 50 year old woman. In both maxilla and mandible there is diffuse involvement of the entire gingival mucosa. There are areas of erythema and areas of ulcerations covered by fibrin, especially in the mandible. These clinical manifestations are similar to those observed in patients with benign mucous membrane pemphigoid (Fig. 10-40). The atrophic (ulcerative) lichen planus is histologically characterized by a very thin epithelium. Often the epithelium is only ⅕ of its normal thickness, and it is easy to understand that the mucosa in these areas assumes a red color, as the many small vessels from the inflamed areas shine through. The bullous type is very seldom met with and rarely affects the gingiva. The plaque type may also involve the gingiva. Clinically it appears as white, homogeneous areas which in a number of cases may be conceived as a superimposed leukoplakia as these patients

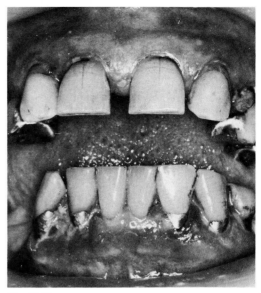

Fig. 10-52.

frequently smoke. The atrophic and ulcerative types of lichen planus, also including the gingival manifestations, are often accompanied by marked pain, which necessitates treatment. An electrogalvanic influence from metal restorations ought to be excluded first. As most of the patients with ulcerative lesions have a superimposed Candida albicans infection, this complication should be treated either before or at the same time as the steroid treatment of the lichen planus is carried out. It is often necessary to treat a patient for several months in order to arrive at a satisfactory result.

Diseases of the musculoskeletal system

Dermatomyositis

Fig. 10-53 shows some very delicate gingival changes in a 9 year old girl suffering from dermatomyositis. The marginal gingiva, especially in the maxilla, is slightly edematous and the seat of slight telangiectatic

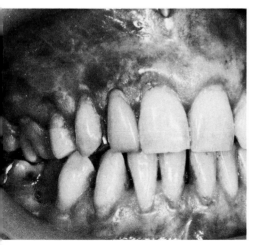

Fig. 10-51.

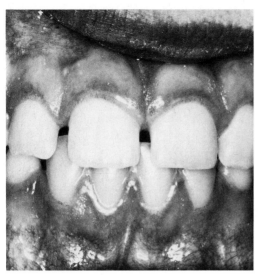

Fig. 10-53.

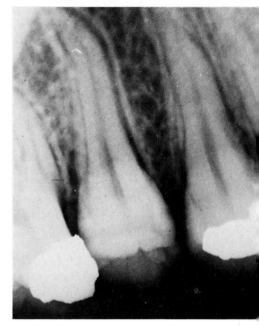

Fig. 10-55.

changes which irradiate from the marginal gingiva, giving the mucosa a faint reddish-bluish color. For 3 years the girl suffered from dermatomyositis, a rare disease which primarily affects the skin and skeletal muscles. The disease belongs to the so-called "connective tissue diseases of unknown etiology". In the early stages cutaneous edema is observed, which later turns into a telangiectatic erythema. It appears reason-

able to assume that this tendency to form telangiectasias, is reflected in the gingival reaction illutrated in Fig. 10-53.

Osteitis deformans

Fig. 10-54 is a radiograph of 28 in a 70 year old man referred because of delayed healing after extraction of 2 molars in the right side of the maxilla. As radiography disclosed a peculiar bone structure of the "ground glass" type, an additional radiographic examination of the entire skeleton was undertaken. This revealed pathologic changes in the skull, characteristic of osteitis deformans or Paget's disease. Biopsy of the jaw bone showed a mosaic-like structure, and there was a marked increase in alkaline phosphatases, thus the diagnosis of osteitis deformans was made. In patients with osteitis deformans, hypercementosis is often reported, a change which can be seen in Fig. 10-54 which also discloses a blurring of the periodontal membrane.

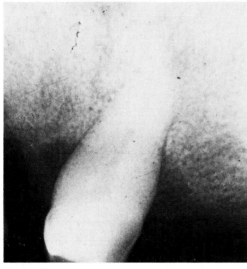

Fig. 10-54.

Scleroderma

Fig. 10-55 is a radiograph of 16, 15, 14 in a 21 year old man, suffering from diffuse scleroderma. He experienced toothache-like symptoms from 15, which is intact, but in traumatic occlusion and articulation. Radiography disclosed a marked widening of the periodontal membrane of 15 and most of the other teeth. Concurrently with the widening of the periodontal membrane there is a thickening of the lamina dura of the alveolar bone. Widening of the periodontal membrane in patients with scleroderma has been reported by several investigators, but the frequency of the changes varies from 7-40%. Diffuse scleroderma is a chronic disease characterized by diffuse fibrosis of the skin and other organs. The etiology is unknown, but immunologic factors appear to play a part. In the present case the tooth-ache-like symptoms are explicable by the traumatic load which 15 has been exposed to, due to extrusion of the tooth resulting from the edema of the periodontal membrane. When the tooth was relieved by grinding, the symptoms disappeared. Fig. 10-56 shows the histologic changes in the widened periodontal membrane of a 24 in a 43 year old woman with diffuse sclerodermia. The normal straight course of the Sharpey's fibers is replaced by a collagenous tissue without orientation of the fibers and with focal hyalinization.

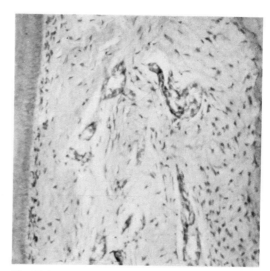

Fig. 10-56.

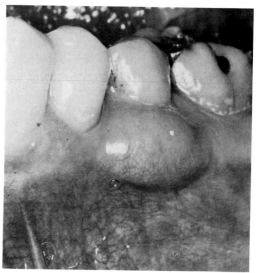

Fig. 10-57.

Congenital anomalies

Recklinghausen's neurofibromatosis

Fig. 10-57 illustrates a localized gingival enlargement in a 35 year old woman, who for 20 years had a recognized neurofibromatosis of Recklinghausen. She has had neurofibromas and café-au-lait spots on back and stomach. The tongue presented a single tumor, removed together with the gingival enlargement, which is a most unusual man-

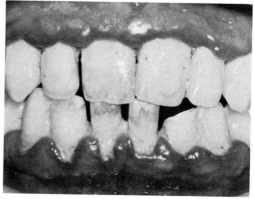

Fig. 10-58.

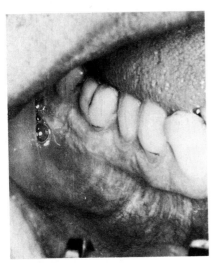

Fig. 10-59.

heart disease after infancy. As the blood does not carry sufficient oxygen, a cyanosis arises. This change may be manifest at birth but in lighter cases it occurs in early childhood and has a tendency to progress. The cyanotic color of the gingiva corresponds to the general cyanotic color of the patient. Considering that the patient in Fig. 10-58 is only 29 years of age, the severe periodontal destruction has developed because of insufficient supply of oxygen.

ifestation of Recklinghausen's neurofibromatosis. In both instances the histologic examination showed the characteristic structures of a neurofibroma.

Fallot's tetralogy

Fig. 10-58 shows the gingival conditions in a 29 year old man suffering from Steno-Fallot's tetralogy, the most prevalent cyanotic

White sponge nevus

Fig. 10-59 illustrates a gingival manifestation of white sponge nevus (nævus albus spongiosus, white folded gingivostomatosis) in a 33 year old man. The disease, which is symptomless, is a congenital disturbance in the differentiation of the epithelium genetically transmitted by an autosomal dominant mode of inheritance. It manifests itself early in childhood and increases throughout life. The affected oral mucosa appears white or gray, thickened, deeply folded and spongy. Some patients also have manifestations in vagina and/or rectum. The condition may show variations in intensity and may be mistaken for leukoplakia, but the case history,

Fig. 10-60.

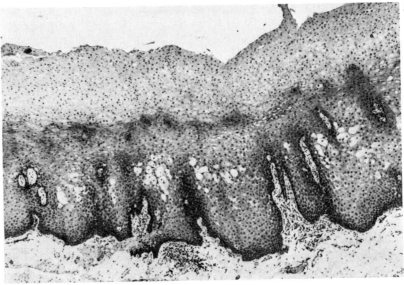

in the early appearance of the disease, will validate the diagnosis of leukoplakia. Malignant transformation has not been reported. Fig. 10-60 is a photomicrograph of a biopsy from the buccal mucosa of a patient with white sponge nevus. There is a very pronounced increase in the superficial layers of the epithelium characterized by heavy parakeratosis. In the spinal cell layers there are many large, bright, vacuolated cells, often called nevus cells.

Drug stomatitis

Cytostatics

Fig. 10-61 illustrates some irregular and asymmetric gingival lesions in the form of small localized necroses at 11, 21 and 43, 42, 41 and 31 in a 42 year old man, who received immunosuppressive treatment with azathioprine in connection with a kidney transplantation. Azathioprine belongs to the group of cytostatics which are also being used in the treatment of malignant systemic diseases. Many patients treated with these compounds develop a drug stomatitis characterized by erythemas and ulcerations.

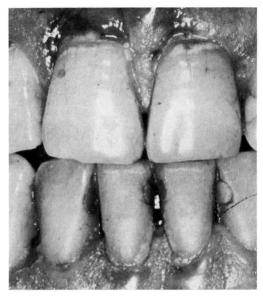

Fig. 10-61.

Hydantoin derivatives

For 40 years phenytoin (5.5-diphenylhydantoin (DPH), Dilantin®, Epanutin®) has been the preferred medication for epilepsy. However, in the last 10 years phenytoin has to a certain extent been replaced by carbamazepine because it has fewer side effects.

Fig. 10-62.

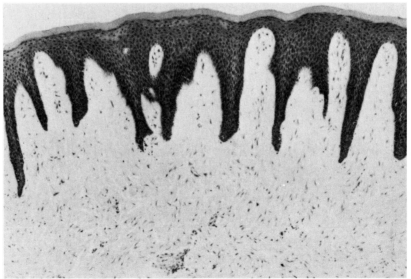

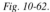

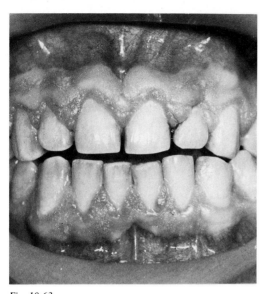

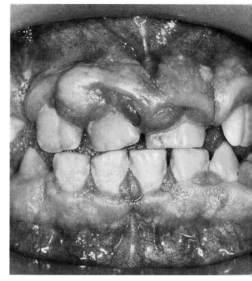

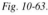

Fig. 10-63.   Fig. 10-64.

The side effects of phenytoin are varied and comprise, besides the well known gingival enlargement, disturbances of the nervous system, blood forming tissues, bone, skin, liver, endocrine glands and the immune system.

The gingival enlargement has been designated as hyperplasia gingivae diphenyl hydantoinea, diphenylhydantoin gingival overgrowth, Dilantin® hyperplasia, etc. The gingival enlargement in phenytoin treatment is not due to either hypertrophy or hyperplasia of fibroblasts and/or collagenous fibers. The number of these elements per unit tissue is normal, but the growth is uncontrolled, consequently the term gingival overgrowth. The reported incidence of gingival hyperplasia in patients receiving phenytoin varies from 3-62%; there is no sex predilection.

A number of histologic studies have tried to elucidate the pathogenesis of the gingival enlargement. By means of autoradiography an increased mitotic activity has been demonstrated in fibroblasts from biopsies from phenytoin conditioned gingival changes. Tissue cultures of fibroblasts have been tre-

ated with phenytoin and an increased mitotic activity was found. However, the activity decreased under the influence of ascorbic acid. The pathogenesis is still an unsolved problem. An excellent review is provided by Hassell (1981).

A characteristic feature of the fibrous overgrowth is hyperplasia of the covering squamous cell epithelium, which sends long and slender projections into the connective tissue (Fig. 10-62). The gingival enlargement begins as an overgrowth of the interdental papillae followed by a spreading in the other regions of the gingiva. Fig. 10-63, from an 18 year old man, shows a slight increase in volume of several interdental papillae. This epileptic patient was treated with phenytoin for several years. Fig. 10-64 illustrates an enlargement which is quite monstrous. The patient, a 15 year old boy, received 300 mg phenytoin daily for 2 years on account of epileptic seizures. Despite the marked enlargement, the gingiva has maintained its normal stippling and color in contrast to idiopathic gingival fibromatosis, where the color is red and the surface glossy (Figs. 10-27, 10-28). In later stages, where the fibrous overgrowth has led to the formation of deep pseudopockets, an inflammation develops whereby the stippling is lost.

There is a correlation between degree of gingival enlargement and daily dosage of phenytoin, oral hygiene and other local irritants (Aas 1963). The incidence of gingival enlargement is higher in younger persons. Although the increase in volume affects the vestibular as well as the lingual gingivae, the vestibular changes are the most pronounced. Inexplicable is the definite predilection for the anterior gingiva. It is characteristic that the fibrous overgrowth does not appear on the edentulous alveolar ridge.

The most severe cases of gingival enlargement must be treated by gingivectomy. Several studies have demonstrated that it is possible to prevent the development of marked lesions by an intense effort comprising removal of calculus and plaque every third month, combined with careful tooth brushing and use of dental floss. Despite these precautions a small increase in gingival volume may develop in the anterior segment within the first 6 months, a change which is not aggravated in the following months.

Industrial intoxications

Lead

Fig. 10-65 shows a typical lead line in a 45 year old man who worked in a battery plant for many years. Besides the gingival lead line (halo saturninus) the patient suffers from fatigue, lead colic, and a grayish color of the skin, characteristic symptoms of lead intoxication. As lead is widely used in industry, lead intoxication is still an important industrial hazard. In a number of cases lead intoxication has been recognized by a gingival lead line. The line is bluish-black, a few mm wide and follows the marginal gingiva. The lead line is due to deposits of insoluble lead sulfide in the endothelial cells of the capillaries and in the histiocytes. In some cases it may be difficult to distinguish between a lead line and subgingival calculus.

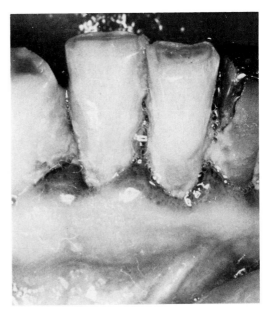

Fig. 10-65.

Mercury

Fig. 10-66 illustrates a gingival change in the form of prominent edema of the marginal gingivae and interdental papillae. The gingivae are loosened from the teeth; at 41 and 31

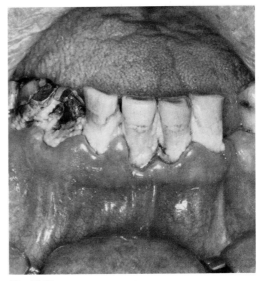

Fig. 10-66.

there is a fibrin covered ulceration. The gingival mucosa bleeds easily. The patient is a 48 year old man who has worked in direct contact with mercury. After 1 week he suffered from general malaise, sore throat, and bleeding gingivae. Later, severe stomatitis developed with yellowish, annular, slightly elevated lesions on the tongue and buccal mucosae. The patient was referred because of the stomatitis which turned out to be the key to recognizing mercury intoxication. An investigation of the Hg content in the urine showed 11000 γ/l, a concentration which is times higher than the highest so far reported in patients with industrial mercury intoxication. The patient was treated successfully with dimercaprol.

References

Aas, E. (1963) Hyperplasia gingivae diphenylhydantoinea. *Acta Odontologica Scandinavica,* Supplement 34.

Adams, D., Carney, J. S. & Dicks, D. A. (1974). Pregnancy gingivitis: a survey of 100 antenatal patients. *Journal of Dentistry* 2, 106-110.

Bernick, S. M., Cohen, D. W., Baker, L. & Laster, L. (1975) Dental disease in children with diabetes mellitus. *Journal of Periodontology* 46, 241-246.

Cohen, W. D., Friedman, L. A., Shapiro, J., Kyle, C. G. & Franklin, S. (1970) Diabetes mellitus and periodontal disease: two year longitudinal observations. I. *Journal of Periodontology* 41, 709-712.

Cohen, W. D., Shapiro, J., Friedman, L., Kyle, C. G. & Franklin, S. (1971) A longitudinal investigation of the periodontal changes during pregnancy and fifteen months postpartum. II. *Journal of Periodontology* 42, 653-657.

Faulconbridge, A. R., Bradshaw, W. C. L., Jenkins, P. A. & Baum, J. D. (1981) The dental status of a group of diabetic children. *British Dental Journal* 151, 253-255.

Hassell, T. M. (1981). *Epilepsy and the oral manifestations of phenytoin therapy.* Monographs in Oral Science. New York: S. Karger.

Hugoson, A. (1970) Gingival inflammation and female sex hormones. A clinical investigation of pregnant women and experimental studies in dogs. *Journal of Periodontal Research* 5 Supplement 5.

Lindhe, J. & Attström, R. (1967). Gingival exudation during the menstrual cycle. *Journal of Periodontal Research* 2, 194-198.

Löe, H. & Silness, J. (1963). Periodontal disease in pregnancy. I. Prevalence and severity. *Acta Odontologica Scandinavica* 21, 533-551.

McCullen, J. A., Van Dyke, T. E., Horoszewicz H. & Genco, R. J. (1981) Neutrophil chemotaxis in individuals with advanced periodontal disease and a genetic predisposition to diabetes mellitus. *Journal of Periodontology* 52, 167-173.

Pankhurst, C. L., Waite, I. M., Hicks, K. A. Allen, Y. & Harkness, R. D. (1981) The influence of oral contraceptive therapy on the periodontium – duration of drug therapy. *Journal of Periodontology* 52, 617-620.

Pindborg, J. J. (1980). *Atlas of diseases of the oral mucosa.* 3rd ed. Copenhagen: Munksgaard.

Tiililä, I. (1962) Epulis gravidarum. Thesis. *Suom. Hammaslaeaek. Toim.* 58, Supplement 1.

CHAPTER 11

Tumors and Tumor-like Lesions Originating from the Periodontium

Epulides
    Peripheral giant cell granuloma
    Gingival fibroma
    Pyogenic granuloma

Benign neoplasms of oral mucosa
    Neurilemoma
    Capillary hemangioma
    Calcifying epithelial odontogenic tumor

Cysts
    Gingival cyst

Malignant tumors
    Squamous cell carcinoma
    Malignant melanoma
    Osteoblastic osteosarcoma
    Chondroblastic osteosarcoma
    Metastasis from an adenocarcinoma of colon
    Metastasis from lung carcinoma
    Kaposi's sarcoma
    Histiocytic lymphoma

22 and 23, which have become separated by the pressure exerted by the tumor. It is from a 58 year old man who for 6 months has had a swelling between 22 and 23. The tumor, which is bluish in color, is soft, well defined and the seat of an ulceration. Tumor-like lesions, originating from the gingiva, are called epulides, a term which is occasionally conceived as a synonym for a giant cell containing process. This is an erroneous concept, as the term epulis, verbally translated from Greek, only means "arisen from the gingiva". Many different pathologic proces-

The present descriptions of tumors and tumor-like lesions do not pretend to be a complete account of such lesions related to the periodontal tissues. They should serve as characteristic examples and emphasize, partly that the periodontal tissues may be the origin of such lesions, partly that the reaction of these tissues may differ from reactions observed at other locations. The author distinguishes between a tumor and a neoplasm.

Epulides

Peripheral giant cell granuloma

Fig. 11-1 shows a rather large tumor between

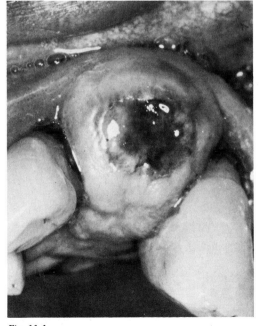

Fig. 11-1.

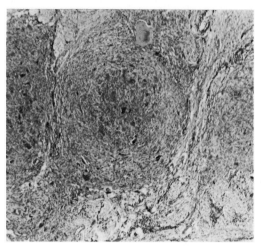

Fig. 11-2.

ses may appear clinically as epulides. The peripheral giant cell granuloma, most often seen in younger individuals, is more frequent in women than in men, and the mandible is more often affected than the maxilla. The predominant location is facially in the anterior regions. Fig. 11-2 is a photomicrograph of the peripheral giant cell granuloma in Fig. 11-1. In the low power magnification, numerous giant cells can be identified. They occur in granuloma-like formations separated by septae of collagenous fibers. At the bottom of the picture osteoid tissue can be noticed. These 2 features: connective tissue septae and osteoid are characteristic of giant cell granulomas. Between the giant cells there is a vivid proliferation of endothelial cells leading to the formation of numerous small capillaries. In these areas many hemorrhages are seen, causing the typical color of the lesion. The giant cell granuloma has great growth potential as can be observed from Fig. 11-1. It is characteristic that the giant cell granuloma has a marked tendency for recurrence.

Gingival fibroma

Fig. 11-3 is from a 25 year old man who lacks

the molars in the right side of the mandible In contrast to the giant cell granuloma, the lesion illustrated in Fig. 11-3 is firm and o the same color as the adjacent mucosa. As the lesion contains fibrous tissue, it is ofter called a "fibrous epulis", a term whick should be replaced by "gingival fibroma" These fibromas may vary in size, although it is quite rare to see such a large lesion as in Fig. 11-3. The fibroma occours more often in women than in men and more frequently in the maxilla than in the mandible. The majority of these lesions is found in the anterior region. The gingival fibroma possesses considerable force and is able to separate the teeth from each other. Chronic irritation may play a part in the development of a gingival fibroma. Fig. 11-4 is a photomicrograph of such a fibroma, which is covered by squamous cell epithelium, slightly keratinized and shows some variations in the length of the epithelial ridges. The major part of the lesion consists of cell poor, collagenous tissue where the fiber bundles can be recognized. As the histologic structure is the same as in fibromas at other locations of the oral mucosa it is difficult to understand why the gingival fibroma is associated with a

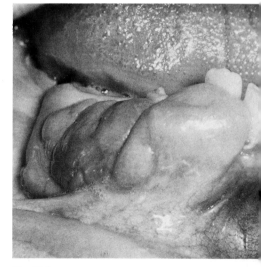

Fig. 11-3.

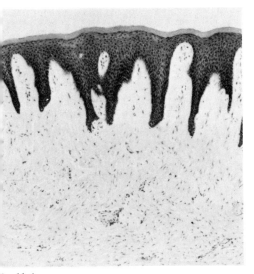

Fig. 11-4.

high rate of recurrence, not found at other locations.

Pyogenic granuloma

Fig. 11-5 illustrates a lesion in a 30 year old woman, between 22 and 21 which have become separated due to pressure from the lesion which is fiery red with small ulcerations. The appearance is characteristic of a pyogenic granuloma, sometimes called a telangiectatic granuloma. The pyogenic granuloma may occur in all areas of the oral mucosa, but is most frequently found on the marginal gingiva. The granuloma may be conceived as an exaggerated reaction to minor trauma without it having been possible to demonstrate a definite infectious organism. Due to its red color, which may sometimes turn to a cyanotic hue, the pyogenic granuloma may be mistaken for a giant cell granuloma. Fig. 11-6 is a photomicrograph of the lesion shown in Fig. 11-5. To the right in the picture there is a squamous cell epithelium; the rest of the surface is a fibrin covered ulceration. Just below the surface there is heavy acute inflammation. After that follows massive proliferation of endothelial cells characterized by numerous, very small and thin walled lumina. The content of erythrocytes in these luminae is responsible for the red color of the lesion. As is the case with the giant cell granuloma and the gingival fibroma, the pyogenic granuloma has a high potential for recurrence.

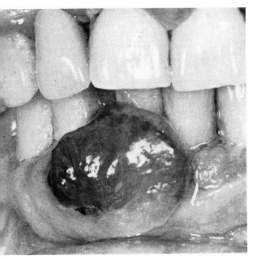

Fig. 11-5.

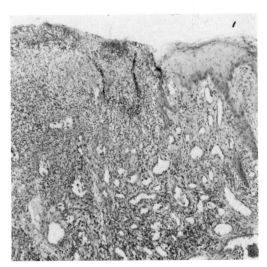

Fig. 11-6.

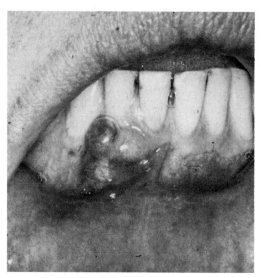

Fig. 11-7.

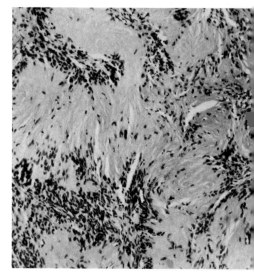

Fig. 11-8.

Benign neoplasms of oral mucosa

Neurilemoma

Fig. 11-7 shows an epulis (i.e. a tumor originating from the gingiva) in a 19 year old man who has had the lesion for the past 6 months. It originated suddenly as a soft, well defined tumor in the gingiva of 43. Since then, the lesion has become somewhat harder and 2 more lesions have appeared as can be seen in the illustration. The tumor extends down to the bottom of the labial groove. A radiographic examination does not reveal any osseous destruction. The "epulis" is surgically removed and the histologic examination shows a well encapsulated neoplasm. The fine structure is characterized by fusiform cells arranged as palisades and a cell free zone with delicate fibers as seen in Fig. 11-8. The combination of cell free zones and palisading cells is called a Verocay body, which is typical of a neurilemoma of the Antoni type A. The type B is characterized by microcystic degenerations. The neurilemoma is a benign tumor arising from the sheaths of peripheral nerves. When the neoplasm occurs in the mouth it is supposed to stem from branches of the fifth cranial nerve, the trigeminal. Clinically, the neoplasm is found in the superficial soft tissues as a firm, nodular tumor. The consistency may be softer when a cystic degeneration has taken place. In contrast to the neurofibroma (p. 279), the neurilemoma is almost always surrounded by a capsule and thus easy to remove.

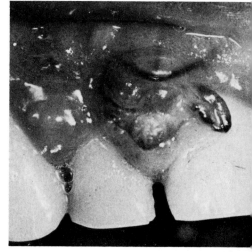

Fig. 11-9.

Capillary hemangioma

After fibromas, pyogenic granulomas and verruca vulgaris hemangiomas are the most frequent tumors of the oral mucosa. Several authors doubt whether hemangiomas are true neoplasms and suggest they be classified as developmental anomalies. That may apply for the capillary, but not for the cavernous hemangiomas. The later are the second type of hemangiomas to be found in the mouth.

Fig. 11-9 shows a capillary hemangioma which not only affects the gingiva but also the corresponding area of the upper lip. The patient is a 20 year old man who has had the lesion as long as he can remember. It is deep red in color, slightly lobulate and often causes bleeding at tooth brushing. Fig. 11-10 is a photomicrograph of the hemangioma from Fig. 11-9. Two areas of intense endothelial proliferation can be seen with formation of small, thin walled vessels. Between the 2 areas there is a band of cell poor collagenous tissue. When Fig. 11-10 is compared with Fig. 11-6, depicting a pyogenic granuloma, it is evident that the endothelial proliferation of the pyogenic granuloma is complicated by a strong inflammatory reaction which is not observed in the capillary hemangioma. When planning the treatment of capillary hemangiomas it should be kept in mind that a spontaneous regression may occur.

Calcifying epithelial odontogenic tumor

Odontogenic tumors seldom originate from the periodontal tissues. It is often debated whether gingival fibromas with islands of odontogenic epithelium should be classified as odontogenic tumors. Some authors call these lesions odontogenic epithelial hamartomas. The following entities may occur as an "epulis": ameloblastoma, dentinoma, adenomatoid odontogenic tumor, calcifying odontogenic cyst and calcifying epithelial odontogenic tumor. The peripheral ameloblastoma presenting as a gingival tumor is by

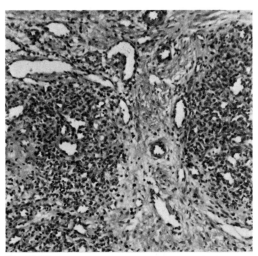

Fig. 11-10.

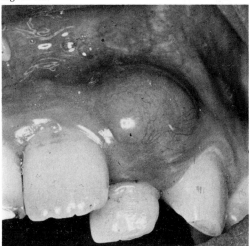

Fig. 11-11.

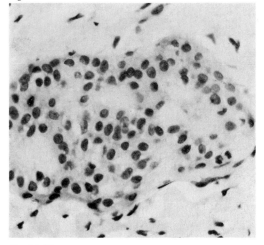

Fig. 11-12.

some authors conceived as the so-called "gingival basal cell carcinoma".

Fig. 11-11 is an example of a peripheral type of calcifying epithelial odontogenic tumor found in a 29 year old woman. The tumor manifests itself as a gingival swelling, firm and well demarcated. The lesion does not arise from the marginal gingiva for which reason it is not a true "epulis". The lesion has been present for 5 years and not caused any symptoms. There are no osseous changes. Fig. 11-12 is a photomicrograph of the neoplasm in Fig. 11-11. The picture is dominated by a large island of epithelial odontogenic tumor: intracellular degeneration with swelling of the cytoplasm. In the illustration there are no calcifications, but they were found in other sections. An extraosseous location of the calcifying epithelial odontogenic tumor is rare; in an analysis of 113 cases only 5 were extraosseous.

Cysts

Gingival cyst

Fig. 11-13 shows a well demarcated, soft and fluctuating swelling on the alveolar gingiva between 44 and 43 in a 75 year old woman.

The presumed cyst is surgically removed and studied histologically. Fig. 11-14 illustrates that the specimen is covered by squamous cell epithelium. The picture is dominated by a cyst, partially filled with erythrocytes. The wall of the cyst is a very thin, squamous cell epithelium, often only 2 layers thick, and nonkeratinized. Gingival cysts are most often found between the lateral incisor and first premolar on the facial aspect. Some cases are diagnosed clinically, whereas some are recognized histologically in biopsies from the gingiva. Clinically recognizable cysts are most frequent in the mandible. A gingival cyst may arise from (1) rests of the dental lamina, enamel organ, or the islands of Malassez, (2) degenerative, cystic changes in proliferating epithelial ridges from the gingival epithelium, or (3) from traumatic implantation of surface epithelium into the connective tissue. Gingival cysts are more prevalent than was hitherto thought.

Malignant tumors

Squamous cell carcinoma

Fig. 11-15 shows an ulcerated neoplasm in a

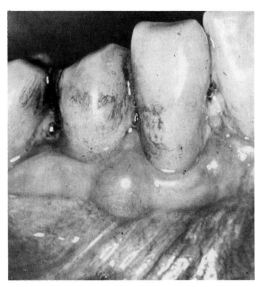

Fig. 11-13.

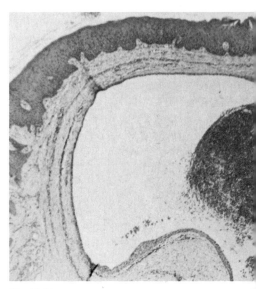

Fig. 11-14.

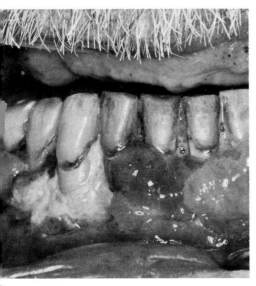

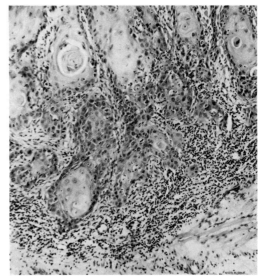

Fig. 11-15.

Fig. 11-16.

79 year old man, an ardent smoker, who for 1 month experienced symptoms from the gingiva. The neoplasm extends from 46 to 32 and is characterized by indurated margins and a fibrin covered ulceration appearing red on the picture. All 4 mandibular incisors are very loose and a radiograph reveals destruction of the osseous part of the periodontium. A biopsy is taken and Fig. 11-16 shows the results: a highly differentiated squamous cell carcinoma with horn pearl formation. The carcinoma is infiltrating the cross striated muscles at the bottom of the picture. The carcinoma has elicited a strong immunologic reaction illustrated by a massive accumulation of lymphocytes. In the literature it is rare to see a distinction maintained between a gingival cancer and a cancer developed on the edentulous alveolar ridge. Thus, many reports deal with cancer of the "gums". In most of these cases men have dominated, and only older people are affected. In recent years a marked shift in male/female ratio has been observed. In England the ratio was 5:1 in 1932-39, but in 1960-69 it was 1:1. Most gingival cancers affect the maxilla and 60% are located posteriorly to the premolars. In an American

study it has been shown that dentists play an important part in the early recognition of gingival cancer; 60% of these patients are first seen by a dentist. Gingival cancer begins as an ulceration, often associated with leukoplakia, and infiltrates rapidly in depth, with osseous involvement. In another American study gingival cancer had exceeded 3 cm at admission in 44% of the referred cases.

Malignant melanoma

Fig. 11-17 shows a large malignant melanoma originating from the gingiva in a dark skinned individual from Kerala in South India. Besause of the growth of the neoplasm, the teeth in the affected area have been lost. In contrast to the carcinoma there is no induration at the periphery of the melanoma. Fig. 11-18 is a photomicrograph of a biopsy from a malignant melanoma similar to the neoplasm seen in Fig. 11-17. The surface epithelium is atrophic and a direct transition from epithelium to tumor tissue can be seen in the form of junctional activity. The tumor cells are large and very irregular in shape. There are many cells with abnor-

291

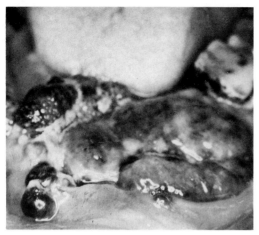

Fig. 11-17.

appear to be equally affected. The palata mucosa is the favorite site for developmen of melanomas, followed by gingiva and ton gue. The degree of pigmentation varies great deal; in some cases the tumor is color less, an amelanotic melanoma. Usually, th tumor is recognizable by a swelling which bleeds easily even after small traumas. Th prognosis is worse for oral melanomas than for cutaneous melanomas. The 5 year survi val rate is only 20% for oral melanomas. Th prognosis is most severe in cases where th tumor arises suddenly and becomes substan tial within a few weeks. In the early stages o a melanoma an amalgam tattoo may be rele vant in the differential diagnostic considera tions.

mal accumulation of chromatin, and the mitotic activity is high. The black and white reproduction does not allow the recognition of the many melanin granules which are present in the cytoplasm of the tumor cells. The tumor originates from the melanocytes present in the basal layer of the oral epithelium. During this development – the junctional activity – the borderline between tumor and epithelium becomes blurred. Several authors are of the opinion that people with dark skin are more disposed to develop melanomas than are Caucasoids. Both sexes

Osteoblastic osteosarcoma

Fig. 11-19 shows a round, well demarcated firm swelling on the alveolar gingiva be tween 43 and 42 in a 26 year old woman. It i also evident that 42 is tilted against 43. Two months before admission, the patien noticed soreness of 42, and for 5 days ther had been a feeling of swelling in the affecte region. A radiograph (Fig. 11-20) reveal that the periodontal membrane distally to 4 is much widened. Mesially on 43 there is lesser, but evident, widening of th

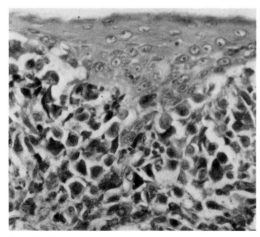

Fig. 11-18.

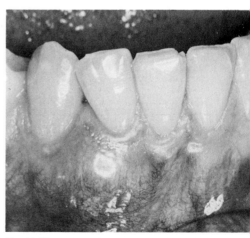

Fig. 11-19.

periodontal membrane. As these changes have only been reported in patients with osteosarcoma this diagnosis appears likely. A biopsy shows a typical osteoblastic osteosarcoma, and a resection of the area where the tumor is located is carried out with retention of the base of the mandible. Fig. 11-21 is a photomicrograph of the surgical specimen; to the right in the picture, the root surface of 42 can be seen. The periodontal membrane is very wide and most of the Sharpey's fibers are replaced by tumor tissue which consists partly of cellular tissue with tumor cells, partly of bone produced by the tumor cells. As these are similar to osteoblasts the tumor is designated as an osteoblastic osteosarcoma. In a 7 year follow-up period there has been no recurrence.

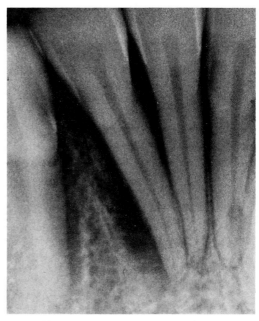

Fig. 11-20.

Chondroblastic osteosarcoma

Fig. 11-22 is a radiograph of the area between 21 and 22 in a 26 year old woman who 3 months before admission noticed a swelling of the affected region. Clinically, there is an elongation of 21, which is slightly tilted. There is a marked widened periodontal membrane with an irregular contour comprising small radiopaque bodies. A biopsy shows that the lesion is a chondroblastic osteosarcoma. After resection of the area containing the tumor the patient was fol-

Fig. 11-21.

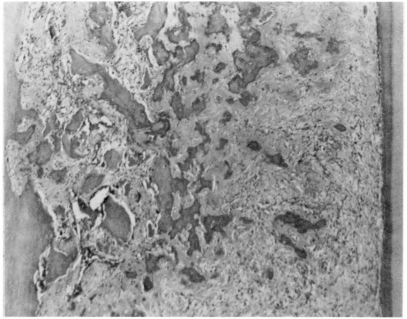

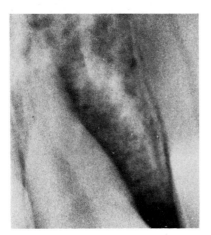

Fig. 11-22.

lowed for 8 years without any signs of recurrence. A Danish study has shown that there is 1 jaw osteosarcoma per year per million population. In U.S.A. a study has found 0.07 cases of jaw osteosarcoma per 100.000 population per year. ⅙ of the jaw sarcomas encountered are osteosarcomas. In recent years it has been recognized that a number of jaw osteosarcomas will have, as their first manifestation, a widening of the periodontal membrane as described ind the 2 cases above. When the first symptoms of a jaw osteosarcoma appear the patients are, on average, 30 years old, a decade older than for osteosarcomas in other bones. The mandible is more often affected than the maxilla. Although trauma may occasionally be present in the case history, the majority of patients give no information of trauma. In contrast to carcinomas, swellings associated with osteosarcomas are rarely ulcerated.

Metastasis from an adenocarcinoma of colon

Fig 11-23 is a radiograph of the area 43-31 in a 60 year old man who has an indolent swelling of the gingiva, an epulis, corresponding to 43-31, recognized by the patient 2 weeks before admission. The radiograph reveals an osseous destruction between 43 and 42. Two weeks later the 2 teeth are extracted due to marked purulent exudation from the pockets. As the swelling has not disappeared weeks after the extractions, a biopsy is taken showing an adenocarcinoma. The past history of the patient reveals that 5 years ago h was operated on for an adenocarcinoma o the colon. Three years later there are lun metastases and then, after a further 2 years the gingival metastasis develops. Fou months after gingival biopsy the patient die from extensive metastases. Fig. 11-24 show that the gingival biopsy is covered by slightly atrophic, squamous cell epithelium The connective tissue is dominated by strongly stainable tumor tissue with numer ous ductal imitations. There are many mi oses and a number of hyperchromatic nuclei The histologic picture is typical of a adenocarcinoma. In a Finnish analysis of 33 metastases to the oral tissues 8% were from carcinoma of the colon and rectum. Of th 26 cases, 22 were found in the mandible an only 3 in the maxilla. In 2 instances metas tases to the soft tissue of the mouth could b demonstrated.

Metastasis from lung carcinoma

Fig. 11-25 shows a large "epulis" originatin from the gingiva between 24 and 25 in a 6

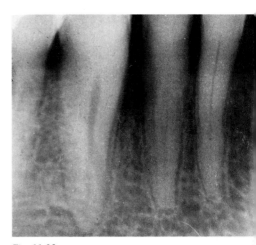

Fig. 11-23.

year old woman who, for 4 months, has had a pain in the left side of the mandible. Two weeks before admission the patient noticed a swelling of the gingiva corresponding to the premolars in the left side of the maxilla. The tumor is soft, fiery red, and, in the incisal third, the seat of a fibrin covered ulceration. The entire tumor is removed surgically and studied histologically (Fig 11-26). The microscopic diagnosis is a low differentiated carcinoma with suspected of metastasis. As the patient has been operated on 3 months previously for a lung carcinoma, it is concluded that the "epulis" most likely is a metastasis from the primary lung tumor. The photomicrograph shows that the surface is covered by an atrophic epithelium. Just below the surface epithelium, tumor tissue is present without a capsule. A certain nuclear pleomorphism can be recognized even at the low power magnification. Among the metastases to the oral regions, the lung cancer occupies the second place after metastases from mammary cancers. Whereas the majority of metastases are to the osseous part of the mandible, a number of lung metastases will occur in the form of an "epulis", a fact which emphasizes the need for a histologic examination of all "epulides". In a recent study of metastases to the oral regions it turned out that there is an increase in a number of reported cases of metastases from lung tumors, due most likely to the explosive increase of smoking related lung cancers. In an analysis of 18 cases of metastases to the soft tissues of the mouth, not less than 50% occur as an "epulis". In a Finnish analysis of soft tissue metastases to the mouth, 30% were localized to the gingiva.

Kaposi's sarcoma

Fig. 11-27 shows a deep red and soft lesion on the alveolar gingiva in a 40 year old man. A short while before the oral changes occurred the patient received a kidney transplantation and was therefore treated by the immunosuppressive drug azathioprine. Re-

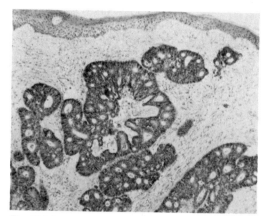

Fig. 11-24.

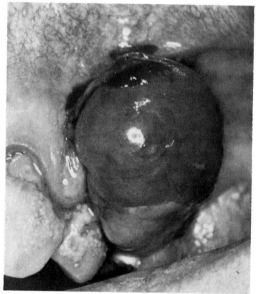

Fig. 11-25.

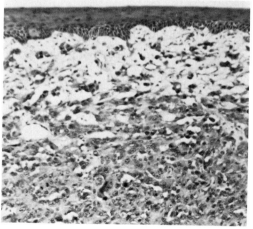

Fig. 11-26.

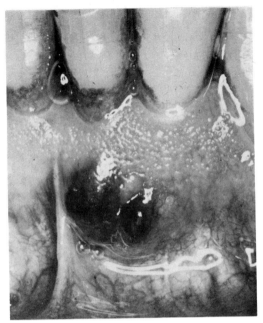

Fig. 11-27.

lated to this medication a herpetic gingivostomatitis developed with manifestations in several areas of the oral mucosa. Some weeks after that attack, a Kaposi's sarcoma was diagnosed on the left crus and a few days later red, elevated, angioma-like, well

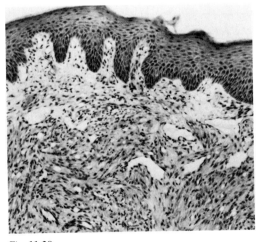

Fig. 11-28.

demarcated lesions develop. A biopsy is taken from the lesion in Fig. 11-27. The histologic examination confirms the clinical suspicion of a Kaposi's sarcoma. Fig. 11-28 shows that the surface is covered by nonkeratinized squamous epithelium. Just below the epithelium there is a cell rich tumor tissue characterized by small and fusiform cells. In several areas small, thin walled vessels are formed. At a higher magnification an increased number of mitoses can be seen. Kaposi's sarcoma is a neoplastic disease probably derived from the reticuloendothelial system and characterized by multiple skin tumors and occasional visceral manifestations. The disease is most prevalent among Negroes and mostly affects men. Recent years have seen several outbreaks of Kaposi's sarcoma among homosexual men; several of these cases have been diagnosed by the oral manifestations. However, in the majority, the oral manifestations will appear after the cutaneous lesions.

Histiocytic lymphoma

Fig. 11-29 shows a large and soft tumor in the incisor region of a 73 year old man, who 3 years previously has been operated on for a histiocytic lymphoma in the stomach. Two years after the operation, the patient has a lymphoma on the neck and after that the gingival lesion appears. The tumor is ulcerated but not indurated. After the diagnosis has been established from biopsy, the tumor is treated with cobolt irradiation, but with only temporary relief. His general condition becomes worse and the patient dies 2 months after the gingival lesion was diagnosed. Previously, the histiocytic lymphoma was called a reticulosarcoma. It is a malignant tumor consisting of large cells with rather bright nuclei. Many mitoses are present and in a number of cases a reticulum stain will disclose fine argyrophilic fibrils around the tumor cells. Fig. 11-30 is a photomicrograph of an oral histiocytic lymphoma. The arrows indicate 3 mitotic figures. The primary histiocytic lymphoma is rare in the oral cavity.

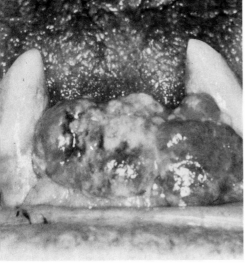

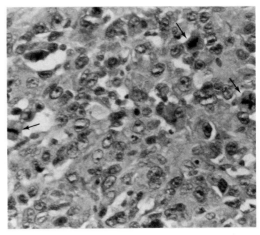

Fig. 11-30.

Fig. 11-29.

When it occurs, the diagnosis may be quite difficult to arrive at as the first manifestations may resemble a nonspecific periodontal disease or a pericoronitis. The histiocytic lymphoma may also arise intraosseously in the jaws, a location which appears to have a better prognosis than if the tumor arises in the soft tissues. The histiocytic lymphoma may affect all age groups. The soft tissue derived lymphomas are most often seen in old people, whereas the osseous type is observed in the young. The dominant symptom is a swelling, which may be confused with an inflammatory process. Also the biopsy may be difficult to interpret and repeated biopsies may be necessary.

CHAPTER 12

Examination of Patients with Periodontal Disease

The gingiva
The periodontal ligament – the root cementum
  Pocket depth measurements
  Attachment level measurements
  Errors inherent in periodontal probing
  Assessment of furcation involvements
  Assessment of tooth mobility
The alveolar bone
  Radiographic analysis
  Sounding
Diagnosis of the periodontal lesions
  1. Gingivitis
  2. Periodontitis levis
  3. Periodontitis gravis
  4. Periodontitis complicata
Oral hygiene
  References

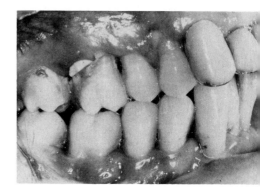

a

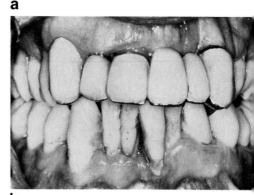

b

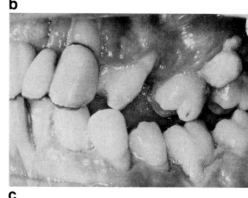

c

Clinically, periodontal disease is characterized by color and texture alterations of the gingiva, e.g. redness and swelling, as well as an increased tendency for bleeding on probing in the gingival sulcus/pocket area (Figs. 12-1 a-c). In addition, the periodontal tissues may exhibit a reduced resistance to probing (increased depth of the clinical pocket) and/or tissue recession. Advanced stages of the disease are also frequently associated with increased tooth mobility and drifting of teeth.

In the radiograph, periodontal disease may be recognized by reduced height of the alveolar bone (Fig. 12-2). If bone loss has progressed at a similar rate in a certain part of the dentition, the crestal contour of the remaining bone is in the radiograph even: "horizontal" bone loss. Angular bony defects are the result of bone loss which has developed at different rates around different teeth/tooth surfaces: "vertical" bone loss.

Figs. 12-1 a-c. Clinical status of a patient suffering from advanced periodontal disease. Note the presence of different signs of periodontal disease such as texture alterations of the gingiva, gingival recessions (in the region of teeth 23 and 31), crowding of teeth (the mandibular front teeth), pus formation (tooth 14) and drifting of the premolars and molars.

298

In the histological section, periodontal disease is characterized by the presence of an inflammatory cell infiltrate (Fig. 12-3) within an area of the gingival connective tissue adjacent to the bacterial deposits on the tooth or root surface. Within the infiltrated area there is a pronounced loss of collagen. In more advanced forms of periodontal disease, loss of connective tissue attachment and apical downgrowth of dentogingival epithelium along the affected root surface are important findings.

Results from clinical and animal research have demonstrated that most forms of periodontal disease 1) have a progressive character and, if left untreated, in many cases may result in tooth loss, 2) can be arrested or even cured following proper therapy. This means that the recognition of periodontal disease and its involvement in various parts of the dentition is of utmost importance.

Examination of a patient with respect to periodontal disease must not only identify sites with inflammatory alterations in the dentition but also the extent of tissue breakdown in these sites. The examination should therefore include all parts of the dentition and describe the periodontal conditions at all buccal, lingual and approximal tooth surfaces present. Since periodontal disease includes inflammatory alterations of the gingiva and a progressive loss of periodontal ligament and alveolar bone, the examination must include measures describing such pathological alterations.

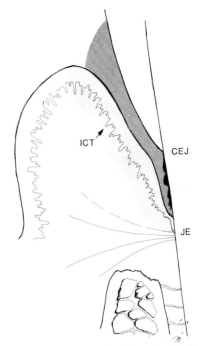

Fig. 12-3. Schematic drawing illustrating the histological features of periodontal disease. Note the infiltrated connective tissue area (ICT).

The gingiva

Clinical signs of gingival inflammation include changes in color and texture of the gingiva and an increased tendency for bleeding on probing.

Various index systems have been developed to facilitate the description of presence and degree of gingivitis in epidemiological and clinical research (for a

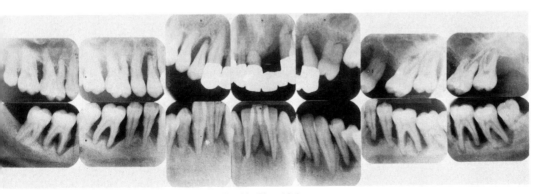

Fig. 12-2. Radiographic status of the patient described in Figs. 12-1 a-c.

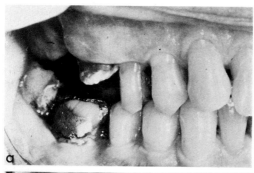
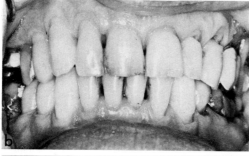
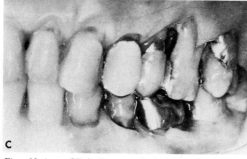

Figs. 12-4 a-c. Clinical status of a 55 year old male with periodontal disease.

cation of the apical extent of the gingival lesion is made in conjunction with *pocket depth measurements*. This means that in sites where "shallow" pockets are present inflammatory lesions residing in the over portion of the gingiva are distinguished by probing in the superficial marginal tissue. When the infiltrate resides in sites with deepened pockets and attachment loss, the inflammatory lesion in the apical part of the pocket should be identified by probing to the bottom of the deepened pocket and not by probing in the marginal portion of the gingiva.

Fig. 12-4 a-c illustrates the clinical status of a 55 year old male with periodontal disease. The examination procedures used in evaluating the location and extension of periodontal disease will be demonstrated by using this case as an example.

Bleeding on probing: a blunt periodontal probe is inserted to the "bottom" of the gingival pocket and is moved gently along the tooth (root) surface (Fig. 12-5). If bleeding is provoked from the apical area of the pockets by this instrumentation the site examined is considered inflamed.

Fig 12-6 illustrates the chart used to identify gingival sites which at the initial examination were found to bleed on probing. Each tooth in the chart is represented by a square and each tooth surface by a triangle. The upper triangle represents the buccal gingival unit, the bottom triangle the lingual unit and the remaining fields the 2 approximal gingival units. A cross is inserted in those fields of the chart which correspond to the inflamed gingival units. The mean gingivitis score is given as a percentage figure. In the present patient (Fig. 12-4 a-c) 27 out of a total number of 52 gingival units in the maxilla bled on probing. The gingivitis score for the maxillary dentition is thus 50%. The corresponding score for the mandibular dentition is 59%. This method of charting not only serves as a means of illustrating areas of health and disease in the dentition but similar chartings during the course of therapy will disclose sites which do not heal properly following therapy.

detailed presentation of these indices the reader is referred to Chapter 2). In the individual patient, refined and qualitative distinctions between various forms of gingivitis, i.e. initial, early and established gingival lesions (Page & Schroeder 1976), serve no meaningful purpose since the correct diagnosis can be made only in the histological section. Since, however, the symptom "bleeding on probing" to the bottom of the gingival sulcus/pocket is associated with the presence of an inflammatory infiltrate in this area, the occurrence of such bleeding is an important indicator of disease. The identifi-

The periodontal ligament – the root cementum

In order to evaluate the amount of tissue lost in periodontal disease and also to identify the apical extension of the inflammatory lesion the following parameters should be recorded:

a) pocket depth (probing depth)
b) attachment level (probing attachment level)
c) furcation involvement
d) tooth mobility

Pocket depth measurements

The pocket depth, i.e. the distance from the gingival margin to the bottom of the gingival pocket, is measured by means of a graduated probe (Fig. 12-7). The pocket depth should be assessed at each surface of all teeth in the dentition. In the periodontal chart (Fig. 12-9) it may be sufficient to identify only the deepest value recorded at each tooth sur-

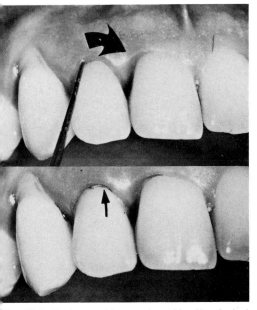

Fig. 12-5. Pocket probing used to identify gingival inflammation. A site is considered inflamed if bleeding is provoked by gentle probing to the bottom of the pocket.

SITES WITH GINGIVITIS

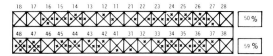

Fig. 12-6. The gingivitis chart of the patient seen in Fig. 12-4.

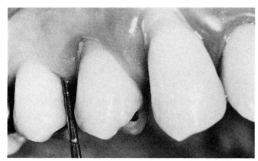

Fig. 12-7. Measurement of probing depth. Note the gingival recessions at the buccal aspect of teeth 14 and 13.

face. Pocket depth values of < 4 mm may be excluded from the chart since such pockets can be regarded as falling within normal variations.

Results from pocket depth measurements only in rare situations (when the gingival margin coincides with the cementoenamel junction) give proper information regarding the extent of loss of attachment. For example, an inflammatory edema may cause a swelling of the free gingiva resulting in a coronal displacement of the gingival margin without a concomitant migration of the dentogingival epithelium to a level apical to the cementoenamel junction. In such a situation a pocket depth exceeding 3-4 mm represents a so-called "pseudopocket". In other situations, an obvious loss of attachment may have occurred without a concomitant increase of the pocket depth. A situation of this kind is shown in Fig. 12-7 at the buccal aspect of 14 and 13 where recessions of the gingiva can be seen.

301

Attachment level measurements

Attachment levels may be assessed by means of the graduated probe and expressed as the distance in mm from the cemento-enamel junction to the bottom of the gingival pocket. The largest distance for each tooth surface is recorded and may be included in the periodontal chart.

Errors inherent in periodontal probing

The distances recorded in a periodontal examination using a periodontal probe have generally been assumed to represent a fairly accurate estimate of the pocket depth or attachment level at a given site. In other words, the tip of the probe has been assumed to identify the level of the most apical cells of the dentogingival epithelium. Results from recent research have demonstrated, however, that this is seldom the case (Saglie et al. 1975, Listgarten et al. 1976, Armitage et al. 1977, Ezis & Burgett 1978, Spray et al. 1978, Robinson & Vitek 1979, van der Velden 1979, Magnusson & Listgarten 1980, Polson et al. 1980). Listgarten (1980) listed a variety of factors which influence the result of a measurement made with a periodontal probe. These factors include 1) the thickness of the probe used, 2) malposition of the probe due to anatomic features such as the contour of the tooth surface, 3) the pressure applied on the instrument during probing, 4) the degree of inflammatory cell infiltration in the soft tissue and accompanying loss of collagen, etc. Listgarten suggested that "a distinction should be made between the histological and the clinical pocket depth to differentiate between the depth of the actual anatomic defect and the measurement recorded by the probe".

Measurement errors depending on factors such as the thickness of the probe, the contour of the tooth surface and improper angulation of the probe can be reduced or avoided by the selection of a proper instrument and careful management of the exami-

nation procedure. More difficult to avoid however, are errors resulting from variations in probing force and the extent of inflammatory alterations of the periodontal tissues. As a rule, the greater the probing force, the deeper is the penetration of the tip of the probe into the tissue. In this context it should be realized that in investigations designed to disclose the force used by different clinicians, the probing force was found to range from 3-130 g (Gabathuler & Hassel 1971, Hassell et al. 1973), and also to differ by as much as 2:1 for the same dentist from one examination to another. In order to exclude measurement errors related to the effect of variations in probing force, so-called pressure sensitive probes have been developed. Such probes will enable the examiner to probe with a predetermined force (van der Velden & de Vries 1978, Vitek et al. 1979, Polson et al. 1980). However over- and underestimation of the "true" pocket depth or attachment level may occur also when this type of probing device is employed (Armitage et al. 1977, Robinson & Vitek 1979, Polson et al. 1980). Thus, when the connective tissue subjacent to the pocket epithelium is infiltrated by inflammatory cells, the periodontal probe will most certainly penetrate beyond the apical termination of the dentogingival epithelium. This results in an overestimation of the "true" depth of the pocket. Conversely, when the inflammatory infiltrate decreases in size, following successful periodontal treatment and a concomitant deposition of new collagen takes place within the previously inflamed tissue area, the dentogingival tissue will become more resistant to penetration by the probe. The tip of the probe may now fail to reach the apical termination of the epithelium. This results in an underestimation of the "true" pocket depth or attachment level. The magnitude of the difference between the probing measurement and the histologic "true" pocket depth may range from fractions of a mm to several mm (Listgarten 1980)

From this discussion it should be understood that reduction of pocket depths fol-

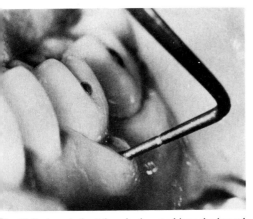

ig. 12-8. A periodontal probe inserted into the buccal urcation area of a mandibular molar. A furcation nvolvement of degree 2 was diagnosed.

owing periodontal treatment and/or gain of ttachment, assessed by periodontal prob-ng, are not necessarily signs of formation of new connective tissue attachment in the ottom of the previous pocket. Rather, such change may merely represent a resolution of the inflammatory process without an accompanying attachment gain. In this con-ext it should be realized that the terms "poc-ket depth" and "gain and loss of attachment" n modern literature have often been changed to the more adequate terms "prob-ng depth" and "gain and loss of *clinical* attachment" or "probing pocket depth" and "probing attachment level".

Current knowledge of the histopathology of periodontal lesions and healing of such esions has thus resulted in an altered con-cept regarding the significance of periodon-al probing. However, despite difficulties in nterpreting the proper significance of pock-et depth and attachment level measure-ments, such determinations still give the clinician a useful estimation of the degree of disease involvement and particularly so when the information obtained is related to other findings of the examination procedure such as "bleeding on probing", alveolar bone height alterations, etc.

Assessment of furcation involvements

In the progression of periodontal disease around 2- or multirooted teeth the destructi-ve process may involve the supporting struc-tures of the furcation area (Fig. 12-8). Elaborate therapeutic techniques must often be used to properly treat such *furcation involvements*. Therefore, the precise iden-tification of the presence and extension of periodontal tissue breakdown within the fur-cation area of each multirooted tooth is of importance for the proper diagnosis and treatment planning.

Furcation involvements may be classified into:

Degree 1: horizontal loss of supporting tis-sues not exceeding ⅓ of the width of the tooth.

Degree 2: horizontal loss of supporting tis-sues exceeding ⅓ of the width of the tooth, but not encompassing the total width of the furcation area.

Degree 3: horizontal "through-and-through" destruction of the sup-porting tissues in the furcation.

The degree of furcation involvement is presented in the periodontal chart (Fig. 12-9) together with a description of on which tooth surface the involvement has been iden-tified (e.g. tooth 26: 2m,b,d; tooth 48: 2 b; tooth 36: 2b,l, etc.). A detailed discussion regarding diagnosis of furcation involve-ments and treatment of furcation involved teeth is presented in Chapter 18.

Assessment of tooth mobility

The continuous loss of the supporting tissues in progressive periodontal disease may result in increased tooth mobility. Increased tooth mobility may be classified in the fol-lowing way:

Degree 1: Movability of the crown of the tooth 0.2-1 mm in horizontal direction

Degree 2: Movability of the crown of the

Periodontal chart

Tooth	Pocket depth				Furcation involvement	Tooth mobility
	m	b	d	l		
16	4	4	4		3	
15	4		6			1
14	5		6	4		
13	4		4			
12	4		6	6		
11						
21			6	5		
22	6		7	4		
23	4		8	5		
24	6					
25		4	7			1
26	6		4		m,b,d 2	
27	4	4	8	8	3	
48	8	8	4	4	b 2	2
47	6	14	8	4	3	1
~~46~~						
45	4		6	4		
44			6	4		
43			4			
42	6					
41			4			
31			4			
32			4			
33	6					
34			4			
35	5		6	6		1
36	10		8		b,l 2	
37	6	4	10	6	b 2	

Fig. 12-9. Periodontal chart including the data obtained from the examination of the patient presented in Fig. 12-4.

tooth exceeding 1 mm in horizontal direction

Degree 3: Movability of the crown of the tooth in vertical direction as well.

In this context it should be realized that plaque associated periodontal disease is not the only cause of increased tooth mobility. For instance, overloading of teeth and trauma may result in tooth hypermobility. Increased tooth mobility can frequently be observed also in conjunction with periapical osteitis, immediately following periodonta surgery, etc. From a therapeutic point c view it is important not only to assess th degree of increased tooth mobility but als the cause of the observed hypermobility (se Chapter 8).

All data collected in conjunction wit measurements of pocket depths and attach ment levels and from the assessments of fu cation involvements and tooth mobility ar included in the *periodontal chart.* (Fig. 1: 9). The various teeth are in this cha denoted according to the two-digit syste adopted by FDI in 1970.

The alveolar bone

Radiographic analysis

The height of the alveolar bone and the ou line of the bone crest are examined in th radiographs (Fig. 12-10). The X-ray imag provides information of the height and con figuration of the interproximal alveola bone. Covering structures (bone tissue teeth) often make it difficult to properl identify the outline of the buccal and lingua alveolar bone crest. The analysis of th radiographs must therefore be combine with a detailed evaluation of the pocke depth and attachment level data in order t arrive at a correct diagnosis concernin "horizontal" and "vertical" bone loss.

Following active treatment, the patient must be enrolled in a follow-up and mainte nance care program aimed at preventin recurrence of periodontal disease. Thi program includes regular reexaminations t study the periodontal conditions. Such reex aminations often require repeated radio graphic analyses of teeth and jaws with cer tain time intervals. To enable meaningfu comparative analyses, a radiographic tech nique should be used which produce periodic reproducible roentgenograms. A technique of this kind has been described b Eggen (1969) and others.

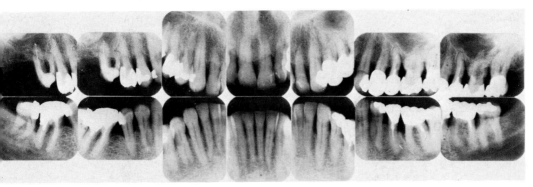

Fig. 12-10. Radiographic status of the patient presented in Fig. 12-4.

Sounding

In order to arrive at a correct diagnosis with respect to the alveolar bone level, the presence of angular bony defects and interdental osseous craters etc., a particular method, called "sounding", is often used. Following local anesthesia the periodontal probe is inserted into the pocket. The tip of the probe is forced through the supraalveolar connective tissue to make contact with the bone and the distance from the cementoenamel junction to the bone level is assessed in mm.

Diagnosis of the periodontal lesions

The information regarding the condition of the various periodontal structures (the gingiva, the periodontal membrane – the root cementum and the alveolar bone) which has been obtained by the examination procedures presented, should form the basis for the proper diagnosis of periodontal disease (Fig 12-11). It is often to advantage to give each tooth in the dentition an individual diagnosis. Four different diagnoses may be used:

DIAGNOSIS OF THE PERIODONTAL LESION

DIAGNOSIS	CRITERIA	
	Periodontal charting	Miscellaneous
	Radiographic analysis	
Gingivitis	No loss of supporting tissues (pseudopockets)	Bleeding on probing
Periodontitis levis	"Horizontal" loss of supporting tissues < 1/3 of the root length	Bleeding on probing
Periodontitis gravis	"Horizontal" loss of supporting tissues > 1/3 of the root length	Bleeding on probing
Periodontitis complicata	Angular bony defects:	Bleeding on probing
	interdental craters	
	infrabony pockets	
	Furcation involvement 2, 3	
	Mobility 3	

Fig. 12-11. The conditions of the periodontal tissues around each individual tooth in the dentition are described using different criteria (periodontal charting, radiographic analysis) and diagnoses.

1. Gingivitis

This diagnosis is used when one or several gingival units around a particular tooth are found to bleed on probing. Pocket depth and attachment level measurements and radiographic analysis fail to indicate loss of supporting tissues. "Pseudopockets" may be present.

2. Periodontitis levis

The pocket depth and attachment level measurements and the radiographic analysis indicate an even ("horizontal") loss of sup-

305

DIAGNOSIS:			16	15	14	13	12	11	21	22	23	24	25	26	27	
Gingivitis																
Parodontitis levis						✗		✗			✗	✗				
Parodontitis gravis				✗	✗		✗		✗	✗			✗			
Parodontitis compl.			✗				✗						✗	✗	✗	

			48	47		45	44	43	42	41	31	32	33	34	35	36	37	
Gingivitis																		
Parodontitis levis							✗	✗	✗			✗	✗	✗				
Parodontitis gravis						✗				✗	✗				✗	✗	✗	
Parodontitis compl.	✗	✗														✗	✗	

Fig. 12-12. Chart of diagnosis describing the patient in Fig. 12-4.

Tooth	Symptom	Diagnosis	Tooth	Symptom	Diagnosis
			48	furcation involvement (2)	complicata
			47	furcation involvement (3)	complicata
16	furcation involvement (3)	complicata			
15	"horizontal" loss of supporting tissues > 1/3 of the root length	gravis	45	"horizontal" loss of supporting tissues > 1/3 of the root length	gravis
14	"horizontal" loss of supporting tissues > 1/3 of the root length	gravis	44	"horizontal" loss of supporting tissues < 1/3 of the root length	levis
13	"horizontal" loss of supporting tissues < 1/3 of the root length	levis	43	"horizontal" loss of supporting tissues < 1/3 of the root length	levis
12	angular bony defect (bottom of the defect located on "gravis level")	gravis et complicata	42	"horizontal" loss of supporting tissues < 1/3 of the root length	levis
11	"horizontal" loss of supporting tissues < 1/3 of the root length	levis	41	"horizontal" loss of supporting tissues > 1/3 of the root length	gravis
21	"horizontal" loss of supporting tissues > 1/3 of the root length	gravis	31	"horizontal" loss of supporting tissues > 1/3 of the root length	gravis
22	"horizontal" loss of supporting tissues > 1/3 of the root length	gravis	32	"horizontal" loss of supporting tissues < 1/3 of the root length	levis
23	"horizontal" loss of supporting tissues < 1/3 of the root length	levis	33	"horizontal" loss of supporting tissues < 1/3 of the root length	levis
24	"horizontal" loss of supporting tissues < 1/3 of the root length	levis	34	"horizontal" loss of supporting tissues < 1/3 of the root length	levis
25	angular bony defect (bottom of the defect located on "gravis level")	gravis et complicata	35	"horizontal" loss of supporting tissues > 1/3 of the root length	gravis
26	furcation involvement (2)	complicata	36	angular bony defect (bottom of the defect located on "gravis level") furcation involvement (2)	gravis et complicata
27	furcation involvement (3)	complicata	37	angular bony defect (bottom of the defect located on "gravis level") furcation involvement (2)	gravis et complicata

porting tissues not exceeding ⅓ of the length of the root. Inflammation should be recognized by "bleeding on probing" to the "bottom of the pocket".

SITES WITH PLAQUE

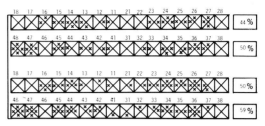

SITES WITH GINGIVITIS

Fig. 12-13. The plaque and gingivitis chart of the patient presented in Fig. 12-4.

3. Periodontitis gravis

Pocket depth and attachment level measurements and the radiographic analysis indicate an even ("horizontal") loss of supporting tissues exceeding ⅓ of the length of the root. "Bleeding on probing" to the "bottom of the pocket" must be present.

4. Periodontitis complicata

This diagnosis is used 1) when an angular bony defect (infrabony pocket, interdental osseous crater) is present adjacent to a tooth, 2) when a tooth exhibits a "degree 3 mobility" and 3) for a multirooted tooth in which furcation involvements of degree 2 or 3 have been identified. "Bleeding on probing" to the "bottom of the pocket" must be present.

When an angular bony defect is present, the level of the root surface on which the bottom of the defect is located should also be defined. Hence, a tooth with this kind of osseous defect is often given a combined diagnosis: *periodontitis levis et complicata* when the apical termination of the angular bony defect is located on the "levis level" on the root surface, and *periodontitis gravis et complicata* when it is located on the "gravis level".

A chart of diagnosis is shown in Fig. 12-12. This particular chart refers to the patient whose clinical status is shown in Figs. 12-4 a-c, periodontal chart in Fig. 12-9 and radiographic status in Fig. 12-10. The various teeth have received the diagnoses indicated.

Oral hygiene

In conjunction with examination of the periodontal tissues, the patient's oral hygiene standard must also be evaluated. *Absence* or *presence* of plaque on each tooth surface in the dentition is recorded. The bacterial deposits may be stained with a disclosing solution to facilitate their detection. The presence of plaque is marked in appropriate fields in the plaque chart shown in Fig. 12-13. The mean plaque score for the dentition is given as a percentage value in correspondence with the system used for gingivitis.

Alterations with respect to the presence of plaque and gingival inflammation are illustrated in a simple way by the repeated use of the combined plaque and gingivitis chart (Fig. 12-13) during the course of treatment.

In addition to the assessment of plaque, retention factors for plaque, such as supra- and subgingival calculus, defective margins of dental restorations, etc., should also be identified and included in the periodontal chart.

The methods described above for the examination of patients with respect to periodontal disease provide a thorough analysis of the presence, extent and severity of the disease in the dentition. The correct diagnosis for each individual tooth should form the basis for the treatment planning of the individual case.

References

Armitage, G. C., Svanberg, G. K. & Löe, H. (1977) Microscopic evaluation of clinical measurements of connective tissue attachment level. *Journal of Clinical Periodontology* **4**, 173-190.

Eggen, S. (1969) Standardiserad intraoral röntgenteknik. *Sveriges Tandläkareförbunds Tidning* **17**, 867-872.

Ezis, I. & Burgett, F. (1978) Probing related to attachment levels on recently erupted teeth. *Journal of Dental Research* **57**, Special Issue A 307, Abstract No. 932.

Gabathuler, H. & Hassell, T. (1971) A pressure-sensitive periodontal probe. *Helvetica Odontologica Acta* **15**, 114-117.

Hassell, T. M., Germann, M. A. & Saxer, V. P. (1973) Periodontal probing: Investigator discrepancies and correlations between probing force and recorded depth. *Helvetica Odontologica Acta* **17**, 38-42.

Listgarten, M. A. (1980) Periodontal probing: What does it mean? *Journal of Clinical Periodontology* **7**, 165-176.

Listgarten, M. A., Mao, R. & Robinson, P. J. (1976) Periodontal probing and the relationship of the probe tip to periodontal tissues. *Journal of Periodontology* **47**, 511-513.

Magnusson, I. & Listgarten, M. A. (1980) Histological evaluation of probing depth following periodontal treatment. *Journal of Clinical Periodontology* **7**, 26-31.

Page, R. C. & Schroeder, H. E. (1976) Pathogenesis of chronic inflammatory periodontal disease. A summary of current work. *Laboratory Investigations* **33**, 235-249.

Polson, A. M., Caton, J. G., Yeaple, R. N. & Zander, H. A. (1980) Histological determination of probe tip penetration into gingival sulcus of humans using an electronic pressure-sensitive probe. *Journal of Clinical Periodontology* **7**, 479-488.

Robinson, P. J. & Vitek, R. M. (1979) The relationship between gingival inflammation and resistance to probe penetration. *Journal of Periodontal Research* **14**, 239-243.

Saglie, R., Johansen, J. R. & Flötra, L. (1975) The zone of completely and partially destructed periodontal fibers in pathological pockets. *Journal of Clinical Periodontology* **2**, 198-202.

Spray, J. R., Garnick, J. J., Doles, L. R. & Klawitter, J. J. (1978) Microscopic demonstration of the position of periodontal probes. *Journal of Periodontology* **49**, 148-152.

van der Velden, U. (1979) Probing force and the relationship of the probe tip to the periodontal tissues. *Journal of Clinical Periodontology* **6**, 106-114.

van der Velden, U. & de Vries, J. H. (1978) Introduction of a new periodontal probe: the pressure probe. *Journal of Clinical Periodontology* **5**, 188-197.

Vitek, R. M., Robinson, P. J. & Lautenschlager, E. P. (1979) Development of a force-controlled periodontal instrument. *Journal of Periodontal Research* **14**, 93-94.

Treatment Planning

Introduction

Caries and periodontal disease, the most prevalent disorders of the dentition, have until recently been treated mainly by symptomatic (reparative) measures. This mode of treatment could be considered appropriate as long as the etiology of these 2 disorders remained obscure. At the present time, however, important aspects of the etiology and pathogenesis of both caries and periodontal disease are properly understood and therapeutic methods are available by which the causative factors can be eradicated or controlled and their recurrence prevented.

Caries and periodontal disease are infectious disorders associated with bacterial colonization of the surfaces of teeth. Factors such as bacterial specificity and pathogenicity as well as the disposition of the individual for the disease, e.g. local and general resistance, may influence the initiation, rate of progression and clinical character of the plaque associated dental disorders. Findings from animal experiments and longitudinal studies in humans, however, have conclusively demonstrated that treatment including the elimination or control of the plaque infection and the introduction of careful plaque control measures in most, if not all, cases results in dental and periodontal health. Even if health cannot always be achieved and maintained, the *arrest of desease progression* following treatment must be the goal of modern dental care.

Treatment of patients suffering from caries and periodontal disease including symptoms of associated pathological conditions such as pulpitis, periapical osteitis, marginal abscess, tooth migration, etc., should from a didactic point of view be divided into 3 different classes:

1. *Cause related measures:* the objective of this treatment is the removal or control of the various plaque infections.

2. *Corrective measures:* including tradiional therapeutic measures such as periodontal surgery, endodontic therapy, restorative and prosthetic treatment. The volume of corrective therapy required and the selection of means for the restorative and prosthetic therapy should be determined only when the *level of success* of the causative therapy can be properly evaluated. The patients' ability to co-operate in the overall therapy must determine the content of the corrective treatment. If this ability is failing or lacking it is often not worth initiating treatment procedures which only in the fully cooperative patient will improve the results of therapy. The validity of this statement can be exemplified by the results of studies aimed at assessing the relative value of different types of surgical methods in the treatment of periodontal disease. Thus, a number of clinical

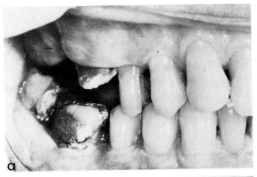

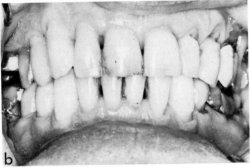

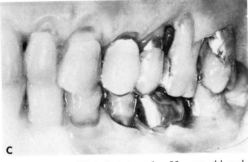

Figs. 13-1 a-c. Clinical status of a 55 year old male (U.N.) with periodontal disease.

recurrence. For each individual patient a recall system must be designed which includes 1) the outline of self performed but professionally monitored plaque control programs, 2) scaling and root planing measures, 3) fluoride application, etc. In addition, this treatment involves the regular control of fillings and other restorations made during the corrective phase of therapy.

In a textbook chapter it is obviously impossible to discuss all the different symptoms of disease which may be encountered in each individual patient. The aim of this presentation is to explain the overall objectives of the treatment planning for patients with moderately advanced and advanced periodontal disease and to describe the logical order of the use of different means of therapy.

Information preceding treatment planning

The basis for the treatment planning described in this chapter is established by the clinical data collected from the examination of the patient presented in Chapter 12. This particular patient (U.N., male, 55 years of age) was examined with respect to his periodontal conditions, i.e. gingival sites displaying signs of *bleeding on probing* were assessed, *pocket depths* and *furcation involvements* were measured and graded, *tooth mobility* was assessed and the radiographs were analyzed to determine the *height* and *outline* of the *alveolar bone crest*.

The clinical characteristics of the dentition of this patient are shown in Figs. 13-1 a-c. The periodontal chart, and the radiographs are presented in Fig. 13-2. Based on these findings, each tooth in the dentition was given a proper periodontal diagnosis (Fig. 13-2). In addition to the examination of the periodontal conditions, detailed assessments of primary and recurrent *caries* were made for all tooth surfaces in the dentition. Furthermore, the patient was also examined with respect to endodontic problems, occlusal problems, temporomandibular joint dysfunction, etc. (Fig. 13-3).

The present patient exhibited signs of secondary caries lesions adjacent to several

trials (Lindhe & Nyman 1975, Nyman et al. 1975, 1977, Rosling et al. 1976 a, b, Nyman & Lindhe 1979) have demonstrated that gingivectomy and flap procedures performed in patients with proper plaque control levels often result in gain of alveolar bone and clinical attachment, while surgery in plaque infected dentitions may cause additional destruction of the periodontium.

3. *Maintenance measures:* the aim of this treatment is the prevention of disease

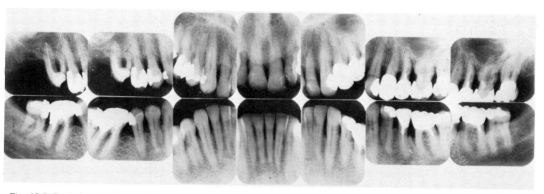

Fig. 13-2. Periodontal chart and radiographs relating to patient U.N. described in Fig. 13-1.

restorations, particularly in the molar regions (Fig. 13-1a), and root caries in the distal surface of 25 (Fig. 13-2) and the mesial surface of 26 (Fig. 13-1c). (It should be observed that in a patient with a large number of caries lesions an additional number of examination procedures, e.g. assessments of secretion rate and buffering capacity of the saliva, number of lactobacilli, *Streptococcus mutans,* etc., will facilitate the selection of therapeutic measures.) In addition, periapical osteitis was diagnosed in 47 and several defective root fillings could be found (Fig. 13-2).

Periodontal chart							Diagnosis			
Tooth	Pocket depth				Furcation involvement	Tooth mobility	Gingivitis	Parodontitis levis	Parodontitis gravis	Parodontitis compl.
	m	b	d	l						
16	4	4	4		3					x
15	4		6			1		x		
14	5		6	4				x		
13	4		4				x			
12	4		6	6				x	x	
11							x			
21			6	5				x		
22	6		7	4				x		
23	4		8	5			x			
24	6						x			
25		4	7			1			x	x
26	6		4		m,b,d 2					x
27	4	4	8	8	3					x
48	8	8	4	4	b 2	2				x
47	6	14	8	4	3	1				x
46										
45	4		6	4				x		
44			6	4			x			
43			4				x			
42	6						x			
41			4					x		
31			4					x		
32			4				x			
33	6						x			
34			4				x			
35	5		6	6	b,l 2	1		x		
36	10		8		b,l 2			x	x	
37	6	4	10	6	b 2				x	x

Plaque score: 47 %   Gingivitis score: 55 %

Treatment planning

Initial treatment plan

Not until a detailed diagnosis of all pathological conditions has been made, have proper prerequisites been established for an appropriate tentative treatment plan. At this early stage in the management of a patient it is in most instances impossible to make a definite decision regarding all aspects of the corrective therapy, because:

1. *The degree of success of the cause related treatment remains unknown:* The result of the cause related treatment of an individual case forms the basis for the selection of means for corrective therapy. The degree of disease elimination that can be reached depends on the efficacy of e.g. subgingival scaling and root planing, but also to a certain extent on the patient's ability to adopt proper dietary habits and plaque control techniques.

2. *The patient's "subjective" need for treatment is not known:* When the dentist has completed the examination of the patient

311

Examination

of

1. Periodontal disease

2. Caries

3. Endodontic problems

4. Occlusal problems   Diagnoses

5. Temporomandibular

dysfunction

etc.

Fig. 13-3.

and an inventory has been made regarding periodontal disease, caries, pulpal disease, temporomandibular joint disease, etc., he/she presents "the case" for his/her patient. During the case presentation it is important to find out if the patient's subjective need for dental therapy coincides with the dentist's professional appreciation of the kind of therapy required. It is important that the dentist understands that the main objective of dental therapy, besides *elimination of pain, is to satisfy the patient's demands regarding esthetics and chewing function* (comfort), demands which certainly vary considerably from one individual to another.

3. *The result of certain parts of the treatment cannot be predicted:* In patients exhibiting advanced forms of caries and periodontal disease it is often impossible to anticipate if all teeth which are present at the initial examination can be successfully treated or to predict the result of certain parts of the intended therapy. In other words, critical and difficult parts of the treatment must be performed first and the result must be evaluated before

all aspects of the definitive corrective treatment can be properly anticipated and described.

Case presentation

The "Case presentation" is an essential component of the initial treatment and must include a description for the patient of different therapeutic goals available. At the case presentation for the present patient the following treatment plan was described:

The teeth in the dentition from 15-24, and from 45-35 ought not to present any therapeutic problems. For the remaining teeth in the dentition, however, the treatment involves a number of difficult therapeutic measures:

48 and 47 extraction: cannot be treated due to the advanced loss of supporting tissue at the buccal aspect of the teeth in combination with deep furcation involvements and periapical osteitis as far as 47 is concerned (Fig. 13-2).

16 extraction: even if it is possible, from a therapeutic point of view, to preserve the palatal root, the maintenance of this root does not improve esthetics or chewing comfort; the tooth has no antagonist after extraction of 47 (Fig 13-2).

25 and 27 extraction: 25 cannot be treated due to advanced root caries in combination with advanced loss of periodontal tissue support at the distal aspect of the tooth; 27 has a periodontal pocket communicating with periapical lesions in combination with furcation involvement of degree 3 (Fig. 13-2).

26, 36 and 37 present a number of difficult problems from a therapeutic point of view: 26 shows signs of deep and extended root caries on the mesiobuccal root in combination with furcation involvement of degree 2 m,b,d (Figs. 13-1 c and 13-2). Note also the unfavorable root- and root canal anatomy of the buccal roots with respect to endodontic treatment. However, the palatal root of 26 can be maintained; in 36 there is a deep angular bony defect on the mesial aspect and furcation involvement of degree 2 b,l; 37 has a deep infrabony pocket at the distal surface (10 mm, see the periodontal chart) and furcation involvement of degree 2 b. The distal root 36 or the mesial root 37 (or both) are available for treatment.

Alternative treatment
Two different alternatives for treatment were presented to the patient:

Alternative 1. Extraction of 25 and all molars and the maintenance of a dentition comprising 15 – 24 and 45 – 35. This alternative may be adequate with respect to "chewing comfort" but may be questionable from an esthetic point of view.

Alternative 2. Extraction of the molars in the right side of the upper and lower jaws (16, 48, 47) and also of 25 and 27; root separation of 26 with the maintenance of the palatal root of this tooth to be used as abutment for a 3-unit bridge to replace the extracted 25; root separation of one of the molars 36 or 37 with the maintenance of one root to be used as abutment for a 3-unit bridge to obtain occlusal contact with the maxillary bridge.

It should be observed that *alternative 2* involves a considerably larger volume of therapy than *alternative 1*. In a situation like this, expected benefits inherent in a certain treatment versus obvious disadvantages should always be explained to and discussed with the patient. His/her attitude to the alternatives presented must guide the dentist in the design of a proper plan for the overall treatment. In the present case the patient preferred the treatment described as alternative 2.

Initial (cause related) therapy
The treatment was initiated and included the following measures to eliminate or control the plaque infection:
1. *Instruction* in oral hygiene measures with subsequent check-ups and reinstruction.
2. *Scaling* and *root planing* in combination with removal of retention factors for plaque.

3. *Excavation* and restoration of carious lesions.
4. *Endodontic treatment* 26 (palatal root) and 37 (mesial root). Endodontic treatment was carried out at an early stage to allow a proper evaluation of healing before the restorative treatment was initiated.
5. *Extraction* of 16, 48, 47. Temporary prosthetic replacement (for esthetic and functional reasons) of teeth which, during this initial phase of the treatment, have to be extracted should preferably be made in the form of removable partial dentures. The use of a removable prosthesis allows the dentist to eventually choose between a removable partial denture and a fixed bridge as permanent prosthetic therapy. If, on the other hand, the temporary prosthetic reconstruction is made in the form of a fixed bridge, the permanent prosthetic therapy must inevitably include fixed bridgework. Such an alternative may, however, during the course of treatment appear to be contraindicated. In the present patient, temporary prosthesis was not indicated.

Reexamination
The initial phase of therapy is terminated with a thorough analysis (Examination 2) of the results obtained with respect to the elimination or degree of control of the dental diseases. This implies that a reevaluation of the patient's caries activity must be performed as well as new assessments of gingival conditions, pocket depths, tooth mobility, etc. The result of this reevaluation forms the basis for the selection of therapeutic measures that should be included in the phase of definite treatment.

Planning of corrective therapy (definitive treatment plan)

If the results from the reexamination, made at the termination of the initial treatment phase, show that caries and periodontal disease have been brought under proper con-

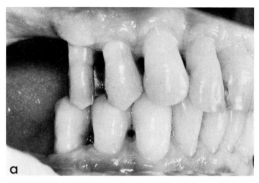

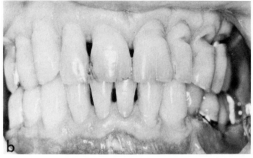

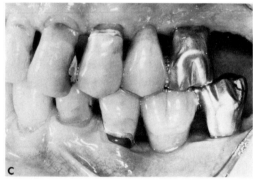

Figs. 13-4 a-c. Clinical status of patient U.N. after periodontal and restorative treatment. Compare with Fig. 13-1.

3. *Periodontal surgery:* The planning of the type and extent of surgical treatment should be based on the pocket depth and "bleeding on probing" measurements made at the end of the initial phase of treatment. Periodontal surgery should be limited to those areas of the dentition where the inflammatory lesions in pockets of >4 mm could not be resolved by scaling and root planing.

4. *Definitive restorative and prosthetic treatment* including permanent restorative therapy (crown and bridge, removable partial dentures, etc.).

Corrective therapy
The present patient after initial therapy displayed low plaque and gingivitis values (5-10%) and no active carious lesions. The corrective treatment therefore included the following components:

1. *Periodontal surgery* around teeth, where pockets (>4 mm) persisted which bled on probing.

2. *Root separation* 37 and extraction of the distal root.
   Root separation 26 and extraction of the buccal roots.

3. *Extraction* 36, 25 and 27.

4. Preparation and installation of *fixed bridges* 24, [25,] 26 (palatal root) and 35, [36,] 37 (mesial root).
   The result of the overall treatment is shown in Figs. 13-4 a-c and Fig. 13-5.

Planning of maintenance therapy

Following completion of *cause related* and *corrective therapy* the patient must be enrolled in a recall system which aims at preventing the recurrence of disease. The time interval between the recall appointments should always be related to the ability of the patient to maintain a proper oral hygiene standard. Findings reported from several long-term clinical trials have suggested that a maintenance program based on recall appointments once every 3 months is, in most patients, effective in preventing disease recurrence. At the various recall visits the

trol, the corrective treatment may be carried out in the following sequence:

1. *Extractions* of teeth that cannot be maintained. If such extractions include teeth which must be replaced for esthetic or functional reasons, a temporary removable partial denture or a temporary fixed bridge must be inserted.

2. *Additional endodontic treatment*

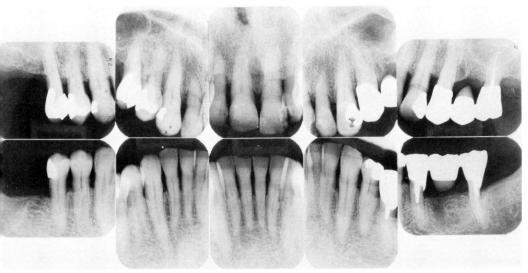

ig. 13-5. Radiographs of patient U.N. after periodontal and restorative treatment. Compare with Fig. 13-2.

ollowing procedures should be carried out:
. Evaluation of the oral hygiene standard.
. Scaling and polishing of teeth (if indicated).
Once a year an examination should be
performed including assessments of 1) caries
urfaces, 2) gingivitis, 3) pathologically
leepened pockets, 4) furcation involve-
nents, 5) tooth mobility and 6) alterations of
he alveolar bone level.
· The patient used in this chapter to
lescribe the guiding principles of treatment
planning, was during the first 6 months after
he active treatment recalled once every 2
nonths, during the next 6 months once every
3 months, and subsequently only once every
5 months. The clinical and radiographic
tatus respectively 8 and 11 years after active
reatment are shown in Fig. 13-6 and 13-7. In
he course of this 11 year period there were
10 signs of recurrence of caries or periodon-
al disease. The buccal cusp of the crown of
ooth 15 was fractured approximately 5 years
after active therapy and the tooth restored
by a gold crown with a porcelain facing.
The large variety of treatment problems
hat different patients may present may
obviously require that deviations are made

from the sequence of treatment steps (initial
therapy, corrective therapy, maintenance
therapy, etc.) discussed above. Such deviations may be accepted as long as the fundamental principles regarding the overall
therapy are understood (Fig. 13-8: flow
chart).
Three patients will be presented below
together with a brief description of their
specific dental problems and the treatment
delivered in order to demonstrate the
rationale behind such variations in the sequence of therapy.

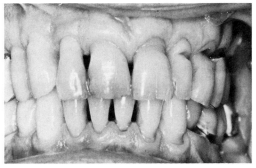

Fig. 13-6. Clinical status of patient U.N. 8 years after
active treatment.

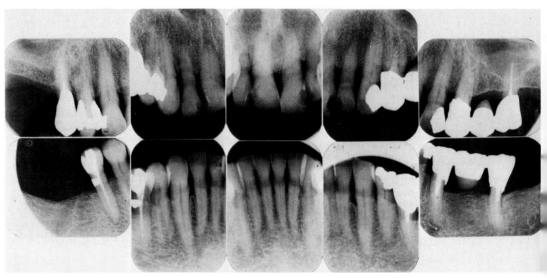

Fig. 13-7. Radiographs of patient U.N. obtained 11 years after active treatment.

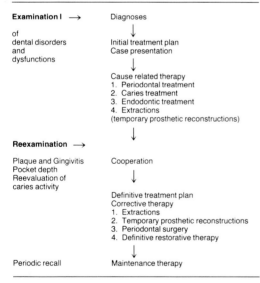

Examination I →	Diagnoses
of	↓
dental disorders	Initial treatment plan
and	Case presentation
dysfunctions	↓
	Cause related therapy
	1. Periodontal treatment
	2. Caries treatment
	3. Endodontic treatment
	4. Extractions
	(temporary prosthetic reconstructions)
	↓
Reexamination →	
Plaque and Gingivitis	Cooperation
Pocket depth	
Reevaluation of	↓
caries activity	
	Definitive treatment plan
	Corrective therapy
	1. Extractions
	2. Temporary prosthetic reconstructions
	3. Periodontal surgery
	4. Definitive restorative therapy
	↓
Periodic recall	Maintenance therapy

Fig. 13-8. Flow chart describing the sequence of delivery of various treatment procedures in the over-all therapy.

Case reports

Patient K. A. (female, 29 years old)

Initial examination

The periodontal status (pocket depths, furcation involvements, tooth mobility, radiographs and diagnoses) from the initial examination of patient K. A. is shown in Fig. 13-9. The data obtained from this examination disclosed the presence of an advanced destruction of the supporting tissues in most parts of the dentition and presence of a large number of angular bony defects. The teeth 14, 12, 11, 21, 22, 23, 24, 25, 43, 42, 41, 31, 32, 33, 37 exhibited increased mobility. The plaque and gingivitis scores were 75 and 70% respectively.

Treatment planning

In the planning of the treatment of this case it seemed reasonable to anticipate the extraction of some teeth in this severely diseased dentition, namely 14, 11, 21 and 31 (see radiograph: Fig. 13-9). The extraction of these teeth calls for extensive prosthetic therapy. Should additional teeth be

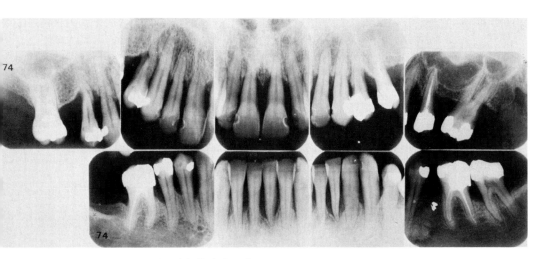

Fig. 13-9. Case K.A. (29 year old female). Periodontal chart and radiographs prior to therapy.

Periodontal chart						Diagnosis				
						Gingivitis	Parodontitis levis	Parodontitis gravis	Parodontitis compl.	
Tooth	Pocket depth				Furcation	Tooth				
	m	b	d	l	involvement	mobility				
16					b l		x			
15										
14	8		8	7	m,d l	2		x	x	
13			5	5				x		
12	8		5			1		x		
11	8		5	5		2		x	x	
21	8		7	6		2		x	x	
22	6		6	5		1		x		
23			4	5		1		x		
24	6		8	4	m,d l	1		x	x	
25			5			1		x		
26										
27			6		b,d l			x		
46	5		5		b l			x		
45			7					x	x	
44	8		8	4				x	x	
43	8		6	6		1		x	x	
42	6		5			1		x		
41	4					1		x		
31	6		6	6		2		x	x	
32	4		5			1		x		
33	8		7	5		1		x	x	
34								x	x	
35										
36			5		b l			x		
37	7		7	6	b l	1		x		

Plaque score: 75   Gingivtis score: 70

scheduled for extraction on "prosthetic" indications? The neighboring teeth of 11, 21 and 31 also exhibited advanced loss of supporting structures and showed signs of increased mobility. It could be questioned therefore if these teeth (12, 22, 41, 32) could serve as proper abutments for fixed bridge reconstructions. The extraction of tooth 31 would most likely motivate the extraction of the remaining 3 mandibular incisors too, and consequently a therapy be anticipated which included the preparation and installation of a fixed bridge from tooth 44 to tooth 34. Extraction of 11 and 21 would motivate the extraction of 12, 22, 14 and 24 as well, and call for a bridge construction from tooth 16 to 25 or 26.

The prerequisites for a proper prognosis for the prosthetic therapy described above are 1) optimal self performed oral hygiene, 2) proper healing of the periodontal tissues following cause related and corrective therapy and 3) a carefully monitored maintenance care program. If these prerequisites can be met, it may, on the other hand, be possible to avoid all anticipated tooth extractions in this patient. If this attempt is success-

ful, prosthetic therapy can be entirely avoided. As stated above most of the teeth had increased mobility. This mobility, however, did not disturb the chewing comfort of this patient. The tooth mobility *per se*, therefore, was not regarded as an indication for splinting.

317

Conclusions: In a case of this character extensive efforts should be made to properly treat inflammatory periodontal disease in the entire dentition *before* decisions are made to extract one or several teeth. Decisions regarding possible extractions should not be taken until after the healing of periodontal surgery.

Treatment

Subsequent to initial examination, the patient was given a detailed "Case presentation" and information regarding alternative goals of and prerequisites for the overall

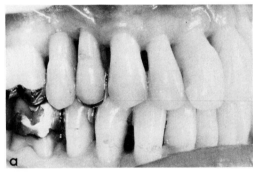

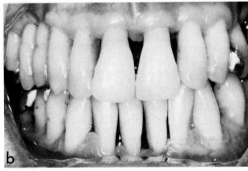

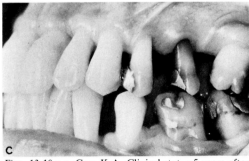

Figs. 13-10 a-c. Case K.A. Clinical status 5 years after initial treatment.

treatment. This information included a description of the role of dental plaque in the etiology of periodontal disease and the significance of optimal plaque control for a successful therapeutic result. A treatment program was subsequently planned which aimed at maintaining all teeth, thereby avoiding extensive prosthetic therapy. The overall treatment was performed in the following sequence:

Initial therapy

Oral hygiene instruction and plaque control evaluation. Scaling and root planing. Adjustment of improper amalgam restorations.

Corrective therapy (following reevaluation at Examination 2)

Periodontal surgery involving careful removal of subgingival soft and hard deposits and root planing. All teeth in the dentition could be maintained and the furcation involvements in the premolar and molar areas could be treated successfully with furcation plasty.

After healing, a fixed bridge (16, [15,] 14) was fabricated and inserted on esthetic indications.

Maintenance therapy

During the first 6 months after completion of the initial and corrective therapy the patient was recalled for maintenance care every ? weeks. This interval between the recall appointments was then gradually extended to 3 months.

Concluding remarks

The result of the treatment is shown in Figs 13-10 a-c (clinical status 5 years after initial treatment), Fig. 13-11 (radiographs 8 years after treatment) and Fig. 13-12 (periodontal chart 8 years after treatment). There has been no recurrence of periodontal disease during the period of maintenance.

The planning of the overall treatment and the sequence of the different treatment procedures used in this case were selected for presentation in order to illustrate the following principle: In patients exhibiting a generalized advanced breakdown of the periodontal tissues, but with an intact number of teeth, considerable efforts should

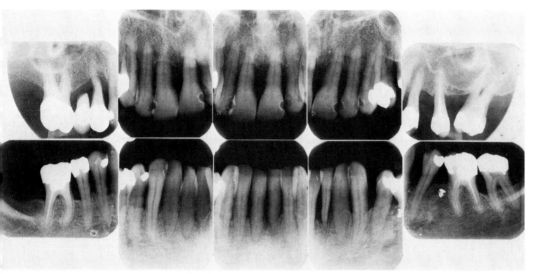

Fig. 13-11. Case K.A. Radiographs obtained 8 years after treatment.

Periodontal chart					
Tooth	Pocket depth			Furcation	Tooth
	m	b	d	l	involvement	mobility

Tooth	Pocket depth (m b d l)	Furcation involvement	Tooth mobility
16			
15			
14			
13			
12			1
11			
21			1
22			1
23			
24			
25			
26			
27			
46			
45			
44			
43			
42			1
41			1
31			2
32			1
33			
34			
35			
36			
37			

Fig. 13-12. Case K.A. Periodontal chart from recordings made 8 years after treatment.

be made to maintain all teeth if this is technically possible. Extraction of one single tooth in such a dentition will frequently also mean the extraction of several others for "prosthetic reasons". The end result could be an extensive prosthetic rehabilitation which would have been entirely unneccessary if the treatment planning had been properly done.

Patient B. H. (female, 40 years old)

Initial examination

The periodontal status (pocket depths, furcation involvements, tooth mobility, radiographs) from the initial examination is shown in Fig. 13-13. The data obtained from this examination disclosed essentially shallow pockets in most parts of the dentition except for isolated areas (the region 11-24) where some pockets exhibited probing depths varying between 4 and 7 mm. It should be observed that, particularly in the maxillary front region, pronounced gingival recessions prevailed. This means that even the moderate probing depth values obtained reflected advanced loss of the supporting tissues. This was further confirmed by the

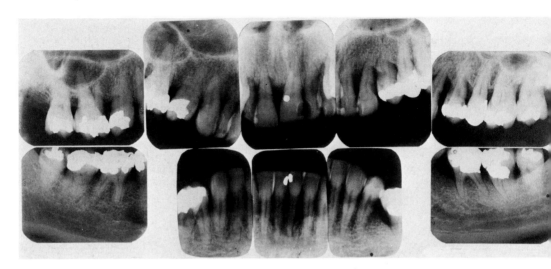

Fig. 13-13. Case B.H. (40 year old female). Periodontal chart and radiographs from the initial examination.

severe loss of alveolar bone (see radio-graphs: Fig. 13-13) in this region where some of the teeth exhibited increased mobility (tooth 11: degree 2 in combination with elongation; tooth 23: degree 3 and tooth 24: degree 2). In the posterior tooth regions there was a loss of the periodontal tissues varying between ⅓ and ½ of the length of the roots. In the mandibular front tooth region the destruction was severe particularly around tooth 31. This tooth was found to be non-vital and exhibited a mobility of degree 2. The plaque and gingivitis scores were 25 and 30% respectively.

Treatment

In discussing with the patient different alternatives of treatment it was first suggested that tooth 23 had to be extracted. Not more than 2-3 mm of the apical portion of the root was still invested in supporting bone. The tooth exhibited a degree 3 mobility in conjunction with premature occlusal contact in the intercuspal position and on laterotrusive movement of the mandible. The question arose, however, of what consequences extraction of tooth 23 would have on the overall therapy. For instance: the neighboring teeth (22 with advanced periodontal des-

Periodontal chart

Tooth	Pocket depth				Furcation involvement	Tooth mobility
	m	b	d	l		
17	4					
16	4			4		
~~15~~						
14			4			
13				4		
12						
11	6			4		2
21	4					
22			4			
23	5		6	5		3
24	4		7			2
25						
26				5	d 1	
27	6	4				
48						
47						
46						
45	4		4			
44			4			
43						
42						
41						
31						2
32						
33	4					
34	4					
~~35~~						
36	4				b 1	
37	4				b 1	
38						

Plaque score: 25 %   Gingivitis score: 30 %

ruction at the distal aspect, and 24 with severe loss of supporting tissue including increased mobility) could not be considered as proper abutment teeth for a 3-unit bridge replacing tooth 23. The demand for proper abutment teeth would therefore require a further extension of the bridge restoration to include teeth 21 and 25 (following extraction also of 24). This extension of the bridge construction implies, however, that tooth 11 will be the first nonsplinted neighboring tooth. Considering the small amount of periodontium which persisted around this tooth, possible recurrence of disease following treatment would almost certainly result in loss of tooth 11. It may, therefore, appear to be necessary to extract 11 as well, and to extend the bridge to tooth 13, since tooth 12 may also be considered improper as the terminal abutment tooth on the right side of the jaw.

From this discussion it is apparent that extraction of one single tooth (23) in this dentition will lead to extraction of a number of additional teeth to exclude their incorporation in the permanent reconstruction. The result is, thus, an extensive bridge therapy which can be avoided if only the critical tooth (23) can be maintained. Therefore it was decided to treat all teeth and postpone the decision of tooth extractions until the result of the periodontal treatment could be properly evaluated.

Initial therapy
Oral hygiene instruction and plaque control evaluation. Scaling and root planing. Occlusal adjustment of 11, 23 and 24. Correction of improper amalgam restorations.

Corrective therapy (following reevaluation at Examination 2)
Periodontal surgery in the region of 11-24. Extraction of 28 and 48 (semi-impacted molars).
Endodontic treatment of 31.

Six months following this part of the corective treatment, a new evaluation including measurements of tooth mobility showed that no pathologically deepened pockets were present and that the mobility had decreased in all initially hypermobile teeth (11: from degree 2 to 1; 23: from degree 3 to

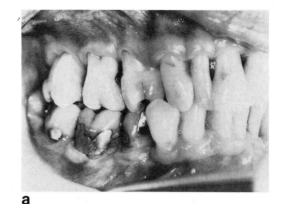

a

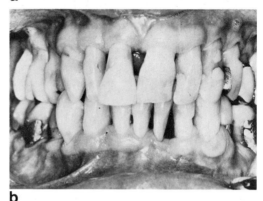

b

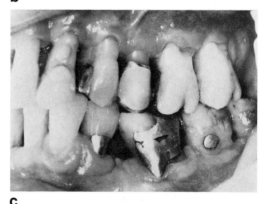

c

Figs. 13-14 a-c. Case B.H. Clinical status 12 years after treatment.

2; 24: from degree 2 to 0; 31: from degree 2 to 1). All teeth could thus be maintained and there were no indications for additional tooth extractions. The treatment was completed by preparation and insertion of a crown restoration in tooth 25.

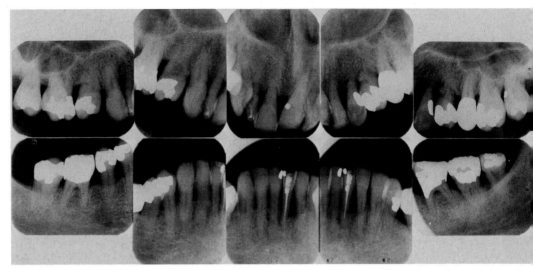

Fig. 13-15. Case B.H. Radiographs obtained 12 years after active therapy. Note that no loss of alveolar bone has occurred during the 12 years of maintenance. Compare with Fig. 13-13.

Maintenance therapy
During the first year after completion of the corrective therapy the patient was enrolled in a maintenance care program with recall appointments once every 3 months and thereafter once every 6 months.

The result of the treatment (12 years after) is shown in Figs. 13-14 a-c (clinical status) and Fig. 13-15 (radiographs). No further loss of supporting tissues had occurred during this observation period.

Figs. 13-16 a-c. Case P.O.S. (30 year old male). Clinical status prior to therapy.

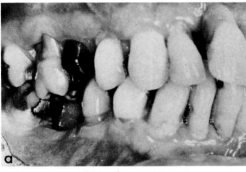

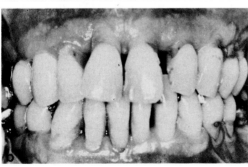

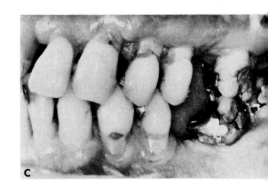

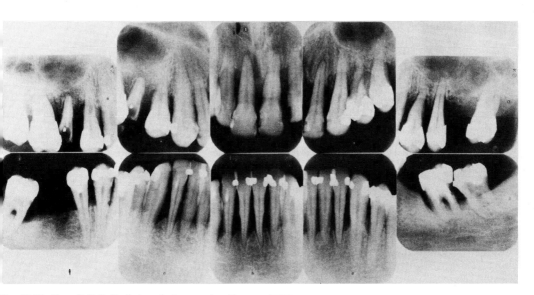

Fig. 13-17. Case P.O.S. Periodontal chart and radiographs from the initial examination.

Patient P.O.S. (male, 30 years)

Initial examination

The clinical status of this patient is illustrated in Figs. 13-16 a-c and the periodontal status (pocket depths, furcation involvements, tooth mobility, radiographs and diagnoses) from the initial examination in Fig. 13-17. The dentition was characterized by severe destruction of the supporting apparatus including advanced loss of the interradicular periodontal tissues in all molars and the 2 first maxillary premolars. Most teeth were markedly mobile particularly the incisors in both jaws. The plaque and gingivitis scores were 100%.

Treatment planning

A thorough analysis of the periodontal conditions in this patient revealed that certain teeth could no longer be treated and maintained but had to be extracted. Hence, it was decided to extract teeth 14 and 24 (furcation involvement of degree 2 from both mesial and distal aspects) and 12, 11, 21, 22 (loss of the supporting tissues to a level close to or beyond the apices in combination with a mobility of degree 3). In the mandible, 42, 41, 31, 32 and 37 could not be maintained.

Tooth	Pocket depth m	b	d	l	Furcation involvement	Tooth mobility	Gingivitis	Parodontitis levis	Parodontitis gravis	Parodontitis compl.
17	9		8	6	m,d 2	1				x
16	8		8		m,b,d 2	2				x
15	8		7	4		1			x	
14	8	4	8	5	m,d 2	2				x
13	6		5	4		1		x		
12	8	4	7	8		3			x	x
11	10	8	10			3			x	x
21	7		10	8		3				x
22	8	5	7	5		3				x
23	8		10	6		2			x	x
24	9		10	7	m,d 2	2				x
25	8	6	8	7		2			x	
26										
27	10	8	8	4	m,d 2, d 1	2				x
47	10	5	8	7	3	1				x
48										
45	8		7	5				x		
44	8		8	7		1		x		
43	7		8	5		1		x	x	
42	7	4	7	7		3				x
41	7	4	7	7		3				x
31	7	4	7	7		3				x
32	7	4	7	7		3				x
33	8		5	6		1		x		
34	10		6	7		1			x	x
35	5		4					x		
36										
37	10	7	8	7	3	2				x
38	6	8	9	8	b,1 2	2				x

Plaque score: 100 %   Gingivitis score: 100 %

The overall treatment of this patient, therefore, had to include prosthetic replacement of a number of teeth.

Alternative 1

Mandible: In the planning phase it was anti-

323

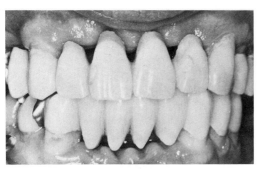

Fig. 13-18. Case P.O.S. Clinical status of the front tooth region at completion of the initial, cause related treatment.

cipated that the prosthetic rehabilitation of the mandibular dentition ought not to involve any technical difficulties since 33 and 43 as well as 34, 35 and 44, 45 were available for periodontal therapy and, hence, could be used as abutment teeth for a cross-arch fixed bridge. It did not seem reasonable to maintain the furcation involved molars 47 and 38, so these teeth were also scheduled for extraction. In this context it should be understood that if 47 and 38 were maintained, the treatment would have included not only endodontic measures but also root separation and periodontal surgery, production of posts and cores and the incorporation of the preserved roots as abutments in the cross-arch bridge construction.

Maxilla: The maxillary dentition presented more difficult therapeutic problems. If the patient was to be rehabilitated with a fixed bridge, it was considered pertinent to maintain the 2 maxillary canines (teeth 13 and 23) and at least 1 tooth in the premolar (molar) regions on both sides of the jaw (15 and 25) and/or one or more roots of 17, 16 and 27.

Definitive prosthetic treatment of the maxillary dentition by means of a removable, partial denture was not considered appropriate since the various abutment teeth for such denture displayed a markedly increased mobility. For the same reason it was considered inappropriate to *temporarily* replace the extracted teeth by means of a provisional removable partial denture. The provisional prosthesis had to be fabricated in the form of a fixed bridge in order to enable proper stabilization (splinting) of the hypermobile 13, 23 and 25 prior to periodontal surgery. In the present case the temporary bridge should not include tooth 15 and the maxillary molars. Tooth 15 was to be left uncovered in order to facilitate endodontic therapy and the preparation and insertion of a post and core. In addition, the maxillary molars had to be accessible for periodontal therapy including endodontic treatment and root separation. In order to facilitate the surgical procedures and also to avoid the risk of a further increase of the tooth mobility, the extractions of 14, 12, 11, 21 and 22 and the insertion of the temporary bridge had to be

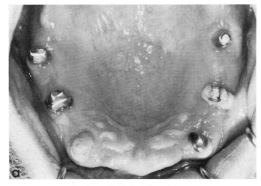
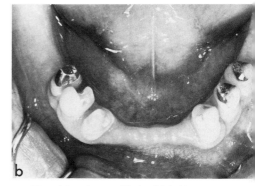

Figs. 13-19 a, b. Case P.O.S. The abutment teeth used for a maxillary (a) and a mandibular (b) bridge.

carried out *prior* to the start of the surgical phase of treatment.

Alternative 2

The alternative treatment to the one outlined above is a complete denture in the maxillary jaw and a removable partial denture in the mandible with the use of 45, 44, 43 and 33, 34, 35 as abutment teeth.

Treatment

The clinical and radiographical symptoms of the advanced disease present as well as the therapeutic alternatives were thoroughly discussed with the patient. This discussion included a detailed explanation of the role of optimal plaque control for the long-term good prognosis. The treatment was performed according to alternative 1 and in the following sequence:

Initial therapy

Instruction regarding oral hygiene measures. Scaling and root planing. Evaluation of the ability of the patient to maintain a high standard of oral hygiene.
Extraction of 14, 12, 11, 21, 22. Temporary acrylic bridge [14,] 13, [12, 11, 21, 22,] 23, 24, 25; (24 was temporarily maintained in order to ensure proper stability of the temporary bridge).
Extraction of 47, 42, 41, 31, 32, 37, 38. Temporary acrylic bridge 44, 43, [42, 41, 41, 32,] 33, 34, 35; (45: because the tooth was non-vital it was not incorporated in the bridge to facilitate endodontic treatment). Endodontic treatment 15, 45. The clinical status at the completion of initial treatment is seen in Fig. 13-18.

Corrective therapy

Periodontal surgery around the teeth which at the reevaluation of the case after initial therapy still exhibited pathologically deepened pockets which bled on probing. The palatal roots of 17 and 27 were maintained and the buccal roots were extracted following separation.
Extraction of 16 and 24.
Following healing after surgery, posts and cores were inserted in 17, 15, 27 and 45 (Figs. 13-19a,b) and permanent fixed bridges were

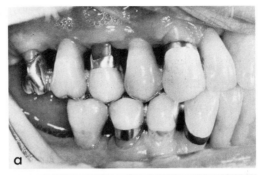

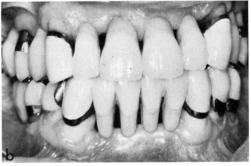

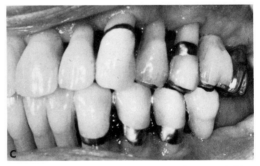

Figs. 13-20 a-c. Case P.O.S. Clinical photograph illustrating the result of treatment after 8 years of maintenance.

designed and fabricated with the following outline:
maxilla: 17 (palatal root), [16,] 15, [14,] 13, [12, 11, 21, 22,] 23, [24,] 25, [26,] 27 (palatal root).
mandible: [46,] 45, 44, 43, [42, 41, 31, 32,] 33, 34, 35, [36].

Maintenance therapy

After completion of active treatment this patient was enrolled in a maintenance care

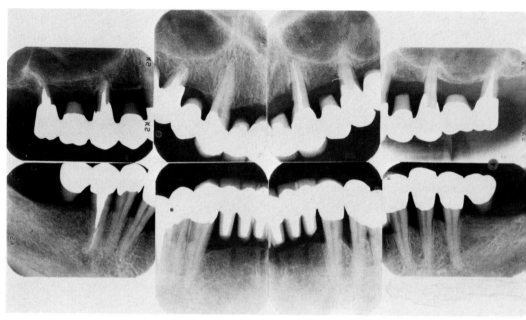

Fig. 13-21. Case P.O.S. Radiographs obtained 8 years after completion of active therapy. Note that no further loss of alveolar bone has occurred during the 8 years of maintenance.

program including recall appointments once every 3 months. Clinical photographs (Figs. 13-20 a-c) and radiographs (Fig. 13-21) illustrate the result of the treatment at the 8 year control. No further loss of supporting tissues occurred during the maintenance period.

References

Lindhe, J. & Nyman, S. (1975) The effect of plaque control and surgical pocket elimination on the establishment and maintenance of periodontal health. A longitudinal study of periodontal therapy in cases of advanced disease. *Journal of Clinical Periodontology* **2**, 67-79.

Nyman, S. & Lindhe, J. (1979) A longitudinal study of combined periodontal and prosthetic treatment of patients with advanced periodontal disease. *Journal of Periodontology* **50**, 163-169.

Nyman, S., Lindhe, J. & Rosling, B. (1977) Periodontal surgery in plaque-infected dentitions. *Journal of Clinical Periodontology* **4**, 240-249.

Nyman, S., Rosling, B. & Lindhe, J. (1975) Effect of professional tooth cleaning on healing after periodontal surgery. *Journal of Clinical Periodontology* **2**, 80-86.

Rosling, B., Nyman, S. & Lindhe, J. (1976a) The effect of systematic plaque control on bone regeneration in infrabony pockets. *Journal of Clinical Periodontology* **3**, 38-53.

Rosling, B., Nyman, S., Lindhe, J. & Jern, B. (1976b) The healing potential of the periodontal tissues following different techniques of periodontal surgery in plaque-free dentitions. A 2-year clinical study. *Journal of Clinical Periodontology* **3**, 233-250.

CHAPTER 14

The Cause Related Phase of Periodontal Therapy

Introduction

The complete treatment of patients suffering from periodontal disease and caries including associated pathologic conditions (e.g. pulpitis, periapical osteitis, tooth migration, tooth loss) can, for didactic purposes, be divided into 3 different, but frequently overlapping, phases (see Chapter 13):

1 *The cause related* (initial) *phase,* the objective of which is the arrest of progressive periodontal disease by the removal (or control) of the microbial plaques.

2 *The corrective phase,* the main objective of which is the restoration of function and esthetics.

3 *The maintenance phase,* which is aimed at preventing recurrence of periodontal disease.

In this chapter therapeutic and preventive measures will be described which are commonly used in the cause related (initial) phase of therapy.

Objectives of cause related therapy

The measures used in the cause related phase of therapy with respect to *periodontal disease* aim at the elimination and the prevention of recurrence of supra- and subgingivally located bacterial deposits from the tooth surfaces. This is accomplished by:

* Motivating the patient to combat dental disease (*patient information*).
* Giving the patient *instruction* in proper oral hygiene techniques (*self performed plaque control methods*).
* *Scaling and root planing.*
* *Removing* additional *retention factors* for plaque such as overhanging margins of restorations, ill-fitting crowns, etc.

Means of cause related therapy

Patient information

Most people brush their teeth at fairly regular intervals but fail to clean their teeth thoroughly enough to prevent the development of dental disease. A common reason for the inadequate standard of self performed oral hygiene is lack of proper knowledge of periodontal disease and caries and motivation to combat them.

In most cases, therefore, the cause related phase of therapy must be initiated by a demonstration to the patient of symptoms of dental disease found in her/his mouth. This can be accomplished by allowing the patient to participate in the professional examination of her/his oral cavity (e.g. by the use of a magnifying hand-mirror). Areas of the dentition exhibiting dental and periodontal health should be identified by the dentist as well as sites displaying symptoms of disease. The patient should learn to recognize a carious lesion, to distinguish between a healthy and inflamed gingival unit and to appreciate the difference between a normal and an increased probing depth.

The Bleeding Index chart illustrating the patient's gingival condition as well as the Probing Depth chart showing the result of the probing depth examinations should be presented and explained (see Chapter 12). The results of the radiographic examination should also be reported; areas of the dentition with normal height of alveolar bone should be outlined as well as sites with varying degrees of bone loss. The radiographic findings can subsequently be compared with the probing depth data and the relationship between the 2 parameters explained. In other words, patients must be given the opportunity to familiarize themselves with their own dentition.

The *second stage* of this information may include a description of the reasons for the presence and the particular location of disease. It is important that the dentist emphasizes that bacteria which colonize the tooth surfaces are the main cause of both periodontal disease and caries. The patient should learn to realize that bacteria which have formed dental plaques can reduce not only the plaque pH – and produce caries lesions – but also release substances which initiate and maintain inflammatory alterations of the gingiva and cause breakdown of the attachment apparatus.

The *third stage* may involve the illustration

of the location of plaque in the dentition. First the plaque stained with a disclosing solution. Then the patient and the dentist in collaboration examine the tooth surfaces, one by one, for the presence of plaque. Areas in the dentition without plaque and without signs of pathology should be identified, as well as those with plaque and associated signs of periodontal disease and caries. The patient should now be made aware that active participation in the treatment is essential to a successful result.

In summary: detailed information must be given to the patient regarding personal, dental status and the relationship between the presence of dental plaque and calculus in the mouth and the location of sites showing dental disease. This information is aimed at motivating the patient to cooperate in the treatment. The subsequent instruction in proper oral hygiene techniques will only be effective if the patient recognizes oral health as a valuable asset and goal. The information that patients must receive concerning the cause and symptoms of periodontal disease can be delivered in many different ways. The "step by step system" described above has been used for many years and in a large number of clinical trials performed at the Department of Periodontology, University of Gothenburg, Sweden (Lindhe & Nyman 1975, Rosling et al. 1976, Lindhe et al. 1982).

Self performed plaque control methods

Tooth brushing methods
A variety of tooth brushing methods or techniques have been described in the literature. These methods can be classified in different categories with respect to the pattern of motion that the brush performs:
roll: "Rolling Stroke", "Modified Stillman"
vibratory: "Stillman", "Charters", "Bass"
circular: "Fones"
vertical: "Leonard"
horizontal: "Scrub-brush".
A number of studies have been carried out in

1) The Bass' method

A soft, multitufted brush is applied with its head at an angle of 45° to the long axis of the teeth (Fig. 14-1) and pressed in an apical direction against the gingival margin. The brush is moved in an anterior-posterior direction with short strokes in a vibrating motion. When the lingual surfaces of the anterior teeth are cleaned,

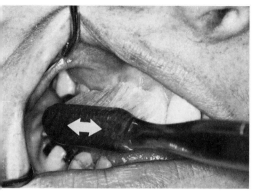

Fig. 14-1. The Bass method of toothbrushing. In this illustration the head of the toothbrush is placed against the buccal surfaces of the posterior teeth of the right maxilla. Note the angulation of the bristles against the tooth and the direction (arrows) of the motion.

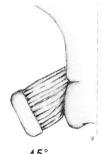

45°

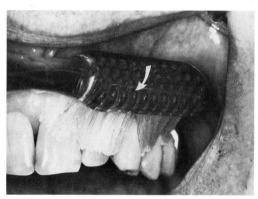

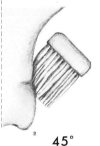

45°

Fig. 14-2 a. The Charters' method of tooth brushing. The head of the toothbrush is placed in the left maxilla. Note the angulation of the bristles against the buccal tooth surfaces. The bristles are forced into the interproximal areas.

order to compare the toothcleaning effect accomplished by brushing using some of the above presented techniques. So far, however, no one method of tooth brushing has been shown to be clearly superior to the others.

More important than the selection of a certain method of tooth brushing for the establishment of proper home-care habits is the willingness and to some extent the ability of individual patients to properly clean their teeth. The control of the results of self performed tooth cleaning, preferably with the use of *plaque disclosing agents* (see below) is also more important for the institution of proper home-care habits than the instruction and practice in a particular method of brushing.

Since, however, the Bass' (Bass 1954) and the Charters' (Charters 1948) methods of tooth brushing are probably the most commonly recommended techniques in dental practice, a description of these methods seems justified:

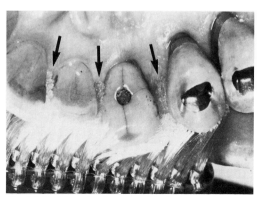

Fig. 14-2b. The palatal aspect of the incisor region in the maxilla illustrating the penetration of the bristles through the interproximal spaces (arrows).

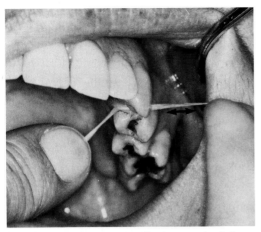

Fig. 14-3a. Dental floss is used for interproximal cleaning. The floss is carefully guided through the contact point between teeth 23 and 24. When contact has been established between the floss and the distal/mesial tooth surface the floss is moved, by minute sawing movements, against the surface for cleaning.

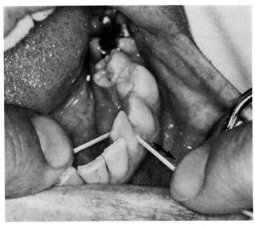

Fig. 14-3 b. The dental floss is guided through the interdental contact point between teeth 33 and 32 by the two index fingers.

the brush has to be turned into a vertical position to obtain proper access to the gingival area of the teeth. The Bass' method, properly used, is effective for the removal of soft deposits located immediately above and below the gingival margin.

2) The Charters' method
   The head of the brush is applied to the teeth at an angle of approximately 45° to

the occlusal plane (Fig. 14-2). The bristles of the toothbrush are directed towards the occlusal/incisal surfaces and the brush is moved back and forth in a rotatory motion. This method of tooth cleaning is effective particularly in cases with receded interdental papillae, i.e. when the interdental spaces are open and thus accessible for the penetration of the brush bristles.

Interdental cleaning
Tooth cleaning using an ordinary toothbrush will not properly eliminate plaque in the interdental areas (Lövdal et al. 1958). Adjunctive instruments, therefore, have to be used for interproximal plaque removal. Depending upon the shape of the interproximal space *dental floss* or *tape, toothpicks, interproximal brushes* and/or *single-tufted brushes* should be used.

Dental floss and tape
In cases where the interdental papillae completely fill the interdental spaces, effective removal of plaque from the interproximal tooth surfaces may be accomplished by flossing. In the daily plaque control program the dental floss can, without causing damage to the gingiva and periodontal ligament, be brought 2-3.5 mm below the tip of the papilla (Waerhaug 1981). Several types of floss (waxed, unwaxed) have been introduced but no differences in the cleansing potential of different brands of floss have so far been reported (Keller & Manson-Hing 1969). The correct technique for applying the dental floss is illustrated in Fig. 14-3. When properly used, almost all parts of the interproximal surfaces can be cleaned with the floss (O'Leary 1970). However, this method of interdental cleaning has some limitations:
1. For some patients with inadequate dexterity the technique is difficult to master.
2. Flossing may be more time consuming than interproximal cleansing with picks (Gjermo & Flötra 1970).
3. Improper use of the floss can cause damage to the interdental gingival tissue (Thoma & Goldman 1960).

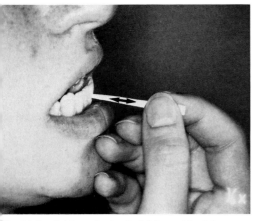

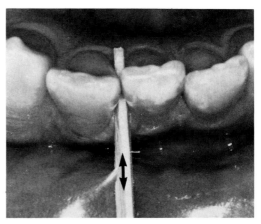

Fig. 14-4 a. A triangular toothpick is used for interprox-mal tooth cleaning. The toothpick is secured in its posi-ion with "finger rest" on the cheek for stabilization of movements.

Fig. 14-4 b. The tooth pick is properly inserted in an interproximal site in the lower front tooth region.

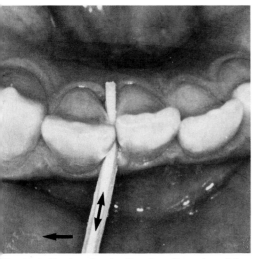

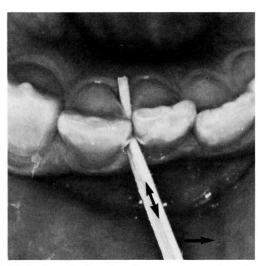

Fig. 14-4c. By changing the direction of insertion of the toothpick the 2 proximal tooth surfaces are properly cleaned.

Toothpicks

In sites where the interdental papillae are receded the toothpick is an excellent substi-tute to dental floss for interproximal clean-ing. The tooth pick should be made of soft wood, and have a triangular shape to fit the interdental space (Waerhaug 1959). The proper use of the toothpicks is illustrated in Fig. 14-4.

Interproximal brush

In cases with wider interdental spaces an interproximal brush (bottle neck brush) is often effective for the removal of plaque from the approximal surfaces. The inter-proximal brushes are manufactured in dif-ferent sizes (Fig. 14-5) and should be selected to fit, as closely as possible, the indi-vidual interdental space (Fig. 14-6). Small inter-proximal brushes can be inserted into handles, (Fig. 14-7) which may facilitate the cleaning of the interproximal areas in the posterior parts of the dentition.

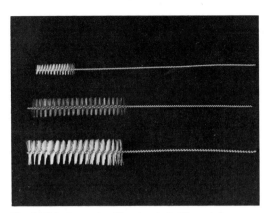

Fig. 14-5. Interproximal brushes in 3 different sizes.

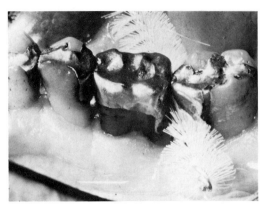

Fig. 14-6. An interproximal brush has been inserted in a wide interdental space between teeth 46 and 47. Lingual view.

Single-tufted brush

A single-tufted brush often has to be used in regions of the dentition which are not easily reached with other oral hygiene instruments, e.g. furcation areas, distal surfaces of the most posterior molars and buccal or lingual tooth surfaces with an irregular gingival margin (Fig. 14-8).

Adjunctive aids

Disclosing agents

Dental plaque is difficult to detect, particularly to the untrained eye. Disclosing agents should be used, therefore, to demonstrate the presence and location of plaque and to evaluate the efficacy of the patient's home-care technique (Fig. 14-9). As a rule, the disclosing agent should be applied after tooth brushing and interdental cleaning. The patient can hereby identify the sites where the oral hygiene technique is inadequate. Substances aimed at staining dental plaque have been used in dentistry for many years (Arnim 1963, Ten 1981). Examples of such substances are *erythrocin, fuchsin* and more recently a *fluorescin containing* dye for visualization of plaque when exposed to an ultraviolet light (Plack-lite®). Erythrocin containing *tablets* or *wafers* are available as "over the counter products". The disclosing

tablets should be used by the patient in the home-care program and the wafers by the dentist for plaque assessments (Fig. 14-10).

Intraoral mirror

As stated above, an important step in the patient's self performed home-care is the nonprofessional control of the efficacy of tooth cleaning procedures. Bathroom lights are often inadequate for intraoral illumination, which is why a mirror-light combina-

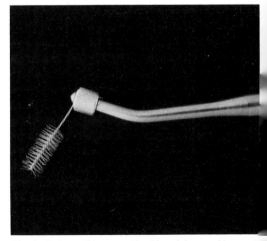

Fig. 14-7. A small interproximal brush inserted in a custom-made handle.

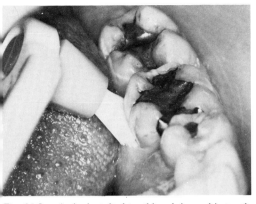

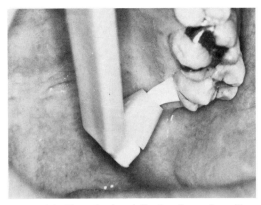

Fig. 14-8 a. A single-tufted toothbrush is used in tooth regions where cleaning by means of an ordinary toothbrush is difficult to master. The lingual surfaces of lower molars are cleaned.

Fig. 14-8 b. The palatal and distal surfaces of maxillary molars are cleaned by means of a single-tufted toothbrush.

tion can for some patients be a useful adjunct for the detection of residual plaque (Fig. 14-11).

Irrigation devices

The use of water irrigating devices has been recommended as a valuable supplement to mechanical plaque control measures. Many investigators have tried to determine the potential of such devices to assist in the removal of dental plaque but the findings reported from such clinical trials are inconclusive. Studies by Matsuzaki et al. (1974) and Hugoson (1978) failed to demonstrate significant reduction of plaque and gingivitis scores in patients using water irrigators. However, in special cases the use of a device for the irrigation of antiseptics (chlorhexidine) may be an excellent adjunct to mechanical tooth cleaning for the removal of both food debris and plaque (Lang & Räber 1981).

Dentifrices

A dentifrice should be used in combination with tooth brushing for the purpose of 1) facilitating plaque removal and 2) applying agents to the tooth surfaces for therapeutic or preventive purposes. The abrasive material of the dentifrice should have a particle size and composition which prevents wear of tooth substances but facilitates plaque removal. The question remains how abra-

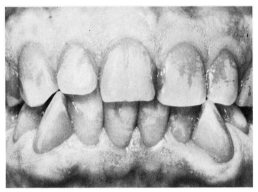

Fig. 14-9a. Disclosing agents are used to disclose the presence of dental plaque. Note remaining dental plaque on the buccal tooth surfaces after staining.

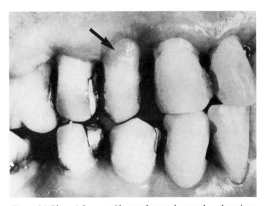

Fig. 14-9b. After self performed tooth cleaning, remaining plaque can be identified by the patient following rinsing with a disclosing solution (arrow).

333

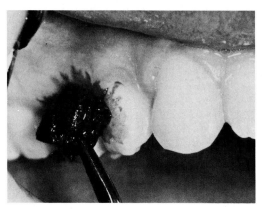

Fig. 14-10. Wafers containing disclosing solutions are often used to identify plaque.

sive a dentifrice should be to assist in the removal of plaque without damage. Studies comparing the effect of abrasive and nonabrasive dentifrices regarding their potential as adjuncts for plaque removal have failed to disclose an obvious benefit of toothpastes. The establishment of a stained pellicles seems, however, to be favored in subjects using nonabrasive dentifrices (Bergenholtz et al. 1971). The dentifrice is also an excellent vehicle for the administration of substances to the tooth surfaces such as *fluorides, antiseptics* (e.g. chlorhexidine), *enzymes* (e.g. amyloglucosidase, glucose oxidase) or other substances (e.g. for desensitization of hypersensitive tooth surfaces).

Plaque control program for the periodontal patient

The system used to teach the patient a proper tooth cleaning technique may of course vary from one dentist/hygienist to another. Below one system is presented which has been used in clinical trials (Lindhe & Nyman 1975, Rosling et al. 1976, Lindhe et al. 1982).

First session
1. Ask the patient to clean her/his teeth using own traditional technique.
2. Explain to the patient the use of disclosing agents to identify plaque at sites where the tooth cleaning technique has

been inadequate. Apply the disclosing solution to the teeth. Use disclosing wafers. Demonstrate the result for the patient; use a hand-mirror – and ask the patient to identify all sites where plaque remains.
3. Ask the patient to clean her/his teeth once more and stress the importance of removing plaque from the stained sites. Discuss the possibility of altering her/his traditional tooth brushing technique.
4. Check the result of the second tooth cleaning practice together with the patient. Are there still areas harboring stained material? Discuss the need for adjunctive aids for interproximal cleaning, e.g. toothpicks, dental floss, interproximal brushes.
5. Allow the patient under careful supervision to practice the use of dental floss or toothpick. Discuss the result obtained.

Second session (2-4 days later)
1. Apply the disclosing solution to the teeth and ask the patient to evaluate the result of her/his home-care program. All sites harboring stained material should be identified on a chart.
2. Discuss the result and adjust the technique, if necessary.

Third session (1-2 weeks later)
Apply the disclosing solution to the teeth and evaluate the result of the home-care pro-

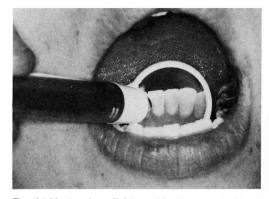

Fig. 14-11. A mirror-light combination may facilitate for the patient the detection of plaque on the lingual tooth surfaces.

gram. All sites harboring stained material are identified on a chart. Discuss the result of the self performed tooth cleaning by means of a plaque chart (Fig. 14-12) and, if needed, adjust the technique and the armamentarium.

Depending on the ability of the patient to learn how to practice proper oral hygiene measures, the time required for the instruction may vary considerably. Thus, additional oral hygiene sessions may be required. It is important, however, to point out that the efficacy of self performed plaque control should be evaluated and presented to the patient at each appointment during both the active and the maintenance phase of therapy (see Chapter 25).

Lesions produced by oral hygiene measures

Damage of hard and soft tissues caused by extensive tooth brushing or the use of adjunctive oral hygiene aids is sometimes seen in periodontal patients. In rare cases the damage may be extensive. The buccal aspects of canines and premolars and the approximal surfaces of lower incisors are sites in which this type of damage most frequently occurs (Fig. 14-13). Factors contributing to such damage can include 1) too stiff bristles of the toothbrush, 2) too extensive tooth brushing and interdental instrumentation and 3) the use of a highly abrasive dentifrice during brushing and interdental cleaning.

Findings from clinical and laboratory research have demonstrated that damage of *hard tissue* is mainly due to the abrasive component of the dentifrice used, while lesions in the gingiva can be produced by tooth brushing or flossing also without the use of a dentifrice. It is important to realize that as soon as hard and soft tissue damage is identified, the oral hygiene technique has to be changed in order to arrest the progression of the lesions.

Chemical plaque control measures

The proper removal of dental plaque by mechanical means is for most individuals

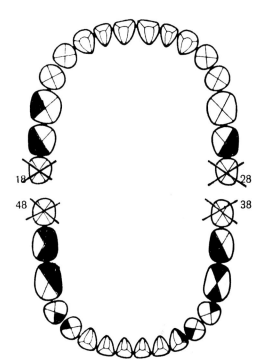

Fig. 14-12. A chart illustrating the teeth and tooth surfaces in the upper and lower jaws. The distribution of tooth surfaces with dental plaque (shadowed areas) is identified. In this case the plaque score is 17%.

both a time demanding and, from a technical aspect, difficult procedure to master. Considerable interest has been directed, therefore, towards the use of drugs to assist or substitute mechanical plaque control measures. The drugs used have been directed either exclusively against the *supragingival plaque* or against both the *supra- and subgingival microbiota*. Varying degrees of *supragingival plaque control* have been accomplished mainly by the use of *antiseptics* but also different *enzyme preparations* and *tensioactive agents* (e.g. fluorides) have been incorporated in mouthwashes, dentifrices, chewing gums and other vehicles. In attempts to combat the *subgingival microbiota* 1) *antiseptics* or *antibiotics* have been introduced in the periodontal pockets by different local delivery devices or 2) *antibiotics* have been administered to periodontal patients via the systemic route.

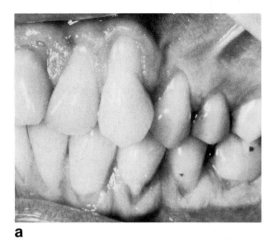

a

Fig. 14-13 a. Soft tissue damage as a result of extensive tooth brushing. Note gingival recession on the buccal gingival surface of e.g. tooth 23.

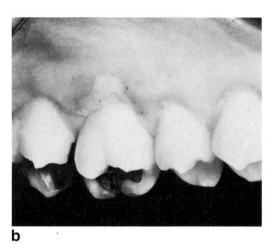

b

Fig. 14-13 b. Note multiple ulcerations of the buccal gingival margin in the right maxilla.

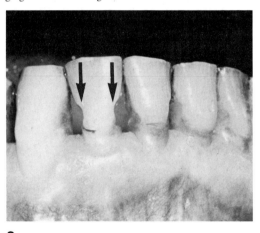

c

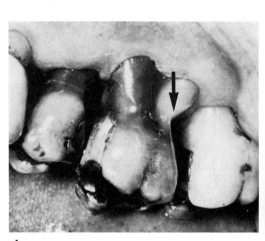

d

Figs. 14-13c,d. Hard tissue damage (arrows) has resulted after extensive use of interdental brushes.

Antiseptics

The possibility of suppressing the oral microflora by antiseptics has been tested ever since Miller (1890, 1896) suggested that caries may be prevented by the use of antibacterial substances. In an article entitled "Prophylaxis and Pyorrhea" Hartzell in 1932 stated that pyorrhea "is the result of the activity of a heavy coat of germ life clinging to the sides and necks of human teeth" and that "local prophylaxis of the oral cavity, when intelligently practiced can and will absolutely prevent bacterial destruction of the tissues of the teeth and their investing processes". He continued "for cleansing processes, no one has yet discovered anything more effective than soap" and recommended a soap made by "boiling sodium hydrate and castor oil together, the technical name of which is *sodium ricinoleate*". Thirty years later Dossenbach & Mühlemann (1961) tested the effect of such a sodium ricinoleate preparation in a clinical trial and noted that topical application of this soap to human volunteers leads to almost complete inhibition of calculus formation.

Hanke (1940) postulated "If plaques consist largely of living microorganisms, it should be possible to remove them with a suitable germicide; and that this can be done has not previously been demonstrated". He subsequently reported the result from a clinical trial which showed that plaques can be eliminated if the mouth is carefully rinsed once or twice daily with antiseptic solutions containing organic mercurials.

In more recent years plaque inhibition *in vitro* and *in vivo* has been demonstrated following administration of antiseptics such as *chloramin T, cetylpyridinium chloride, benzalkonium chloride, chlorhexidine* (Strålfors 1961, Schroeder 1969, Löe & Rindom Schiött 1970). An excellent review on this topic was published by Schroeder (1969) to which the reader is referred for detailed information.

The antiseptic which during the last decade has received most attention is *chlorhexidine digluconate* or *acetate*. Schroeder (1969) noted a 73% reduction in the formation of dental calculus in humans who regularly rinsed their mouths with a solution of 0.1% chlorhexidine acetate. In a classic paper from 1970, Löe & Rindom-Schiött reported observations demonstrating that young dental students who refrained from mechanical tooth cleaning measures but twice daily, for 3 weeks, rinsed with a 0.2% solution of chlorhexidine, did not develop microbial plaques and related signs of gingivitis. They also observed that individuals who had been on a "no oral hygiene regimen" for 17 days and who during this period had accumulated large amounts of plaque, lost their supragingivally located plaques after a 6 day period of chlorhexidine rinsings. The experiments reported thus reveal that it is not only possible to prevent plaque formation by rinsing the mouth with chlorhexidine but also to remove or disperse established microbial aggregates. Other experiments have documented that chlorhexidine, used in a mouthwash, may prevent not only gingivitis but also caries (Löe et al. 1970).

Why is chlorhexidine effective? Rindom-

Schiött et al. (1970) showed that 2 daily rinses with chlorhexidine digluconate reduced the number of salivary bacteria by 85-95%. But since several other antibacterial substances are equally or even more effective than chlorhexidine against oral bacteria *in vitro* (Gjermo et al. 1970), and since oral bacteria rapidly multiply (Strålfors 1961) it was assumed that, with chlorhexidine, factors other than the antibacterial properties *per se* were important for its pronounced plaque inhibitory effect. Such a factor may be the adsorption to and subsequent slow release of chlorhexidine from tooth surfaces, pellicle substances or oral mucous membranes. An antimicrobial milieu is thus established in the oral cavity for a period of several hours after one rinsing with this drug.

When should chlorhexidine be used? Chlorhexidine should be used in situations where mechanical plaque control measures are difficult to exercise but an ideal oral hygiene is required. This means that chlorhexidine mouth rinsing should be employed by patients following periodontal surgery to ensure ideal conditions for wound healing (e.g. Hirst 1972, Asboe-Jörgensen et al. 1974, Hamp et al. 1975, Addy & Dolby 1976, Davies 1977, Westfelt et al. 1982) and, in addition, in patients suffering from acute necrotizing gingivitis.

Chlorhexidine is, however, of limited value in the treatment of advanced periodontal disease with deep periodontal pockets. The reason for this is the apparent inability of the drug, used in a mouthwash, to reach the apical portions of the periodontal pockets (Flötra et el. 1972). More recently data have been reported demonstrating that chlorhexidine, by the use of so called subgingival washings, may reach the apical portions of the periodontal pockets and interfere with the subgingival microbiota. Further studies are needed, however, to assess how effective such washings are in patients with advanced periodontal disease.

The clinical use of chlorhexidine has revealed some side effects. Discolorations of teeth, silicate fillings and the dorsum of the tongue are almost always seen in patients using the drug on a regular basis (Eriksen & Gjermo 1973). Some patients also complain about the bitter taste of the drug and interference with the sense of taste (Löe 1969, Schroeder 1969, Löe & Rindom-Schiött 1970).

Antibiotics

The use of antibiotics as an adjunct to periodontal therapy has been discussed for many years. However, long-term trials in humans describing the effect of such adjunctive therapy is still, with a few exceptions, lacking. Studies of the composition of the subgingival plaque in advanced periodontal lesions in humans have revealed that the microbiota from such sites is dominated by Gram negative, anaerobic or capnophilic rods. This finding, together with *in vitro* assessments of the susceptibility of potential periodontopathic micro-organisms to antibiotics, has prompted the use of mainly *tetracycline* and *minocycline* (a semisynthetic tetracycline) in periodontal therapy. Tetracycline and minocycline are not only effective against the proposed periodontal pathogens but, if administered via the systemic route, the drugs are concentrated in the gingival fluid at levels higher than in serum. Clinical trials performed in humans with adult forms of periodontal disease, however, have failed to reveal an additional effect of tetracycline above what can be accomplished by scaling and root planing. Tetracycline used alone, i.e. without concomitant mechanical debridement, had no prolonged therapeutic effect (Listgarten et al. 1978).

In patients with juvenile periodontitis, however, a treatment program including administration of tetracycline, root instrumentation and soft tissue curettage, resolved the lesions and, in 90% of cases, prevented disease recurrence (Lindhe 1982).

Other drugs such as *metronidazole* (active against the anaerobic segment of the microbiota), *spiramycin, clindamycin* have also been tested but additional studies are required to assess the efficacy of these compounds in periodontal therapy.

Based on available information it seem reasonable to suggest that in most forms o human periodontal disease:

* Antibiotic therapy cannot substitute conventional treatment including scaling and root planing.
* Antibiotics used as adjuncts to conventional measures of therapy offer no obvious advantage.
* Tetracycline (250 mg × 4 per day for 2 weeks) should be used as an adjunctive measure in the treatment of juvenile periodontitis.
* In patients with systemic disease, antibiotic therapy may be considered to protect the individual against spread of the infection during subgingival instrumentation.
* In rare cases where repeated mechanical therapy has failed to resolve the inflammatory lesion antibiotics may be tried to prevent disease progress.

Before the use of antibiotics can be recommended in periodontal therapy much research needs to be performed to assess 1 which drug should be administered in a given situation, 2) the potential hazards of this type of adjunctive therapy.

Scaling and root planing

Definitions

Scaling is a procedure which aims at the removal of plaque and calculus from the tooth surface. Depending on the location of the deposits scaling has to be performed by supragingival or subgingival instrumentation. The objective of supragingival scaling is the removal of deposits from the clinical crown of the teeth. Root planing denotes a technique of instrumentation by which the "softened" cementum is removed and the root surface is made "hard" and "smooth". Subgingival scaling and root planing (root curettage) are performed as either closed or open procedures. The *closed* procedure implies subgingival instrumentation without intentional displacement of the gingiva, i.e.

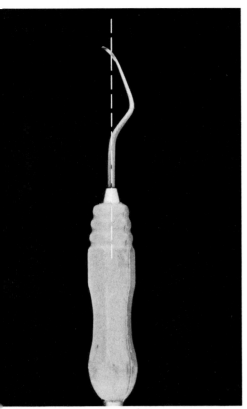

Fig. *14-14*. A double-ended, hand instrument with cool-
ip. The cutting edges of the blades are centered over
e long axis of the handle.

he root surface is not accessible for direct
isual inspection. The *open* procedure calls
or exposure of the affected root surface by
easures which displace the gingival tissue.
he gingivae are thus incised and reflected
o facilitate access for the instrument and vis-
ility for the operator in the field of opera-
on.

struments and instrumentation
nstruments used for scaling and root plan-
ng are classified as:

. **Hand instruments**
 Curettes, sickles, hoes, chisels, files
. **Ultrasonic instruments**
. **Rotating instruments**

1. Hand instruments

A hand instrument is composed of 3 parts:
The *working part* (the blade), the *shank* and
the *handle*. The cutting edges of the blade
are centered over the long axis of the handle
in order to obtain proper balance of the
instrument (Fig. 14-14). The blade is often
made of *carbon steel, stainless steel* or *tungsten carbide.*

Curettes (Fig. 14-15)
Curettes are instruments used for both
supra- and subgingival scaling and root planing. The working part of the curette is the
spoon shaped blade which has 2 curved cutting edges. The 2 edges are united by the
rounded toe. The curettes are usually made
"double ended" with mirror-turned blades.
The length and angulation of the shank as
well as the dimensions of the blade differ
between different brands of the instrument
(Fig. 14-16).

Sickles (Fig. 14-17)
The sickle is manufactured with either a
curved or a straight blade which has a triangular cross-section and 2 cutting edges. The
"facial" surface between the 2 cutting edges
is flat in lateral direction but may be curved
in the direction of its long axis. The "facial"
surface converges with the 2 lateral surfaces
of the blade. The sickles are mainly used for
supragingival debridement or scaling in shallow pockets. The instrument is also manufactured with angulated shanks (Fig. 14-
18).

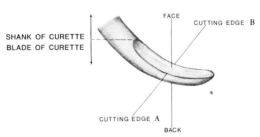

Fig. *14-15*. Schematic illustration of the design of the
blade of a curette.

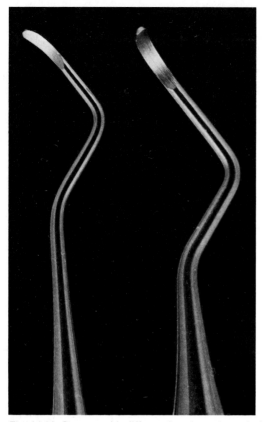

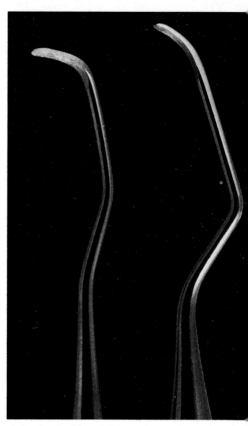

Fig. 14-16. Curettes with different lengths and angulations of the shank. (a) and (b) are curettes used for supr gingival and (c) and (d) curettes for subgingival instrumentation. Increased angulation of the shank (b and d) of th curettes permits proper instrumentation in posterior tooth regions.

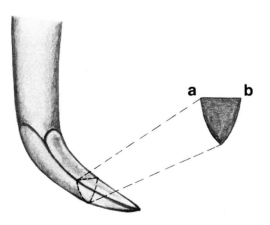

Fig. 14-17. Schematic illustration of the cross-section of the blade of a sickle. The cutting edges are positioned at (a) and (b).

Hoes (Fig. 14-19)
The hoe has only 1 cutting edge. The blade turned at a 100° angle to the shank with th cutting edge bevelled at a 45° angle. Th blade can be positioned at 4 different inclina tions in relation to the shank: facial, lingua distal and mesial. The hoe is mainly used fo supragingival scaling but is an excellei instrument for root planing during periodoi tal surgery.

Chisels (Fig. 14-20)
The periodontal chisel is probably not con monly used nowadays. The straight or bei chisel may be used for the rapid dislodge ment of heavy masses of calculus, located o the approximal and lingual surface of mai dibular anterior teeth.

Files (Fig. 14-21)

A periodontal file has multiple cutting edges lined up as a series of miniature hoes on a round or rectangular base. A flat and small file can be used for planing root surfaces in narrow pockets or furcation areas which may be inaccessible with other instruments.

Instrumentation

Supragingival scaling: The debridement of the dentition of a patient with periodontal disease is almost always initiated by supragingival scaling. To facilitate subgingival instrumentation supragingival calculus and gross overhangs of amalgam restorations or metal crowns should be eliminated first (see below; Fig. 14-22). This initial phase of the debridement can be performed by means of hand instruments or ultrasonic instruments (see below). When hand instrumentation is preferred for the initial debridement a curette, a sickle, or a chisel may be used to split off calculus from its attachment to the enamel and/or the exposed part of the root. Following hand instrumentation the clinical crowns should be polished with rubber cups, and first pumice and subsequently more fine grained (2-3 /um) polishing pastes should be used. In most cases supragingival scaling may be completed in one session to allow the patient thereafter to properly exercise the self performed plaque control program.

Subgingival scaling and root planing: Performed with hand instruments, these treatment procedures aim at removing not only soft and hard deposits from the root surface but also small amounts of tooth substance. Root cementum and dentine are removed in the shape of small chips which carry the deposits and which during the cutting operation are curled up at the front side (in the cutting direction) of the blade of the instrument. This method of instrumentation is denoted "orthogonal cutting" which implies the removal of tooth substance by means of an edge which to a varying extent penetrates the hard substance of the root. The result of the cutting operation is dependent on the material and geometry of the edge, the sharpness of the edge and the forces used

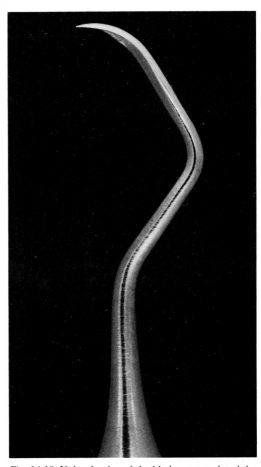

Fig. 14-18. If the shank and the blade are angulated the sickle will have properties similar to those of a curette.

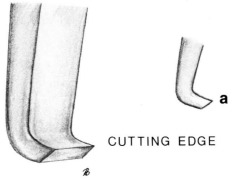

CUTTING EDGE

Fig. 14-19. The cross-section of a hoe. Note the position of the cutting edge (a).

341

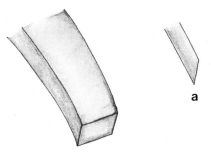

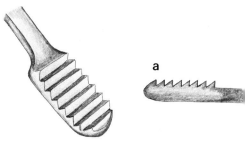

Fig. 14-20. The cross-section of a chisel. Note the position of the cutting edge (a)

Fig. 14-21. The cross-section of a file. Note the position of the cutting edges (a).

during instrumentation (Lindhe 1964). Even if subgingival scaling and root planing are often regarded as 2 separate procedures with different objectives (see definition) in clini-

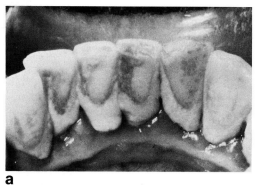

a

Fig. 14-22a. Photograph illustrating the lingual aspect of the mandibular front tooth region with supragingival plaque and calculus.

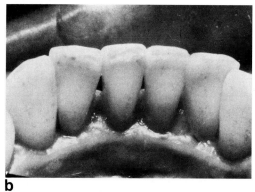

b

Fig. 14-22b. The same tooth region 3 weeks after supragingival scaling and institution of proper oral hygiene.

cal work they cannot always be separate from one another. As stated above subging val instrumentation aims at resolving th inflammation in the gingiva and arresting th progressive destruction of the attachme apparatus by removing the microbiota of th gingival pocket. Coupled with supragingiv plaque control, therefore, subgingiv debridement is the most important measu in the treatment of plaque associate periodontal diease. *In many cases it is th only therapeutic measure that needs to be pe formed* (Fig. 14-23).

Prior to the start of the subgingiv instrumentation the degree of gingiv inflammation and breakdown of the su porting apparatus in all parts of the dentiti must have been properly assessed (se

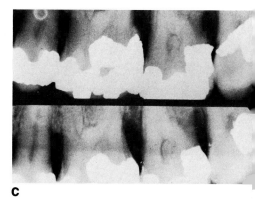

c

Fig. 14-22c. Radiographs of the maxillary left ja before and after removal af calculus and amalgam ove hangs.

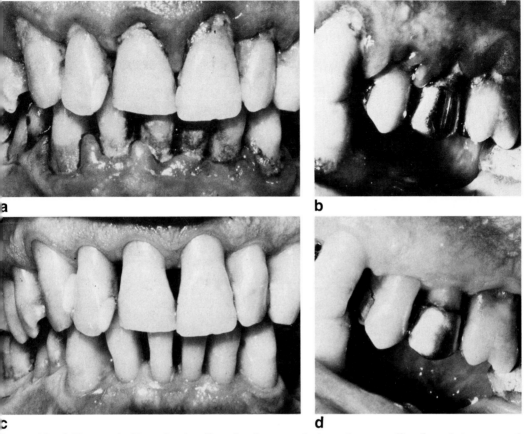

Figs. 14-23 a-d. Photographs illustrating the effect of scaling, root planing and proper self performed plaque control on the gingival tissues. Note gingival recession and the stippled outer surface of the gingiva after treatment (c,d) compared to the status before treatment (a,b).

Chapter 12). Depending on the severity of the case and the skill of the operator the number of teeth that may be included in each session of subgingival scaling and root planing varies. As a general rule, however, each session should not involve the treatment of more than 4-6 teeth.

The subgingival instrumentation is often performed under local anesthesia. The root surface of the diseased site is first explored with a probe to identify (1) the probing depth (2) the anatomy of the root surface (irregularities, root furs, open furcations, etc), (3) the location of the calcified deposits.

When the characteristics of all surfaces selected for treatment have been assessed, the instrument, almost always a curette, is inserted into the first pocket. The instrument is held in a so-called *modified pen grasp* and with a *finger rest* – fourth finger rest or third finger rest – with the face of the blade parallel to, but in only light contact with, the root surface (Fig. 14-24). It is important that all root surface instrumentation is performed with a proper finger rest. This implies that 1 finger – the third or the fourth, should act as a fulcrum for the movement of the blade of the instrument. A proper finger rest should fulfill the following require-

343

ments: (1) provide a stable fulcrum, (2) permit optimal angulation of the blade, (3) enable the use of wrist-forearm motion. In addition, the finger rest should be secured as close as possible to the particular root surface selected for treatment to enable careful instrumentation.

After the base of the periodontal pocket has been identified with the distal edge of the blade, the instrument is turned into a proper "cutting" position (Fig. 14-25). The grasp of the instrument is tightened, the force between the cutting edge and the root surface is increased, and the blade is moved in a firm stroke (working stroke) in coronal direction. Due to the structural and chemical composition of root cementum and dentine, the cutting operation *should always be initiated at the bottom of the pocket and be guided in coronal direction.* In this movement the edge penetrates, to some extent, the root surface and removes, in the form of a chip, root substance with attached calculus. The working stroke is followed by a finishing stroke the objective of which is to produce a smooth root surface (root planing). After the working and finishing strokes have been made, the probe is inserted in the pocket again and the surface characteristics of the root surface reassessed. Working and finishing strokes must be made in different directions to cover all aspects of the selected root surface (crosswise, back and forth) but, as stated above, the strokes should always start from an apical position and be guided in coronal direction.

Instrument sharpening: The hand instruments must have proper cutting edges in order to make subgingival instrumentation a precise and efficient procedure. In order to remove calculus and tooth substance a curette with *a blunt cutting edge* has to be *pressed* against the root surface with a larger force than is required with a sharp instrument. The tactile sensitivity is hereby impaired. Scaling with instruments with blunt cutting edges often results in an incomplete removal of calculus but in the establishment of a "smoothened" root surface. Remaining calculus on such a

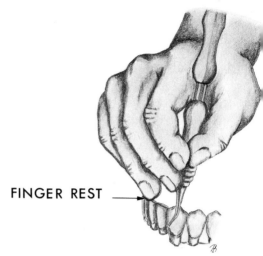

FINGER REST

Fig. 14-24. Schematic illustration demonstrating the proper "third finger rest" using a modified pen grasp in the molar region in the right lower jaw.

"smoothened" root surface is difficult to detect even with a periodontal probe. The cutting edge of the hand instrument, therefore, has to be controlled repeatedly during scaling, by testing it on e.g. a plastic stick (Fig. 14-26). During the course of the scaling session sharpening stones should therefore be frequently used to maintain the cutting edges in proper condition.

The sharpening of hand instruments can be performed by means of either "rotating" (cylindrical or cone shaped) stones or "plain" stones (India or Arkansas stones). Curettes and sickles are sharpened by grinding the lateral surfaces and/or the face of the blade. It is important that the original geometry of the instrument is not changed by the sharpening procedure (Fig. 14-27).

The root surface should not be considered properly treated until the operator, using a periodontal probe, finds the surface " smooth" and "hard". *It is not the intention of this textbook chapter to describe in detail the technique for subgingival instrumentation. Clinical training under careful supervision is the only way by which the proper technique*

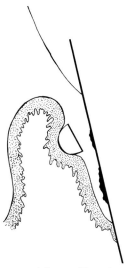

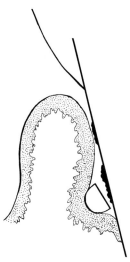

Fig. 14-25a. The curette is inserted into the periodontal pocket. Note the close to zero degree angulation of the face of the curette against the root surface.

Fig. 14-25b. The bottom of the periodontal pocket is identified with the distal edge of the blade of the curette.

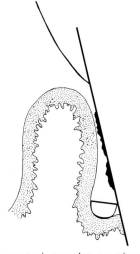

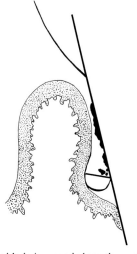

Fig. 14-25c. The curette is turned to a cutting position for scaling.

Fig. 14-25d. The blade is moved along the root surface in a scaling stroke to remove calculus.

for subgingival scaling and root planing can be learned.

2. Ultrasonic instruments

For many years ultrasonic instruments (e.g. Cavitron®, Amdent®, Odontoson®) have been used for removal of plaque, gross deposits of calculus and stains. Scaling with ultrasonic instruments often results in the establishment of an uneven root surface. It

has been suggested, therefore, that ultrasonic scaling should be supplemented by hand instrumentation to establish a smooth root surface (Björn & Lindhe 1962). Recent clinical studies, however, have evaluated the effect of scaling with ultrasonic vs hand instruments (Torafson et. al. 1979, Badersten et al. 1981). They found that debridement of 4-7 mm pockets with ultrasonic instrumentation was equally suc-

345

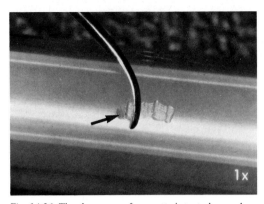

Fig. 14-26. The sharpness of a curette is tested on a plastic stick. A chip (arrow) is easily produced by a sharp instrument.

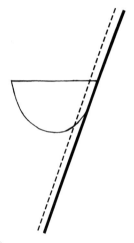

Fig. 14-27. Schematic drawing illustrating the sharpening of a curette. The original geometry of the cutting edge must be maintained during the sharpening procedure.

cessful for healing of diseased periodontal sites as scaling with hand instruments (curettes). It has also been questioned whether indeed *a smooth* root surface after treatment in subgingival areas is important for successful healing (Rosenberg & Ash 1974). Waerhaug (1956) found that a junctional epithelium readapted and formed a normal "epithelial cuff" also on uneven root surfaces. Properly used, ultrasonic instrumentation, therefore must be regarded as a valuable substitute (not only as an adjunct) to conventional scaling with hand instruments.

Instrumentation

The removal of plaque and calculus by ultrasonic instrumentation is accomplished by a) the vibration of the tip of the instrument, b) the spraying and cavitation effect of the fluid coolant. The vibrations (amplitude ranging from 0.006-0.1 mm) are produced by a metal core which can change its dimension in an electromagnetic field with an operating frequency between 25.000 and 42.000 HZ. During the generation of the ultrasonic vibrations heat is produced, which is why the tip always has to be cooled with water or saline during instrumentation.

Prior use the instrument must be adjusted as regards the power (tuning) and waterspray according to the manual (Fig. 14-28). The tip should be applied to the tooth surface with very light pressure and be moved back and forth over the surface in sweeping movements and in such a way that its pattern

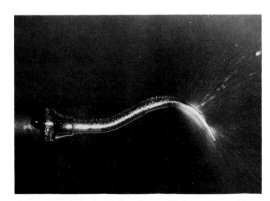

Fig. 14-28. The tip of the ultrasonic instrument. Note the spraying and cavitation of the fluid used for cooling.

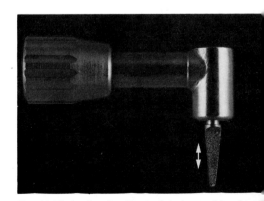

Fig. 14-29. A tringular diamond tip inserted in a hand piece. Arrows indicate the directions of the movement.

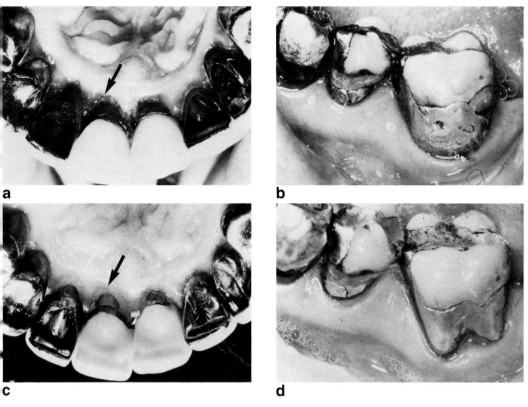

Figs. 14-30 a-d. Amalgam restorations before (a, b) and after (c, d) the adjustment of the overhangs. The buccal restoration in tooth 36 is prepared in order to reduce the degree of furcation involvement. Note the recession of the healed gingiva in (c) and the excellent oral hygiene status.

of vibration is parallel to the tooth surface to prevent damage to the tooth. A periodontal probe should be used to check the root surface characteristics after ultrasonic instrumentation.

3. Rotating instruments
Root furs and furcation areas create certain technical problems for proper debridement using hand instruments and ultrasonic instruments. In these areas rotating instruments like fine grained diamonds may be used. Care should be taken, however, that excessive amount of tooth substance is not removed during this cutting operation.

Removal of plaque retention factors

In an epidemiological study Björn et al. (1969, 1970) observed that ill-fitting artificial crowns and fillings were associated with a reduced height of the periodontal bone level. Jeffcoat & Howell (1980) reported that marginal bone loss was more pronounced around teeth with overhanging amalgam restorations than around teeth without restorations. Rodrigues-Ferrer et al. (1980) concluded that "the presence of a subgingival overhanging defective margin may be the only important clinically significant feature of an amalgam restoration related to the pathogenesis of inflammatory periodontal disease". It is not the overhang of the restoration *per se,* which causes or maintains periodontal disease. Waerhaug (1960) pointed out that the more advanced gingival inflammation, observed in sites with ill-fitting restorations, was the result of extensive plaque accumulation and not of mechanical irritation by the filling material. Thus, overhangs of restorations must be removed to (1) facilitate the removal of plaque and calculus and (2) to establish an anatomy of the restoration which facilitates self performed tooth cleaning.

Overhanging margins of dental restorations can be removed using a flame shaped diamond stone mounted on a handpiece for rotatory movements or a flat diamond stone mounted on a handpiece for horizontal reciprocal movements (Eva-system®, Fig. 14-29). The overhang should be removed and the restoration should be given a proper form and surface. The instrumentation should always be completed by the use of flame shaped finir burs and a polishing paste (grain size 40-2 μm). After polishing, fluorides should be applied (in solutions or in a varnish) in order to reinstitute the fluoride concentration of the adjacent tooth surface.

The adjustment of an improperly designed filling or artificial crown is often a difficult and time consuming procedure. It is often more convenient to remove the improper filling (crown) and insert a new one with a proper marginal fit. Fig. 14-30 illustrates the effect on the periodontal tissues of the adjustment of amalgam overhangs.

Evaluation of the effect of cause related therapy

Since cause related therapeutic measures constitute the most significant part of the overall treatment of periodontal disease, the meticulous assessment of the result obtained by these measures is of utmost importance. Hence, the clinical examination performed towards the end of this phase of treatment

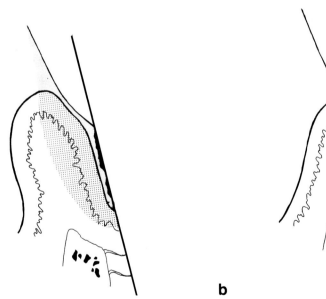

a   b

Figs. 14-31 a-b. Schematic drawing of a gingival unit before (a) and after (b) cause related therapy. Clinical signs such as reduced plaque and gingivitis scores and reduced probing depth values as a result of recession indicate healing after the cause related therapy. Remaining plaque and calculus in the apical part of the root surface of the pocket area (b) may, however, maintain the inflammatory lesion (shadowed area) in the apical part of the pocket. Probing to the bottom of the pocket will result in bleeding.

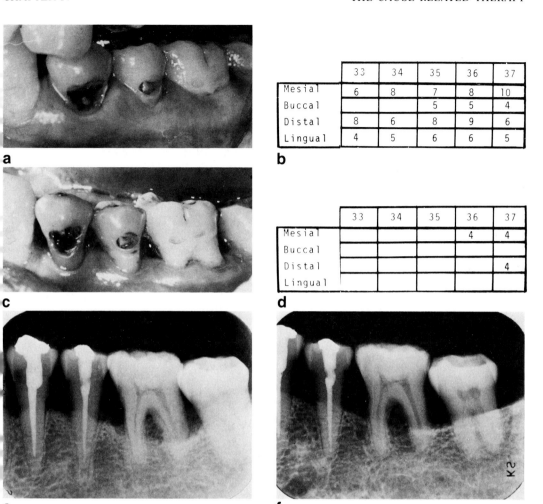

	33	34	35	36	37
Mesial	6	8	7	8	10
Buccal			5	5	4
Distal	8	6	8	9	6
Lingual	4	5	6	6	5

	33	34	35	36	37
Mesial				4	4
Buccal					
Distal					4
Lingual					

Figs. 14-32 a-f. Photographs illustrating the buccal surfaces of premolars and molars before (a) and 1 year after cause related periodontal therapy (c). Note the recession of the gingival margin following therapy. The reduction of probing depths and absence of bleeding on probing from the bottom of the pockets after treatment (b, d) indicate resolution of gingivitis. A comparison between the radiographs obtained before (e) and after (f) scaling and root planing demonstrates that treatment has also changed the outline of the alveolar bone crest.

must include assessments of the effect of the professional procedures as well as of the patient's home-care standard. The result of the therapeutic measures should be described in terms of (1) degree of resolution of gingival inflammation, (2) degree of reduction of probing depth and alterations of clinical attachment levels and (3) improvement of tooth mobility and (4) improvement of the self performed oral hygiene.

The observations made at this reexamination form the basis for the selection of therapeutic measures which should be included in the definitive, corrective phase of treatment. It is usually possible, with the data obtained from this examination, to classify the patient into one of the following categories:

1. The data from the reexamination may describe a patient who has a proper standard of oral hygiene, but in whom a number of

gingival sites still bleed on probing and in whom a significant reduction of the probing depths at these sites has not been achieved. In such a patient the phase of definitive treatment should include periodontal surgery in order to gain access to those root surfaces on which subgingival scaling and root planing have evidently failed to remove plaque and calculus (Fig. 14-31).

2. The reexamination may describe a patient with a proper oral hygiene standard, no gingival inflammation (no bleeding on probing), in whom the probing depths have been markedly reduced and the clinical attachment levels improved. In such a patient, no further periodontal treatment may be indicated even if, in some areas, deepened pockets may persist (Fig. 14-32).

3. The reexamination may recognize a patient, who despite repeated instructions in tooth cleaning measures during the course of initial therapy, has a poor standard of oral hygiene. This patient evidently lacks motivation or ability to exercise proper home-care and should not be regarded as a candidate for periodontal surgery. This does not preclude, however, restorative treatment measures on aesthetic and functional indications, but the patient should be made aware of the fact that even though the professional scaling and root planing may have been performed to perfection, reinfection of the periodontal pockets may sooner or later result in recurrence of destructive periodontal disease.

References

Addy, M. & Dolby, A. E. (1976) The use of chlorhexidine mouthwash compared with a periodontal dressing following gingivectomy procedures. *Journal of Clinical Periodontology* **3**, 59-65.

Arnim, S. S. (1963) The use of disclosing agents for measuring tooth cleanliness. *Journal of Periodontology* **34**, 227-245.

Asboe-Jörgensen, V., Attström, R., Lang, N. P. & Löe, H. (1974) Effect of a chlorhexidine dressing on the healing after periodontal surgery. *Journal of Periodontology* **45**, 13-17.

Badersten, A., Nilvéus, R. & Egelberg, J. (1981) Effect of non-surgical periodontal therapy. I. Moderately advanced periodontitis. *Journal of Clinical Periodontology* **8**, 57-72.

Bass, C. C. (1954) An effective method of personal oral hygiene. *Journal of Louisiana Medical Society* **106**, 100-112.

Bergenholtz, A., Lignell, L. & Öberg, G. (1971) Quantitative evaluation of the plaque-removing ability of four commercial dentifrices. Personal communication.

Björn, A.-L., Björn, H. & Grkovic, B. (1969) Marginal fit of restorations and its relation to periodontal bone level. I. Metal fillings. *Odontologisk Revy* **20**, 311-322.

Björn, A-L., Björn, H. & Grkovic, B. (1970) Marginal fit of restorations and its relation to periodontal bone level. II. Crowns. *Odontologisk Revy* **21**, 337-346.

Björn, H. & Lindhe, J. (1962) The influence of periodontal instruments on the tooth surface. A methodological study. *Odontologisk Revy* **13**, 355-369.

Charters, W. J. (1948) Proper home care of the mouth. *Journal of Periodontology* **19**, 136-139.

Davies, R. M. (1977) Use of Hibitane following periodontal surgery. *Journal of Clinical Periodontology* **4**, 129-135.

Dossenbach, W. F. & Mühlemann, H. R. (1961) Effect of penicillin and ricinoleate on early calculus formation. *Helvetica Odontologica Acta* **5**, 25-28.

Eriksen, H. M. & Gjermo, P. (1973) Incidence of stained tooth surfaces in students using chlorhexidine-containing dentifrices. *Scandinavian Journal of Dental Research* **81**, 533-537.

Flötra, L., Gjermo, P., Rölla, G. & Waerhaug, J. (1972) A 4-month study on the effect of chlorhexidine mouth-washes on 50 soldiers. *Scandinavian Journal of Dental Research* **80**, 10-17.

Gjermo, P., Baastad, K. L. & Rölla, G. (1970) The plaque-inhibiting capacity of 11 antibacterial compounds. *Journal of Periodontal Research* **5**, 102-109.

Gjermo, P. & Flötra, L. (1970) The effect of different methods of interdental claeaning. *Journal of Periodontal Research* **5**, 230-236.

Hamp, S.-E., Rosling, B. & Lindhe, J. (1975) Effect of chlorhexidine on gingival wound healing in the dog. A histometric study. *Journal of Clinical Periodontology* **2**, 143-152.

Hanke, M. T. (1940) Studies on the local factors in dental caries. I. Destruction of plaques and retardation of bacterial growth in the oral cavity. *J. Am. Dent. Ass.* **27**, 1379-1393.

Hartzell, T. B. (1932) Prophylaxis and pyorrhea. *Journal of the American Dental Association* **19**, 260-263.

Hirst, R. (1972) Chlorhexidine: A review of the literature. *Periodontal Abstracts* **20**, 52-58.

Hugoson, A. (1978) Effect of the Water Pik® device on plaque accumulation and development of gingivitis. *Journal of Clinical Periodontology* **5**, 95-104.

Jeffcoat, M. K. & Howell, T. H. (1980) Alveolar bone destruction due to overhanging amalgam in periodontal disease. *Journal of Periodontology* **51**, 599-602.

Keller, S. E. & Manson-Hing, L. R. (1969) Clearance studies of proximal tooth surfaces. III and IV. *In vivo* removal of interproximal plaque. *Alabama Journal of Medical Science* **6**, 399-405.

Lang, N. P. & Räber, K. (1981) Use of oral irrigators as vehicle for the application of antimicrobial agents in chemical plaque control. *Journal of Clinical Periodontology* **8**, 177-188.

Lindhe, J. (1964) Orthogonal cutting of dentine. *Odontologisk Revy* **15**, Supplement 8.

Lindhe, J. (1982) Treatment of localized juvenile periodontitis. In *Host-Parasite Interactions in Periodontal Diseases*, ed. Genco, R.J. & Mergenhagen, S.E., pp. 382-394. Washington, D.C.: American Society for Microbiology.

Lindhe, J. & Nyman, S. (1975) The effect of plaque control and surgical pocket elimination on the establishment and maintenance of periodontal health. A longitudinal study of periodontal therapy in cases of advanced disease. *Journal of Clinical Periodontology* **2**, 67-79.

Lindhe, J., Westfelt, E., Nyman, S., Socransky, S. S., Heijl. L. & Bratthall, G. (1982) Healing following surgical/non-surgical treatment of periodontal disease. *Journal of Clinical Periodontology* **9**, 115-128.

Listgarten, M. A., Lindhe, J. & Helldén, L. (1978) Effect of tetracycline and/or scaling in human periodontal disease. *Journal of Clinical Periodontology* **5**, 246-271.

Löe, H. (1969) Present day status and direction for future research on the etiology and prevention of periodontal disease. *Journal of Periodontology* **40**, 678-682.

Löe, H., von der Fehr, F.R. & Rindom-Schiött, C. (1970) Inhibition of experimental caries by plaque prevention. The effect of chlorhexidine mouthrinses. *Scandinavian Journal of Dental Research* **80**, 1-9.

Löe, H. & Rindom-Schiött, C. (1970) The effect of mouthrinses and topical application of chlorhexidine on the development of dental plaque and gingivitis in man. *Journal of Periodontal Research* **5**, 79-83.

Lövdal, A., Arnö, A. & Waerhaug, J. (1958) Incidence of clinical manifestations of periodontal disease in light of oral hygiene and calculus formation. *Journal of the American Dental Association* **56**, 21-23.

Matsuzaki, A., Sugano, K., Tachibana, T., Katano, Y. & Nahamura, J. (1974) The effects of toothbrushing and water-jetting on oral hygiene. *Japanese Journal of Conservative Dentistry* **17**, 150-153.

Miller, W. D. (1890) *The Micro-organisms of Human Teeth*. Philadelphia: S. S. White Dental Mfg. Co.

Miller, W. D. (1896) *Lehrbuch der Konservierenden Zahnheilkunde*. Leipzig: George Thieme.

O'Leary, T. J. (1970) Oral hygiene agents and procedures. *Journal of Periodontology* **41**, 625-629.

Rindom-Schiött, C., Löe, H., Jensen, S. B., Kilian, M., Davies, R. M. & Glavind, K. (1970) The effect of chlorhexidine mouthrinses on the human oral flora. *Journal of Periodontal Research* **5**, 84-89.

Rodrigues-Ferrer, H. J., Strahan, J. D. & Newman, H. N (1980) Effect on gingival health of removing overhanging margins of interproximal subgingival amalgam restorations. *Journal of Clinical Periodontology* **7**, 457-462.

Rosenberg, R. M. & Ash Jr., N. N. (1974) The effect of root roughness on plaque accumulation and gingival inflammation. *Journal of Periodontology* **45**, 146-150.

Rosling, B., Nyman, S. & Lindhe, J. (1976) The effect of systematic plaque control on bone regeneration in infrabony pockets. *Journal of Clinical Periodontology* **3**, 38-53.

Schroeder, H. E. (1969) *Formation and Inhibition of Dental Calculus*, p. 145. Berne-Stuttgart-Vienna: Hans Huber Publishers.

Strålfors, A. (1961) Disinfection of dental plaques in man. In *Caries Sympposium*, Zürich. Proc. Int. Symp. Nov. 2 and 3, ed. Mühlemann, H. R. & König, G., pp 154-161. Berne: Hans Huber Publishers.

Ten, A. (1981) Disclosing agents in plaque control. *Journal of Western Society of Periodontology*, Periodontal abstracts **29**, 81-86.

Thoma, K. H. & Goldman, H. M. (1960) *Oral Pathology*. 5th ed., p. 20g. St. Louis: C. V. Mosby Co.

Torafson, T., Kiger, R., Selvig, K. A. & Egelberg, J. (1979) Clinical improvement of gingival conditions following ultrasonic versus han instrumentation of periodontal pockets. *Journal of Clinical Periodontology* **6**, 165-176.

Waerhaug, J. (1956) Effect of rough surface upon gingival tissue. *Journal of Dental Research* **35**, 323-325.

Waerhaug, J (1959) Periodontittprofylaxe. I *Nordisk Klinisk Odontologi*, Ch. 14/11:1 Copenhagen: A/S Forlaget for Faglitteratur.

Waerhaug, J. (1960) Histologic consideration which govern where the margin of restoration should be located in relation to the gingiva. *Dental Clinics of North America* 167-176.

Waerhaug, J. (1981) Healing of the dento-epithelial junction following the use of dental floss. *Journal of Clinical Periodontology* **8**, 144-150.

Westfelt, E., Nyman, S., Lindhe, J. & Socransky, S. (1982) Use of chlorhexidine as a plaque control measure following surgical treatment of periodontal disease. *Journal of Clinical Periodontology* **10**, 22-36.

Periodontal Surgery: Objectives & Indications

for the various surgical techniques. Even if some uncertainty still persists concerning general indications for surgical treatment as well as special merits offered by various techniques there are, however, straightforward and detailed objectives described for the various surgical methods used in periodontal therapy.

Since most forms of periodontal disease are plaque associated disorders it is obvious that surgical treatment can only be considered as an adjunct to cause related therapy. Therefore the various surgical methods should be evaluated on the basis of their potential to contribute to plaque control and thereby to the long-term preservation of the periodontium.

Introduction

In this chapter the term "periodontal surgery" will be used to describe surgical manipulations of periodontal soft tissues and bone. Although scaling and root planing are considered by many authors as surgical procedures, this type of root instrumentation will not be discussed here.

Over the years a number of different surgical techniques have been described and used in periodontal therapy. A superficial review of the literature in this area may give the reader a somewhat confusing apprehension of the specific objectives and indications

Objectives of periodontal surgery

Historically, periodontal surgery has been performed for a number of reasons. In the early days, curing of periodontitis was attempted by excising diseased gingival tissue and removing "necrotic" bone. When it became clear that periodontal disease did not result in necrosis of the alveolar bone and that gingival inflammation represented a defense reaction rather than the disease itself, this rationale was abandoned.

Pocket elimination then became the main objective of periodontal therapy. The removal of the pocket by a gingivectomy incision became the dominating aim of a surgical procedure which served two purposes: (1) the pocket which was considered a crucial element in the sequence of events leading to progression of periodontal disease was eliminated, and (2) the root surface was made accessible for scaling and self performed tooth cleaning.

While these objectives cannot be entirely discarded today, the necessity for pocket elimination in periodontal therapy has been challenged. During recent years our understanding of the biology of the periodontal tissues, the pathogenesis of periodontal disease, and the healing capacity of the periodontium has markedly increased. New information has thus formed the basis of a more broadly differentiated appraisal of the part played by periodontal surgery in the preservation of teeth.

Traditionally, *increased pocket depth* has been the main criterion in determining whether periodontal surgery should be performed. However, pocket depth is no longer as unequivocal a concept as it used to be. The *probing depth,* i.e. the distance from the gingival margin to the point where the periodontal probe is stopped by tissue resistance, may only rarely correspond to pocket depth. It has been demonstrated that heavily inflamed gingival tissue allows the probe to penetrate apically to the termination of the pocket epithelium whereas the probe may not reach this area when the gingiva is healthy. This is a fact which speaks in favor of the recommendation that the pocket depth value used as an indicator for surgical treatment should be the value obtained at the end of cause related therapy, i.e. after the resolution of gingival inflammation.

It must be understood, however, that regardless of the accuracy with which pockets can be measured, there is no established correlation between pocket depth and the presence or absence of active disease. This means that symptoms other than increased probing depth should be present to justify surgery. These include clinical signs of inflammation, especially exudation and bleeding on probing (to the bottom of the pockets), as well as improper gingival morphology. Finally, the fact that proper plaque control maintained by the patient is a decisive factor for a good prognosis, must be considered prior to the initiation of surgery.

In conclusion, the main objective of periodontal surgery is to contribute to the preservation of the periodontium by facilitating plaque removal and plaque control, and periodontal surgery can serve this purpose by:

1. securing that professional scaling and root planing is performed effectively
2. establishing gingival contours that are optimal for the patient's self-performed plaque control

In addition to this, periodontal surgery may aim at the

3. regeneration of periodontal attachment lost due to destructive disease.

Create access for scaling and root planing

The complete removal of soft and hard deposits from the root surfaces is necessary for the successful treatment of periodontal disease. The depth of a pocket markedly influences the effectiveness with which professional debridement and root planing can be performed, but no definite mm limit for successful subgingival debridement has yet been established. Suggestions as to pocket depths which can be cleaned properly, range from 3-5 mm, but factors other than the pocket depth *per se* should also be considered. These include root fissures and concavities and root furcations (Fig. 15-1). The presence of such conditions may jeopardize the debridement of even shallow pockets.

It should be emphasized that subgingival scaling and root planing are difficult procedures to master and the possibility of achieving proper results by a "blind" approach should not be overestimated. A frequent cause of treatment failure, manifested in persisting inflammation and progression of attachment loss, is the insufficient removal of plaque and calculus from the subgingival root surfaces.

In cases where it is unlikely that scaling and root planing alone will result in complete subgingival debridement, the root surfaces *should be exposed* by surgical means to obtain full accessibility.

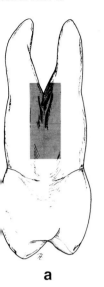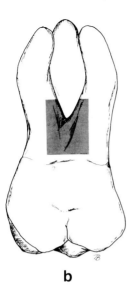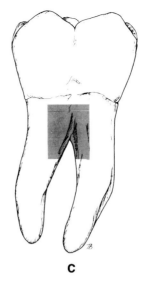

a   b   c

Figs. 15-1a-c. Examples of root surfaces (shaded areas) where morphologic conditions impede debridement. (a) Proximal surface on upper first premolar. (b). Facial surface on upper first molar. (c) Lingual surface on lower first molar. These conditions may be associated with comparatively shallow pockets.

Facilitate the patient's self performed plaque control

Since supragingival plaque may be reestablished soon after thorough tooth cleaning and since plaque may cause inflammatory changes in the gingiva already a few days after its formation, the patient's daily home-care efforts are of utmost importance for the maintenance of periodontal health after treatment. Most patients consider effective plaque control a difficult task. Therefore this effort should be facilitated by establishing optimal conditions for self performed tooth cleaning. These include absence of gingival contours which impede plaque removal by home-care techniques. While it is established that deviations from "physiological" gingival contours *per se* do not cause periodontal disease, it is also known that major aberrations such as gingival hyperplasia, and gingival craters, and recessions may promote plaque retention. (Fig. 15-2). These aberrations can be corrected by surgical means.

Facilitate regeneration of periodontal tissues

Ideally, the treatment of destructive periodontal disease would aim at the regeneration of the lost attachment tissues (principal fibers, alveolar bone and root cementum). Surgical procedures which claim to achieve such regeneration have been described as *new attachment* or *re-attachment operations*. Recent research, however, has questioned whether such operations may in fact lead to the establishment of a new periodontal ligament in root areas previously exposed to periodontal pockets. It appears that healing by a long epithelial attachment is a more likely outcome. New attachment procedures in periodontal therapy are discussed in Chapter 19.

The fact that periodontal therapy often fails to promote true regeneration of supporting tissues, destroyed by periodontal disease, implies that the major objectives of periodontal therapy are (1) to obtain access for proper debridement and (2) to establish a gingival morphology which facilitates home-care.

355

General guidelines for periodontal surgery

The overall treatment of periodontal disease may be divided into different phases (see Chapter 13):

. Examination; including medical and dental history, *temporary treatment planning*, and treatment of acute conditions when indicated

. Cause related phase; comprising removal of tooth deposits, and establishing of proper home-care techniques. Tooth extractions, placement of temporary fillings and prostheses, endodontic treatment (when indicated)

. Evaluation of patient cooperation and tissue response; The time lapse between termination of the cause related phase of therapy and this evaluation is usually from 1-6 months

. Definitive treatment phase;
Periodontal surgery
Restorative/functional treatment

. Maintenance phase.

In accordance with this sequence, the final decision concerning type and extent of periodontal surgery to be performed should be made after the effect of cause related therapy has been evaluated. This practice has the following advantages:

1. the removal of calculus and bacterial plaque has eliminated or markedly reduced the gingival inflammation (edema hyperemia, flabby tissue consistency) thereby making assessment of the "true" gingival contours and pocket depth possible

2. the resolution of gingival inflammation has made the tissue firmer which facilitates surgical treatment. The propensity for bleeding is reduced making inspection of the field of operation easier

3. a better basis for the prognosis has been established. The tissue reaction to scaling and home-care efforts gives information on the patient's "resistance". The effectiveness of the patient's home-care is of decisive importance for the long-term prognosis. Lack of effective home-care will often mean that the patient should be excluded from surgical treatment.

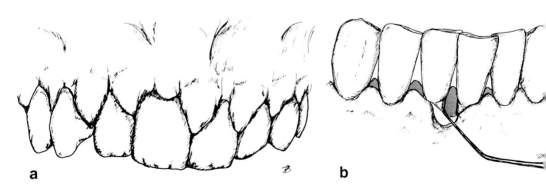

Figs. 15-2 a, b. Examples of gingival aberrations which favor plaque retention and thereby impede the patient' plaque control. (a) Gingival hyperplasia. (b) Gingival craters.

Indications for surgical treatment

Improper access for scaling and root planing

As discussed above, scaling and root planing are methods of therapy which are difficult to master. The difficulties in accomplishing proper debridement increase proportionately to (1) increasing depth of the periodontal pockets, (2) increasing width of the tooth surfaces, (3) the presence of root fissures, root concavities, furcations, and defective margins of dental restorations in the subgingival area.

Provided a correct technique and suitable instruments are used (Chapter 14), it is usually possible to properly debride pockets up to 5 mm of depth. However, this mm limit cannot be considered a universal rule of thumb. Reduced accessibility and the presence of the above mentioned impeding conditions may prevent proper debridement of shallow pockets whereas in sites with good accessibility and favorable root morphology proper debridement can be accomplished even in deeper pockets.

It is often difficult to ascertain by clinical means whether subgingival instrumentation has been properly performed. Following scaling, the root surfaces should be smooth and hard – roughness will often indicate the presence of remaining subgingival calculus. It is also important to monitor carefully the gingival reaction to sub-gingival debridement. If inflammation persists or if bleeding is elicited by gentle probing in the subgingival area, the presence of subgingival deposits should be suspected. If such symptoms are not resolved by repeated subgingival instrumentation, then surgical treatment should be performed to expose the root surfaces for proper cleaning.

Impaired access for self performed plaque control

The level of plaque control which can be maintained by patients is determined not only by the patient's interest and dexterity but also, to some extent, by the morphology of the dentogingival area.

The patient's responsibility in a plaque control program must obviously include the cleansing of the supragingival tooth surfaces and the marginal part of the gingival sulcus which can be reached by toothbrush, toothpick or other devices. This means that the tooth area coronal to the gingival margin and at the entrance of the gingival sulcus should be the target for the patient's home-care efforts.

Pronounced gingival hyperplasia and gingival craters are examples of morphology aberrations which may impede proper home-care. Likewise, the presence of restorations with defective marginal fit or adverse contour and surface characteristics at the gingival margin may seriously compromise plaque removal.

By the professional treatment of periodontal disease, the dentist prepares the dentition for the patient in such a way that home-care can be effectively managed. After treatment the following objectives should have been met:

. no sub- or supragingival dental deposits
. no pathological pockets (no bleeding on probing to the bottom of the pockets)
. no plaque retaining aberrations of gingival morphology
. no plaque retaining parts of restorations in relation to the gingival margin
. a relationship of the gingival margin to root concavities and entrances to furcations, which makes plaque removal possible

These requirements lead to the following indications for periodontal surgery:

. accessibility for proper scaling and root planing
. pocket depth reduction
. correction of gross gingival aberrations
. shift of the gingival margin to a position apically to plaque retaining restorations
. establishment of a morphology of the gingival margin conducive to plaque control, also in furcations

357

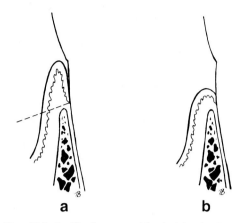

Figs. 15-3a,b. Gingivectomy. The incision is directed towards the bottom of the pocket (a) and the part of the gingiva enclosing the pocket is removed. Healing takes place from the level of incision (b).

elimination or recontouring of furcation involvements by root resection.

Indications for various surgical techniques

Attempts have been made to classify different surgical modalities used in the treatment of periodontal disease. Distinctions between methods involving the marginal tissues and those involving the mucogingival area have been made, and, further between tissue eliminating/resective varieties and tissue preserving/reconstructive types. Such classifications appear less meaningful since several techniques are often combined in the treatment of individual cases, and since there is no clear-cut relationship between disease characteristics and selection of surgical methods.

In the following, the general *indications* for the various surgical methods will be presented. The techniques are outlined in Chapter 17.

Gingivectomy

The obvious indication of gingivectomy is the presence of deep supraalveolar pockets

(Fig. 15-3). In addition, the gingivectomy technique can be used to reshape abnormal gingival contours such as gingival craters and gingival hyperplasias (Fig. 15-4). In such cases the technique is often termed *gingivoplasty*. Gingivectomy is not considered suitable in situations where the incision will lead to the removal of the attached gingiva. This is the case when the bottom of the pocket to be excised is located at, or below, the mucogingival junction. Furthermore, since the gingivectomy procedure is aimed at the complete elimination of the periodontal pocket this procedure can not be used in periodontal sites when infra-bony lesions or bony craters are present.

These limitations, combined with the development in recent years of surgical methods which have a broader field of application, provide better healing conditions and make the postoperative period less unpleasant to the patients, have led to less frequent use of gingivectomy.

Gingivectomy is, however, the treatment of choice in situations where measures are needed to (1) recontour the gingiva so that the margins of subgingival restorations become supragingivally located and (2) recontour the gingiva to facilitate restorative therapy.

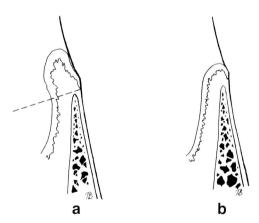

Figs. 15-4a,b. Elimination of gingival hyperplasia. The bottom of the pocket is at the cementoenamel junction and the gingival margin has shifted coronally (pseudopocket, coronal pocket). The principles of incision (a) and healing (b) are identical to those of gingivectomy.

CHAPTER 15

Curettage

Curettage, which was formerly used extensively, is defined as the removal, by means of a curette, of the inner surface of the soft tissue wall of the pocket. The rationale behind this includes that:
. the removal of pocket epithelium and inflamed connective tissue results in new attachment of connective tissue and/or epithelium to the tooth surface (see Chapter 19)
. tissue shrinkage following curettage (Fig. 15-7) contributes to pocket reduction.

The reasons why curettage is no longer frequently used are:
. the procedure is technically difficult to master and, in addition, time consuming
. the results of healing are similar after curettage and flap surgery
.. the complete removal of subgingival deposits by scaling and root planing results in optimal healing without curettage
. if removal of pocket epithelium and adjacent connective tissue is attempted, more effective methods are available (reverse bevel incision).

Flap operations

The advantages of flap operations include that:
. by the use of a reverse bevel incision (Fig. 15-8) existing attached gingiva is preserved
. the root surfaces are exposed, whereby scaling and root planing can be carried out effectively
. the marginal alveolar bone will be exposed whereby the morphology of bony defects can be identified and the proper treatment secured
. furcation areas will be exposed, the degree of involvement and the "tooth-bone" relationship can be identified
. the flap can be repositioned at its original level or shifted apically, thereby making it possible to adjust the gingival margin to the local conditions
. the flap procedure preserves the oral epithelium and often makes the use of surgical dressings superfluous
.. the postoperative period is usually less unpleasant to the patient when compared to gingivectomy.

Flap operations can be used in all cases where surgical treatment of periodontal dis-

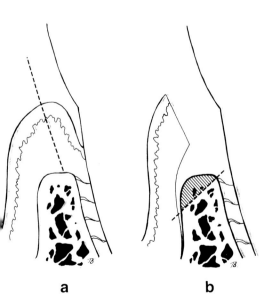

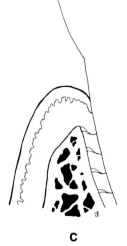

Figs. 15-5a-c. Osteoplasty used for the recontouring of bony ledge. (a) Reverse bevel incision. (b) Deflection of a mucoperiosteal flap and removal of excess bone which does not support principal fibers. (c) Healing with tight flap adaptation and appropriate gingival contour.

a   b   c

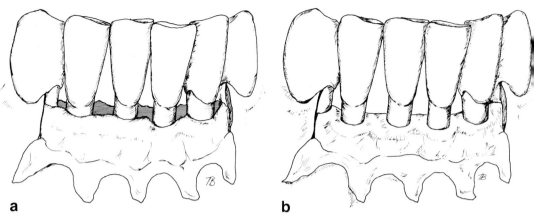

a　　　　　　　　　　　　　　　　　　　　　　**b**

Fig. 15-6a,b. Osteoplasty in connection with interdental bony craters. (a) Craters enclosed by uneven facial and lingual bone edges. (b) Recontouring ensures tight flap adaptation and promotes optimal healing.

ease is indicated. Flap procedures are *particularly* useful where pockets extend beyond the mucogingival border and/or where treatment of bony lesions and furcation involvements is needed.

Osseous surgery

The removal of alveolar bone in surgical procedures may involve 2 different types of bone structures: bone in which principal periodontal fibers insert, and bone without such fibers. The removal of the first type of bone structure has been termed *ostectomy,* and of the second type *osteoplasty.*

Ostectomy and osteoplasty have previously been used on the assumption that recontouring of alveolar bone to conform to "physiologic" form would improve the prognosis of the overall treatment. Results from longitudinal clinical studies have failed to confirm this assumption. As a general rule, therefore, care must be exercised when supporting bone, i.e. bone directly involved in the attachment of the tooth, is to be removed (*ostectomy*).

Osteoplasty may be used in cases where bony ledges or edges prevent close adaptation of the flaps after surgery. Often in cases of advanced periodontal disease bone ledges are present on the buccal and lingual aspects of the alveolar bone margin in the molar and premolar regions of the dentition. When flap operations are indicated in such areas for other reasons, such ledges should be recontoured (Fig. 15-5). A similar procedure is recommended in the treatment of buccal furcation involvements.

Bony craters are to a large extent surrounded by bone tissue not involved in tooth attachment. The facial and lingual edges of such craters may be recontoured to allow for close interdental adaptation of the flaps (Fig. 15-6.).

Mucogingival surgery

The presence of a zone of attached gingiva has been considered a part of the defense mechanisms of the periodontal tissues. Periodontal disease or a traumatic tooth brushing technique may result in loss of the zone of attached gingiva (gingival recession; Fig. 15-9). As a consequence, the gingival margin may be located at or near the bottom of the vestibular fornix which may jeopardize proper tooth cleaning by the patient.

There are descriptions of surgical techniques which aim at the reestablishment or widening of the zone of attached gingiva

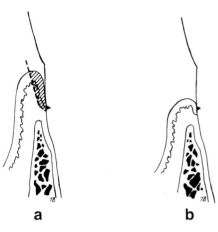

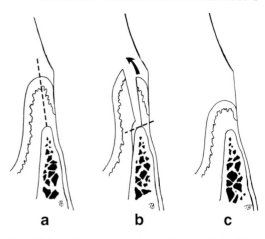

Figs. 15-7.a,b. Gingival curettage. (a) The shaded area comprising pocket epithelium and adjacent connective tissue is removed by a curette. (b) Healing with pocket reduction.

Fig. 15-8a-c. Reverse bevel technique. (a). Incision from the gingival margin to the crest of the alveolar bone. (b) Deflection of the flap and removal of the soft tissue wall of the pocket after its release from the periodontal ligament. (c) Healing.

such as *gingival transplantation, deepening of the vestibular fold, frenectomy* (see Chapter 18), but the indications for these procedures have undergone revision in recent years. It has been established that the absence of attached gingiva can be compatible with periodontal health, and thus, the mere existence of this condition does not constitute an indication for surgical intervention. Rather, the need for treatment should be evaluated individually. The persistence of inflammation in areas without attached gingiva following cause related therapy and in patients who otherwise practice effective home-care, could justify surgical correction of the condition.

Conclusions

The objectives of surgical treatment of periodontal disease are to support the causative therapy by: (1) making subgingival root surfaces accessible for thorough scaling and root planing; (2) establishing gingival contours which facilitate the patient's home-care; (3) providing conditions for healing of periodontal lesions which preserve the maximum of supporting tissue.

Whether surgical treatment should be performed at all, and if so, what kind of technique should be used, is usually decided after the results of cause related therapy have been evaluated with regard to tissue response and patient cooperation. As a general rule surgical modalities of therapy which preserve or induce the formation of periodontal tissue should be preferred to those which resect or eliminate tissue.

As stated previously, postoperative plaque control is the most important variable in determining the net result of

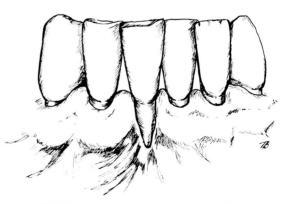

Fig. 15-9. Recession of the gingiva. Absence of the zone of attached gingiva means that the facial-gingival margin is comprised of movable alveolar mucosa.

361

periodontal surgery. Provided proper post-operative plaque control levels are established, most surgical treatment techniques will result in conditions which favor the long-term maintenance of the periodontium. If post-operative hygiene fails, progressive loss of supporting tissue will take place regardless of the surgical technique used.

Contraindications for periodontal surgery

Patient cooperation

Since optimal postoperative plaque control is decisive for the success of periodontal treatment, a patient who fails to cooperate during cause related therapy should not be exposed to surgical treatment.

Even though short-term postoperative plaque control entails frequent professional treatments, the long-term responsibility for maintaining good oral hygiene must rest with the patient. Theoretically, even the poorest oral hygiene performance by a patient may be compensated for by frequent dental visits (e.g. once a week), but it is unrealistic to imagine larger groups of patients handled in this manner. A typical recall schedule for periodontal patients involves 3-monthly professional consultations. Patients who cannot maintain satisfactory oral hygiene over this period should normally be considered unsuited for periodontal surgery.

Cardiovascular disease

Arterial hypertension does not normally preclude periodontal surgery. The patient's medical history should be checked for previous untoward reactions to local anesthesia. Local anesthetics, free from or low in adrenaline should be used, and an aspirating syringe should be adopted to safeguard against intravascular injection.

Angina pectoris does not normally preclude periodontal surgery. The medicines used

and the number of episodes of angina may indicate the severity of the disease. Pre medication with sedatives, and local anesthetics low in adrenaline are often recommended. Safeguards should be adopted against intravascular injection.

Heart infarction-patients should not be subjected to periodontal surgery in the month immediately following hospitalization, and thereafter only on strong indications and in cooperation with the physician in charge.

Anticoagulant treatment implies increased propensity for bleeding. Periodontal surgery should be scheduled after consultation with the physician. Salicylates should not be used for postoperative pain control since they increase bleeding tendency.

Rheumatic endocarditis, congenital heart lesions, heart and vascular implants involve risks for transmission of bacteria to heart tissues and heart implants during the transient bacteremia which follows manipulation of infected periodontal pockets. Treatment of patients with these conditions should be preceded by antiseptic mouthrinsing (0.2% chlorhexidine) and an appropriate antibiotic should be prescribed, starting a few hours before the operation.

Blood disorders

If the medical history includes blood disorders, their exact nature should be disclosed.

Patients suffering from acute leukemias, agranulocytosis and lymphogranulomatosis must *not* be subjected to periodontal surgery.

Anemias in mild and compensated forms do not preclude surgical treatment. More severe and less compensated forms may entail lowered resistance to infection and increased propensity for bleeding. In such cases periodontal surgery should only be performed after consultation with the patient's physician.

Hormonal disorders

Diabetes mellitus entails lowered resistance to infection, propensity for delayed wound healing and predisposition to arteriosclerosis. Well compensated patients may be subjected to periodontal surgery provided precautions are taken not to disturb dietary and insulin routines.

Adrenal function may be impeded in patients receiving large doses of corticosteroids over an extended period. These conditions involve reduced resistance to physical and mental stress, and doses of corticosteroid may have to be altered during the period of periodontal surgery. The patient's physician should be consulted.

Neurological disorders

Epilepsy is often treated with *phenytoin* which, in approximately 50% of the cases, may mediate the formation of gingival hyperplasia. These patients may without special restrictions be subjected to periodontal surgery for correction of the hyperplasia. There is, however, a strong propensity for recurrence of the hyperplasia, which in many cases can be counteracted by intensifying the plaque control.

Multiple sclerosis and Parkinson's disease may in severe cases make ambulatory periodontal surgery impossible. Paresis, impaired muscular function, tremor, and uncontrollable reflexes may necessitate treatment under general anesthesia.

References

Reviews of periodontal surgical procedures:

Barrington, E. P. (1981) An overview of periodontal surgical procedures. *Journal of Periodontology* **52**, 518-528.

Robinson, P. J. (1977) Evaluation of therapy – Advances in periodontal therapy 1966-1977. In *International Conference on Research in the Biology of Periodontal Disease*, ed. Klavan, B., pp. 378-427. Chicago.

The efficacy of periodontal surgical procedures (1980) Session II. In *Efficacy of Treatment Procedures in Periodontics*, ed. Shanley, D. B., pp. 83-151. Quintessence Publishing Co.

Periodontal probing and assessment of disease activity:

Caton, J., Greenstein, G. & Polson, A. M. (1981) Depth of periodontal probe penetration related to clinical and histologic signs of gingival inflammation. *Journal of Periodontology* **52**, 626-629.

Hancock, E. B. (1981) Determination of periodontal disease activity. *Journal of Periodontology* **52**, 492-499.

Listgarten, M. A. (1980) Periodontal probing: What does it mean? *Journal of Clinical Periodontology* **7**, 165-176.

Effectiveness of calculus removal:

Rabbani, G. M., Ash, M. M. & Caffesse, R. G. (1981) The effectiveness of subgingival scaling and root planing in calculus removal. *Journal of Periodontology* **52**, 119-123.

Evaluation of different surgical techniques:

Caffesse, R. G. (1980) Longitudinal evaluation of periodontal surgery. *Dental Clinics of North America* **24**, 751-766.

Dorfman, H. S., Kennedy, J. E. & Bird, W. C. (1980) Longitudinal evaluation of free autogenous gingival grafts. *Journal of Clinical Periodontology* **7**, 316-324.

Hall, W. B. (1981) The current status of mucogingival problems and their therapy. *Journal of Periodontology* **52**, 569-575.

Hangorsky, U. & Bissada, N. F. (1980) Clinical assessment of free gingival graft effectiveness on the maintenance of periodontal health. *Journal of Periodontology* **51**, 274-278.

Hill, R. W., Ramfjord, S. P., Morrison, E. C., Appleberry, E. A., Caffesse, R. G., Kerry, G. J. & Nissle, R. R. (1981) Four types of periodontal treatment compared over two years. *Journal of Periodontology* **52**, 655-662.

Knowles, J., Burgett, F., Morrison, E., Nissle, R. & Ramfjord, S. (1980) Comparison of results following three modalities of periodontal therapy related to tooth type and initial pocket depth. *Journal of Clinical Periodontology* **7**, 32-47.

Knowles, J. W., Burgett, F. G., Nissle, R. R., Shick, R. A., Morrison, E. C. & Ramfjord, S. P. (1979) Results of periodontal treatment related to pocket depth and attachment level. Eight years. *Journal of Periodontology* **50**, 225-233.

Lindhe, J. & Nyman, S. (1975) The effect of plaque control and surgical pocket elimination on the establishment and maintenance of periodontal health. A longitudinal study of periodontal therapy in cases of advanced disease. *Journal of Clinical Periodontology* **2**, 67-79.

Matter, J. (1982) Free gingival grafts for the treatment of gingival recession. *Journal of Clinical Periodontology* **9**, 103-114.

Newell, D. H. (1981) Current status of the management of teeth with furcation invasions. *Journal of Periodontology* **52**, 559-568.

Rosling, B., Nyman, S., Lindhe, J. & Jern, B. (1976) The healing potential of the periodontal tissues following different techniques of periodontal surgery in plaque-free dentitions. *Journal of Clinical Periodontology* **3**, 233-250.

Wirthlin, M. R. (1981) The current status of new attachment therapy. *Journal of Periodontology* **52**, 529-544.

Zamet, J. S. (1975) A comparative clinical study of three periodontal surgical techniques. *Journal of Clinical Periodontology* **2**, 87-97.

Periodontal tissue reactions and healing:

Caton, J., Nyman, S. & Zander, H. (1980) Histometric evaluation of periodontal surgery. II. Connective tissue attachment levels after four regenerative procedures. *Journal of Clinical Periodontology* **7**, 224-231.

Kantor, M. (1980) The behavior of angular bony defects following reduction of inflammation. *Journal of Periodontology* **51**, 433-436.

Karring, T., Nyman, S. & Lindhe, J. (1980) Healing following implantation of periodontitis affected roots into bone tissue. *Journal of Clinical Periodontology* **7**, 96-105.

Moghaddas, H. & Stahl, S. S. (1980) Alveolar bone remodelling following osseous surgery. *Journal of Periodontology* **51**, 376-381.

Page, R. C. & Schroeder, H. E. (1981) Current status of the host response in chronic marginal periodontitis. *Journal of Periodontology* **52**, 477-491.

Tagge, D. L., O'Leary, T. J. & El-Kafrawy, A. H. (1975) The clinical and histological response of periodontal pockets to root planing and oral hygiene. *Journal of Periodontology* **46**, 527-533.

Effect of plaque control and maintenance care:

Axelsson, P. & Lindhe, J. (1981) Effect of controlled oral hygiene procedures on caries and periodontal disease in adults. *Journal of Clinical Periodontology* **8**, 239-248.

Axelsson, P. & Lindhe, J. (1981) The significance of maintenance care in the treatment of periodontal disease. *Journal of Clinical Periodontology* **8**, 281-294.

Rosling, B., Nyman, S. & Lindhe, J. (1976) The effect of systematic plaque control on bone regeneration in infrabony pockets. *Journal of Clinical Periodontology* **3**, 38-53.

Tabita, P. V., Bissada, N. F. & Maybury, J. E. (1981) Effectiveness of supragingival plaque control on the development of subgingival plaque and gingival inflammation in patients with moderate pocket depth. *Journal of Periodontology* **52**, 88-93.

Waerhaug, J. (1981) Effect of Toothbrushing on subgingival plaque formation. *Journal of Periodontology* **52**, 30-34.

Effect of non-surgical therapy:

Badersten, A., Nilvéus, R. & Egelberg, J. (1981) Effect of nonsurgical periodontal therapy. I. Moderately advanced periodontitis. *Journal of Clinical Periodontology* **8**, 57-72.

Lindhe, J., Westfelt, E., Nyman, S., Socransky, S. S., Heijl, L. & Bratthall, G. (1982) Healing following surgical/non-surgical treatment of periodontal disease. *Journal of Clinical Periodontology* **9**, 115-128.

CHAPTER 16

Periodontal Surgery: Instruments Used for Periodontal Surgery

General considerations
The instrument tray
Surgical instruments
Knives
Scalers and curettes
Instruments for bone removal
Instruments for handling flaps
Additional equipment

General considerations

Surgical procedures used in periodontal therapy often involve the following measures:

Incision and excision
Deflection and readaptation of mucosal flaps
Removal of adherent fibrous and granulomatous tissue
Scaling and root planing
Removal of bone tissue
Root sectioning
Suturing
Application of wound dressing

Instruments used for these purposes include:

Periodontal knives
Periosteal elevators
Tissue scissors
Soft tissue and bone rongeurs
Scalers and curettes
Bone chisels and files
Burs
Sutures and needle holders
Suture scissors
Plastic instruments

The set of instruments used for the various periodontal surgical procedures should have a comparatively simple design. As a general rule, the number and variety of instruments should be kept to a minimum. In addition to particular instruments used for periodontal treatment modalities, equipment and instruments generally used in oral surgery are often needed.

Within each category of surgical instruments used for periodontal therapy there are usually several brands available varying in form and quality, leaving ample opportunity for individual preferences.

In the selection of instruments, e.g. scalers and curettes, with blades of different sizes, it should be realized that the accessibility to the root surfaces of deep pockets is often limited. In such sites gracile instruments are therefore to be preferred.

The instruments should be stored in sterile "ready-to-use" packs or trays. Handling, storing and labeling of surgical instruments and equipment must be managed in such a way that interchanging of sterile and non-sterile items is prevented.

It is also important that the instruments are kept in good working condition. The maintenance routine should ensure that scalers, curettes, knives, etc. with fixed blades are sharp and the hinges of scissors, rongeurs and needle holders are properly lubricated. Spare instruments (sterile) should always be available to replace instruments found to be defective or accidentally contaminated.

The instrument tray

Instrument trays for periodontal surgery may be arranged in several ways. Different

365

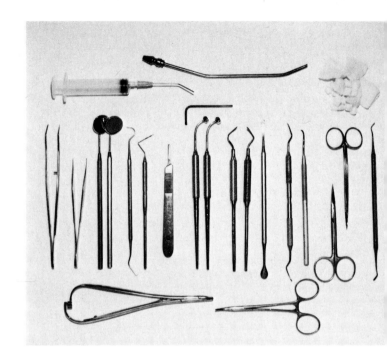

Fig. 16-1. Instruments used for periodontal surgery; included in a standard tray.

trays can be used for different procedures or a standard tray can be used for all procedures supplemented with the particular instruments that are needed for a specific procedure.

A commonly used standard tray combines the basic set of instruments used in oral surgery with a few periodontal instruments. The instruments listed below are often found on such a standard tray (Fig. 16-1):

    Cotton pliers
    Tissue pliers (a.m. Ewald)
    Mouth mirrors
    Explorer (a.m. Maillefer)
    Graduated periodontal probe
    Handles for disposable surgical blades:
    a) Bard-Parker handle
    b) Blakes handles with screw-key
    Waerhaug knives (No. 1 and 2)
    Mucoperiosteal elevator
    Curettes (e.g. Columbia No. 2R/2L, Sandviken Coromant No. 2)
    Suture scissors
    Tissue scissors
    Plastic instrument

    Hemostat
    Needle holder
    Syringe for irrigation
    Aspirator tip

Additional equipment may include:
    Drapings for the patient
    Rubber gloves
    Physiological saline
    Syringe for local anesthesia

Surgical instruments

Knives

Knives are available with fixed or replaceable blades. The advantage of the fixed blade versions is that the blade can be given any shape and orientation in relation to the handle which is considered appropriate. A disadvantage is that such instruments need frequent resharpening.

Knives with fixed blades are predominantly used for gingivectomy and Fig. 16-2 gives examples of such knives.

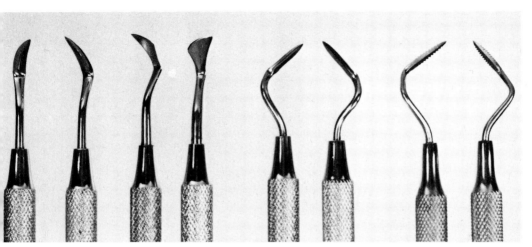

Fig. 16-2. Examples of paired gingivectomy knives. From left to right: Crane-Kaplan ¾, Kirkland ¹⁵/₁₆, Orban ½, Waerhaug ½.

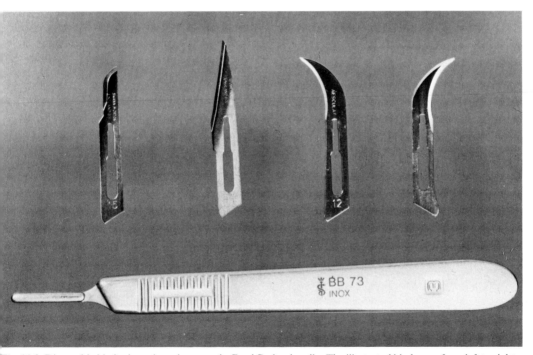

Fig. 16-3. Disposable blades in various shapes and a Bard-Parker handle. The illustrated blades are from left to right: No. 15, No. 11, No. 12, No. 12d

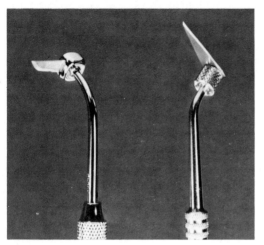

Fig. 16-4. Special handles for disposable blades.
Left: Detsch handle
Right: Blake handle

curettes and scalers with durable cutting
edges are often used when access is no
problem.

Instruments for bone removal

Sharp bone chisels or bone rongeurs (Fig.
16-6) cause least tissue damage and should
be employed whenever access permits. With
reduced access, surgical burs or files may be
used. The burs should operate at low speed
and ample rinsing with sterile physiological
saline should ensure cooling and removal of
tissue remnants.

New disposable blades are always sharp.
They can be rapidly replaced if found defective. The cutting edge of the blades normally
follows the long axis of the handle, a fact
which limits their use. However, knives with
disposable blades fitted in angulation in relation to the handle are also available.

The disposable blades are manufactured
in different shapes (Fig. 16-3). When
mounted in ordinary handles (Bard-
Parker®), they are used for releasing incisions in flap operations and mucogingival
surgery and for reverse bevel incisions where
access is obtainable. Special handles (Fig.
16-4) make it possible to mount blades in
positions which facilitate the use of such
knives for both gingivectomy excisions and
reverse bevel incisions.

Scalers and curettes

Scaling and root planing in conjunction with
periodontal surgery take place on exposed
root surfaces. Therefore access to the root
surfaces for debridement may be obtained
also by means of comparatively sturdy
instruments (Fig. 16-5). Tungsten carbide

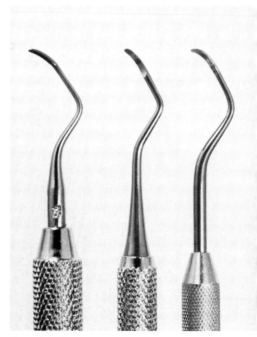

Fig. 16-5. Curettes which may be used in conjunction
with periodontal surgery.
From left to right:
Tungstencarbide curette (Ash ¹³/₁₄)
Goldman-Fox ¾
Columbia ¹³/₁₄.
These instruments are double ended. Only one end of
each instrument is illustrated.

Instruments for handling flaps

Proper healing of the periodontal wound is critical for the success of the operation. It is therefore important that the manipulation of the soft tissue flaps is performed with a minimum of tissue damage. Thus, care should be exercised in the use of periosteal elevators when flaps are deflected. Plastic instruments may be used as periosteal elevators and tissue retractors. Surgical pliers and tissue retractors which pierce the tissues should not be applied in the marginal area of the flaps. Needle holders with small beaks and atraumatic sutures should be used.

Additional equipment

Hemorrhage is rarely a problem in periodontal surgery. The characteristic oozing type of bleeding can normally be controlled by a pressure pack (sterile gauze moistened with saline). Bleeding from small vessels can be stopped by clamping and tying using a hemostat and resorbable sutures. If the vessel is surrounded by bone, bleeding may be stopped by crushing the nutrient canal in which the vessel runs with a blunt instrument.

Sterile physiological saline is used for rinsing and moistening the field of operation and for cooling when burs are employed. The saline solution may be kept in a sterile metal cup on the instrument tray and may be applied to the wound by means of a sterile

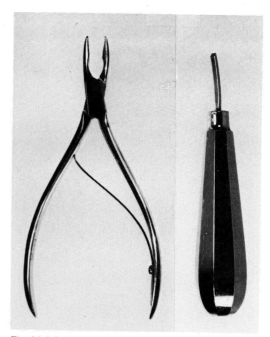

Fig. 16-6. Bone rongeur and bone chisel.

disposable plastic syringe and a needle with rounded tip.

Visibility of the field of operation is secured by using effective suction. The lumen of the aspirator tip should have a smaller diameter than the rest of the tube in order to prevent clogging.

The head of the patient may be covered by autoclaved cotton drapings or sterile disposable plastic/paper drapings. The operator and the assistant should wear sterile rubber gloves.

CHAPTER 17

Periodontal Surgery: Techniques for Periodontal Pockets

Introduction

It is a matter of historical interest that early descriptions of surgical techniques in periodontal therapy were aimed at attaining access to the diseased root surfaces. This could be accomplished without excision of the soft tissue pocket ("open-view operations"). Later procedures were described by which the "diseased gingiva" was excised (gingivectomy procedures). The concept that not only inflamed soft tissues, but also "infected and necrotic bone", had to be eliminated called for the development of surgical techniques by which the alveolar bone could be exposed and resected (flap procedures). Other concepts such as (1) the importance of maintaining the mucogingival complex (i.e. a wide zone of attached gingiva) and (2) the possibility for regeneration of periodontal tissues have also prompted the introduction of "tailor-made" surgical techniques.

In the following, surgical procedures will be described which represent important steps in the development of the surgical component of periodontal therapy.

Gingivectomy procedures

The surgical approach as an alternative to subgingival scaling for pocket therapy was already recognized in the latter part of the 19th century, when Robicsek (1884) pioneered the so-called "*gingivectomy*" procedure. Gingivectomy was later defined by Grant et al. (1979) as being "the excision of the soft tissue wall of a pathologic periodontal pocket". The surgical procedure which aimed at *pocket elimination* was usually combined with recontouring of the diseased gingiva to restore physiological form.

Robicsek (1884) and later Zentler (1918) described the gingivectomy procedure in the following way:
The line to which the gum is to be resected is determined first. Following a straight

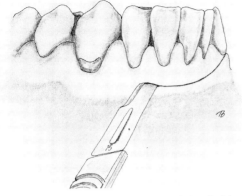

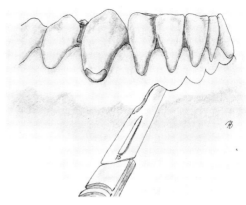

Fig. 17-1. Gingivectomy. The straight incision technique.

Fig. 17-2. Gingivectomy. The scalloped incision technique.

(Robiscek; Fig. 17-1) or scalloped (Zentler; Fig. 17-2) incision, first on the labial and then on the lingual surface of each tooth, the diseased tissue could be loosened and lifted out by means of a hook shaped instrument. After elimination of the soft tissue, the exposed alveolar bone could be scraped. The area could then be covered by some kind of antibacterial gauze or be painted with disinfecting solutions. The result obtained would show an eradication of the deepened periodontal pocket and a local condition which could be kept clean more easily.

Technique

The gingivectomy procedure as it is employed today was described in 1951 by Goldman. When the dentition in the area scheduled for surgery has been properly anesthetized, the depths of the pathological pockets are identified either with pocket marking forceps (e.g. ad modum Crane-Kaplan; Fig. 17-3a) or by means of a conventional periodontal probe (Figs. 17-3b, c). At the level of the bottom of the pocket the gingiva is pierced with the blade of the forceps (probe) and a bleeding point is produced on

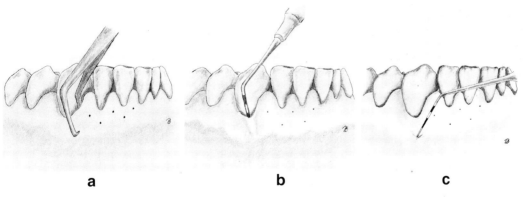

a   b   c

Figs. 17-3.a-c. Gingivectomy. Pocketmarking. (a) When pocket marking forceps are used the probing beak of the instrument is placed parallel to the long axis of the tooth. This gives a correct orientation for the perforating beak to indicate the "bottom" of the pocket. (b) An ordinary periodontal probe can also be used to identify the bottom of the deepened pocket. (c) When the depth of the pocket has been assessed an equivalent distance is delineated on the outer aspect of the gingiva. The tip of the probe is then turned horizontally and used to produce a bleeding point at the level of the pocket bottom.

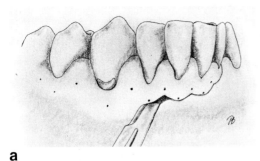

a

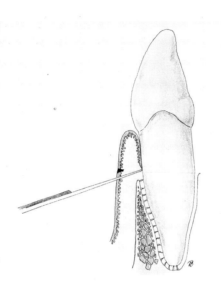

b

Figs. 17-4a,b. Gingivectomy. (a) The primary incision. (b) The incision is terminated at a level apical to the "bottom" of the pocket and is angulated to give the cut surface a distinct bevel.

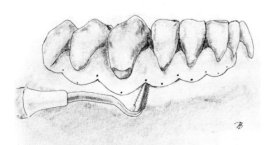

Fig. 17-5. Gingivectomy. The secondary incision is performed by means of a Waerhaug knife.

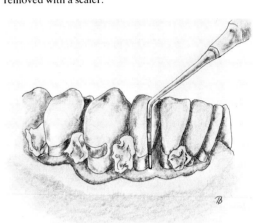

Fig. 17-6. Gingivectomy. The detached gingiva is removed with a scaler.

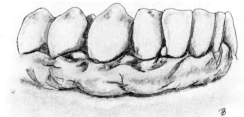

Fig. 17-7. Gingivectomy. Probing for residual pockets. Note that gauze packs have been placed in the interproximal spaces to control bleeding.

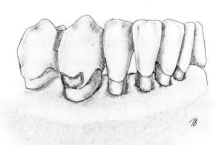

Fig. 17-8. Gingivectomy. The periodontal dressing has been applied and properly secured.

Fig. 17-9. Gingivectomy. The postoperative appearance of the surgically treated area.

he outer surface of the soft tissue. The pockets are probed and bleeding points produced at several location points around each tooth in the area. The series of bleeding points produced describes the depth of the pockets in the area scheduled for treatment and is used as a guideline for the incision.

The primary incision (Fig. 17-4) which may be made by a scalpel (blade No. 12B or 5; Bard-Parker®) in either a Bard-Parker handle or a Blake's handle or a Kirkland knife No. 15 or 16, should be planned to give a thin and properly festooned margin of the remaining gingiva. Thus, in areas where the gingiva is bulky, the incision must be placed at a level more apical to the level of the bleeding points than in areas with a thin gingiva, where a less accentuated bevel is needed. The beveled incision is directed towards the base of the pocket or to a level slightly apical to the apical extension of the junctional epithelium. In areas where the interdental pockets are deeper than the buccal or lingual pockets, additional amounts of buccal and/or lingual (palatal) gingiva must be removed in order to establish a "physiologic" contour of the gingival margin. This is often accomplished by initiating the incision at a more apical level.

Once the primary incision is completed on the buccal and lingual aspects of the teeth, the interproximal soft tissue is separated from the interdental periodontium by a secondary incision using an Orban knife (No. 1 or 2) or a Waerhaug knife (No. 1 or 2; a saw-toothed modification of the Orban knife; Fig. 17-5).

The incised tissues are carefully removed by means of a curette or a scaler (Fig. 17-6). Remaining tissue tabs are removed with a curette or a pair of scissors. Pieces of gauze packs often have to be placed in the interdental areas to control bleeding. When the field of operation is properly prepared, the exposed root surfaces are carefully scaled and planed.

Following meticulous debridement, the dentogingival regions are probed again to detect any remaining pockets (Fig. 17-7). The gingival contour is checked and, if needed, corrected by means of knives or rotating diamond stones.

To protect the incised area during the period of healing, the wound surface must be covered by a periodontal dressing (Fig. 17-8). The dressing should be closely adapted to the buccal and lingual wound surfaces as well as to the interproximal spaces. Care should be taken not to allow the dressing to become too bulky, since this is not only uncomfortable for the patient, but also facilitates the dislodgement of the dressing. The dressing should remain in position for 10-14 days.

After removal of the dressing the teeth must be cleaned and polished. The root surfaces are carefully checked and remaining calculus removed with a curette. Excessive granulation tissue is eliminated with a curette. The patient is instructed to properly clean the operated segments of the dentition which now have a different morphology as compared to the preoperative situation (Fig. 17-9).

Healing and dimensional changes following gingivectomy

Within a few days following excision of the inflamed gingival soft tissues coronal to the base of the periodontal pocket, epithelial cells start to migrate over the wound surface. The epithelialization of the gingivectomy wound is usually complete within 7-14 days following surgery (Engler et al. 1966, Stahl et al. 1968). During the following weeks a new dentogingival unit is formed (Fig. 17-10). The fibroblasts in the supraalveolar tissue adjacent the tooth surface proliferate (Waerhaug 1955) and new connective tissue is laid down. If this regeneration occurs in the vicinity of a plaque free tooth surface a free gingival unit will form which has all the characteristics of a normal free gingiva (Hamp et al. 1975). This regeneration occurs in coronal direction and appears clinically as a gain of marginal height (Fig. 17-10c). The height of the newly formed free gingival unit may vary not only between different parts of the dentition, but also from one tooth surface to another.

The reestablishment of a new, free gingival unit by coronal regrowth of tissue from the line of the "gingivectomy" incision implies that sites with so-called "zero pockets" only occasionally occur following gingivectomy. Complete healing of a gingivectomy wound takes 4-5 weeks, although the surface of the gingiva by clinical inspection may already appear healed after approximately 14 days (Ramfjord et al. 1966). Minor remodeling of the alveolar bone crest may also occur during the healing phase.

Flap procedures

The original Widman flap

One of the first detailed descriptions of the use of a flap procedure for pocket elimination was published in 1918 by *Leonard Widman*. In his article "The operative treatment of pyorrhea alveolaris" Widman described a mucoperiosteal flap design, aimed at removing the pocket epithelium and the inflamed connective tissue, thereby facilitating optimal cleaning of the root surfaces. Sectional releasing incisions were first made to demarcate the area scheduled for surgery (Fig. 17-11). These incisions were made from the midbuccal gingival margins of the 2 peripheral teeth of the treatment area and were continued several mm out into the alveolar mucosa. The 2 releasing incisions were connected with a gingival incision which followed the outline of the gingival margin and *separated the pocket epithelium and the inflamed connective tissue from the noninflamed gingiva*. Similar releasing and gingival incisions were, if needed, made on the lingual aspect of the teeth.

A mucoperiosteal flap was elevated to expose at least 2-3 mm of the marginal alveolar bone. The collar of inflamed tissue around the neck of the teeth was removed with curettes (Fig. 17-12) and the exposed root surfaces were carefully scaled. Bone recontouring was recommended to achieve an ideal anatomical form of the underlying alveolar bone (Fig. 17-13).

Following careful debridement of the teeth in the surgical area, the buccal and lingual flaps were laid back over the alveolar bone and secured in this position with interproximal sutures (Fig. 17-14). Widman pointed out the importance of placing the soft tissue margin at the level of the alveolar bone crest, so that no pockets would remain. The surgical procedure resulted in the exposure of root surfaces. Often the interproximal areas were left without soft tissue coverage of the alveolar bone.

The main advantage of the *"original Widman flap"* procedure in comparison to the gingivectomy procedure included according to Widman (1918), (1) less discomfort for the patient, since healing mainly occurred by primary intention and further (2) that it was possible to reestablish a proper contour of the alveolar bone in sites with angular bony defects.

The Neumann flap

Only a few years later *Neumann* (1920, 1926) suggested the use of a flap procedure which in some aspects was different from that originally described by Widman. According to the technique suggested by Neumann an intracrevicular incision was made through the base of the gingival pockets and the entire gingiva (and part of the alveolar mucosa) was elevated in a mucoperiosteal flap. Following its elevation, the inside of the flap was curetted to remove the pocket epithelium and the granulation tissue. The root surfaces were subsequently carefully "cleaned". Any irregularities of the alveolar bone were corrected to give the bone crest a horizontal outline. The flaps were then trimmed to allow both an optimal adaptation to the teeth and a proper coverage of the alveolar bone on both the buccal/lingual (palatal) and the interproximal sites. With regard to pocket elimination, Neumann pointed out the importance of removing the soft tissue pockets i.e. placing the flap at the crest of the alveolar bone.

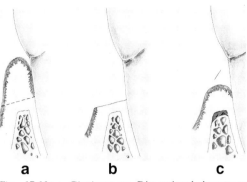

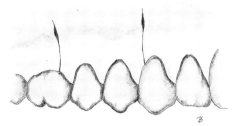

Fig. 17-11. *Original Widman flap.* Two releasing incisions demarcate the area scheduled for therapy.

Figs. 17-10a-c. *Gingivectomy.* Dimensional changes as a result of therapy. (a) Illustrates the preoperative dimensions. The broken line indicates the location of the primary incision. (b) The suprabony pocket has been eliminated. (c) Dimensions following proper healing. Minor resorption (shadowed area) of the alveolar bone crest as well as some loss of connective tissue attachment has occurred.

The modified flap operation

In a publication from 1931 *Kirkland* described a surgical procedure to be used in the treatment of "periodontal pus pockets". The procedure was called the *"modified flap operation"*. In this procedure incisions were made intracrevicularly through the bottom of the pocket (Fig. 17-15) on both the labial and lingual aspects of the interdental area. The incisions were extended in mesial and distal directions. The gingiva was retracted labially and lingually to expose the diseased root surfaces (Fig. 17-16) which were carefully debrided (Fig. 17-17). Angular bony defects were curetted. Following the elimination of pocket epithelium and granulation tissue from the inner surface of the flaps these were *replaced* in their original position and secured with interproximal sutures (Fig. 17-18). Thus, no attempt was made to reduce the preoperative depth of the pockets.

In contrast to the *"original Widman flap"* as well as the *"Neumann flap"*, the *"modified flap operation"* did not include (1) extensive sacrifice of noninflamed tissues and (2) apical displacement of the gingival margin. Since the root surfaces were not markedly exposed hereby, the method could for esthetic reasons, be useful in the anterior regions

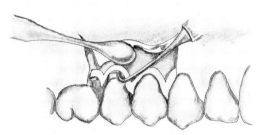

Fig. 17-12. *Original Widman flap.* The collar of inflamed gingival tissue is removed following the elevation of a mucoperiosteal flap.

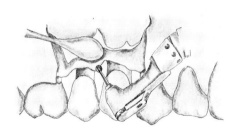

Fig. 17-13. *Original Widman flap.* By bone recontouring a "physiologic" contour of the alveolar bone may be reestablished.

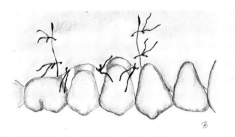

Fig. 17-14. *Original Widman flap.* The coronal ends of the buccal and lingual flaps are placed at the alveolar bone crest and secured in this position by sutures.

375

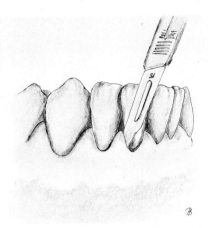

Fig. 17-15. *Modified flap operation.* Intracrevicular incision.

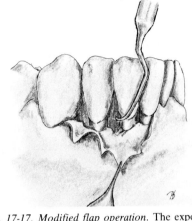

Fig. 17-17. *Modified flap operation.* The exposed root surfaces are subjected to mechanical debridement.

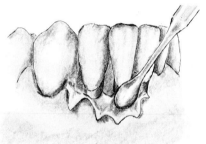

Fig. 17-16. *Modified flap operation.* The gingiva has been retracted to expose the "diseased" root surfaces.

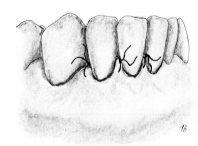

Fig. 17-18. *Modified flap operation.* The flaps are replaced to their original position and sutured.

of the dentition. Another advantage with the "modified flap operation" included the potential for bone regeneration which according to Kirkland (1931), in fact, frequently occurred.

The main objectives of the flap procedures so far described, were to (1) facilitate the debridement of the root surfaces as well as the removal of the pocket epithelium and the inflamed connective tissue, (2) eliminate the deepened pockets (the original Widman flap and the Neumann flap) and (3) cause a minimal amount of discomfort and trauma to the patient.

The apically repositioned flap

In the 50ies and 60ies new surgical techniques for the removal of soft and, when indicated, hard tissue periodontal pockets were described in the literature. The import-

ance of maintaining after surgery *an adequate zone of attached gingiva* was now emphasized. One of the first authors to describe a technique for the preservation of a zone of attached gingiva following surgery was *Nabers* (1954). The surgical technique developed by Nabers was originally denoted *"repositioning of attached gingiva"*, and was later modified by *Ariaudo & Tyrrell* (1957). In 1962 *Friedman* proposed the term *"apically repositioned flap"* to describe more appropriately the surgical technique introduced by Nabers. Friedman emphasized the fact that at the end of the surgical procedure, the entire complex of the soft tissues (gingiva and alveolar mucosa) rather than the gingiva alone was displaced in an apical direction. Thus, rather than excising the amount of gingiva, which would be in excess *after* osseous surgery (if performed), the whole mucogingival complex was maintained and apically

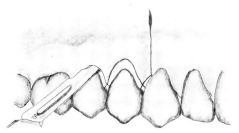

Fig. 17-19. Apically repositioned flap. Following a vertical releasing incision the reverse bevel incision is made through the gingiva and the periosteum.

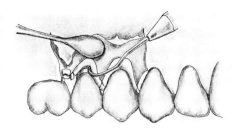

Fig. 17-20. Apically repositioned flap. A full thickness mucoperiosteal flap is raised and the tissue collar, including the pocket epithelium and the inflamed connective tissue, is removed with a curette.

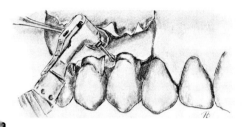

a

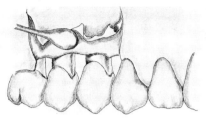

b

Figs. 17-21a,b. Apically repositioned flap. Osseous surgery is performed by means of a rotating bur (a) to recapture the physiologic contour of the alveolar bone (b).

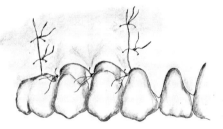

Fig. 17-22. Apically repositioned flap. The flaps are repositioned in apical direction, to the level of the recontoured alveolar bone crest and retained in this position by sutures.

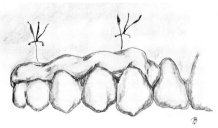

Fig. 17-23. Apically repositioned flap. A periodontal dressing is placed over the surgical area to ensure that the flaps remain in the correct position during healing.

repositioned. This surgical technique was used on buccal surfaces in both upper and lower jaws and on lingual surfaces in the lower jaw. According to Friedman (1962) the technique should be performed in the following way:

A reverse bevel incision is made using a scalpel with a Bard-Parker blade (No. 12B or No. 15). How far from the buccal/lingual gingival margin the incision should be made is dependent on the pocket depth as well as the thickness and the width of the gingiva (Fig. 17-19). If the gingiva preoperatively is

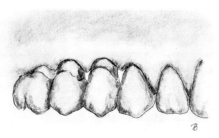

Fig. 17-24. Apically repositioned flap. The postoperative appearance of the surgically treated region of the dentition.

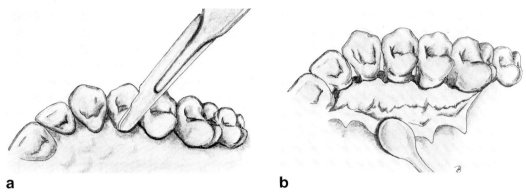

a   **b**

Figs. 17-25a,b. Bevelled flap. A primary incision is made through the periodontal pockets (a) and a conventional mucoperiosteal flap is elevated (b).

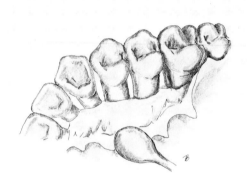

Fig. 17-26. Beveled flap. Scaling, root planing and osseous recontouring have been performed in the surgical area.

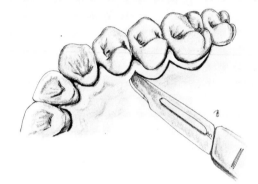

Fig. 17-27. Beveled flap. The palatal flap is replaced and a secondary, scalloped, reverse bevel incision is made to adjust the length of the flap to the height of the remaining alveolar bone.

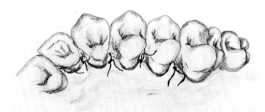

Fig. 17-28. Beveled flap. The shortened flap is placed over the alveolar bone and in close contact with the root surfaces.

hin and only a narrow zone of attached ging-
va is present, the incision should be made
close to the tooth. The beveling incision
should be given a scalloped outline to ensure
maximal interproximal coverage of the
alveolar bone, when the flap is subsequently
repositioned. Vertical releasing incisions
extending out into the alveolar mucosa (i.e.
past the mucogingival junction) are made at
each of the end points of the reverse bevel
incision, thereby making possible the apical
repositioning of the flap.

A full thickness, mucoperiosteal flap
including buccal/lingual gingiva and alveolar
mucosa is raised by means of a
mucoperiosteal elevator. The marginal collar of tissue including pocket epithelium and
granulation tissue is removed with curettes
(Fig. 17-20). The root surfaces are carefully
scaled and planed.

The alveolar bone crest is recontoured
with the objective of recapturing the normal
form of the alveolar process but at a more
apical level (Fig. 17-21). The osseous
surgery is performed using burs (Fig. 17-21a)
and/or bone chisels.

Following careful adjustment the buc-
cal/lingual flap is repositioned to the level of
the newly recontoured alveolar bone crest
and secured in this position (Fig. 17-22). The
incisional and excisional technique used,
makes it not always possible to obtain proper
soft tissue coverage of the denuded interproximal alveolar bone. A periodontal dressing should therefore be applied to protect
the exposed bone and to retain the soft tissue
at the level of the bone crest (Fig. 17-23).
After healing an "adequate" zone of
attached gingiva is preserved and no residual
pockets should remain (Fig. 17-24).

To handle periodontal pockets on the
palatal aspect of the teeth *Friedman*
described a modification of the "apically
repositioned flap", which he termed the
"*beveled flap*". Since there is no alveolar
mucosa present on the palatal aspect of the
teeth, it is not possible to reposition the flap
in apical direction. In order to prepare the
tissue of the gingival margin to follow properly the outline of the alveolar bone crest, a

conventional mucoperiosteal flap is first
reflected (Figs. 17-25a, b). The tooth surfaces are debrided and osseous recontouring
is performed. The palatal flap is subsequently replaced and the gingival margin is
prepared and adjusted to the alveolar bone
crest by a secondary scalloped and beveled
incision (Figs. 17-26, 17-27). The flap is secured in this position with inter-proximal
sutures (Fig. 17-28).

Among a number of suggested advantages
of the "*apically repositioned flap*" procedure, the following have been emphasized:

. Minimum pocket depth postoperatively.
. If optimal soft tissue coverage of the
  alveolar bone is obtained, the postsurgical
  bone loss is minimal.
. The postoperative position of the gingival
  margin may be controlled and the entire
  mucogingival complex may be maintained.

The sacrifice of periodontal tissues by bone
resection and the subsequent exposure of
root surfaces (which may cause root
hypersensitivity) were regarded as the main
disadvantages of this technique.

The modified Widman flap

Ramfjord & Nissle (1974) described the
"*modified Widman flap*" technique which is
also recognized as the "*open flap curettage*"
technique. It should be observed that while
the "*original Widman flap*" technique
included both apical displacement of the
flaps and osseous recontouring (elimination
of angular bony defects) to obtain proper
pocket elimination, the "*modified Widman
flap*" technique does not intend to meet
these objectives. Ramfjord & Nissle (1974)
described the "modified Widman flap"
technique:

The *initial incision* (Fig. 17-29) which may
be performed with a Bard-Parker knife (No.
11) should be parallel to the long axis of the
tooth and placed approximately 1 mm from
the buccal gingival margin in order to properly separate the pocket epithelium from the

379

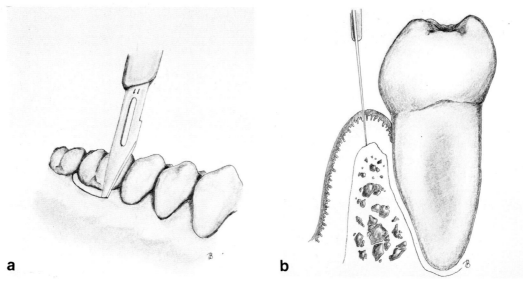

Figs. 17-29a,b. Modified Widman flap. The initial incision is placed 0.5-1 mm from the gingival margin (a) and parallel to the long axis of the tooth (b).

flap. If the pockets on the buccal aspects of the teeth are less than 2 mm deep, or if esthetic considerations are important, an intracrevicular incision may be made. Furthermore, the scalloped incision should be extended as far as possible in between the teeth, to allow maximum amounts of the interdental gingiva to be included in the flap.

A similar incision technique is used on the palatal aspect. Often, however, the scalloped outline of the initial incision may be accentuated by placing the knife a distance of 1-2 mm away from the midpalatal surface of the teeth. By extending the incision as far as possible in between the teeth, sufficient amounts of tissue can be included in the

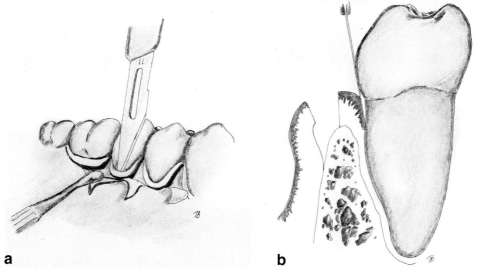

Figs. 17-30a,b. Modified Widman flap. Following careful elevation of the flaps a second intracrevicular incision (a) is made to the alveolar bone crest (b).

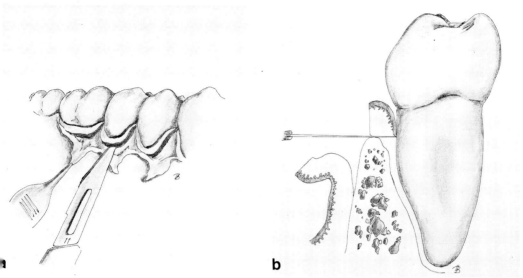

Figs. 17-31a,b. Modified Widman flap. The third incision is made in a horizontal direction (a) and close to the surface of the bone crest (b), thereby separating the soft tissue collar from the root surfaces and the alveolar bone.

palatal flap to allow for proper coverage of the interproximal bone when the flap is sutured. Vertical releasing incisions are not usually required.

Buccal and palatal full thickness flaps are carefully elevated with a mucoperiosteal elevator. The flap elevation should be limited and allow only a few mm of the alveolar bone crest to become exposed. To facilitate the gentle separation of the collar of pocket epithelium and granulation tissue from the root surfaces an intracrevicular incision (Fig. 17-30) is made around the teeth *(second incision)* to the alveolar crest.

A *third incision* (Fig. 17-31) made in a horizontal direction and in a position close to

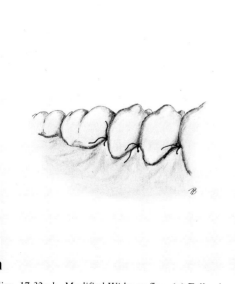

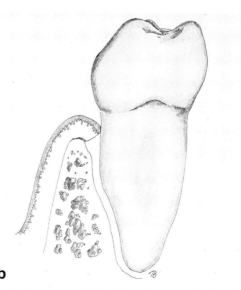

Figs. 17-32a,b. Modified Widman flap. (a) Following curettage the flaps are carefully adjusted to cover the alveolar bone and sutured. (b) Complete coverage of the interproximal bone as well as a close adaptation of the flaps to the tooth surfaces should be accomplished.

381

the surface of the alveolar bone crest, separates the soft tissue collar of the root surfaces from the bone. The pocket epithelium and the granulation tissues are removed by means of curettes. The exposed roots are carefully scaled and planed, except for a narrow area close to the alveolar bone crest in which remnants of attachment fibers may be

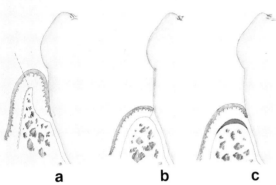

a   **b**   **c**

Figs. 17-33a-c. Apically repositioned flap. Dimensional changes. (a) Illustrates the preoperative dimensions. The broken line indicates the site from which the mucoperiosteal flap is reflected. (b) Bone recontouring has been completed. (c) Dimensions following proper healing. Minor resorption of the marginal alveolar bone has occurred (shadowed area) as well as some loss of connective tissue attachment.

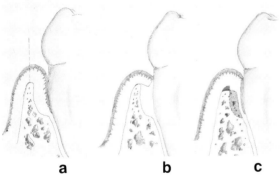

a   **b**   **c**

Figs. 17-34a-c. Modified Widman flap – dimensional changes. (a) Illustrates the preoperative dimensions. The broken line illustrates the site from which the mucoperiosteal flap is reflected. (b) Surgery (including curettage of angular bony defects) is completed. (c) Dimensions following proper healing. Osseous repair (dotted area) as well as a small amount of crestal bone resorption (shadowed area) have occurred. Note the presence of a long junctional epithelium interposed between the regenerated bone tissue and the root surface.

preserved. Angular bony defects are carefully curetted.

Following curettage, the flaps are trimmed and adjusted to the alveolar bone to obtain complete coverage of the interproximal bone (Fig. 17-32). If this adaptation cannot be achieved by soft tissue re-contouring some bone may be removed from the outer aspects of the alveolar process in order to facilitate the allimportant flap adaptation The flaps are sutured together with individual interproximal sutures. Surgical dressing may be placed over the area to ensure close adaptation of the flaps to the alveolar bone and the root surfaces. The dressing a well as the sutures are removed after 1 week

The main advantages of the *"modified Widman flap"* technique, in comparison with other procedures previously described are (1) the possibility of obtaining a close adaptation of the soft tissues to the root surfaces and (2) the minimum of trauma to which the alveolar bone and the soft connective tissues are exposed (Ramfjord & Nissl 1974). The technique also results in less exposure of the root surfaces, which from a esthetic aspect is an advantage in the treatment of anterior segments of the dentition.

Dimensional changes following flap surgery

The apically repositioned flap (Fig. 17-33) following osseous surgery for elimination of bony defects and the establishment of "physiologic contours" and repositioning of th soft tissue flaps to the level of the alveolar bone, healing will occur primarily by first intention, especially in areas where proper soft tissue coverage of the alveolar bone has been obtained. During the initial phase of healing bone resorption of varying exten almost always occurs in the crestal area of the alveolar bone (Ramfjord & Costic 1968). The extent of the reduction of th alveolar bone height, resulting from thi resorption, is related to the thickness of th bone in each specific site (Wood et al. 1972 Karring et al. 1975).

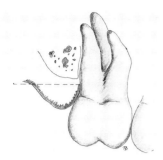

Fig. 17-35. Distal wedge procedures. A simple gingivectomy incision (broken line) is used to eliminate the soft tissue pocket and the fibrous tissue pad behind a second maxillary molar.

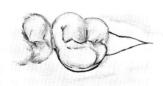

Fig. 17-36. Distal wedge procedures. Buccal and lingual vertical incisions are made through the retromolar pad behind a mandibular second molar.

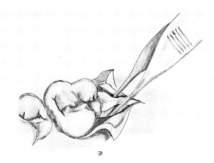

Fig. 17-37. Distal wedge procedures. The triangular shaped wedge of tissue, prepared by the vertical incisions, is dissected from the underlying bone and removed.

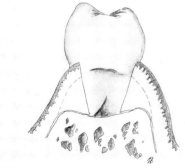

Fig. 17-38. Distal wedge procedures. The walls of the buccal and lingual flaps are reduced in thickness by undermining incisions (broken lines).

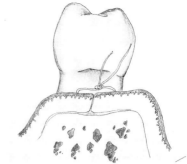

Fig. 17-39. Distal wedge procedures. The flaps, which have been trimmed and shortened to avoid overlapping wound margins, are sutured.

During the phase of tissue regeneration and maturation a new dentogingival unit will form by coronal growth of the connective tissue. This regrowth occurs in a manner similar to that which characterized healing following gingivectomy.

The "modified Widman flap" (Fig. 17-34): if a "modified Widman flap" is carried out in an area with a deep infrabony lesion, bone repair may occur within the boundaries of the lesion (Rosling et al. 1976, Polson & Heijl 1978). However, a small amount of crestal bone resorption is also seen. The amount of bone fill obtained is dependent upon (1) the anatomy of the osseous defect (e.g. a 3-walled infra-bony defect often provides a better mold for bone repair than 2- or 1-walled defects), (2) the amount of crestal bone resorption and (3) the extent of chronic inflammation which may occupy the area of healing. However, interposed between the regenerated bone tissue and the root surface a long junctional epithelium is always found (Caton & Zander 1976, Caton et al. 1980). The apical cells of the newly formed junctional epithelium are found at a level on the root, which closely coincides with the presurgical attachment level.

Distal wedge procedures

In many cases the treatment of periodontal pockets on the distal surface of distal molars is complicated by the presence of bulbous tissues over the tuberosity or by a prominent retromolar pad. The most direct approach to pocket elimination in such cases in the maxillary jaw is the gingivectomy procedure. The incision is started on the distal surface of the tuberosity and carried forward to the base of the pocket of the distal surface of the molar (Fig. 17-35).

However, when there are only limited amounts of attached gingiva present or none at all, or if a distal angular bony defect has been diagnosed, the bulbous tissue should be reduced in size rather than being removed *in toto*. This may be accomplished by the *"distal wedge procedure"* (Robinson 1966). This technique facilitates access to the osseous defect and makes it possible to preserve sufficient amounts of attached gingiva and mucosa.

Technique

Buccal and lingual incisions are made in vertical direction through the tuberosity or retromolar pad to form a triangular wedge (Fig. 17-36). The facial and lingual incisions should be extended in a mesial direction along the buccal and lingual surfaces of the distal molar to facilitate flap elevation.

The facial and lingual walls of the tuberosity or retromolar pad are deflected and the incised wedge of tissue is dissected and separated from the bone (Fig. 17-37).

The walls of the facial and lingual flaps are then reduced in thickness by undermining incisions (Fig. 17-38). Loose tags of tissue are removed and the root surfaces are scaled and planed. If necessary, the bone is recontoured.

The buccal and lingual flaps are replaced over the exposed alveolar bone, the edges trimmed to avoid overlapping wound margins. The flaps are secured in this position with interrupted sutures (Fig. 17-39). The sutures are removed after approximately 1 week.

The distal wedge procedure may be modified according to individual requirements. One such modification of the original distal

wedge procedure is depicted in Figs. 17-40 to 17-45.

Osseous surgery

The principles of osseous surgery in periodontal therapy were outlined by Schluger (1949) and Goldman (1950). They pointed out that alveolar bone loss caused by inflammatory periodontal disease often results in an uneven outline of the bone crest. Since, according to these authors the gingival contour is closely dependent on the contour of the underlying bone as well as the proximity and anatomy of adjacent tooth surfaces, the elimination of soft tissue pockets often has to be combined with osseous reshaping and the elimination of osseous craters and angular bony defects to establish and maintain shallow pockets and optimal gingival contour after surgery.

Osseous recontouring and eradication of angular bony defects and craters are excisional techniques which should be used with caution and discrimination. Sometimes deep bony defects may, for their complete elimination, require such an advanced resection of alveolar bone that the periodontal tissue support of adjacent teeth, which primarily are not so seriously involved in the disease process, may have to be compromised. In such cases bone resection should be avoided.

Osteoplasty

The term *osteoplasty* was introduced by Friedman in 1955. The purpose of osteoplasty is to create a physiological form of the alveolar bone *without* removing any "supporting" bone. Osteoplasty therefore is a technique analogous to gingivoplasty. Examples of osteoplasty are the thinning of thick osseous ledges and the establishment of a scalloped contour of the buccal (lingual and palatal) bone crest (Fig. 17-46). The leveling of interproximal craters and the elimination of bone walls of circumferential

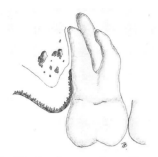

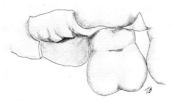

Fig. 17-42. *Distal wedge procedures*. Buccal and palatal flaps have been elevated.

Fig. 17-40. Distal wedge procedures. Illustrates a deep periodontal pocket combined with an angular bony defect at the distal aspect of a second maxillary molar.

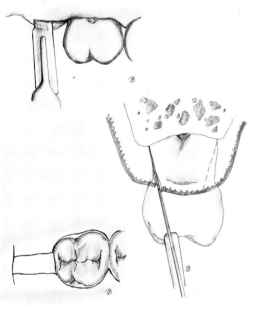

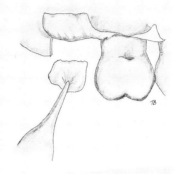

Fig. 17-43. *Distal wedge procedures*. The rectangular wedge is dissected from the underlying bone and removed.

Figs. 17-41a-c. Distal wedge procedures. (a, b) Two parallel reverse bevel incisions, one buccal (indicated by broken line in Fig. 17-41b) and one palatal, are made from the distal surface of the second maxillary molar to the posterior part of the tuberosity. (c) A buccolingual incision is then made to connect the two parallel incisions. The buccal and palatal incisions are extended in mesial direction along the buccal and palatal surfaces of the second and first maxillary molars to facilitate flap elevation.

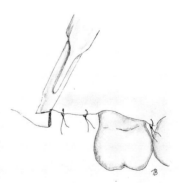

Fig. 17-44. *Distal wedge procedures*. Following bone recontouring the flaps are trimmed and shortened to avoid overlapping wound margins and sutured. The remaining fibrous tissue pad, distal to the buccolingual incision line, is "leveled" by means of a gingivectomy incision.

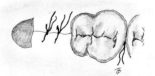

Fig. 17-45. *Distal wedge procedures*. The distal wedge procedure is completed. Note that a close soft tissue adaptation has been accomplished to the distal surface of the second maxillary molar.

osseous defects are often referred to as osteoplasty since usually no resection of supporting bone is required (Figs. 17-47, 17-48).

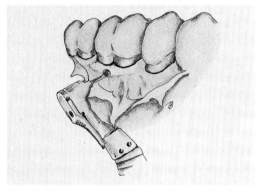

Fig. 17-46. Osteoplasty. Thick osseous ledges in a mandibular molar area are eliminated by means of a round bur.

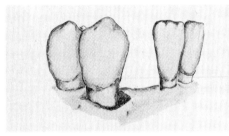

Fig. 17-47. Osteoplasty. An infrabony defect is present at the mesiobuccal aspect of the mandibular right canine.

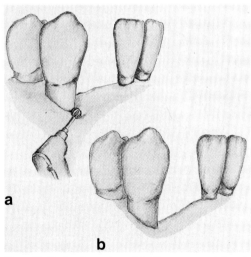

a

b

Figs. 17-48a,b. Osteoplasty (a) The osseous defect is removed by osseous recontouring. A rotating bur is used. (b) The osteoplasty is completed. Note that no supporting bone has been resected.

Ostectomy

Ostectomy is considered to be an important part of surgical technique aimed at pocket elimination. However, the therapist is often faced with the dilemma of deciding whether to eliminate an angular bony defect in situations where osseous resection may compromise the periodontal tissue support of a neighboring tooth. The alternatives are (1) to maintain the area without osseous resection, (2) to compromise the amount of bone removal and accept that a certain pocket depth will remain or (3) to extract the involved tooth if the bony defect is too advanced.

After exposing the alveolar bone by the elevation of a flap, buccal and/or lingual crater walls are reduced to the base of the osseous defect using a round bur or a diamond stone under continuous saline irrigation (Fig. 17-49). Bone chisels, files and rongeurs can also be used. If bone resection has been carried out in the interdental area, the buccal and lingual/palatal bone margins may subsequently have to be recontoured to compensate for discrepancies in bone height resulting from the interdental bone resection (Fig. 17-50). It is considered important to remove the small peaks of bone, which often remain in the area of the line angles. The objective of bone surgery is thus to establish a "physiologic" anatomy of the alveolar bone, but at a more apical level. The soft tissue flaps are recontoured and adapted to the newly created bone margin.

Suturing

When a flap procedure has been employed it is important to ensure that, at the end of surgery, the flaps are placed in the intended position and that they are properly adapted to each other and the tooth surfaces. Preferably full coverage of the buccal/lingual (palatal) and interdental alveolar bone should be obtained with the soft tissue flaps. If this can be achieved healing by first intention results and the postoperative bone

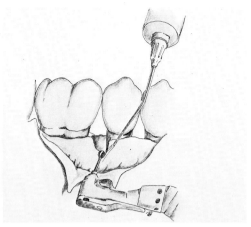

Fig. 17-49. Ostectomy. An osseous defect on the distal surface of a mandibular second bicuspid has been exposed following reflection of mucoperiosteal flaps. The bone walls are reduced to the base of the defect using a rotating round bur under continuous saline irrigation.

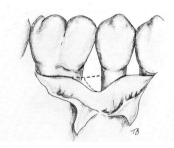

Fig. 17-50. Ostectomy. The osseous recontouring procedure is completed. Note that in this illustration some supporting bone has been removed from the buccal aspect of both the second bicuspid and the first molar.

resorption becomes minimal. Therefore, prior to suturing, the flap margins should be trimmed to properly fit the buccal and lingual (palatal) bone margin as well as the interproximal areas; excessive soft tissue must be removed. If the amount of flap tissue present is insufficient to cover the interproximal bone, the flaps at the buccal or lingual aspects of the teeth must be re-contoured and, in some cases, even coronally displaced.

Following proper trimming, the flaps are secured in correct position by sutures. The materials most commonly used as sutures in periodontal surgery are fabricated of silk

and various synthetic materials. The dimensions usually preferred are 3-0 or 4-0. These materials are nonresorbable and should be removed after 7-14 days.

Since the flap tissue following the final preparation is thin, nontraumatic needles (eyeless), either curved or straight, with a small diameter should be used. Such needles are available as rounded (noncutting) or with different cutting edges.

Technique

The 3 most frequently used sutures in periodontal flap surgery are (1) interrupted interdental sutures, (2) suspensory sutures and (3) continuous sutures.

The *interrupted interdental suture* (Fig. 17-51) provides a close interdental adaptation between the buccal and lingual flaps with equal tension on both units. This type of suture is therefore not recommended when the buccal and lingual flaps are repositioned at different levels. When this technique of suturing is employed, the needle is passed through the buccal flap from the external surface, across the interdental area and through the lingual flap from the internal

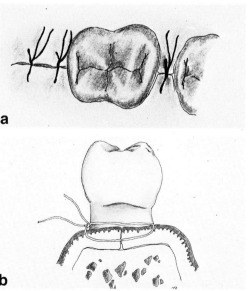

a

b

Figs. 17-51a,b. Suturing. Interrupted interdental suture

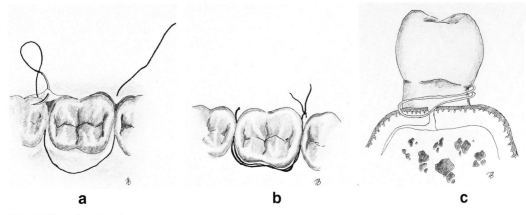

Figs. 17-52a-c. Suturing. Suspensory suture.

surface, or vice versa. When closing the suture, care must be taken to avoid tearing of the flap tissues.

The *suspensory suture* (Fig. 17-52) is used primarily when the surgical procedure is of limited extension and involves only the tissue of the buccal or lingual aspect of the teeth. It is also the suture of choice when the buccal and lingual flaps are repositioned at different levels. The needle is passed through the buccal flap from its external surface at the mesial side of the tooth, placed around the lingual surface of the tooth and passed through the buccal flap on the distal side of the tooth (Fig. 17-52a). The suture is brought back to the starting point via the lingual surface of the tooth and tied (Figs. 17-52b, c). If a lingual flap has been elevated as well, this is secured in the intended position using the same technique.

The *continuous suture* (Fig. 17-53) is commonly used when flaps involving several teeth should be apically repositioned. When flaps have been elevated on both sides of the teeth, one flap at a time is secured in its proper position. The suturing procedure is started at the mesial/distal aspect of the buccal flap by passing the needle through the flap and across the interdental area. The suture is laid around the lingual surface of the tooth and returned to the buccal side

through the next interdental space. The procedure is repeated tooth by tooth until the distal/mesial end of the flap is reached. Thereafter the needle is passed through the lingual flap (Fig. 17-53a), with the suture laid around the buccal aspect of each tooth and through each interproximal space. When the suturing of the lingual flap is completed and the needle has been brought back to the first interdental area, the positions of the flaps are adjusted and secured in their proper positions by closing the suture (Fig. 17-53b). Thus, only one knot is needed.

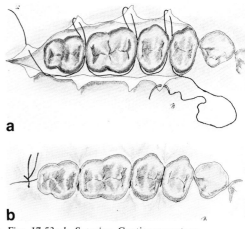

Figs. 17-53a,b. Suturing. Continuous suture.

Periodontal dressings

Periodontal dressings are used mainly (1) to protect the wound prepared during surgery, (2) to obtain and maintain a close adaptation of the mucosal flaps to the underlying bone (especially when a flap has been apically repositioned) and (3) for the comfort of the patient. In addition, periodontal dressings can, during the initial phase of healing, prevent postoperative bleeding and, if properly placed in the operated segment (especially interproximally), prevent the formation of excessive granulation tissue.

The periodontal dressing should have the following properties:
1. The dressing should be soft, but still have enough plasticity and flexibility to facilitate its placement in the operated area and to allow proper adaptation.
2. The dressing should set within a reasonable time.
3. After setting, the dressing should have sufficient rigidity to prevent fracture and dislocation.
4. The dressing should also have a smooth surface after setting to prevent irritation to the cheeks and lips.
5. The dressing should preferably have proper bactericidal effect to prevent excessive plaque formation.
6. The dressing must not detrimentally interfere with healing.

It has been suggested that antibacterial agents should be incorporated in periodontal dressings to prevent bacterial growth in the wound area during healing. Results from clinical studies and *in vitro* evaluation of the antibacterial properties of various periodontal dressings, however, suggest that the antibacterial activity of most commercial dressings is probably exhausted long before the end of the 7-14 day period during which the dressing is frequently maintained in the operated segment (O'Neil 1975, Haugen et al. 1977).

Mouth rinsing with antibacterial agents such as chlorhexidine does not prevent the formation of plaque *under* the dressing (Plüss et al. 1975), and should therefore not be regarded as a means to improve or shorten the period of wound healing.

The periodontal dressings most commonly used may be devided into 2 groups: *eugenol containing* and *noneugenol containing* dressings.

Eugenol dressings

These dressings have a zinc oxide eugenol basis. The dressing is supplied as a powder and a liquid, which are mixed together. Zinc oxide which is used as setting material, forms, when mixed with eugenol, a hardened mass. The powder also contains rosin, tannic acid, cellulose fibers and zinc acetate, while the liquid in addition to eugenol may contain vegetable oils, thymol and color additives. Zinc oxide can be substituted by other similar materials such as magnesium oxide. The setting involves both chemical and physical processess and is influenced by moisture, proportions of powder and liquid used, mixing time and temperature. The addition of a metallic salt such as zinc acetate accelerates setting. The rosin reacts with the zinc oxide to give the dressing better rigidity. Tannic acid has been used to improve wound healing, but its use has been prohibited in some countries because of the risk of liver damage. On account of its suggested beneficial effects on wound healing, however, tannic acid is still a constituent in several commercial dressings. Cellulose fibers are incorporated in order to improve the setting of the dressing material. Eugenol is weakly antiseptic and has a slight sedative effect. The vegetable oils, which are added to the liquid in order to dissolve the eugenol, will also increase the plasticity of the dressing and reduce some tissue irritation caused by the eugenol. Thymol is a weak antiseptic. Sensitivity reactions sometimes occur when zinc oxide eugenol dressings are used and it is usually the eugenol which provokes this kind of reaction.

Noneugenol dressings

Since several reports have been published

indicating adverse effects of eugenol and since eugenolcontaining dressings have an unpleasant taste to many patients, eugenol free dressings have been developed. Several such dressings are available, e.g. Coe-Pak® and Peripac®.

Coe-Pak® which is frequently used in periodontal surgery, is supplied in 2 tubes. One tube contains oxides of various metals (mainly zinc oxide) and lorothidol (a fungicide). The second tube contains non-ionizing carboxylic acids and chlorothymol (a bacteriostatic agent). Equal parts from both tubes are mixed together immediately prior to insertion. The setting time can be prolonged by adding a retarder. Other typical noneugenol dressings are supplied as powder and liquid, which are mixed.

Cyanoacrylates have also been used as periodontal dressings with varying success. Dressings of the cyanoacrylate type are applied in a liquid directly onto the wound or sprayed over the wound surface. Although the application of this kind of dressing is simple, its properties often do not meet clinical demands, which is why its use, at present, is rather limited.

It should be noted that noneugenol dressings may also provoke hypersensitivity reactions.

Application technique

Following gingivectomy periodontal dressings are used primarily to protect the wound, while following flap surgery the dressing is often used to keep the flaps in close contact with the underlying bone.

When bleeding from the operated tissues has ceased, the dressing material is inserted. Frequently the interproximal areas are filled with the pack material first. Thin rolls of the dressing, adjusted in length to cover the entire field of operation, are then placed against the buccal and lingual surfaces of the teeth. The rolls are pressed against the tooth surfaces and the dressing material forced into the interproximal areas. The surface of the dressing is subsequently smoothed. The

dressing should not cover more than the apical third of the tooth surfaces (Figs. 17-8, 17-23). Coe-Pak® may also be applied to the wound surfaces by means of a plastic syringe.

It is important to ensure that dressing material is never introduced between the flap and the underlying bone or root surface. To avoid such faulty placement of the pack, the wound surface may occasionally be protected with for example tin foil prior to the insertion of the dressing. Tin foil applications are recommended in sites where an insufficient adaptation of the flap to the bone or the root has been accomplished. Furthermore, interference of the dressing with mucogingival structures (e.g. the vestibular fold, frenula) should be carefully checked.

Local anesthesia in periodontal surgery

The pain experienced by the periodontal patient during surgical procedures may not only be caused by the mechanical instrumentation in the preparation of the wound area but may also emanate from the teeth. Thus pain of varying intensity can be elicited from the teeth, especially in cases of exposed root dentin, by such factors as cold, heat, vibration, drying, etc.

In order to prevent the patient from suffering an unpleasant pain sensation during the course of surgical treatment the entire area of the dentition scheduled for surgery, the teeth as well as the periodontal tissues, should be properly blocked by a locally applied anesthetic drug.

Local anesthesia in the maxilla

The presence of porosities in the external lamina of the alveolar bone of the maxilla permits an anesthetic solution, deposited in the buccal oral mucosa, to penetrate the alveolar bone and reach the apex of the

390

arget tooth. Thus, local analgesia of the pulp and buccal periodontal tissues of the maxillary dentition can easily be accomplished by a series of injections in the mucogingival fold of the treatment area.

After the administration of 0.5-1 ml of the anesthetic solution as a deposit in the buccal fold, pulpal analgesia will be accomplished in the tooth close to the injection site and in some 80% of cases, also in the neighboring teeth. Thus, if larger areas of the dentition are scheduled for treatment, repeated injections (in the buccal fold) have to be performed, e.g. at the central incisor, canine, second premolar and second molar.

In the posterior maxillary regions the number of injection sites may be reduced by using a tuberosity injection which is made to block the superior alveolar branches of the maxillary nerve as they descend on the zygomatic surface of the maxilla and which, consequently, provides analgesia in a larger area. Because of the risk involved in intravascular injections, however, in most instances this type of block anesthesia should be avoided.

The palatal nerves are blocked by an injection made at a right angle to the mucosal surface, approximately 10 mm apical to the gingival margin. If the treatment area on the palatal aspect of the jaw is wide in apicocoronal direction, around 1 ml of the anesthetic solution should be placed close to the major palatine foramen. This injection will block the anterior and accessory palatine nerves and produce analgesia of all soft and hard tissues from the area of the third molar to the canine. Analgesia of the palatal tissues of the front tooth region is accomplished by an injection made at the site of the incisive papilla. In order to prevent unnecessary pain by this injection, and to avoid a deposition of the anesthetic solution in the vessels emerging from the incisor canal a lateral injection approach should be preferred. The pain produced by injections into the nonresilient palatal tissue can, in cases of advanced bone loss, be minimized if the injections are made from the buccal aspect, i.e. through the interdental gingiva.

In order to obtain proper ischemia in the gingival tissues small amounts of the anesthetic solution can also be injected into the interdental papillae. Such injections should be performed after proper analgesia has been accomplished by buccal and palatal infiltration.

If the anesthetic solution (2% solution of lidocaine, containing 10-12.5 mg adrenaline/ml) is distributed in the upper jaw, in the way proposed above, in the vast majority of the cases proper analgesia will be accomplished for a period of at least 60 min.

Local anesthesia in the mandible

In the front tooth region of the lower jaw an infiltration with an anesthetic solution in the buccal fold will produce proper analgesia in many cases, especially in young patients. The anesthetic effect is the result of the penetration of the drug through porosities in the mandible, similar to those present in the maxilla. In older patients, however, such pores often have reduced dimensions. Consequently, the rate and degree of penetration of the anesthetic solution towards the apices of the mandibular front teeth are reduced and the anesthetic effect obtained by injections in the buccal fold is therefore insufficient. As a rule, analgesia of the teeth and the soft and hard tissues of the mandible should be obtained by a mandibular blockade injection made on the side scheduled for surgery, supplemented by an infiltration anesthesia at the mental foramen of the contralateral side.

The periodontal tissues on the buccal side of the mandible are anesthetized by blocking the buccal nerve with an injection made at the lateral side of the mandible, preferably at the level of the second or third molar. The lingual periodontal tissues are anesthetized by blocking the lingual nerve, either by a blockade close to the mandibular foramen, often made in connection with the mandibular blockade, or by an injection in the floor of the mouth close to the site of operation. Supplementary injections to obtain proper ischemia of the gingival tissues may be made in the interdental papillae. It should be observed that the lag time between the injection and the establishment of proper analgesia after a mandibular blockade is significantly longer (about 3-5 min) than following infiltration injections in the maxillary jaw.

Local anesthetic solutions used in periodontal surgery

All local anesthetic procedures should aim at using the lowest dose of the least concentrated solution. Proper analgesia for periodontal treatment procedures can almost always be obtained with a 2% solution of lidocaine containing 10-12.5 mg adrenaline/ml. Some clinicians may advocate the use of a higher epinephrine concentration (20 mg/ml) but such a highly concentrated solution may only result in a marginal increase of the duration of the analgesia. The high epinephrine content may, however, increase the risk for side effects, especially if the solution is inadvertently injected intravascularly in a patient with circulatory disorders.

Provided proper lege artis measures are followed a 2% lidocaine solution (epinephrine concentration 10-12.5 mg/ml) can be safely used in all healthy patients. Prior to

injection of any anesthetic solution carefu aspiration must be performed. The injec tions must be made slowly so that an adverse systemic effects induced by the dru can be observed and counteracted before th entire dosage has been administered.

Concluding remarks

Many of the technical problems experiencee in periodontal surgery stem from the dif ficulties in assessing accurately the degre and type of breakdown that has occurree prior to surgery. Furthermore, at the time o surgery, previously undiagnosed defect may be recognized or some defects may hav a more complex outline than initially antici pated. Since each of the surgical procedure described above is designed to deal with specific situation or to meet a certain objec tive, it must be understood that no singl standardized technique alone can be appliee when periodontal surgery is undertaken in given patient. Therefore, in each surgica field, different techniques are often used an combined in such a way that the overa objectives of the surgical part of th periodontal therapy are met. The relativ importance of surgical therapy in the overa treatment of periodontal disease as well a the outcome of the various techniques is dis cussed in Chapter 24.

References

Ariaudo, A. A. & Tyrrell, H. A. (1957) Repositioning and increasing the zone of attached gingiva. *Journal of Periodontology* **28**, 106-110.

Caton, J., Nyman, S. & Zander, H. (1980) Histometric evaluation of periodontal surgery. II. Connective tissue attachment levels after four regenerative procedures. *Journal of Clinical Periodontology* **7**, 224-231.

Caton, J. G. & Zander, H. A. (1976) Osseous repair of an infrabony pocket without new

attachment of connective tissue. *Journal o Clinical Periodontology* **3**, 54-58.

Engler, W. O., Ramfjord, S. P. & Hiniker, J. J (1966) Healing following simple gingivectomy A tritiated thymidine radioautographic study I. Epithelialization. *Journal of Periodontolog* **37**, 298-308.

Friedman, N. (1955) Periodontal osseous surge ry: Osteoplasty and ostectomy. *Journal o Periodontology* **26**, 257-269.

Friedman, N. (1962) Mucogingival surgery. The apically repositioned flap. *Journal of Periodontology* **33**, 328-340.

Goldman, H. M. (1950) Development of physiologic gingival contours by gingivoplasty. *Oral Surgery, Oral Medicine and Oral Pathology* **3**, 879-888.

Goldman, H. M. (1951) Gingivectomy. *Oral Surgery, Oral Medicine and Oral Pathology* **4**, 1136-1157.

Grant, D. A., Stern, I. B. & Everett, F. G. (1979) *Periodontics in the Tradition of Orban and Gottlieb.* 5th ed. St. Louis: C.V. Mosby Co.

Hamp, S-E., Rosling, B. & Lindhe, J. (1975) Effect of chlorhexidine on gingival wound healing in the dog. A histometric study. *Journal of Clinical Periodontology* **2**, 143-152.

Haugen, E., Gjermo, P. & Ørstavik, D. (1977) Some antibacterial properties of periodontal dressings. *Journal of Clinical Periodontology* **4**, 62-68.

Karring, T., Cumming, B. R., Oliver, R. C. & Löe, H. (1975) The origin of granulation tissue and its impact on postoperative results of mucogingival surgery. *Journal of Periodontology* **46**, 577-585.

Kirkland, O. (1931) The suppurative periodontal pus pocket; its treatment by the modified flap operation. *Journal of the American Dental Association* **18**, 1462-1470.

Nabers, C. L. (1954) Repositioning the attached gingiva. *Journal of Periodontology* **25**, 38-39.

Neumann, R. (1920) Die Alveolar-Pyorrhöe und ihre Behandlung. 3rd ed. Berlin: Herman Meusser.

Neumann, R. (1926) The radical surgical treatment of the so-called pyorrhea alveolaris and other diseases of the mouth. *Medical Journal and Record,* 671-673.

O'Neil, T. C. A. (1975) Antibacterial properties of periodontal dressings. *Journal of Periodontology.* **46**, 469-474.

Plüss, E. M., Engelberger, P. R. & Rateitschak, K. H. (1975) Effect of chlorhexidine on dental plaque formation under periodontal pack. *Journal of Clinical Periodontology* **2**, 136-142.

Polson, A. M. & Heijl, L. (1978) Osseous repair in infrabony periodontal defects. *Journal of Clinical Periodontology* **5**, 13-23.

Ramfjord, S. P. & Costich, E. R. (1968) Healing after exposure of periosteum on the alveolar process. *Journal of Periodontology* **38**, 199-207.

Ramfjord, S. P., Engler, W. O. & Hiniker, J. J. (1966) A radioautographic study of healing following simple gingivectomy. II. The connective tissue. *Journal of Periodontology* **37**, 179-189.

Ramfjord, S. P. & Nissle, R. R. (1974) The modified Widman flap. *Journal of Periodontology* **45**, 601-607.

Robicsek, S. (1884) Ueber das Wesen und Entstehen der Alveolar-Pyorrhöe und deren Behandlung. The 3rd Annual Report of the Austrian Dental Association. Reviewed 1965 in *Journal of Periodontology* **36**, 265.

Robinson, R. E. (1966) The distal wedge operation. *Periodontics* **4**, 256-264.

Rosling, B., Nyman, S. & Lindhe, J. (1976) The effect of systemic plaque control on bone regeneration in infrabony pockets. *Journal of Clinical Periodontology* **3**, 38-53.

Schluger, S. (1949) Osseous resection – a basic principle in periodontal surgery? *Oral Surgery, Oral Medicine and Oral Pathology* **2**, 316-325.

Stahl, S. S., Witkin, G. J., Cantor, M. & Brown, R. (1968) Gingival healing. II. Clinical and histologic repair sequences following gingivectomy. *Journal of Periodontology* **39**, 109-118.

Waerhaug, J. (1955) Microscopic demonstration of tissue reaction incident to removal of subgingival calculus. *Journal of Periodontology* **26**, 26-29.

Widman, L. (1918) The operative treatment of pyorrhea alveolaris. A new surgical method. *Svensk Tandläkaretidskrift.* Reviewed 1920 in *British Dental Journal* **1**, 293.

Wood, D. L., Hoag, P. M., Donnenfeld, O. W. & Rosenfeld, L. D. (1972) Alveolar crest reduction following full and partial thickness flaps. *Journal of Periodontology* **42**, 141-144.

Zentler, A. (1918) Suppurative gingivitis with alveolar involvement. A new surgical procedure. *Journal of the American Medical Association* **71**, 1530-1534.

CHAPTER 18

Mucogingival Surgery

Significance of the width of keratinized gingiva for maintenance of periodontal health

For many years the presence of an adequate zone of keratinized and attached gingiva has been considered important for the maintenance of gingival health and for the preclusion of loss of connective tissue attachment (Nabers 1954, Friedman & Levine 1960, Ochsenbein 1960, Carranza & Carraro 1970, Hall 1977, Matter 1982). A narrow zone of gingiva was generally thought incapable of withstanding the frictional forces encountered during mastication, and of dissipating the pull from the muscles of the adjacent alveolar mucosa (Friedman 1957, Friedman & Levine 1960, Ochsenbein 1960). It has also been suggested that a narrow gingiva in association with a shallow vestibular fornix may impede proper oral hygiene and that the accumulation of debris during mastication may be favored in such areas (Gottsegen 1954, Rosenberg 1960, Corn 1962, Carranza & Carraro 1970).

Various opinions have been expressed regarding what should be considered an "adequate" width of gingiva. Some authors hold the opinion that less than 1 mm of attached gingiva is sufficient (Bowers 1963) others have claimed that the width of keratinized gingiva ought to exceed at least 2 mm (Corn 1962). Others again have stated that any width of gingiva which is compatible with gingival health is acceptable (Friedman 1962, De Trey & Bernimoulin 1980).

The various opinions about the need of keratinized or attached gingiva are based mainly on clinical experience rather than scientific evidence. It was the impression that sites with a narrow gingival zone, as seen in Fig. 18-1 were more often inflamed than sites with a wider gingiva. A narrow gingiva may occur generally in a group of teeth, or on the buccal or lingual aspect of single teeth, often in association with localized gingival recession (Fig. 18-2).

A narrow zone of gingiva apical to a gingival recession is often considered as the cause of the recession rather than the effect of its development (for review see Hall 1981). However, it is reasonable to assume that before the development of the recession, the gingiva at such a site had a width that was equal to the depth of the defect or was similar to the width of the gingiva at neighboring teeth where no gingival recession has developed (Fig. 18-2). This means that a narrow zone of gingiva cannot be the etiological factor in the development of localized gingival recessions. Therefore, the rationale for increasing the width of the attached gingiva, apical to a recession, in order to prevent its further regression seems obscure. In this context it should be realized that malalignment of teeth in combination with faulty tooth brushing has been associated with the occurrence of such defects (Woofter 1969).

A few studies have been reported in which attempts have been made to evaluate the sig-

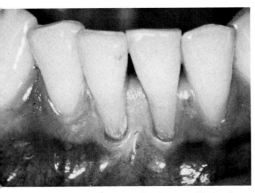

Fig. 18-1. A clinical photograph of a mandibular front tooth region. The gingiva on the buccal aspect of teeth 41 and 31 has an "insufficient" width and shows more inflammation than adjacent gingival units with a wider zone of gingiva.

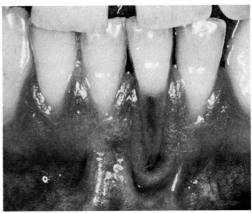

Fig. 18-2. A clinical photograph illustrating a localized gingival recession on the buccal aspect of tooth 41.

nificance of a narrow gingival zone. One of these studies was carried out by Lang & Löe (1972) on dental students who had their teeth professionally cleaned once a day for 6

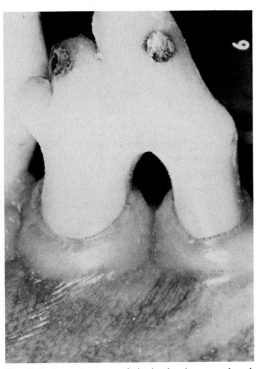

Fig. 18-3. A narrow zone of gingiva has been produced experimentally in a dog by gingivectomy.

weeks. The width of the gingiva of all teeth was then measured and related to the status of the various gingival units. It was found that, in contrast to units with a width of more than 2 mm of keratinized gingiva, units with a width of less than 2 mm of such gingiva (i.e. 1 mm of attached gingiva) were never completely healthy, despite the absence of bacterial plaque. Miyasato et al. (1977) on the other hand, failed to observe any difference in clinical inflammation between areas with a minimal (< 1 mm) and appreciable (> 2 mm) width of keratinized gingiva in 16 experimental subjects exercising proper oral hygiene. When these individuals ceased oral hygiene for a period of 25 days, there was no difference in the development of clinical inflammation between areas with a minimal and those with an appreciable width of the keratinized gingiva.

The role of keratinized gingiva for gingival health has been studied by Wennström et al. (1981, 1982). Following experimentally induced periodontal breakdown around premolar and molar teeth in dogs, the resulting periodontal pockets were eliminated by a gingivectomy or a flap procedure. Healing following the gingivectomy procedure resulted almost consistently in a narrow zone of keratinized gingiva (Fig. 18-3), while the

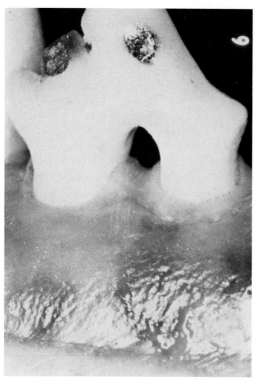

Fig. 18-4. Control site following treatment with a flap procedure. The preoperative width of the gingiva was not significantly altered by the surgical procedure.

flap procedure did not significantly alter the preoperative width of the gingiva (Fig. 18-4). These latter areas were used as representatives for areas with a wide gingival zone,

together with untreated control sites which had not been subjected to periodontal tissue breakdown or surgery.

When after the healing period, plaque was allowed to accumulate freely for 40 days signs of clinical inflammation developed which were more pronounced in tooth regions with a narrow zone of gingiva (Fig. 18-5), than in areas with a wide gingival zone (Fig. 18-6). However, histologic analysis revealed that although areas with a narrow zone of gingiva exhibited more redness than areas with a wide gingival zone, the size of the infiltrated connective tissue portion was similar in the 2 categories of gingiva. The thickness of the free gingiva in buccolingual direction, however, was smaller in specimens with a narrow zone of gingiva than in specimens with a wider gingival zone. The thickness of the keratin layer of the oral epithelium covering the narrow gingiva zones, was also comparatively thinner than that of the wider gingival zones. These observations explained why the narrow gingival zones clinically appeared more inflamed than the wider ones, despite the fact that no differences were observed between the groups regarding the size and extension of the infiltrated zone of the connective tissue. Thus, the results of this study do not lend support to the view that a narrow zone of keratinized gingiva is less resistant to plaque infection than a wide gingival zone. In addi-

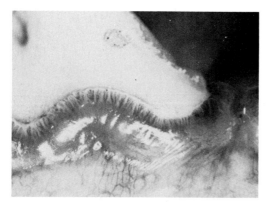

Fig. 18-5. A zone of narrow gingiva showing more pronounced clinical signs of inflammation than a wider zone after 40 days of plaque accumulation.

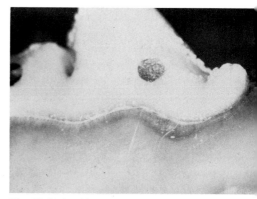

Fig. 18-6. A wide zone of gingiva displaying clinical signs of inflammation after 40 days of plaque accumulation.

tion it was observed that, in the absence of microbial plaque, the gingival units were free from signs of inflammation irrespective of the width of the keratinized gingiva.

Modalities of surgical therapy

The "treatment" of areas with a narrow gingival zone or with localized gingival recession must, like all other conditions associated with destructive periodontal disease, include the removal of hard and soft bacterial deposits from the teeth and be followed by proper plaque control measures. However, on the basis of the assumption that a narrow zone of gingiva is incompatible with gingival health, various surgical techniques have been employed and modified for increasing the width of keratinized gingiva and/or for deepening the vestibular sulcus. These procedures, which are included in the term "mucogingival surgery", are used either in combination with elimination of periodontal pockets which extend beyond the mucogingival junction, or for increasing an "insufficient" width of gingiva in areas without pocket formation. The earliest of these techniques are the "vestibular extension operations" which were designed mainly with the objective of extending the depth of the vestibular sulcus (Bohannan 1962a, b). In recent years, however, the use of pedicle, soft tissue grafts and free gingival grafts have become more common in the management of mucogingival problems (for review see Hall 1981).

Vestibular extension operations

The vestibular extension operations comprise a number of surgical techniques, which have been developed mainly on an empirical basis and without sufficient knowledge about the biology of the involved tissues. The treatment includes the removal of the soft tissue within an area extending from the

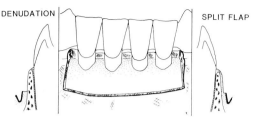

Fig. 18-7. The use of vestibular extension operations for increasing the width of the gingiva involves the production of a wound extending from the gingival margin to a level some mm apical to the mucogingival junction. With the "denudation" technique all soft tissue is removed leaving the alveolar bone exposed. With the "split flap" procedure only the superficial portion of the oral mucosa is removed leaving the bone covered with connective tissue.

gingival margin to a level apical to the mucogingival junction (Fig. 18-7). With the "denudation technique" all soft tissue is removed within the wound area leaving the alveolar bone completely exposed (Ochsenbein 1960, Corn 1962, Wilderman 1964).

Healing following this type of treatment often results in an increased width of the gingival zone, although in some cases only a very limited effect is observed. The exposure of alveolar bone produces severe bone resorption with permanent loss of bone height (Wilderman et al. 1961, Costich & Ramfjord 1968). In addition, the recession of marginal gingiva in the surgical area often exceeds the gain of gingiva obtained in the apical portion of the wound (Carranza & Carraro 1963, Carraro et al. 1964). Due to these complications together with severe postoperative pain for the patient, the use of the "denudation technique" for the management of mucogingival problems can hardly be justified.

With the "periosteal retention" procedure or "split flap" procedure (Fig. 18-7) only the superficial portion of the oral mucosa within the wound area is removed, leaving the bone covered by periosteum (Staffileno et al. 1962, 1966, Wilderman 1963, Pfeifer 1965). Although the preservation of the periosteum implies that less severe bone resorption will occur than following the "denudation technique", loss of crestal bone height has also been observed following this type of operation unless a relatively thick layer of connective tissue is retained on the bone surface (Costich & Ramfjord 1968). If a thick layer is not secured, the periosteal connective tissue tends to undergo necrosis and the subsequent healing will closely resemble that following the denudation technique described above.

Other vestibular extension operations or mucogingival procedures, which have been used for increasing the width of the gingival zone, may in fact be considered as modifications of the "denudation" and "split flap" techniques or combinations of these procedures. The apically repositioned flap procedure (Friedman 1962), for instance, involves the elevation of soft tissue flaps and their displacement during suturing in an apical position, often leaving 3-5 mm of alveolar bone denuded in the coronal part of the surgical area. This involves the same risk for extensive bone resorption as the "denudation technique". It has been reported that a predictable postsurgical result with respect to increase of the width of the gingiva may be obtained following the "apically repositioned flap" technique (Friedman 1962), while other studies have indicated that the presurgical width is retained or becomes only slightly increased (Donnenfeld et al. 1964, Carranza & Carraro 1970).

The use of vestibular extension operations for increasing the width of the gingival zone is based on the assumption that it is the frictional forces encountered during mastication which determine the presence of a keratinized gingiva adjacent to the teeth (Orban 1957, Pfeifer 1963). Therefore, it was believed that by the displacement of muscle attachments and the extension of vestibular depth, the regenerating tissue in the surgical area would be subjected to physical impacts and adapt to the same functional requirements as those met by "normal" keratinized gingiva (Ivancie 1957, Bradley et al. 1959, Pfeifer 1963). Later studies, however, have shown that the characteristic features of the gingiva are determined by some inherent factors in the tissue, rather than the result of functional adaptation and that the differentiation (keratinization) of the gingival epithelium is controlled by morphogenetic stimuli from the underlying connective tissue (see Chapter 1).

Healing

Since the specificity of the gingiva is determined by some inherent factor in the tissues, the postoperative results of vestibular extension procedures depend on the degree to which the various tissues contribute to the formation of granulation tissue in the wound area (Karring et al. 1975). Following the "denudation" or "split flap technique", the wound area is filled with granulation tissue derived from the periodontal ligament, the tissue of the bone marrow spaces, the retained periosteal connective tissue, and the surrounding gingiva and alveolar mucosa (Fig. 18-8). The degree of bone resorption induced by the surgical trauma influences the relative amount of granulation tissue which grows into the wound from these various tissue sources. The resorption of crestal bone exposes varying amounts of the periodontal ligament tissue in the marginal area allowing granulation tissue from the periodontal ligament to fill out the coronal portion of the wound. The greater the bone loss, the greater is the portion of the wound which becomes filled with granulation tissue from the periodontal ligament. This particular tissue possesses the capacity to induce keratinization of the gingival epithelium. This means that the widening of the keratinized gingiva following "denudation" and "split flap" operations is achieved at the expense of a reduced bone height. The "denudation technique" usually results in more bone loss than the "split flap technique". Therefore, a greater amount of granulation tissue capable of inducing a keratinized gingival epithelium develops in the marginal area following the "denudation technique" than following the "split flap technique". This is in accordance with the clinical observation that the "denudation

SPLIT FLAP

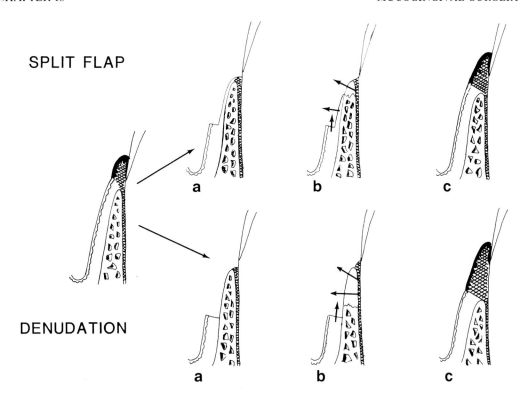

DENUDATION

Figs. 18-8a-c. Schematic drawing illustrating different stages of healing following the "split flap" and "denudation" techniques (a). Cells from the oral mucosa, bone and periodontal ligament (arrows) participate in granulation tissue formation. Due to the difference in the degree of bone resorption (b), a larger area of the coronal portion of the wound is filled with granulation tissue from the periodontal ligament following "denudation" than following the "split flap" technique. Since granulation tissue from the periodontal ligament possesses the ability to induce a keratinized epithelium, "denudation" usually results in a wider zone of keratinized gingiva than is the case following the "split flap" technique (c).

technique" is usually superior to the "split flap technique" in increasing the width of keratinized gingiva (Bohannan 1962a, b).

It is concluded that the success or failure to extend the width of keratinized gingiva by the "denudation" or "split flap" techniques rests with the origin of granulation tissue which is related to the extent of bone loss induced by the surgical trauma. This, in turn, means that the result with respect to increasing the gingival width by methods involving periosteal exposure or denudation of the alveolar bone is unpredictable. The use of such methods is therefore not justified in periodontal therapy. The procedures discussed represent examples on how lack of knowledge about basic biological principles may lead to the development of inappropriate therapeutic methods.

In the study by Wennström et al. (1981), periodontal pockets were produced in dogs. Some of these pockets were eliminated by means of a "gingivectomy" procedure which involved the complete removal of the keratinized gingiva. Following removal of the gingiva, a close adaptation of the alveolar mucosa to the teeth was secured by placing interproximal and inter-radicular sutures (Fig. 18-9). Healing, however, resulted consistently in the reformation of a narrow zone

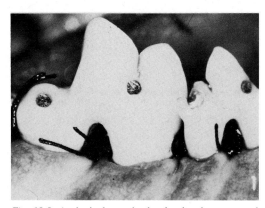

Fig. 18-9. A gingival area in the dog has been treated with gingivectomy involving complete removal of the keratinized gingiva. A close adaptation of the alveolar mucosa to the teeth is ensured by sutures.

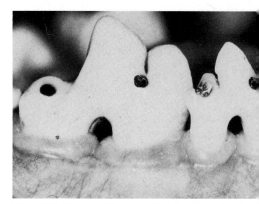

Fig. 18-10. The area illustrated in Fig. 18-9, after heal ing. A narrow zone of gingiva has formed around eac single root.

of keratinized gingiva adjacent to the teeth (Fig. 18-10). Such a gingiva was formed because granulation tissue from the periodontal ligament capable of inducing a keratinized epithelium had proliferated coronally along the tooth surface.

Transplantation of gingiva and palatal mucosa

Studies have shown that gingival and palatal soft tissues maintain their original characteristics after transplantation to areas of the alveolar mucosa (see Chapter 1). Thus, in contrast to vestibular extension operations, the use of transplants offers potential predictability of the postsurgical result following treatment of areas with a narrow gingival zone. For that reason, transplants have become commonly used in the treatment of mucogingival problems in recent years (Haggerty 1966, Nabers 1966, Sullivan & Atkins 1968a, b, Hawley & Staffileno 1970, Edel 1974, Matter 1982). The type of transplant used can be divided into (1) pedicle grafts, which after placement at the recipient site maintain their connection with the donor site and (2) free grafts which are completely deprived of their connection with the donor area.

Pedicle grafts

Laterally repositioned flaps were introduced in periodontal therapy to cover areas with localized gingival recession and to gain keratinized or attached gingiva (Grupe & Warren 1956). This technique involved the reflection of a full thickness flap in a donor area adjacent to the defect and the subse quent displacement of this flap to cover the exposed root surface. More recent modifica tions of this technique (Staffileno 1964 Pfeifer & Heller 1971) utilize a split thick ness flap in order to prevent recession of the gingiva at the donor site.

The surgical procedure is initiated with the preparation of the recipient site (Fig. 18 11). A reverse bevel incision is made al along the gingival margin of the defect (Fig 18-11a). After removal of the dissected poc ket epithelium, the exposed root surface is thoroughly curetted. At a distance o approximately 3 mm from the wound edge which delineates the defect at the side oppo site the donor site, a superficial incision is performed extending from the gingival mar gin to a level approximately 3 mm apical to the defect (Fig. 18-11b). Another superficia incision is then placed horizontally from thi incision to the opposite wound edge (Fig. 18 11b). The epithelium and the outer portion of the connective tissue within the area delineated by these incisions and the wound edges is removed by sharp dissection (Fig. 18-11c). In this way a 3 mm wide recipient bed is created at the one side of the defect, and apically to it (Fig. 18-11c).

After preparation of the recipient site, a tissue flap to cover the recession is dissected in the adjacent donor area. The preparation of this flap is initiated by a vertical superficial incision placed parallel to the wound edge of the adjacent donor site and at a distance which exceeds the width of the recipient bed by approximately 3 mm (Fig. 18-11c). This incision is extended apically to the apical level of the recipient bed and is terminated within the alveolar mucosa with an oblique releasing incision directed towards the gingival recession (Fig. 18-11c). An incision, connecting the vertical incision and the incision previously made around the gingival recession, is placed along the gingival margin of the donor site. A split thickness flap is then prepared by sharp dissection within the area delineated by these incisions (Fig. 18-11d) so that a thin layer of connective tissue is covering the bone in the donor area when the flap is laterally displaced over the denuded root

surface and sutured (Fig. 18-11e). It is important that the oblique releasing incision is made so far apically that the tissue flap can be placed on the recipient bed without being subjected to tearing forces when adjacent soft tissues are moved.

In sites where the gingival recession is deep, the width of keratinized gingiva in the adjacent donor area is often insufficient for preparation of a flap which can cover the entire defect with keratinized tissue. This implies that by laterally repositioning the flap, only the coronal part of the defect would be covered by keratinized gingiva while the remaining apical part becomes covered by alveolar mucosa. If the gingival tissue necrotizes during healing, this may result in a gingival recession with no keratinized gingiva apical to the defect. In order to avoid this complication, it is often appropriate to place the laterally repositioned flap in such a way that it covers only the most apical portion of the defect. However, the prepared tissue flap can also be rotated about 90° when sutured at the recipient bed (Fig. 18-11f). In this way the entire defect becomes covered by keratinized ging-

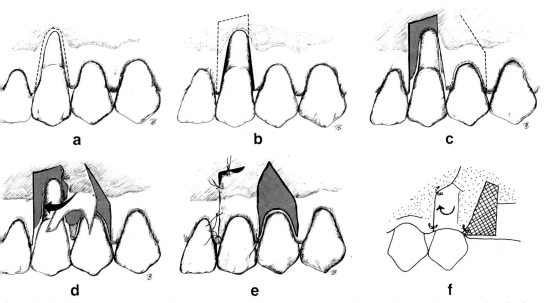

a   b   c

d   e   f

Figs. 18-11a-f. Schematic drawings illustrating the surgical technique for utilizing pedicle grafts to cover localized gingival recessions. Fig. 18-11e illustrates a laterally repositioned flap, and Fig. 18-11f a rotated flap.

iva. Obviously, this rotation of the tissue flap must be prepared during the operation since the width of the tissue flap must in that case be equal to the vertical extension of the defect (Pennel et al. 1965).

After suturing, pressure must be applied against the flap for 2-3 min in order to secure a good adaptation to the underlying recipient bed. Before placement of the periodontal dressing a piece of dry foil is placed over the flap in order to provide a sliding film between the dressing and the graft. This prevents tearing forces being transferred to the graft by movements of the periodontal dressing. The periodontal dressing and the sutures can be removed after 1 week.

Healing

Following the surgical treatment, the laterally repositioned flap is in close contact with the underlying recipient bed only separated from the recipient tissue by a thin fibrin layer. In the areas surrounding the defect, where the recipient bed consists of bone covered by connective tissue, the pattern of healing is similar to that observed following a traditional flap operation. Cells and blood vessels from the recipient bed, as well as from the tissue graft, invade the fibrin layer, which gradually becomes replaced by connective tissue. After 1 week a fibrous reunion is already established between the graft and the underlying tissue.

Healing in the area where the graft is in contact with the denuded root surface has been studied by Wilderman & Wentz (1965) in dogs. According to these authors the healing process can be divided into 4 different stages (Fig. 18-12):

1. The adaptation stage (from 0-4 days).
   The laterally repositioned flap is sepa-

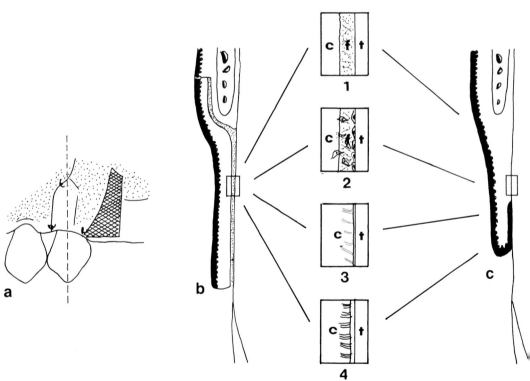

Figs. 18-12a-c. Schematic drawings illustrating healing following treatment of a localized gingival recession with a pedicle graft (a). Fig. 18-12b shows a cross-section through the area immediately after the operation. Fig. 18-12c shows the area after healing. The framed areas (1-4) illustrate the 4 stages into which the healing process can be divided.
c: connective tissue, **f:** fibrin layer, **t:** tooth.

rated from the exposed root surface by a thin fibrin layer. The epithelium covering the transplanted tissue flap starts to proliferate and reaches contact with the tooth surface at the coronal edge of the flap after a few days.

2. The proliferation stage (from 4-21 days).
In the early phase of this stage the fibrin layer between the root surface and the flap is invaded by connective tissue proliferating from the subsurface of the flap. In contrast to areas where healing occurs between 2 connective tissue surfaces, growth of connective tissue into the fibrin layer can only take place from 1 surface. After 6-10 days a layer of fibroblasts is seen in apposition to the root surface. These cells are believed to differentiate into cementoblasts at a later stage of healing. At the end of the proliferation stage, thin collagen fibers are formed adjacent to the root surface, but a fibrous union between the connective tissue and the root has not been observed. From the coronal edge of the wound, epithelium is proliferating apically along the root surface. According to Wilderman & Wentz (1965), the apical proliferation of epithelium may stop within the coronal half of the defect although further downgrowth of epithelium was also frequently observed. Wilderman & Wentz (1965) concluded that it is not the establishment of a fibrous union between the tooth and the flap which arrests the apical migration of the epithelium along the root surface.

3. The attachment stage (from 27-28 days).
During this stage of healing thin collagen fibers become inserted in a layer of new cementum formed at the root surface in the apical portion of the recession.

4. The maturation stage.
This last stage of healing is characterized by continuous formation of collagen fibers. After 2-3 months bundles of collagen fibers are inserting into the cementum layer on the curetted root surface in the apical portion of the recession.

Although there are several publications describing the use of laterally repositioned flaps for the treatment of gingival recession, only a few studies have presented well documented clinical results following this type of therapy (McFull 1968, Sugarman 1969, Guinard & Caffesse 1978). Apparently it is in only a few cases that this type of therapy results in complete coverage of the defect. The possibility of achieving a new connective tissue attachment in the apical portion of the defect seems to be considerably better in narrow gingival recessions than in wider ones. Even if a new connective tissue attachment in all probability fails to form in the entire depth of the defect, the treatment procedure, evidently, rarely, results in the formation of a deep periodontal pocket.

Free grafts

Free grafts of gingiva or palatal mucosa are utilized to increase the zone of gingiva at the buccal or lingual aspect of a single tooth or groups of teeth. In addition, they are used to cover gingival recessions when these are relatively narrow and there is no acceptable donor tissue present in adjacent areas. The principles of utilizing free mucosal grafts were outlined by Sullivan & Atkins (1968a, b).

Like the treatment with pedicle grafts the surgical procedure is initiated with the preparation of the recipient site. A reverse bevel incision is placed at the gingival margin all around the recession (Fig. 18-13a) in order to remove the pocket epithelium (Fig. 18-13b).

After thorough planing of the root surface a 3-4 mm wide recipient bed is prepared around the defect by removing the epithelium, the outer portion of the connective tissue, and muscle fibers (Fig. 18-13c). The free mucosal graft may be obtained from any area having a sufficient quantity of masticatory mucosa (e.g. attached gingiva or palatal mucosa). In order to ensure that a graft of sufficient size and proper contour is removed from the donor area, it is often appropriate to produce a tin foil template over the recipient site. This template is transferred to the donor site where it is out-

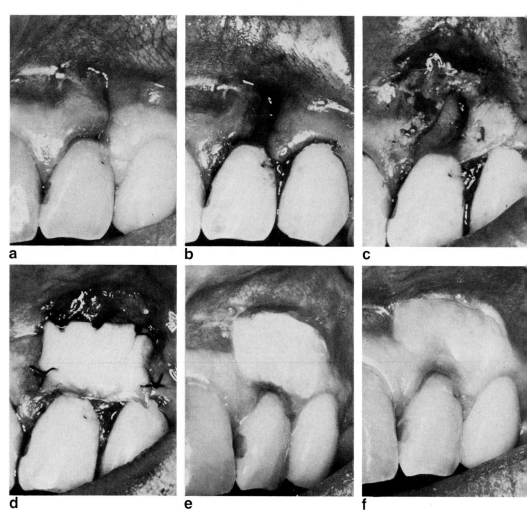

Figs. 18-13a-f. Clinical photographs of a maxillary front tooth region illustrating a narrow gingival recession on the labial aspect of tooth 21 (a). This recession was treated with a free gingival graft. The pocket epithelium all around the defect was removed (b). A recipient bed was then prepared (c). The transplant dissected from the palate was placed in the recipient site and secured by sutures (d). (e) shows the area 14 days and (f) 3 months after treatment.

lined by a shallow incision. A graft with a thickness of 2-3 mm is then dissected from the donor area and placed at the previously prepared recipient bed (Fig. 18-13d). It is advocated that the sutures be placed in the graft before it is cut completely free from the donor area, as this may facilitate its transfer to the recipient site. In order to immobilize the graft at the recipient site, the sutures must be placed in the periosteum or the adjacent attached gingiva (Fig. 18-13d). After suturing, pressure is exerted against the graft for 2-3 min in order to eliminate blood and exudate between the graft and the recipient bed. Before the placement of periodontal dressing a piece of dry foil is placed over the flap. The sutures and periodontal dressing can be removed after 1-2 weeks. A 1-2 week old graft from the palate is shown in Fig. 18-13e immediately after removal of the periodontal dressing. Fig. 18-13f shows the same transplant 3 months after treatment.

Healing

Healing of free gingival grafts placed entirely on a connective tissue recipient bed has been studied in monkeys by Oliver et al. (1968). According to these authors healing can be divided into the following 3 phases (Fig. 18-14):

1. The initial phase (from 0-3 days).
   During these first days of healing a thin layer of exudate is present between the graft and the recipient bed. During this period the grafted tissue survives with an avascular "plasmatic circulation" from the recipient bed. Therefore, it is essential for the survival of the graft that close

contact is established to the underlying recipient bed at the time of operation. A thick layer of exudate or a blood clot may hamper the "plasmatic circulation" and result in the rejection of the graft. The epithelium of the free graft degenerates early in the initial healing phase, and subsequently it becomes desquamated. In placing a graft over a recession, part of the recipient bed will be the avascular root surface. Since the graft is dependent on the nature of its bed for diffusion of plasma and subsequent revascularization, the utilization of free grafts in the treatment of gingival recessions involves

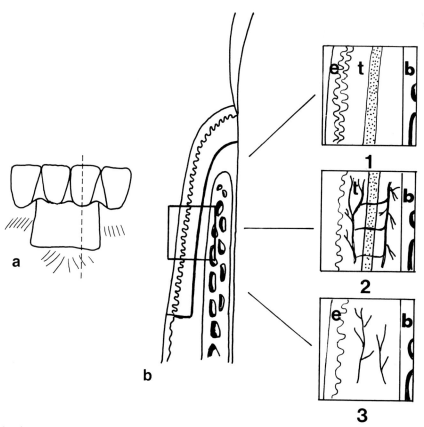

Figs. 18-14a,b. Schematic drawings illustrating healing of a free gingival graft placed entirely on a connective tissue recipient bed (a). A cross-section through the area is shown in (b). The framed areas (1-3) illustrate the 3 phases into which the healing process can be divided.
e: epithelium, t: transplant, b: bone.

a great risk of failure. The area of the graft over the avascular root surface must receive nutrients from the connective tissue bed that surrounds the recession. Thus, the amount of tissue that can be maintained over the root surface is limited by the size of the avascular area. Therefore, it is mainly relatively narrow gingival recessions that can be treated successfully with a free gingival graft.

2. Revascularization phase (from 2-11 days).

After 4-5 days of healing, anastomoses are established between the blood vessels of the recipient bed and those in the grafted tissue. Thus, the circulation of blood is reestablished in the preexisting blood vessels of the graft. The subsequent time period is characterized by capillary proliferation, which gradually results in a dense network of blood vessels in the graft. At the same time a fibrous union is established between the graft and the underlying connective tissue bed. The reepithelialization of the graft occurs mainly by proliferation of epithelium from the adjacent tissues. If a free graft is placed over the denuded root surface, apical migration of epithelium along the root surface may take place at this stage of healing.

3. Tissue maturation phase (from 11-42 days).

During this period the number of blood vessels in the transplant becomes gradually reduced, and after approximately 14 days the vascular system of the graft appears normal. Also, the epithelium gradually matures with the formation of a keratin layer during this stage of healing.

The establishment and maintenance of a "plasmatic circulation" between the recipient bed and the graft during the initial phase of healing is critical to the result of this kind of therapy. Differences between grafts or portions of grafts in their ability to survive transplantation is most probably due to variations in the establishment of an adequate plasmatic diffusion. Therefore, in order to ensure ideal conditions for healing, any

blood lying between the graft and the recipient site must be removed by exerting pressure against the graft following suturing.

The effect of grafting procedures

Although successful treatment of gingival recessions by pedicle grafts or free grafts has been reported in a number of publications (for review see Matter 1982), it is still an open question whether this type of treatment results in the establishment of a new connective tissue attachment to the denuded root surface or a long junctional epithelium facing the root surface.

In a study in dogs, Björn (1961) demonstrated that a new connective tissue attachment could be obtained to the denuded root surface in experimentally produced gingival recessions when infection and migrating epithelial cells were prevented from interfering with healing. Root resorption, however, was also observed.

In a recent study of Nyman et al. (1980) roots deprived of their periodontal ligament tissue and cementum layer were implanted in the jaws of monkeys and dogs in such a way that half their circumference was embedded into bone, while the remaining portion was covered by gingival connective tissue. In this model system, healing never resulted in new attachment formation, but in a passive adaptation of the gingival connective tissue to the root surface. In several specimens considerable resorption had affected the root portions facing the gingival connective tissue. The results of this study were interpreted to indicate that gingival connective tissue cells lack the ability to form a new connective tissue attachment (see Chapter 19). This finding has a particular interest when considering the rationale for the treatment of gingival recessions by free or pedicle gingival grafts. As, in these surgical procedures, gingival connective tissue is placed in contact with a denuded root surface, root resorption should be expected to occur. The reason why this is not a common complication following that type of treatment can be explained by 2 possible events. Either cells from the periodontal ligament migrate coronally, forming a fibrous attachment to the root surface, or epithelial cells proliferate apically, forming a root protective barrier (long junctional epithelium) towards the gingival connective tissue (see Chapter 19). Which type of healing results after treatment of gingival recessions with pedicle grafts or free gingival transplants, is presently not known.

In a recent study, Dorfman et al. (1980) examined the necessity for and effectiveness of, the free gingival grafting procedure in maintaining periodontal attachment. Ninety-two patients with bilateral facial tooth surfaces exhibiting inadequate keratinized gingiva (i.e. less than 2 mm) had a free gingival graft placed on one side, while the opposite side served as the untreated control. Prior to and after surgery, the patients were subjected to scaling and root planing and instruction in oral hygiene measures.

Not surprisingly, the investigators found a significant increase (approximately 4 mm) in the width of keratinized and attached gingiva at the grafted sites. This increased width of gingiva was maintained for a 2 year follow-up period. The attachment level was also maintained throughout this time period. In the control sites the width of keratinized gingiva was less than 2 mm and did not vary significantly during the two years of observation. However, in the ungrafted areas the attachment level was also maintained unchanged during this period. Thus, a narrow zone of gingiva apparently has the same resistance to attachment loss as a wider zone of gingiva. The only result of the grafting procedure was a widening of the gingival zone.

Hangorsky & Bissada (1980) who evaluated the long-term clinical effect of free gingival grafts on the periodontal conditions in 34 patients also failed to observe any difference between grafted and ungrafted sites after from 1-8 years with regard to gingival health and pocket depth. They concluded that "while the free gingival graft is an effective means to widen the zone of the attached and keratinized gingiva, there is no indication that this increase bears direct influence upon periodontal health". This result is in agreement with the findings of De Trey & Bernimoulin (1980), who examined the effect of free gingival grafts in 12 patients with less than 1 mm of attached gingiva on homologous contralateral pairs of mandibular teeth. In this study no significant differences were found in gingival health when test and control sites were compared longitudinally.

Similarly, in a group of 43 patients, monitored for 10-11 years on a careful prophylaxis program, Lindhe & Nyman (1980) found no recession of the gingival margin either in areas where keratinized gingiva was present, or in areas devoid of such tissue. On the contrary, in both types of areas, a small but discernible coronal regrowth of keratinized gingiva occurred.

On the basis of our present knowledge it can be concluded that no scientific data lends support to the hypothesis that neither a narrow zone of gingiva nor localized gingival recessions need further treatment than the control of plaque.

References

Björn, H. (1961) Experimental studies on reattachment. *Dental Practitioner and Dental Records* **11**, 351-354.

Bohannan, H. M. (1962a) Studies in the alteration of vestibular depth. I. Complete denudation. *Journal of Periodontology* **33**, 120-128.

Bohannan, H. M. (1962b) Studies in the alteration of vestibular depth. II. Periosteum retention. *Journal of Periodontology* **33**, 354-359.

Bowers, G. M. (1963) A study of the width of attached gingiva. *Journal of Periodontology* **34**, 201-209.

Bradley, R. E., Grant, J. C. & Ivancie, G. P. (1959) Histologic evaluation of mucogingival surgery. *Oral Surgery* **12**, 1184-1199.

Carranza, F. A. & Carraro, J. J. (1963) Effect of removal of periosteum on post-operative results of mucogingival surgery. *Journal of Periodontology* **34**, 223-226.

Carranza, F. A. & Carraro, J. J. (1970) Mucogingival techniques in periodontal surgery. *Journal of Periodontology* **41**, 294-299.

Carraro, J. J., Carranza, F. A., Albano, E. A. & Joly, G. G. (1964) Effect of bone denudation in mucogingival surgery in humans. *Journal of Periodontology* **35**, 463-466.

Corn, H. (1962) Periosteal separation – Its clinical significance. *Journal of Periodontology* **33**, 140-152.

Costich, E. R. & Ramfjord, S. F. (1968) Healing after partial denudation of the alveolar process. *Journal of Periodontology* **39**, 5-12.

De Trey, E. & Bernimoulin, J. (1980) Influence of free gingival grafts on the health of the marginal gingiva. *Journal of Clinical Periodontology* **7**, 381-393.

Donnenfeld, O. W., Marks, R. M. & Glickman, I. (1964) The apically repositioned flap – a clinical study. *Journal of Periodontology* **35**, 381-387.

Dorfman, H. S., Kennedy, J. E. & Bird, W. C. (1980) Longitudinal evaluation of free autogenous gingival grafts. *Journal of Clinical Periodontology* **7**, 316-324.

Edel, A. (1974) Clinical evaluation of free connective tissue grafts used to increase the width of keratinized gingiva. *Journal of Clinical Periodontology* **1**, 185-196.

Friedman, N. (1957) Mucogingival surgery. *Texas Dental Journal* **75**, 358-362.

Friedman, N. (1962) Mucogingival surgery: The apically repositioned flap. *Journal of Periodontology* **33**, 328-340.

Friedman, N. & Levine, H. L. (1960) Mucogingival surgery: Current status. *Journal of Periodontology* **35**, 5-21.

Gottsegen, R. (1954) Frenulum position and vestibular depth in relation to gingival health. *Oral Surgery* **7**, 1069-1078.

Grupe, J. & Warren, R. (1956) Repair of gingival defects by a sliding flap operation. *Journal of Periodontology* **27**, 290-295.

Guinard, E. A. & Caffesse, R. G. (1978) Treatment of localized gingival recessions. I. Lateral sliding flap. *Journal of Periodontology* **49**, 351-356.

Haggerty, P. C. (1966) The use of a free gingival graft to create a healthy environment for full crown preparation. *Periodontics* **4**, 329-331.

Hall, W. B. (1977) Present status of soft tissue grafting. *Journal of Periodontology* **48**, 587-597.

Hall, W. B. (1981) The current status of mucogingival problems and their therapy. *Journal of Periodontology* **52**, 569-575.

Hangorsky, U. & Bissada, N. B. (1980) Clinical assessment of free gingival graft effectiveness on the maintenance of periodontal health. *Journal of Periodontology* **51**, 274-278.

Hawley, C. E. & Staffileno, H. (1970) Clinical evaluation of free gingival grafts in periodontal surgery. *Journal of Periodontology* **41**, 105-112.

Ivancie, G. P. (1957) Experimental and histological investigation of gingival regeneration in vestibular surgery. *Journal of Periodontology* **28**, 259-263.

Karring, T., Cumming, B. R., Oliver, R. C. & Löe, H. (1975). The origin of granulation tissue and its impact on postoperative results of mucogingival surgery. *Journal of Periodontology* **46**, 577-585.

Lang, N. P. & Löe, H. (1972) The relationship between the width of keratinized gingiva and gingival health. *Journal of Periodontology* **43**, 623-627.

Lindhe, J. & Nyman, S. (1980) Alterations of the position of the marginal soft tissue following periodontal surgery. *Journal of Clinical Periodontology* 7, 525-530.

Matter, J. (1982) Free gingival grafts for the treatment of gingival recession. A review of some techniques. *Journal of Clinical Periodontology* 9, 103-114.

McFull, W. T. (1968) The laterally repositioned flap – criteria for success. *Periodontics* 5, 89-92.

Miyasato, M., Crigger, M. & Egelberg, J. (1977) Gingival condition in areas of minimal and appreciable width of keratinized gingiva. *Journal of Clinical Periodontology* 4, 200-209.

Nabers, C. L. (1954) Repositioning the attached gingiva. *Journal of Periodontology* 25, 38-39.

Nabers, J. M. (1966) Free gingival grafts. *Periodontics* 4, 243-245.

Nyman, S., Karring, T., Lindhe, J. & Plantén, S. (1980) Healing following implantation of periodontitis-affected roots into gingival connective tissue. *Journal of Clinical Periodontology* 7, 394-401.

Ochsenbein, C. (1960) Newer concept of mucogingival surgery. *Journal of Periodontology* 31, 175-185.

Oliver, R. G., Löe, H. & Karring, T. (1968) Microscopic evaluation of the healing and re-vascularization of free gingival grafts. *Journal of Periodontal Research* 3, 84-95.

Orban, B. J. (1957) *Oral Histology and Embryology.* 4th ed., pp. 221-264. St. Louis: C. V. Mosby Company.

Pennel, B. M., Higgison, J. D., Towner, T. D., King, K. O., Fritz, B. D. & Salder, J. F. (1965) Oblique rotated flap. *Journal of Periodontology* 36, 305-309.

Pfeifer, J. S. (1963) The growth of gingival tissue over denuded bone. *Journal of Periodontology* 34, 10-16.

Pfeifer, J. S. (1965) The reaction of alveolar bone to flap procedures in man. *Periodontics* 3, 135-140.

Pfeifer, J. & Heller, R. (1971) Histologic evaluation of full and partial thickness lateral repositioned flaps. A pilot study. *Journal of Periodontology* 42, 331-333.

Rosenberg, N. M. (1960) Vestibular alterations in periodontics. *Journal of Periodontology* 31, 231-237.

Staffileno, H. (1964) Management of gingival recession and root exposure problems associated with periodontal disease. *Dental Clinics of North America,* March, 111.

Staffileno, H., Levy, S. & Gargiulo, A. (1966) Histologic study of cellular mobilization and repair following a periosteal retention operation via split thickness mucogingival surgery. *Journal of Periodontology* 37, 117-131.

Staffileno, H., Wentz, F. & Orban, B. (1962) Histologic study of healing of split thickness flap surgery in dogs. *Journal of Periodontology* 33, 56-69.

Sugarman, E. F. (1969) A clinical and histological study of the attachment of grafted tissue to bone and teeth. *Journal of Periodontology* 40, 381-387.

Sullivan, H. C. & Atkins, J. H. (1968a) Free autogenous gingival grafts. I. Principles of successful grafting. *Periodontics* 6, 121-129.

Sullivan, H. C. & Atkins, J. H. (1968b) Free autogenous gingival grafts. III. Utilization of grafts in the treatment of gingival recession. *Periodontics* 6, 152-160.

Wennström, J., Lindhe, J. & Nyman, S. (1981) Role of keratinized gingiva for gingival health. *Journal of Clinical Periodontology* 8, 311-328.

Wennström, J., Lindhe, J. & Nyman, S. (1982) The role of keratinized gingiva in plaque-associated gingivitis in dogs. *Journal of Clinical Periodontology* 9, 75-85.

Wilderman, M. N. (1963) Repair after a periosteal retention procedure. *Journal of Periodontology* 34, 484-503.

Wilderman, M. N. (1964) Exposure of bone in periodontal surgery. *Dental Clinics of North America,* March, 23-26.

Wilderman, M. N. & Wentz, F. M. (1965) Repair of a dentogingival defect with a pedicle flap. *Journal of Periodontology* 36, 218-231.

Wilderman, M. N., Wentz, F. M. & Orban, B. J. (1961) Histogenesis of repair after mucogingival surgery. *Journal of Periodontology* 31, 283-299.

Woofter, C. (1969) The prevalence and etiology of gingival recessions. *Periodontal Abstracts* 17, 45-49.

Reattachment-New Attachment

Definition

The ultimate goal of periodontal therapy includes not only the arrest of progressive periodontal disease but also the restitution of those parts of the supporting apparatus which have been destroyed, i.e. *restitutio ad integrum.*

Reattachment is a term that has been used to describe the regeneration of tooth supporting structures following therapy. Since, however, the aim of so-called regenerative or reconstructive procedures involves *de novo* formation of connective tissue attachment to root surfaces which during disease progress have lost such attachment, the term *New Attachment* should be preferred (World Workshop in Periodontics 1966).

In this chapter *Reattachment* will be used

to describe *"the reunion of connective tiss* *and root separated by incision or injury"* an *New Attachment* to describe: *"the reunion connective tissue with a root surface whi* *has been pathologically exposed"* (Kalkwa 1974).

New attachment procedures

Root planing and soft tissue curettage

A variety of surgical techniques have be developed and tested for their potential restore periodontal tissues lost in destructi periodontal disease. The first metho describing how to obtain *new attachme* included *scaling* and *root planing* in conjun tion with *soft tissue curettage,* i.e. mechanic removal of the root cementum and the po ket epithelium. Studies in humans (e. Younger 1899, McCall 1926, Beube 194 1952, Orban 1948, Waerhaug 1952, Schaff & Zander 1953, Carranza 1954, 1960) a animals (e.g. Beube 1947, Ramfjord 195 Kon et al. 1969), showed that this type periodontal therapy frequently resulted n only in the establishment of gingival hea but also in a reduction of the initial recorded pocket depths. This decrease in t depth of the periodontal pockets was su gested to be the result partly of shrinkage the initially inflamed gingiva but partly al the effect of the formation of a new conne tive tissue attachment in the apical part the pocket.

Flap procedures

Since the 1950ies, most new attachme attempts, in particular in the treatment angular osseous defects (i.e. infrabony pockets), have besides root planing, also included the elevation of flaps (e.g. Prichard 1957a, b, Patur & Glickman 1962, Wade 1962, 1966, Ellegaard & Löe 1971, Yukna et al. 1976). After elevation of a soft tissue flap (split thickness or full thickness flap) the granulation tissue of the osseous defect is removed and the root surface is carefully scaled and planed. In order to enhance regeneration of bone, small perforations are often made with a bur at several sites of the bony walls. The flap is then sutured to accomplish coverage of the alveolar bone.

Many clinical investigators claimed that new attachment resulted following this type of treatment. Patur & Glickman (1962) reported that bone regeneration and new attachment occurred in 2- and 3-wall infrabony pockets but not in 1-wall pockets. Ellegaard & Löe (1971) presented results from a study comprising 191 lesions in 24 patients with periodontal disease which indicated that after 2-3 years of healing complete regeneration had occurred in around 70% of the 3-wall defects, in 40% of the combined 2- and 3-wall lesions and in 45% of the 2-wall defects. In a study by Rosling et al. (1976) 124 angular bony defects were treated in 12 patients by means of the modified Widman flap procedure (Ramfjord & Nissle 1974). Re-examinations performed 2 years after therapy demonstrated that all osseous defects, irrespective of their initial classification as 2- or 3-wall lesions, were refilled with bone. The authors suggested that this bone fill was indicative of the formation also of new attachment and ascribed the successful healing mainly to the optimal standard of oral hygiene which was accomplished by all patients during healing. (Radiographs illustrating the healing of an infrabony pocket from this study are shown in Fig. 19-1). A similar clinical study with almost identical results (Fig. 19-2) was presented by Polson & Heijl (1978) who concluded: "It appears that infra-bony periodontal defects may predictably remodel throughout their circumferential extent after *surgical debridement and establishment of optimal plaque control".*

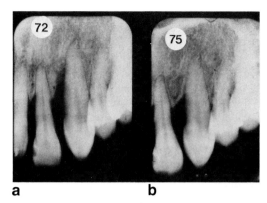

a   **b**

Figs. 19-1a, b. An angular bony defect at the mesial aspect of tooth 23 was in 1972 (a) treated by scaling and root planing in conjunction with a modified Widman flap procedure. Three years after therapy bone repair ("bone fill") had occurred in this site (b).

Grafting procedures

In a number of clinical trials and animal experiments the flap approach has been combined with the insertion of different kinds of implant materials into the curetted bony defects in order to improve healing (e.g. Yuktanandana 1959, Nabers & O'Leary 1965, 1967, Robinson 1969, Schallhorn et al. 1970, Rosenberg 1971, Dragoo & Sullivan 1973a,b, Hiatt & Schallhorn 1973,

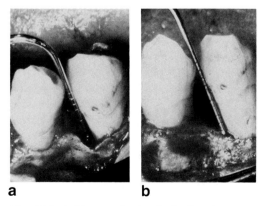

a   **b**

Figs. 19-2a, b. Photographs showing healing of an angular bony defect. The defect at the time of surgery (left) and at reentry after 3 months of healing (right). (From Polson & Heijl 1978).

Froum et al. 1975a,b, 1976, Ellegaard et al. 1976, Hiatt et al. 1978, Dragoo 1981). The various implant materials which have been used so far can be grouped into 4 categories (Gara & Adams 1981):

1. *Autograft:* a graft transferred from one position to another within the same individual:
   a) cortical bone (osseous coagulum)
   b) cancellous bone and marrow obtained either from intra-oral or extra-oral donor sites
   c) combination of cortical and cancellous bone (bone blend).
2. *Allograft:* a graft transferred between genetically dissimilar members of the same species:
   a) viable cancellous bone and marrow
   b) sterilized cancellous bone and marrow
   c) freeze-dried bone.
3. *Heterograft or xenograft:* a graft taken from a donor of another species.
4. Grafts of *bone substitutes* and *synthetic materials.*

The literature suggests that autografts in the form of cancellous bone and hemopoietic marrow establish the most favorable conditions for new attachment during healing after periodontal therapy (Schallhorn 1977, Dragoo 1981). Hiatt et al. (1978) reported that in 66 out of 79 grafted areas new cementum was formed and moved coronally on the root surface while in only 7 out of 21 non-graft cases new cementum was formed. The use of bone and marrow as either autografts or allografts, however, appeared to involve certain risks such as root resorption and ankylosis with the use of fresh material, additional surgical insult to the patient with autografts and possible antigenicity with allografts. Because of such undesired side effects with autografts and allografts, bone substitutes and synthetic materials have been used (Alderman 1969, Levin et al. 1974, Bump et al. 1975, Strub et al. 1979) and reports have been published claiming that healing occurs with the formation of new attachment.

A critical analysis of the literature reveals,

however, that the methods used to induce new attachment are by no means predictable. The inconsistency in the results obtained may be illustrated by the findings of Waerhaug (1952), Schaffer & Zander (1953), Carranza (1954) and Ellegaard & Löe (1971). Waerhaug reported that coronal gain of attachment occurred following subgingival curettage in *only 4 out of 32 treated teeth* while Schaffer & Zander (1953) observed new connective tissue attachment in *5 teeth out of 8.* Carranza (1954) claimed to have obtained new attachment in *41 out of 103 infrabony pockets* following root planing and curettage. Ellegaard & Löe (1971) who used a flap approach claimed that complete regeneration had occurred in *70% of 3-wall pockets,* in *40% of 2- or combined 2- and 3-wall bony lesions,* and that failure resulted in *20-40% of all defects* treated. Also, the effect of grafting procedures in reconstructive therapy shows considerable variation. For extensive review on methods used in new attachment therapy and the results reported, the reader is referred to the review papers by Gara & Adams (1981) and Wirthlin (1981).

Errors inherent in the assessment of new attachment

Clinical means

In recent years criticism has been directed towards the methods which have been used to assess the development of new attachment following therapy. This is particularly the case when the result of treatment has been evaluated by clinical means only, i.e. *attachment level* measurements, *radiographic* analysis and *reentry operations.* The reliability of such clinical methods to determine gain of new attachment is open to criticism.

Periodontal probing
Recent findings by Listgarten et al. (1976), Armitage et al. (1977), van der Velden & de

Vries (1978) and others have demonstrated the inability of periodontal probing to determine accurately the apical termination of the dentogingival epithelium, i.e. the histological or "true" bottom of the pocket. It has been pointed out that improvement of attachment levels following periodontal treatment – assessed by probing – does not necessarily demonstrate the formation of a new connective tissue attachment to the root surface. Rather, improved attachment levels may merely describe the resolution of the inflammatory process within the gingiva without an accompanying "true" gain of attachment, i.e. a connective tissue attachment formed in an area coronal to the level of this attachment before treatment. In other words, the *resolution of the inflammatory lesion in the gingiva will increase the resistance of the tissue to probing*, a phenomenon which clinical probing will identify as an improved attachment level (for a detailed discussion on errors inherent in clinical probing of periodontal pockets see Chapter 12).

Radiograpic analysis – reentry operations
Regeneration of bone tissue ("bone fill"), which frequently occurs within infrabony pockets following so-called reconstructive therapy, has been documented by *measurements* made in *radiographs* obtained in a standardized and reproducible manner and in conjunction with *reentry operations*. Analysis of radiographs obtained of an angular bony defect before and after therapy and inspection of the treated area during a reentry operation can certainly provide evidence for repair of alveolar bone. Such "bone fill", however, does not document the formation of new root cementum and a new periodontal ligament. In fact, it has been demonstrated by Caton & Zander (1976), Moskow et al. (1979) and others that bone regeneration in infrabony pockets can occur opposite a junctional epithelium interposed between the newly formed bone and the curetted root surface. This also means that methods such as radiographic analysis and measurements made at reentry operations are unreliable

for the identification of the formation of new cementum and periodontal ligament tissue.

Histological means

In several studies healing has been analyzed in histological sections of block biopsies obtained after various forms of therapy. In such experiments the location of the attachment level prior to therapy has often been identified by clinical probing. Since it is not possible, however, by clinical means (see above) to identify properly the location of the apical cells of the junctional epithelium, the pretreatment attachment level also in this type of histological material must be regarded as obscure. This means that even combined clinical and histological methods may not be ideal for studying the formation of new connective tissue attachment.

In order to overcome the problem of identifying the attachment level prior to therapy the following method has often been used: after elevation of a soft tissue flap, a notch is prepared in the root surface at the apical level of the periodontal lesion (estimated by clinical inspection). This notch serves as an indicator of the pre-operative attachment level in the biopsy material after therapy. Newly formed cementum and bone present in an area coronal to the notch have been regarded as signs of new attachment (Fig. 19-3). But is this interpretation of such findings correct? For practical reasons, in many studies the notch has not been placed at the apical level of the lesion but at the level of the alveolar bone crest. Will this technique improve the validity of the methods used to identify the pretreatment attachment level?

In a periodontal lesion, accompanied by so-called "horizontal", i.e. even bone loss (Fig. 19-4), there is always an area – around 1 mm high – *between the crest of the supporting alveolar bone and the apical extent of the pocket epithelium* in which the connective tissue fibers are still invested in the root (Waerhaug 1952, 1978). If, following treatment of such a tooth, a connective tissue attachment is found in the biopsy material

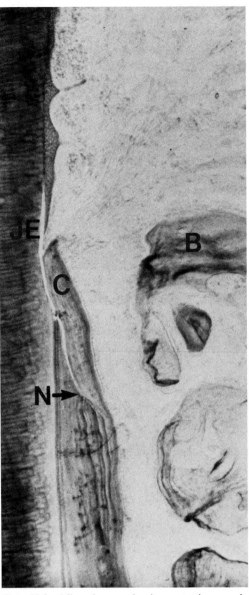

Fig. 19-3. Microphotograph demonstrating newly formed cementum (C) and bone (B) coronal to a notch (N) prepared at the apical level of the periodontal lesion. JE = apical extent of the junctional epithelium. (From Caton & Nyman 1980).

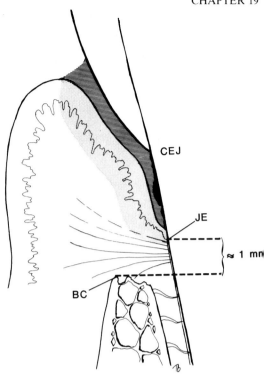

Fig. 19-4. Schematic drawing of a periodontal lesion illustrating the presence of an area with intact connective tissue attachment – ≈ 1 mm high – between the apical extension of the pocket epithelium (JE) and the crest of the supporting alveolar bone (BC).

Further, in sites with infrabony pockets, in which the apical termination of the pocket epithelium is located at some distance apical to the bone crest, a notch prepared in the root surface at the level of the bone crest cannot, of course, serve as a reference for assessments of new attachment within the area of the osseous defect.

From the above discussion it should be understood that most experiments, aimed at assessing the establishment of a new connective tissue attachment following therapy, have suffered from the problem of recognizing properly the attachment level prior to therapy.

within a distance of ≈ 1 mm coronal to the notch this should *not be regarded as a new attachment*. The presence of a connective tissue attachment on the root surface within ≈ 1 mm distance from the bone crest must *be regarded as a reattachment*.

A discriminating animal model

Many efforts have been made to develop research models in which the coronal level of the connective tissue attachment on the root surface both *before* and *after* treatment can be properly assessed. A simple but reliable animal model was finally described (Caton & Zander 1975, Caton & Kowalski 1976), by means of which periodontal lesions of almost identical depth and morphology could be produced around contralateral teeth in the monkey. The periodontal lesions were produced by placing and retaining orthodontic bands of identical size and elasticity around contralateral teeth for the same period of days of undisturbed plaque accumulation (Figs. 19-5 and 19-6). The periodontal lesions, often accompanied by angular bony defects, were treated on one side of the jaw. Healing was studied using the untreated lesions opposite as controls. Hence, in histological sections, differences in the connective tissue attachment levels (measured from the cementoenamel junction) between treated test areas and untreated control areas could be assessed.

Regenerative potential of the periodontal structures

How this model has been used to study the potential of the periodontal tissues to form new attachment will be described below. But first some elementary principles must be outlined regarding wound healing in the periodontium. In 1976, Melcher in a review paper postulated that the cells which repopulate the root surface after surgery determine the nature (quality) of the attachment that will form. This is illustrated in Figs. 19-7a, b.

After a reverse bevel incision and removal of the granulation tissue the curetted root surface may be repopulated by 4 different types of cells namely: epithelial cells, cells from the gingival connective tissue, bone cells and cells from the periodontal ligament.

If the cells from the oral *epithelium* proliferate along the root surface down to the presurgical level of the pocket epithelium, an

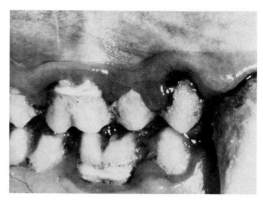

Fig. 19-5. Periodontal tissue breakdown was produced by the placement of orthodontic elastics around the neck of the teeth and by allowing plaque accumulation. Note the swelling of the marginal gingiva. (From Caton & Zander 1975).

epithelial attachment (long junctional epithelium) will result (Fig. 19-8). The contact between the root surface and this long junctional epithelium is maintained by cuticular structures and hemidesmosomes.

If cells from the *gingival connective tissue* populate the root surface, some kind of connective tissue adhesion or attachment between the soft and hard tissue will evidently be established (Fig. 19-9). But do cells from the connective tissue of the gingiva have a

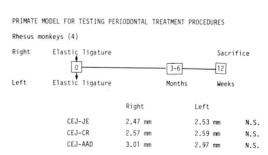

Fig. 19-6. Diagram describing the outline of the experiment. Elastic ligatures (orthodontic elastics) were placed around the teeth on Day 0 and were removed 3-6 months later. The animals were sacrificed 12 weeks after removal of the elastics. Measurements made in histological sections revealed that pockets of almost identical depth and morphology had been produced around contralateral teeth. (From Caton & Kowalski 1976).

415

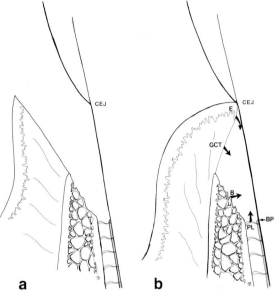

Figs. 19-7a, b. Schematic drawings illustrating the wound after flap elevation and removal of plaque, calculus, pocket epithelium and infiltrated portions of connective tissue (a). The cells which repopulate the wound determine the quality of the attachment (b); epithelial cells (E), gingival connective tissue cells (GCT), bone cells (B), periodontal ligament cells (PL). BP = preoperative bottom of the pocket.

potential to form new cementum and a new fibrous attachment?

If *bone cells* are migrating into contac with the curetted root, surface root resorp tion and ankylosis can occur (Fig. 19-10) But do bone cells have the potential t stimulate the formation of cementum and periodontal ligament fibers?

Ideal conditions of healing may develop i situations where *cells from the periodonta ligament* proliferate in coronal direction t cover the previously diseased root surfac (Fig. 19-11). Such cells have the capacity t form cementum and periodontal ligamen fibers. But is it possible to obtain coloniza tion of such cells on a *root surface* which ha been 1) exposed to a periodontal pocket an 2) instrumented during scaling and roo planing?

Epithelium

The monkey model (Caton & Kowalski 1976) has been used by Caton and coworker (1980) to study the healing of the periodon

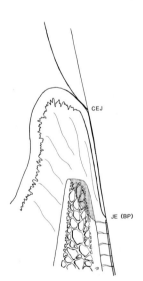

Fig. 19-8. Epithelial attachment — long junctional epithelium — which has formed during healing. JE = apical extent of the junctional epithelium. BP = preoperative level of the pocket epithelium. Shadowed area = bone repair.

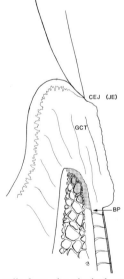

Fig. 19-9. If cells from the gingival connective tissu (GCT) repopulate the root surface, the attachmen occurs in the form of connective tissue adhesion. I addition, root resorption may occur. Shadowed area bone repair.

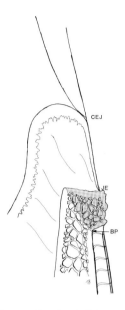

Fig. 19-10. If bone cells migrate into contact with the scaled root surface, root resorption and ankylosis occur. JE = apical extent of the junctional epithelium. BP = preoperative level of the pocket epithelium.

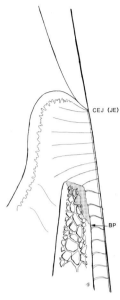

Fig. 19-11. Ideal conditions for healing may develop if cells from the periodontal ligament proliferate to cover the denuded root surface.

tal structures after different modalities of periodontal therapy. The lesions in the test sites were subjected to 1) periodic root planing and soft tissue curettage, 2) root planing in combination with the *modified Widman flap operation without osseous surgery,* 3) root planing in combination with the modified Widman flap operation without osseous surgery but with *implantation into the defects of previously frozen autogenous, red marrow and cancellous bone and* 4) root planing in combination with the modified Widman flap operation without osseous surgery but with *implantation of a bone substitute, beta tricalcium phosphate.*

Histometric measurements made in sections from block biopsies demonstrated that healing following all 4 treatment procedures resulted in the reformation of a long junctional epithelium facing the instrumented root surfaces with *no* sign of new connective tissue attachment. The apical cells of the junctional epithelium were consistently located at or close to their presurgical level in all teeth treated (Figs. 19-12a, b), i.e. at the same level as in the untreated control lesions. This development of a long junctional epithelium occurred in sites with suprabony as well as in sites with infrabony pockets. The findings by Caton & Nyman (1980) and Caton et al. (1980) have been confirmed by Yukna (1976) and Nyman et al. (1981) in similar experiments.

The results of the studies referred to should not, however, be interpreted to mean that the formation of a new connective tissue attachment is impossible. They only demonstrate that new attachment formation is inhibited by the apically migrating dentogingival epithelium. During periodontal wound healing the proliferating epithelial cells reach the presurgical level of the pocket epithelium about 1 week following surgery (Moskow 1964, Kon et al. 1969, Proye & Polson 1982, Karring et al. 1983). This rapid proliferation of the epithelium prevents the gingival con-

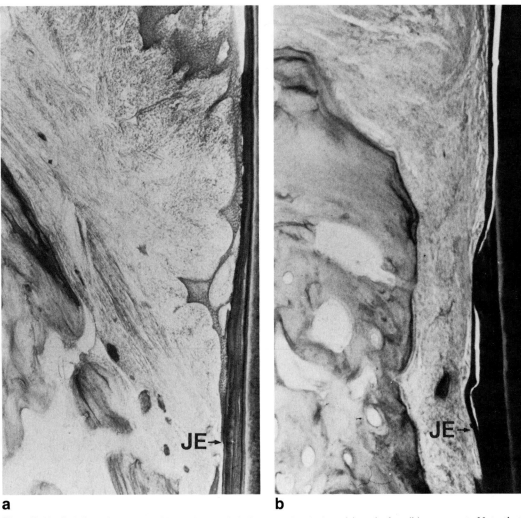

a   b

Figs. 19-12a, b. Microphotographs illustrating an infrabony pocket before (a) and after (b) treatment. Note that "bone fill" has occurred but also that the epithelium has migrated apically to the same level as its apical extension before treatment. JE = apical extent of the junctional epithelium. (From Caton & Nyman 1980).

nective tissue from establishing a close contact with the root surface. *An early contact between the gingival connective tissue and the root has been regarded as the prime prerequisite for the formation of a new attachment* (Björn 1961, Björn et al. 1965, Hiatt et al. 1968). Björn (1961) also claimed that complete new attachment with reorganization of root cementum, periodontal membrane and alveolar bone would be obtained following periodontal therapy provided the epithelium could be excluded from the healing wound, and proper contact between the gingival

connective tissue and the root surface was thereby enabled.

Gingival connective tissue and alveolar bone

In order to evaluate whether the exclusion of the epithelium during healing would in fact result in new attachment, the following experiment was carried out (Nyman et al. 1980). Periodontal tissue breakdown was produced around certain "experimental"

418

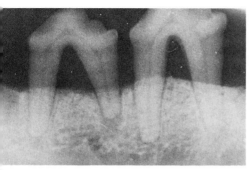

Fig. 19-13. Radiograph of mandibular dog premolars showing destruction of the alveolar bone to approximately half the length of the roots.

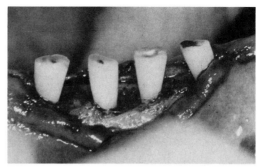

Fig. 19-14. Photograph of experimental roots following separation. Scaling and root planing of the coronal, diseased portions of the separated roots have been carried out.

teeth in monkeys and dogs using the method described by Caton & Kowalski (1976). When the destruction of the supporting tissues had progressed to approximately half the length of the roots (Fig. 19-13), the plaque collecting ligatures were removed. Other teeth in the dentition were extracted to provide space (recipient sites) for subsequent implantation of the diseased roots of the experimental teeth (see below).

Following removal of the ligatures the crowns of the experimental teeth were resected. Full thickness flaps were raised at the facial and oral aspects of the teeth, and the denuded (diseased) parts of the root surfaces were thoroughly scaled and planed (Fig. 19-14). Notches were prepared in the roots at the level of the marginal bone crest.

At each recipient site a full thickness flap was prepared. Grooves, corresponding in size to the roots to be implanted, were prepared in the buccal surface of the jaw bone (Fig. 19-15). The roots of the experimental teeth were extracted and placed in the grooves in the alveolar bone. The flaps were repositioned and sutured to complete coverage of the implanted root and the surrounding bone. With this experimental design, each implanted root was embedded to half its circumference into bone, and the remaining part was covered by the gingival connective tissue of the flap (Fig. 19-16). The epithelium was prevented from migrating into the wound.

After 3 months of healing, the implanted roots with surrounding tissue were harvested and subjected to histological analysis. This analysis revealed the following: in the apical, "nondiseased", portion of the roots, both on the side facing gingival connective tissue and on the side facing bone, there was a fiber reunion between the root surface and the surrounding tissue. The collagen fibers around the root were inserting into newly formed cementum on all of the previously "nondiseased" root surfaces, since this attachment occurred on a root surface from which the connective tissue had been separated by mechanical injury (i.e. by the tooth

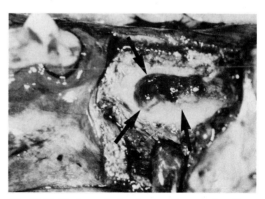

Fig. 19-15. Photograph showing location and size of one groove (arrows) prepared in the buccal surface of the jaw bone. The experimental roots were extracted and placed in grooves of similar design.

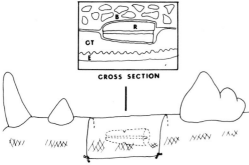

Fig. 19-16. Schematic drawing illustrating the position of a transplanted experimental root. The root (R) is embedded to half its circumference into bone tissue (B). The remaining part is covered by a tissue flap containing gingival connective tissue (CT) and epithelium (E).

extraction), the newly formed attachment was regarded as *re-attachment* (Fig. 19-17). In the coronal, "diseased", portion of the roots (i.e. in areas of the roots which had previously been pathologically exposed) there were no signs of proper regeneration. In the zone of the "diseased" root which faced the gingival connective tissue, collagen fibers were seen with an orientation parallel to the root surface (Fig. 19-17). These fibers

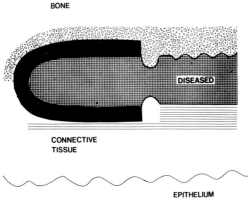

Fig. 19-17. Schematic drawing illustrating the result of healing following root transplantation. In the apical, "nondiseased" portion of the root, a fibrous reunion (reattachment) between the root surface and surrounding tissue was established (black areas). In the coronal, "diseased" root portion new attachment failed to occur.

were in no instance attached to the implanted roots and *de novo* formation of root cementum was never observed. In addition, large resorption lacunae containing multinucleated cells were found along the root surface. In the zone, where the previously "diseased" root surface was facing bone tissue, healing had consistently resulted in extensive root resorption and ankylosis (Fig. 19-17).

This model experiment demonstrated that the formation of a new attachment is not promoted by the mere exclusion of the epithelium from the healing wound. When in a periodontal wound the granulation tissue cells, derived from the gingival connective tissue or from the bone tissue, reach contact with the root surface, a process of *root resorption* is initiated. The experiment thus revealed that *granulation tissue derived from bone or gingival connective tissue lack the ability to establish a new connective tissue attachment to root surfaces which have previously been pathologically exposed.*

The fact that granulation tissue derived from the gingival connective tissue produced root resorption and that granulation tissue derived from the bone produced resorption and ankylosis of roots deprived of their periodontal ligament and root cementum is an interesting finding and concurs with results reported from several studies on reimplantation and transplantation of teeth (Löe & Waerhaug 1961, Andreasen & Hjörting-Hansen 1966, Karring et al. 1980, 1983, Andreasen 1981, Andreasen & Kristerson 1981). On the basis of these findings it may seem surprising that root resorption is not a common complication following periodontal flap surgery, when the soft tissue flap after proper root debridement is normally replaced with its connective tissue in close contact with the curetted root surface. It may also seem surprising that root resorption and ankylosis are rare complications following treatment of infrabony pockets with flap procedures. In fact, since the alveolar bone surrounding the bony defect constitutes a source for granulation tissue formation during healing, resorption and

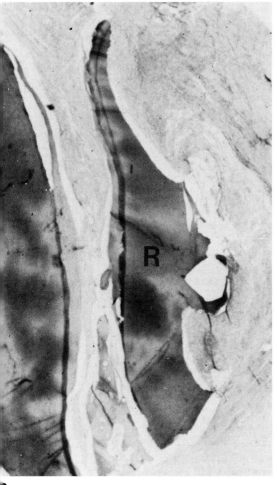 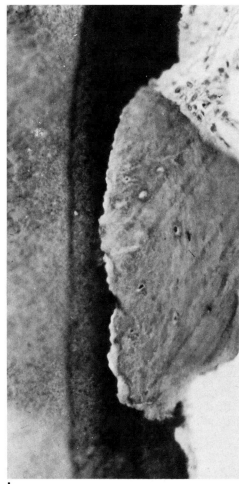

Figs. 19-18a, b. Extensive root resorption (a) and root resorption in conjunction with ankylosis (b) following treatment of advanced periodontal disease in humans using a surgical technique which prevented apical migration of the dentogingival epithelium during healing. R = remaining part of the root. (From Björn et al. 1965).

ankylosis might well be expected to be frequent findings on root surfaces located adjacent to surgically treated infrabony lesions. The reason why such complications do not (or only occasionally) occur is evidently the ability of the epithelial cells to proliferate rapidly to the presurgical location of the pocket epithelium. Hereby, the newly formed epithelial lining acts as a barrier which effectively protects the root against granulation tissue from the alveolar bone and the gingival connective tissue. This conclusion is further supported by the results presented

by Björn et al. (1965) who treated 11 periodontally diseased teeth in 7 human volunteers using a technique which prevented apical migration of the dento-gingival epithelium along the curetted root surface. They reported that root resorption was indeed a common complication following this type of therapy (Figs. 19-18a, b).

From the above description it is obvious that attempts aiming at preventing apical downgrowth of the epithelium along the root surface in order to allow new attachment to form may instead result in root resorption.

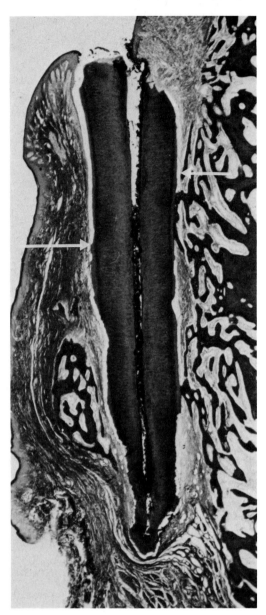

Fig. 19-19. Microphotograph of a transplanted root. The surgical procedure prevented during a 2 week period the epithelium from migrating into the wound. The epithelium has migrated along the coronal, previously periodontitis involved root surfaces down to a level indicated by the arrows. In the areas covered by epithelium there are no signs of resorption. Apical to this level the root surfaces are characterized by root resorption.

In this context a study on the monkey by Karring et al. (1983) should be briefly described. Roots which to half the root length had been exposed to periodontal disease were, following treatment, implanted into bone and gingival connective tissue in a manner similar to that described above (Nyman et al. 1980). After varying time intervals the roots were exposed by a secondary incision through the covering mucosa. The epithelium was thereby enabled to migrate into the wound. If this incision was made within 2 weeks after root implantation, the epithelium migrated into the wound and covered the previously diseased part of the root which showed no signs of resorption or ankylosis (Fig. 19-19). With increasing intervals between implantation of the roots and the secondary incision the migrating epithelium covered the root surface to a diminishing degree and signs of root resorption and ankylosis became more pronounced (Fig. 19-20). Taken together with the data reported previously these findings demonstrate that *the migrating epithelium functions as a protective barrier towards root resorption and ankylosis* during healing following periodontal therapy.

This fact has of course particular interest with respect to the use of bone transplants in the treatment of infrabony pockets (for review see Gara & Adams 1981). The rationale behind such treatment is the concept that bone regeneration in an angular bony defect may favor the formation of new cementum and new connective tissue attachment. The results of the studies discussed above, as well as of other investigations (e.g. Melcher 1970, Atrizadeh et al. 1971, Line et al. 1974, Boyko et al. 1981), demonstrating that granulation tissue derived from bone induces root resorption and ankylosis, however, seem to invalidate the use of bone grafts in periodontal surgery. In fact, when viable bone cells are transferred with fresh iliac bone marrow grafts into infrabony periodontal defects, replacement resorption identified by root resorption and ankylosis often occurs (Schallhorn et al. 1970, Seibert 1970, Sullivan et al. 1971, Burnette 1972

Schallhorn 1972, Dragoo & Sullivan 1973a, b, Dragoo 1981).

Periodontal ligament

A finding in studies on the regenerative potential of the periodontal tissues is that deposition of new cementum with inserting collagen fibers occasionally occurs during healing in the most apical parts of periodontal wounds (Skillen & Lundqvist 1937, Linghorne & O'Connell 1950, Morris 1953, Listgarten 1972, Frank et al. 1974, Caton & Nyman 1980, Cole et al. 1980, Karring et al. 1980, Nyman et al. 1981). This formation of new cementum may be regarded as indicative of the potential for coronal migration (along the root surface) of cells which have the capacity to form a new attachment. In fact, results from experiments (Melcher 1970, Line et al. 1974; for review see Melcher 1976) have provided support for the hypothesis that periodontal ligament cells may possess an ability to produce new cementum.

In order to study if the periodontal ligament cells do indeed have this ability, a research model was developed (Nyman et al. 1982a) by which not only the dentogingival epithelium was prevented from interfering with the wound but by which also granulation tissue, derived from the gingival connective tissue, was inhibited from reaching contact with the root surface during healing. At the buccal aspect of canine teeth in monkeys a U-shaped incision was made through the oral mucosa (Fig. 19-21). A mucoperiosteal flap was raised on the coronal side of the incision to expose the buccal alveolar bone. Within an area extending from a level approximately 3 mm coronal to the apex to a level 2 mm apical to the marginal bone crest, the buccal and the approximal alveolar bone was resected and the root surface thoroughly planed to remove all cementum (Fig. 19-22). By preserving the most marginal portion of the periodontium, wound healing was allowed to occur *without interference from an apically migrating dentogingival*

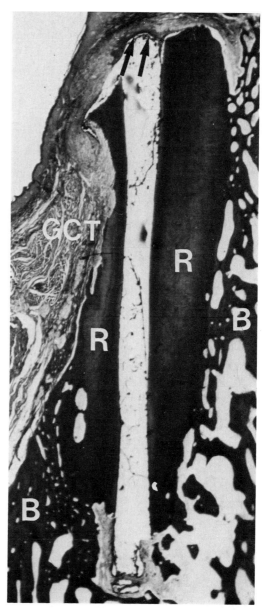

Fig. 19-20. Microphotograph of an implanted root. After 8 weeks of healing the epithelium was allowed to proliferate in apical direction. The epithelium (arrows) covers only part of the coronal, cut root surface. Extensive root resorption is seen on the surface facing the gingival connective tissue (GCT). Resorption and ankylosis characterize the surface facing the bone tissue. R = root, B = bone.

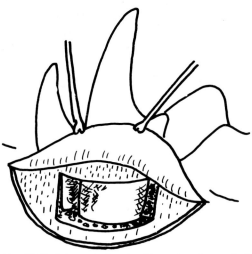

Fig. 19-21. Schematic drawing illustrating the surgical procedure used in the study by Nyman et al. (1982a).

epithelium. In order *to prevent the gingival connective tissue from reaching contact with the root surface* during healing, a Millipore® filter (Millipore Corporation) was placed to cover the fenestration in the alveolar bone (Fig. 19-23). The flap was replaced to the facial surface of the filter and sutured.

The histological analysis of block sections representing 3 months of healing disclosed that new formation of attachment had occurred including newly formed cementum, fibrous attachment and supporting alveolar bone (Fig. 19-24). This finding indicates that the periodontal ligament cells have a considerable potential for producing regeneration. However, this ability of the periodontal ligament cells will manifest itself only if the epithelial cells, the bone cells and the gingival connective tissue cells are prevented from occupying the wound area adjacent to the root during healing.

In the study described above new attachment was obtained on root surfaces which were indeed deprived of their periodontal ligament and cementum but, on the other hand, had not been exposed to plaque or to a periodontal pocket. The *de novo* formation of a functional periodontal apparatus found in these root areas should therefore not be regarded as *new attachment* but rather as *reattachment.* In order to test the hypothesis that new cementum with inserting principal fibers could also be formed on a previously diseased root surface provided cells from the periodontal ligament were enabled to repopulate this portion of the root, the following experiment was recently performed in our laboratory (Nyman et al. 1982b). A male (47 years of age) suffered from advanced periodontal disease of generalized character. A mandibular incisor with deep pockets of long standing and scheduled for extraction was treated using a flap technique. A radiograph of this tooth obtained

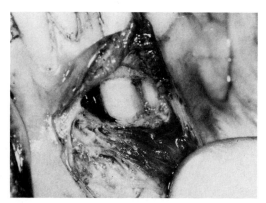

Fig. 19-22. Photograph showing the wound with the denuded part of the root. The cementum layer of this part of the root was removed.

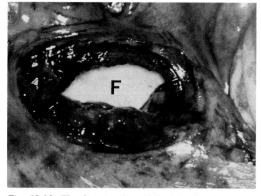

Fig. 19-23. The fenestration of the alveolar bone was covered by a Millipore filter (F) over which the tissue flap was subsequently positioned.

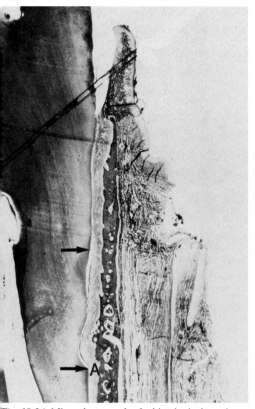

Fig. 19-24. Microphotograph of a histological specimen demonstrating new cementum (between arrows) and regenerated bone along the curetted root surface. A split has occurred between the dentine and the new cementum layer during histological preparation. A = the apical notch prepared in the root surface.

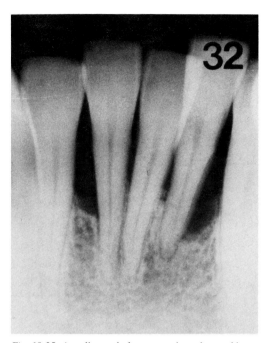

Fig. 19-25. A radiograph demonstrating advanced bone loss in the mandibular incisor part of the dentition of a patient with longstanding periodontal disease.

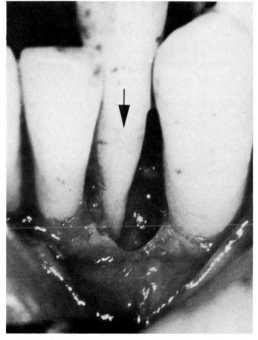

Fig. 19-26. The degree of loss of periodontal tissue in the area of tooth 32 is illustrated after flap elevation. The location of the cementoenamel junction is identified by the arrow. Note the angular bony defect at the buccal and distal aspects of the tooth.

immediately before treatment is shown in Fig. 19-25. The clinical attachment level at the buccal surface of this tooth assessed by probing was found to be located 11 mm apical to the cementoenamel junction (CEJ). Following elevation of soft tissue flaps (Fig. 19-26), a notch was prepared in the buccal root surface at the level of the alveolar bone crest. The distance between the CEJ and this notch was 9 mm. An angular bony defect, 2 mm deep, was found to be present apical to the notch. Following removal of all granulation tissue and careful scaling and root planing (to the bottom of the angular defect), a Millipore® filter (Millipore Corporation)

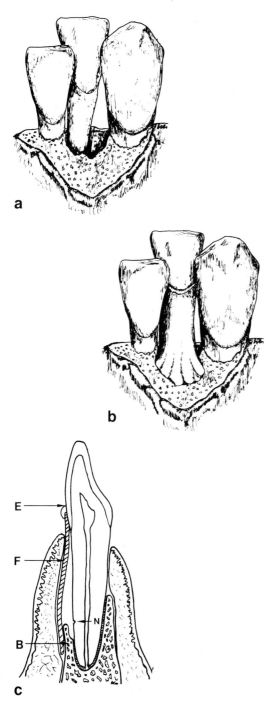

a

b

E

F

N

B

c

Figs. 19-27a-c. Schematic drawings illustrating the root and bone architecture before (a) and after (b) the placement of the Millipore filter (F). Fig. 19-27c demonstrates that the filter (F) covers an area extending from the enamel surface (E) to the alveolar bone (B). A notch (N) was prepared in the root surface at the level of the alveolar bone crest.

was adjusted to cover the buccal and approximal tooth surfaces from a level around 2 mm coronal to the CEJ to a level around 1 mm apical to the bone crest (Figs. 19-27 a-c). The filter was placed in position and adapted to the enamel surface by means of a resin (Concise®). The buccal flap was then replaced to the facial surface of the filter and secured to the lingual flap by interdental sutures. The location of the Millipore filter in relation to the tooth and the surrounding periodontal tissues is illustrated in Fig. 19-27c. With this design of the wound, the filter prevented the gingival connective tissue from contacting the facial and proximal parts of the root during healing. The proliferating oral epithelium was, during healing, thus, guided along the outer surface of the filter rather than along the root surface. The result of treatment after 3 months of healing is shown in Fig. 19-28. This demonstrates that the oral epithelium has proliferated along the facial surface of the Millipore filter. However, in the coronal portion of the gingiva, epithelium from the lingual flap has proliferated into the connective tissue adjacent to the root surface. New cementum with inserting collagen fibers was observed on the facial root surface extending in coronal direction from the apical level of the previous angular bony defect via the notch area to a level 5 mm coronal to the apical border of the notch. Figs. 19-28d, e show the newly formed connective tissue attachment at different levels coronal to the notch.

From this study it can be concluded that a *new attachment* including new cementum and a functional periodontal ligament can in fact become established on a previously diseased root surface.

Figs. 19-28a-d. The upper left microphotogram (a) illustrates the location of the filter (F) in relation to the gingiva and the root surface. Arrow 1 denotes the notch area. Arrows 2 and 3 denote previously exposed root areas coronal to the notch with newly formed cementum and inserting principle fibers. A=artifact. Figs. 19-28b-d = magnifications of the 3 different areas of arrows 1, 2 and 3.

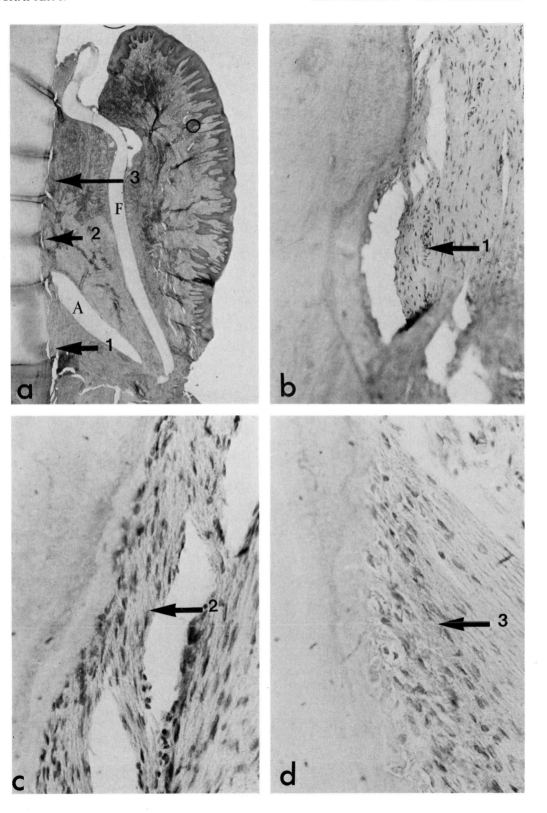

Conclusions

Increasing evidence indicates that *the cells which repopulate the periodontal wound adjacent to the root surface determine the nature of the attachment formed.* Cells which originate from the periodontal ligament possess the ability to form a new attachment (Melcher 1969, 1976, Line et al. 1974, Nyman et al. 1980, 1982a, b, Boyko et al. 1981). However, even if clinical and laboratory research have provided evidence that a new attachment can be formed, no predictable, clinically applicable surgical techniques are presently available by which the periodontal tissues, lost by progressive periodontal disease, can be regained. Regenerative or reconstructive periodontal treatment procedures, used to date, result in a long epithelial attachment with or without accompanying bone fill rather than in the formation of a new connective tissue attachment.

Citric acid – an adjunct for new attachment formation

During recent years, a fresh approach for obtaining new attachment has been developed. Studies on repair of surgical wounds in animals have led to the use of citric acid as a means of promoting new attachment (Register & Burdick 1976, Ririe et al. 1980). Following removal of the root cementum from the periodontitis affected part of the root, citric acid at pH 1 is applied to the dentin surface for 3 min. The superficial zone of the root dentin thereby becomes demineralized which leads to denudation of the collagen fibrils of the dentin matrix. A connective tissue attachment will, according to Ririe et al. (1980), be established by "interdigitation of new and old collagen fibrils at the tooth-gingiva interface". Citric acid conditioning has demonstrated some remarkable success in periodontal defects in dogs (Crigger et al. 1978, Nilvéus 1978) and also enabled the demonstration of new attachment in humans (Cole et al. 1980). However, other studies indicate a limited regeneration following acid conditioning (Cole et al. 1981, Renvert & Egelberg 1981). Therefore, although promising, this method still requires further research before its introduction in clinical practice is recommended.

References

Alderman, N. (1969) Sterile plaster of Paris as an implant in the infrabony environment: A preliminary study. *Journal of Periodontology* **40**, 11-13.

Andreasen, J. O. (1981) Periodontal healing after replantation and autotransplantation of permanent incisors. *International Journal of Oral Surgery* **60**, 54-61.

Andreasen, J. O. & Hjörting-Hansen, E. (1966) Replantation of teeth. II. Histological study of 22 replanted anterior teeth in humans. *Acta Odontologica Scandinavica* **24**, 290-306.

Andreasen, J. O. & Kristerson, L. (1981) The effect of limited drying or removal of the periodontal ligament. Periodontal healing after replantation of mature permanent incisors in monkeys. *Acta Odontologica Scandinavica* **1**, 1-13.

Armitage, G. C., Svanberg, G. K. & Löe, H. (1977) Microscopic evaluation of clinical measurements of connective tissue attachment levels. *Journal of Clinical Periodontology* **4**, 173-190.

Atrizadeh, F., Kennedy, J. & Zander, H. (1971) Ankylosis of teeth following thermal injury. *Journal of Periodontal Research* **6**, 157-159.

Beube, F. E. (1947) A study on reattachment of the supporting structures of the teeth. *Journal of Periodontology* **18**, 55-66.

Beube, F. E. (1952) A radiographic and histologic study on reattachment. *Journal of Periodontology* **23**, 158-164.

Björn, H. (1961) Experimental studies on reattachment. *Dental Practitioner and Dental Reconstruction* **11**, 351-354.

Björn, H., Hollender, L. & Lindhe, J. (1965) Tissue regeneration in patients with periodontal disease. *Odontologisk Revy* **16**, 317-326.

Boyko, G. A., Melcher, A. H. & Brunette, D. M. (1981) Formation of new periodontal ligament by periodontal ligament cells implanted *in vivo* after culture *in vitro*. A preliminary study of transplanted roots in the dog. *Journal of Periodontal Research* **16**, 73-88.

Bump, R. L., Salimeno, T., Hooker, S. P. & Wilkinson, E. G. (1975) The use of woven ceramic fabric as a periodontal allograft. *Journal of Periodontology* **46**, 453-458.

Burnette, E. W. (1972) Fate of an iliac crest graft.

Journal of Periodontology **43**, 88-90.

Carranza, F. A. (1954) A technique for reattachment. *Journal of Periodontology* **25**, 272-277.

Carranza, F. A. (1960) A technique for treating infrabony pockets so as to obtain reattachment. *Dental Clinics of North America*, March, 75-83.

Caton, J. G. & Kowalski, C. J. (1976) Primate model for testing periodontal treatment procedures. II. Production of contralaterally similar lesions. *Journal of Periodontology* **47**, 506-510.

Caton, J. & Nyman, S. (1980) Histometric evaluation of periodontal surgery. I. The modified Widman flap procedure. *Journal of Clinical Periodontology* **7**, 212-223.

Caton, J., Nyman, S. & Zander, H. (1980) Histometric evaluation of periodontal surgery. II. Connective tissue attachment levels after four regenerative procedures. *Journal of Clinical Periodontology* **7**, 224-231.

Caton, J. G. & Zander, H. A. (1975) Primate model for testing periodontal treatment procedures. I. Histologic investigation of localized periodontal pockets produced by orthodontic elastics. *Journal of Periodontology* **46**, 71-77.

Caton, J. & Zander, H. A. (1976) Osseous repair of an infrabony pocket without new attachment of connective tissue. *Journal of Clinical Periodontology* **3**, 54-58.

Cole, R. T., Crigger, M., Bogle, G., Egelberg, J. & Selvig, K. A. (1980) Connective tissue regeneration to periodontally diseased teeth. A histologic study. *Journal of Periodontal Research* **15**, 1-9.

Cole, R. T., Nilvéus, R., Ainamo, J., Bogle, G., Crigger, M. & Egelberg, J. (1981) Pilot clinical studies on the effect of topical citric acid application on healing after replaced periodontal flap surgery. *Journal of Periodontal Research* **16**, 117-122.

Crigger, M., Bogle, G., Nilvéus, R., Egelberg, J. & Selvig, K. A. (1978) The effect of topical citric acid application on the healing of experimental furcation defects in dogs. *Journal of Periodontal Research* **13**, 538-549.

Dragoo, M. R. (1981) *Regeneration of the Periodontal Attachment in Humans.* Philadelphia: Lea & Febiger.

Dragoo, M. R. & Sullivan, H. C. (1973a) A clinical and histological evaluation of autogenous iliac bone grafts in humans. I. Wound healing 2 to 8 months. *Journal of Periodontology* **44**, 599-613.

Dragoo, M. R. & Sullivan, H. C. (1973b) A clinical and histologic evaluation of autogenous iliac bone grafts in humans. II. External root resorption. *Journal of Periodontology* **44**, 614-625.

Ellegaard, B. & Löe, H. (1971) New attachment of periodontal tissues after treatment of intrabony lesions. *Journal of Periodontology* **42**, 648-652.

Ellegaard, B., Nielsen, I. M. & Karring, T. (1976) Composite jaw and iliac cancellous bone grafts in intrabony defects in monkeys. *Journal of Periodontal Research* **11**, 299-310.

Frank, R., Fiore-Donno, G., Cimasoni, G. & Matter, J. (1974) Ultrastructural study of epithelial and connective gingival reattachment in man. *Journal of Periodontology* **45**, 226-235.

Froum, S. J., Ortiz, M., Witkin, R. T., Thaler, R., Scopp, I.W. & Stahl, S. S. (1976) Osseous autografts. III. Comparison of osseous coagulum-bone blend implants with open curettage. *Journal of Periodontology* **47**, 287-294.

Froum, S. J., Thaler, R., Scopp, I. W. & Stahl, S. S. (1975a) Osseous autografts. I. Clinical responses to bone blend or hip marrow grafts. *Journal of Periodontology* **46**, 515-521.

Froum, S. J., Thaler, R., Scopp, I.W. & Stahl, S. S. (1975b) Osseous autografts. II. Histological responses to osseous coagulum-bone blend grafts. *Journal of Periodontology* **46**, 656-661.

Gara, G. G. & Adams, D. E. (1981) Implant therapy in human intrabony pockets: A review of the literature. *Journal of the Western Society of Periodontology, Periodontal Abstracts* **2.**

Hiatt, W. H. & Schallhorn, R. G. (1973) Intraoral transplants of cancellous bone and marrow in periodontal lesions. *Journal of Periodontology* **44**, 194-208.

Hiatt, W. H., Schallhorn, R. G. & Aaronian, A. J. (1978) The induction of new bone and cementum formation. IV. Microscopic examination of the periodontium following human bone and marrow allograft, autograft and nongraft periodontal regenerative procedures. *Journal of Periodontology* **49**, 495-512.

Hiatt, W. H., Stallard, R. E., Butler, E. D. & Badgett, B. (1968) Repair following mucoperiosteal flap surgery with full gingival retention. *Journal of Periodontology* **39**, 11-16.

Kalkwarf, K. I. (1974) Periodontal new attachment without the placement of osseous potentiating grafts. *Periodontal Abstracts* **2**, 53-62.

Karring, T., Nyman, S. & Lindhe, J. (1980) Healing following implantation of periodontitis affected roots into bone tissue. *Journal of Clinical Periodontology* **7**, 96-105.

Karring, T., Nyman, S., Lindhe, J. & Sirirat, M. (1983) Potentials for root resorption during periodontal healing. In press.

Kon, S., Novaes, A. B., Ruben, M. P. & Goldman, H. M. (1969) Visualization of microvascularization of the healing periodontal wound. II. Curettage. *Journal of Periodontology* **40**, 96-105.

Levin, M. P., Getter, L., Adrian, J. & Cutright, D. E. (1974) Healing of periodontal defects with ceramic implants. *Journal of Clinical Periodontology* **1**, 197-205.

Line, S. E., Polson, A. M. & Zander, H. A. (1974) Relationship between periodontal injury, selective cell repopulation and ankylosis. *Journal of Periodontology* **45**, 725-730.

Linghorne, W. J. & O'Connell, D. C. (1950) Studies in the regeneration and attachment of supporting structures of the teeth. I. Soft tissue reattachment. *Journal of Dental Research* **29**, 419.

Listgarten, M. A. (1972) Electron microscopic study of the junction between surgically denuded root surfaces and regenerated periodontal tissues. *Journal of Periodontal Research* **7**, 68-90.

Listgarten, M. A., Moa, R. & Robinson, P. J. (1976) Periodontal probing and the relationship of the probe to the periodontal tissues. *Journal of Periodontology* **47**, 511-513.

Löe, H. & Waerhaug, J. (1961) Experimental replantation of teeth in dogs and monkeys. *Archives of Oral Biology* **3**, 176-184.

McCall, J. O. (1926) An improved method of inducing reattachment of the gingival tissues in periodontoclasia. *Dental Items of Interest* **48**, 342-358.

Melcher, A. H. (1969) Healing of wounds in the periodontium. In *Biology of the Periodontium,* ed. Melcher, A. H. & Bowen, W. H., pp. 497-529. London: Academic Press.

Melcher, A. H. (1970) Repair of wounds in the periodontium of the rat. Influence of periodontal ligament on osteogenesis. *Archives of Oral Biology* **15**, 1183-1204.

Melcher, A. H. (1976) On the repair potential of periodontal tissues. *Journal of Periodontology* **47**, 256-260.

Morris, M. L. (1953) The reattachment of human periodontal tissues following surgical detachment: A clinical and histological study. *Journal of Periodontology* **24**, 220.

Moskow, B. S. (1964) The response of the gingival sulcus to instrumentation: A histological investigation. *Journal of Periodontology* **35**, 112-126.

Moskow, B. S., Karsh, F. & Stein, S. D. (1979) Histological assessment of autogenous bone graft. A case report and critical evaluation. *Journal of Periodontology* **6**, 291-300.

Nabers, C. L. & O'Leary, T. J. (1965) Autogenous bone transplants in the treatment of osseous defects. *Journal of Periodontology* **36**, 5-14.

Nabers, C. L. & O'Leary, T. J. (1967) Autogenous bone grafts: case report. *Periodontics* **5**, 251-253.

Nilvéus, R. (1978) Treatment of periodontal furcation pockets. Experimental studies in dogs. Thesis, Malmö, Sweden.

Nyman, S., Gottlow, J., Karring, T. & Lindhe, J. (1982a) The regenerative potential of the periodontal ligament. An experimental study in the monkey. Journal of Clinical Periodontology **9**, 157-265.

Nyman, S., Karring, T., Lindhe, J. & Plantén, S. (1980) Healing following implantation of periodontitis-affected roots into gingival connective tissue. *Journal of Clinical Periodontology* **7**, 394-401.

Nyman, S., Lindhe, J. & Karring, T. (1981) Healing following surgical treatment and root demineralization in monkeys with periodontal disease. *Journal of Clinical Periodontology* **8**, 249-258.

Nyman, S., Lindhe, J., Karring, T. & Rylander, H. (1982b) New attachment following surgical treatment of human periodontal disease. *Journal of Clinical Periodontology* **9**, 290-296.

Orban, B. (1948) Pocket elimination or re-attachment? *New York Dental Journal* **14**, 227-232.

Patur, B. & Glickman, I. (1962) Clinical and roentgenographic evaluation of the post-treatment healing of infrabony pockets. *Journal of Periodontology* **33**, 164-171.

Polson, A. M. & Heijl, L. (1978) Osseous repair in infra-bony defects. *Journal of Clinical Periodontology* **5**, 13-23.

Prichard, J. (1957a) Regeneration of bone following periodontal therapy. *Oral Surgery* **10**, 247-252.

Prichard, J. (1957b) The infrabony technique as a predictable procedure. *Journal of Periodontology* **28**, 202-216.

Proye, M. & Polson, A. M. (1982) Effect of root surface alterations on periodontal healing. I. Surgical denudation. *Journal of Clinical Periodontology* **9**, 428-440.

Ramfjord, S. P. (1951) Experimental periodontal reattachment in Rhesus monkeys. *Journal of Periodontology* **22**, 67-77.

Ramfjord, S. P. & Nissle, R. R. (1974) The modified Widman flap. *Journal of Periodontology* **45**, 601-607.

Register, A. A. & Burdick, F. A. (1976) Accelerated reattachment with cementogenesis to dentin, demineralized *in situ*. II. Defect repair. *Journal of Periodontology* **47**, 497-505.

Renvert, S. & Egelberg, J. (1981) Healing after treatment of periodontal intraosseous defects. II. Effect of citric acid conditioning of the root surface. *Journal of Clinical Periodontology* **8**, 459-473.

Ririe, C. M., Crigger, M. & Selvig, K. A. (1980) Healing of periodontal connective tissue following surgical wounding and application of citric acid in dogs. *Journal of Clinical Periodontology* **15**, 314-327.

Robinson, R. E. (1969) Osseous coagulum for bone induction. *Journal of Periodontology* **40**, 503-510.

Rosenberg, M. M. (1971) Free osseous tissue autografts as a predictable procedure. *Journal of Periodontology* **42**, 195-209.

Rosling, B., Nyman, S. & Lindhe, J. (1976) The effect of systematic plaque control on bone regeneration in infrabony pockets. *Journal of Clinical Periodontology* **3**, 38-53.

Schaffer, E. M. & Zander, H. A. (1953) Histological evidence of reattachment of periodontal pockets. *Parodontologie* **7**, 101-107.

Schallhorn, R. G. (1972) Postoperative problems associated with iliac transplants. *Journal of Periodontology* **43**, 3.

Schallhorn, R. G. (1977) Present status of osseous grafting procedures. *Journal of Periodontology* **48**, 570-576.

Schallhorn, R. G., Hiatt, W. H. & Boyce, W. (1970) Iliac transplants in periodontal therapy. *Journal of Periodontology* **41**, 566-580.

Seibert, J. S. (1970) Reconstructive periodontal surgery: Case report. *Journal of Periodontology* **41**, 113-117.

Skillen, W. G. & Lundquist, G. R. (1937) An experimental study of periodontal membrane re-attachment in healthy and pathologic tissues. *Journal of the American Dental Association* **24**, 175-185.

Strub, J. R., Gaberthüel, T. W. & Firestone, A. R. (1979) Comparison of tricalcium phosphate and frozen allogenic bone implants in man. *Journal of Periodontology* **50**, 624-629.

Sullivan, H. C., Vito, A. A., Meltzer, A. M. & Rabinowitz, J. L. (1971) A histological evaluation of the use of hemopoietic marrow in intrabony periodontal defects. Program and abstract of papers. *International Association of Dental Research:* meeting.

van der Velden, U. & de Vries, J. H. (1978) Introduction of a new periodontal probe: the pressure probe. *Journal of Clinical Periodontology* **5**, 188-197.

Wade, A. B. (1962) An assessment of the flap operation. *Dental Practitioner and Dental Record* **13**, 11-20.

Wade, A. B. (1966) The flap operation. *Journal of Periodontology* **37**, 95-99.

Waerhaug, J. (1952) The gingival pocket. *Odontologisk Tidsskrift* **60**, Supplement 1.

Waerhaug, J. (1978) Healing of the dento-epithelial junction following subgingival plaque control. I. As observed in human biopsy material. *Journal of Periodontology* **49**, 1-8.

Wirthlin, M. R. (1981) The current status of new attachment therapy. *Journal of Periodontology* **52**, 529-544.

World Workshop in Periodontics (1966) Ed. Ramfjord, S. P., Kerr, D. H. & Ash, M. M. Ann Arbor: American Academy of Periodontology and University of Michigan.

Younger, W. J. (1899) Pyorrhea alveolaris from a bacteriological standpoint with a report of some investigations and remarks on the treatment. *International Dental Journal* **20**, 413-423.

Yukna, R. A. (1976) A clinical and histologic study of healing following the excisional new attachment procedure in rhesus monkeys. *Journal of Periodontology* **47**, 701-709.

Yukna, R. A., Bowers, G. M., Lawrence, J. J. & Fedi, P. F. (1976) A clinical study of healing in humans following the excisional new attachment procedure. *Journal of Periodontology* **47**, 696-700.

Yuktanandana, I. (1959) Bone graft in the treatment of intrabony periodontal pockets in dogs. A histological investigation. *Journal of Periodontology* **30**, 17-26.

CHAPTER 20

Treatment of Furcation Involved Teeth

Objectives

Studies on humans and laboratory animals have documented the decisive part played by bacterial plaque in the etiology of gingivitis and destructive periodontal disease. Consequently, therapeutic measures aimed at eliminating gingival inflammation and arresting progression of periodontal tissue breakdown must include the careful removal of the microbial deposits from the tooth surfaces and the establishment of a home-care program which prevents recurrence of gross amounts of plaque and calculus (for review see Hamp 1973, Rosling 1976).

Treatment of advanced forms of periodontal disease frequently includes surgical procedures. The objectives of these procedures are (see also Chapter 13):

1. to obtain visibility and access to the root surfaces for proper professional debridement
2. to eliminate the pathologically deepened pockets

3. to establish a morphology in the dentogingival region which facilitates proper, self performed, tooth cleaning.

The third of these objectives is particularly valid in the treatment of periodontal disease around multirooted teeth when the destruction of the supporting tissues has involved the furcation areas. The elimination of pathologically deepened pockets and the establishment of a morphology in the furcation areas which facilitates self performed plaque control measures require elaborate therapeutic techniques, since progressive loss of attachment and bone resorption in such sites proceed not only in apical direction along the root surfaces but also in horizontal direction in between the roots.

Anatomical characteristics

The anatomy of the roots and the topography of the alveolar bone in the furcation areas of multirooted teeth in a periodontal patient can be best examined if a mucoperiosteal flap is elevated. Since a surgical approach for diagnostic purposes is only occasionally performed, detailed knowledge regarding the anatomy of the root system of different teeth as well as the natural progress of periodontal disease in such sites is a fundamental prerequisite for the proper interpretation of data obtained by clinical probing and radiographic examination.

General information regarding the anatomy of the furcation areas of multirooted teeth may be gained from *autopsy material*. If the buccal bone plates are removed from an autopsy preparation the

433

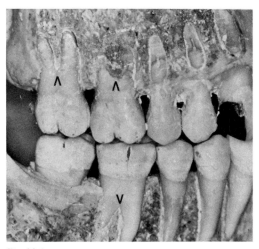

Fig. 20-1a.

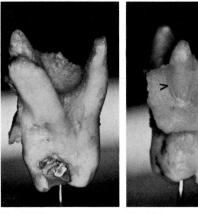

Fig. 20-1b.

Fig. 20-1c.

buccal furcas are exposed (arrows; Fig. 20-1a) as well as the location of the furcas in relation to the cementoenamel junctions. The position and spread of the roots of the maxillary molars often give rise to a large area of interradicular supporting bone (Fig. 20-1b). A thin buccal bone plate is sometimes associated with the presence of fenestrations (arrow; Fig. 20-1c) and/or dehiscences (Fig. 20-1d).

The position and anatomy of the various roots of maxillary and mandibular posterior teeth can also be illustrated in cross-sections of the jaws. Figs. 20-2a and b are schematic drawings from such cross-sections prepared at a distance of a few mm apical to the cementoenamel junction.

In Fig. 20-2a the roots of the *maxillary* second premolar (P2) and the maxillary molars (M1, M2 and M3) are identified as well as the buccal and palatal bone plates. From this drawing it becomes obvious that the mesiobuccal roots of the first and second molars are comparatively wide in buccopalatal direction while the distobuccal roots are of considerably smaller dimension. The palatal roots are often wider in mesiodistal than in buccopalatal direction. The oval shaped mesiobuccal roots usually have marked invaginations while the distobuccal roots generally have a more rounded outline and less frequently exhibit distinct invaginations.

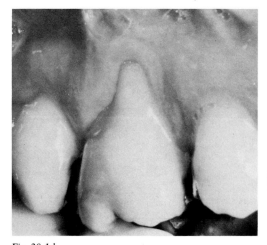

Fig. 20-1d.

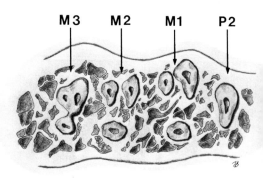

Fig. 20-2a.

In Fig. 20-2b the roots of the *mandibular* molars can be identified. Note the differences in anatomy between the mesial and distal roots. The mesial roots are normally wider in buccolingual direction than the distal roots and frequently have more pronounced root furrows or invaginations. It should also be observed that the buccal alveolar bone plate is thinner adjacent to the roots of the first molars than at the second and, in particular, the third molars.

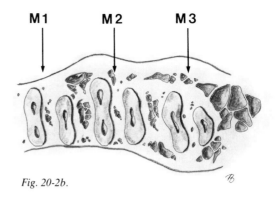

Fig. 20-2b.

The use of *radiographs* to properly identify the structures in the furcation areas is generally of limited value. Hence, in maxillary molars (Fig. 20-3a) frequently only the buccal furca may be properly identified and in mandibular molars (Fig. 20-3b) the images of the buccal and lingual furcas cannot always be distinguished since tooth and bone structures often become superimposed over the furcation areas. It should be noted that the furcation area of the maxillary premolars may be best identified in radiographs obtained by directing the central beam towards the canine (Fig. 20-3c). The information from the radiographs is improved if the radiographic examination includes pictures obtained both by parallelling periapical and traditional bite wing techniques (Figs. 20-3d, e). Fig. 20-3f illustrates a second maxillary molar in which the furcation area is obscured by superimposed hard tissue structures.

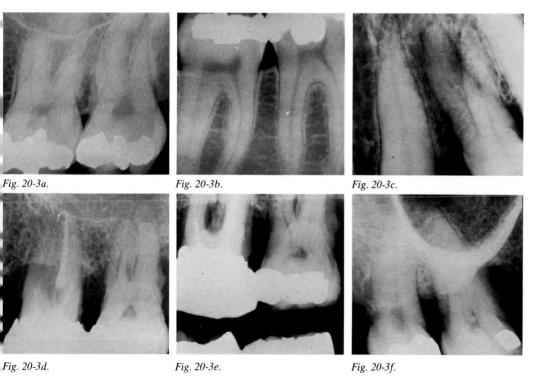

Fig. 20-3a.   Fig. 20-3b.   Fig. 20-3c.

Fig. 20-3d.   Fig. 20-3e.   Fig. 20-3f.

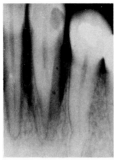
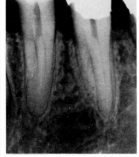
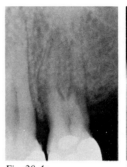
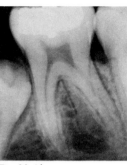

Fig. 20-4a.   Fig. 20-4b.   Fig. 20-4c.   Fig. 20-4d.

The fact that furcas may be present in teeth which normally have only 1 root should also be taken into consideration. Thus, 2-rooted incisors or canines (Fig. 20-4a) and mandibular premolars (Fig. 20-4b) may exist. Occasionally 3-rooted maxillary premolars (Fig. 20-4c) and 4-rooted mandibular molars (Fig. 20-4d) can be found.

Other morphological variations to consider in the diagnosis and treatment of furcation involved teeth are (1) "fusions" between divergent roots (Fig. 20-5a), (2) cervical enamel projections or enamel pearls in the furcation areas (arrow; Fig. 20-5b), (3) presence of accessory pulp canals which communicate with the furcation area, etc.

Rationale for diagnosis

Treatment of periodontal disease around a multirooted tooth should not be initiated until the tooth has been examined for the presence of a furcation involvement. Such an examination should comprise both *clinical probing* and *radiographic analysis*. Graduated periodontal probes, curved explorers or small curettes should be used for the clinical examination. Sometimes the vitality of the affected tooth must be tested in order to differentiate between a plaque associated lesion and a lesion of pulpal origin in the furcation area (see Chapter 9).

Furcation involvements may be *classified* into 3 degrees depending on the extension of the destruction in horizontal direction within the interradicular area:

Degree 1 denotes horizontal loss of periodontal tissue support not exceeding ⅓ of the width of the tooth.

Degree 2 denotes horizontal loss of periodontal tissue support exceeding ⅓ of the width of the tooth but not encompassing the total width of the furcation area.

Degree 3 denotes horizontal "through-and-through" destruction of the periodontal tissues in the furcation area.

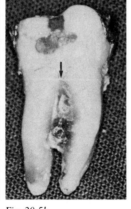

Fig. 20-5a.   Fig. 20-5b.

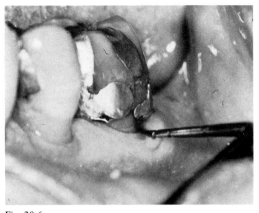

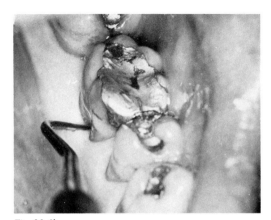

Fig. 20-6a.

Fig. 20-6b.

The buccal furca of the maxillary molars and the buccal (Fig. 20-6a) and lingual (Fig. 20-6b) furcas of the mandibular molars are normally accessible for examination by clinical probing.

The clinical examination of furcas on the approximal tooth surfaces may be more difficult when neighboring teeth are present, and especially if the contact area between the teeth is large. This is particularly the case in maxillary molars. As a rule, however, the furca in the mesial surface of a maxillary molar should be probed from the palatal aspect of the tooth (Fig. 20-7a) while the furca in the distal surface is probed from either the buccal or the palatal aspect (Fig. 20-7b).

Premolars – in particular the first maxillary premolars – often have a varying root anatomy. In addition the roots harbor irregularities such as longitudinal furrows, invaginations (arrow; Fig. 20-8a) or true furcas (Fig. 20-8b) which may open up at different levels from the cementoenamel junction. The clinical examination of maxillary premolars is often difficult due to limited access for probing. It may not always be possible to identify the presence and degree of furcation involvement in such teeth until a flap is raised in an explorative (surgical) procedure in the area.

In addition to *clinical probing*, a *radiographic analysis* should be made as a supplementary examination for possible furca-

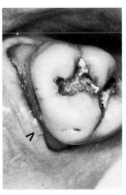
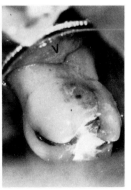
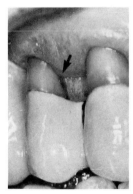
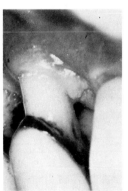

Fig. 20-7a.   *Fig. 20-7b.*   *Fig. 20-8a.*   *Fig. 20-8b.*

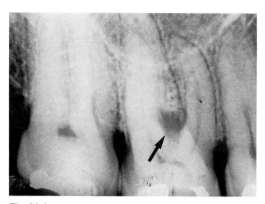

Fig. 20-9a.

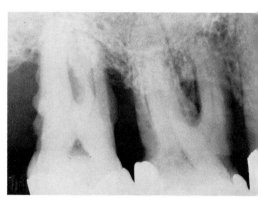

Fig. 20-9b.

tion involvements. The information thus obtained should be related to findings from the clinical examination. Fig. 20-9a (arrow) shows a radiolucency in the buccal furcation area of a maxillary first molar which corresponds to an involvement of *Degree 2* as assessed by clinical probing. No further involvements could be diagnosed in the molar region, either by probing or by radiographic analysis.

In cases of advanced destruction of the supporting apparatus in the molars (Fig. 20-9b), the occurrence of furcation involvements at the mesial and distal aspects of the teeth may be anticipated when the image of the interdental alveolar bone crest in the radiograph is located apically to the "normal" level of the furcas. In the 2 molars (17,

16) illustrated in Fig. 20-9b there were *Degree 3* involvements from the buccal, mesial and distal aspects of the teeth. This diagnosis was confirmed by probing the furcas by means of a curved explorer.

In this context it should be observed that even extensive loss of alveolar bone in the interradicular area of maxillary molars is often not disclosed in the radiograph due to the superimposition of remaining bone structures and of the palatal root (arrows, Fig. 20-10a; Fig. 20-10b).

Different degrees of furcation involvements in mandibular molars are illustrated in Figs. 20-11 a, b. In Fig. 20-11a a through-and-through furcation involvement in tooth 47 can be distinguished already in the radiograph. This diagnosis was further verified by

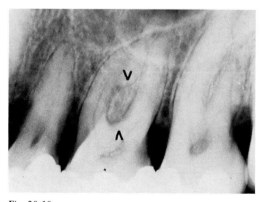

Fig. 20-10a.

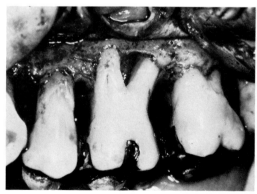

Fig. 20-10b.

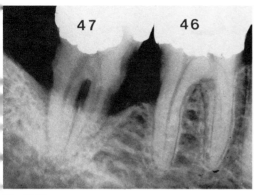

Fig. 20-11a.

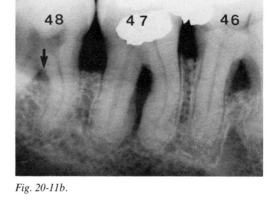

Fig. 20-11b.

the clinical examination which revealed pathologically deepened pockets (8 mm at the buccal and lingual aspects of the tooth), furcation involvement of *Degree 3* and a tooth mobility of Degree 2. On the other hand, it was not possible from the radiograph to detect the *Degree 1* involvements which were probed from both the buccal and lingual aspects of tooth 46. In this radiograph, persisting interradicular alveolar bone in the mid-portion of the furcation area obscured these initial furcation involvements.

In the teeth seen in Fig. 20-11b the clinical assessments of furcation involvements gave the following results: tooth 48 *Degree 1* (from the lingual aspect), tooth 47 *Degree 3* and tooth 46 *Degree 2* (from the buccal aspect). The *Degree 1* involvement in the lingual surface of tooth 48 (arrow) is clearly visible in this radiographic projection, and so is the *Degree 3* involvement in tooth 47. The *Degree 2* involvement at the buccal aspect of tooth 46 is reproduced in a characteristic way. By thorough analysis of the radiograph, the trabecular structure of bone tissue can be detected within the radiolucent zone of the interradicular area; the alveolar bone at the lingual aspect of the tooth is normal in height – no lingual furcation involvement was recorded – and in the radiograph this bone mass is projected over the buccally located lesion in the furcation area.

Rationale for therapy

Since the distance between the cemento-enamel junction and the furcas of multi-rooted teeth – particularly first molars – is often comparatively short, furcation involvements may already develop at initial or moderate stages of breakdown of the attachment apparatus. Proper diagnosis and treatment of periodontal disease at an early stage, i.e. before the furcas have become involved in the destructive process, are therefore important in order to prevent such complications. In cases where furcation involvements have developed, different therapeutic alternatives are available, alternatives which often relate to the different degrees of the involvement:

Degree of involvement	Therapy
Degree 1	Scaling and root planing Furcation plasty
Degree 2	Furcation plasty Tunnel preparation Root resection Tooth extraction
Degree 3	Tunnel preparation Root resection Tooth extraction

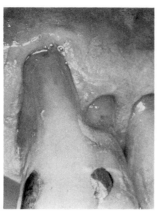
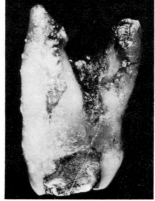
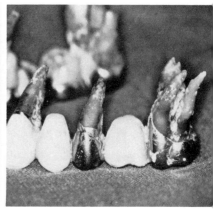

Fig. 20-12a.   Fig. 20-12b.   Fig. 20-12c.

Scaling and root planing

These include the removal of hard and soft bacterial deposits from the tooth and root surfaces, and can be the only procedure used in the treatment of most furcation involvements of *Degree 1*. The successful result of such a simple treatment is illustrated in Fig. 20-12a. In this context it should be borne in mind that healing must result in a morphology in the furcation area which is optimal for self performed plaque control measures. If this demand is not fulfilled, plaque and calculus will again accumulate in the critical area and recurrence of the progressive disease will most likely occur (Figs. 20-12b, c).

If proper conditions for plaque control measures cannot be established by scaling and root planing alone, other therapeutic methods must be used.

Furcation plasty

Includes the following procedures:
. reflection of a mucoperiosteal flap to get proper access to the interradicular area
. removal of soft and hard bacterial deposits and inflammatory soft tissue from the furcation area
. odontoplasty, i.e. removal of tooth substance in the furcation area in order to widen a narrow entrance of the furca and

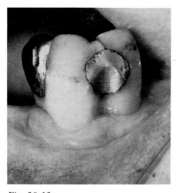
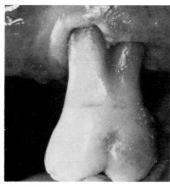
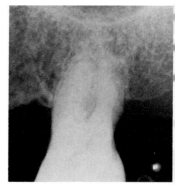

Fig. 20-13a.   Fig. 20-13b.   Fig. 20-13c.

440

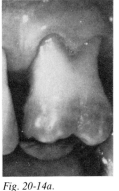
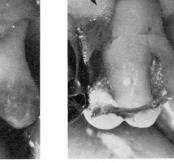
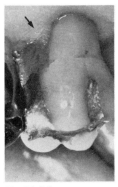
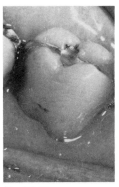
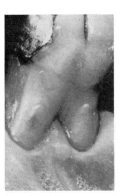

Fig. 20-14a.   Fig. 20-14b.   Fig. 20-14c.   Figs. 20-14d.

to reduce the horizontal depth of the involvement

. osteoplasty, i.e. recontouring of bony defects in the furcation area, if indicated
. repositioning and suturing of the flap.

Furcation plasty is a therapeutic measure preferably used in the treatment of advanced *Degree 1* and initial *Degree 2* involvements. Owing to limitations of access and in securing optimal plaque control, such recontouring encounters difficulties in the areas of proximally located furcas, i.e. in maxillary molars and premolars, when neighboring teeth have approximal contacts. The result of this type of treatment is exemplified in Figs. 20-13a-c and 20-14a-d. The treatment should result in the establishment of a soft tissue papilla which covers the entrance to the interradicular periodontal tissues. It should again be emphasized that the purpose of the procedure is – besides the removal of plaque and calculus – to establish a condition in the dentogingival region which facilitates self performed plaque control measures.

In this context, however, there are reasons to *warn against* too extensive recontouring of the tooth by grinding since this procedure may result in hypersensitivity problems, be detrimental to a vital pulp and further, enhance the risk for root surface caries. In addition, osteoplasty should be performed with caution so that no addi-

tional, unintended, loss of periodontium occurs in the site of operation.

Tunnel preparation

This implies surgical exposure of the entire furcation area. Following elevation of mucoperiosteal flaps at the buccal and lingual aspects of the affected tooth, the root surfaces are scaled and planed and an irregular alveolar bone crest recontoured, if necessary. The flaps are repositioned to the interradicular alveolar bone crest and secured in this position by interdental and interradicular sutures. Surgical packs may be applied to prevent excessive granulation tissue forming in the tunnel space during healing. From a technical aspect the mandibular molars are most suited for this mode of therapy. Fig. 20-15a illustrates the clinical appearance of a mandibular first molar following tunnel preparation. It should be stressed that there is a pronounced risk for caries lesions to develop in the denuded root surfaces within and adjacent to such tunnels (Figs. 20-15b,c) if self performed plaque control is not maintained at a very high level. Consequently, the method should be used with restriction and only in situations where there is space enough between the roots to permit interradicular cleansing by means of an interdental toothbrush (Fig. 20-15d).

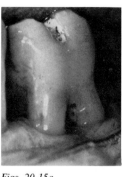
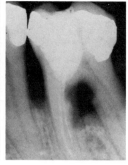
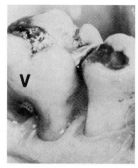
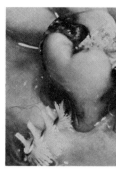

Figs. 20-15a.   *Fig. 20-15b.*   *Fig. 20-15c.*   *Fig. 20-15d.*

Root resection

This is the procedure of choice in cases of deep *Degree 2* and *Degree 3* involvements and includes the removal of one or more roots from a multirooted tooth. The risk of leaving "overhangs" of tooth substance behind during tooth hemisection and root resection (arrow; Fig. 20-16) is an incitement to carry out these procedures after flap elevation which enables proper inspection of the surgically cut dentine surface. A radiograph should also be obtained of the area immediately after surgery to verify that such "overhangs" do not persist.

As a rule, endodontic treatment of the root(s) to be retained following tooth hemisection and root resection should be performed prior to surgery. Hereby information of the result of the endodontic measures will be obtained before extraction of

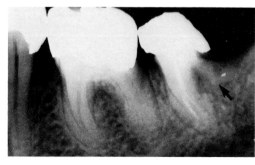

Fig. 20-16.

root(s) which may possibly be maintained as an alternative. In multirooted teeth with advanced destruction of the supporting tissues it may not always be possible to decide, until surgery, which root or roots it is possible or most favorable to preserve. As an alternative to permanent filling of all root canals with guttapercha before surgery, pulpectomy can be performed and the canals be filled with calcium hydroxide. Each of the openings to the root canals is sealed with zinc oxide eugenol cement. Root separation and resection can thus be carried out without risk for bacterial contamination of the root canals. Permanent filling of the root(s) is in such cases performed after surgery.

In the selection of root(s) to be retained following root separation, the following factors should be considered:

. the amount of supporting tissue remaining around the various roots
. the stability of the individual roots
. the root and root canal anatomy with respect to endodontic and restorative treatment procedures
. the periapical condition
. the position of the various roots in the alveolar process in relation to adjacent and opposing teeth.

In a case where, for example, the furcation area of a first mandibular molar is involved to an extent which calls for root resection, it is usually easy to decide which root it is preferable to maintain from the

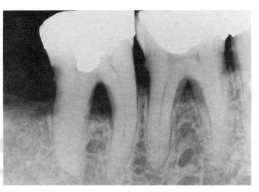

Fig. 20-17a.

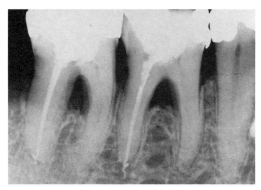

Fig. 20-17b.

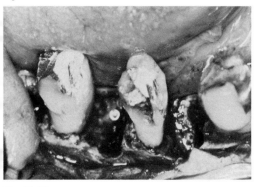

Fig. 20-17c.

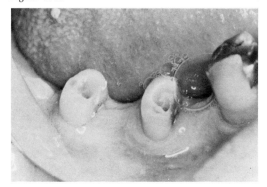

Fig. 20-17d.

periodontal aspect. If the amount of remaining periodontium around the 2 roots is similar, it is often preferable from the endodontic point of view to maintain the distal root. This root has generally only one, wide, root canal and is therefore easily accessible for endodontic treatment. However, the extraction and loss of the mesial portion of the tooth often requires prosthetic replacement by means of a bridge construction. Figs. 20-17a-d demonstrate a case where the 2 mandibular molars on one side of the jaw were furcation involved *(Degree 3)*. The loss of alveolar bone had progressed to, on the average, the same level around all 4 roots (Fig. 20-17a). The distal roots were exposed to endodontic therapy (Fig. 20-17b), tooth hemisection including extraction of the mesial roots was performed (Fig. 20-17c) and, following healing, the mesial portions of the molars were replaced by a fixed bridge, extending from the distal root of the

second molar to the second premolar (Fig. 20-17d). On the other hand, provided the mesial root of a mandibular molar has a root canal anatomy which allows for proper root filling and insertion of a proper post, this root can be preserved and used as an abutment for a single crown. Hereby extensive bridge therapy can be avoided. Such treatment is exemplified in Figs. 20-18a, b.

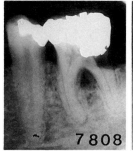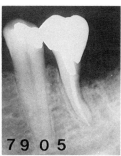

Fig. 20-18a.   Fig. 20-18b.

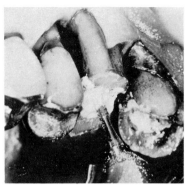
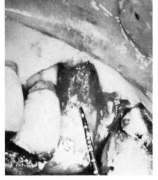
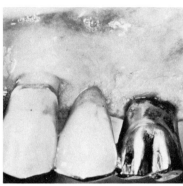

Fig. 20-19a.   Fig. 20-19b.   Fig. 20-19c.

Difficult problems arise when root resection is performed in maxillary molars. Since these teeth often have 3 roots, 1 or 2 roots can be preserved after separation. In spite of careful clinical and radiographic examination, it is often impossible to properly evaluate the extension of the furcation defect until a flap procedure enables direct inspection. In cases of advanced periodontal disease around maxillary molars it is often necessary to separate all 3 roots from each other to obtain access to the interradicular area for assessment of the height of the remaining bone at, for example, the buccal surface of the palatal root and the palatal surfaces of the buccal roots.

The series of photographs presented in Figs. 20-19a-c demonstrate root resection in a first maxillary molar. Fig. 20-19a illustrates how the roots are separated from each other

using a fissure bur. In Fig. 20-19b the alveolar bone crest at the buccal surface of the palatal root is indicated by the tip of the probe after extraction of the 2 buccal roots. Subsequent to the root resection therapy on tooth 26, the two neighboring teeth (25, 27), which could not be treated, were extracted and a 3-unit bridge was inserted (Fig. 20-19c) with the extension 24$\overline{25}$26 (palatal root).

When a maxillary molar suffers furcation involvement from the buccal aspect only, or when the buccal furca and one of the proximal furcas are periodontally involved (e.g. the buccal and the distal furcas), the tooth may be treated as is illustrated in Figs. 20-20a, b. The mesiobuccal and palatal roots were root filled (Fig. 20-20a) and the distobuccal root was resected (Fig. 20-20b). Such a root resection can often be performed without the removal of excessive amounts of tissue from the crown of the tooth, i.e. there may be no need for the placement of an artificial crown following surgery.

Similar treatment of a molar with *Degree 2* involvement in the mesial surface is illustrated in Figs. 20-21 a-d. No involvements were present at the distal and buccal aspects of the tooth. The radiographic analysis (Fig. 20-21a) and the findings during surgery (Fig. 20-21b) disclosed bone loss at the mesial surface down to the apex of the mesiobuccal root. Figs. 20-21 c and d present the result of treatment, i.e. extraction of this root, after 6 months of healing.

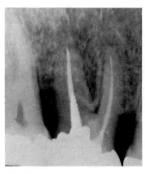
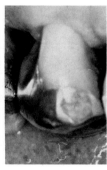

Fig. 20-20a.   Fig. 20-20b.

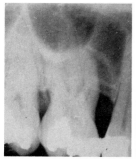

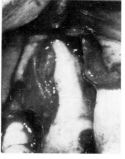

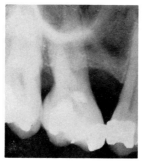

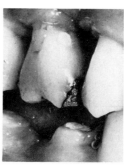

Fig. 20-21a.   *Fig. 20-21b.*   *Fig. 20-21c.*   *Fig. 20-21d.*

Resection of the palatal root might be an unusual way to solve a furcation problem. However, in a situation where the buccal furca is intact but the presence of a mesial and/or a distal furcation involvement is combined with advanced loss of attachment around the palatal root, the removal of this root and the maintenance of the buccal portion of the tooth including the 2 buccal roots can be the procedure of choice. In the case presented in Fig. 20-22a, the second premolar and the second molar were extracted. The root canals of the first premolar and the buccal roots of the first molar were filled. Root resection was carried out in the first molar including extraction of the palatal root. Following healing (Fig. 20-22b) a fixed bridge with the extension 16^{15}14 was inserted (Fig. 20-22c).

Root resection of maxillary first premolars is possible only in rare instances due to the anatomy of the tooth. The furca is often located at such an apical level that the maintenance of 1 root serves no meaningful purpose. In most cases, therefore, a furcation involvement of *Degree 3* in a maxillary first premolar calls for tooth extraction (Figs. 20-23 a, b).

In the selection of roots that can or should be retained in a case with multiple furcation involvements in the maxillary molars, the

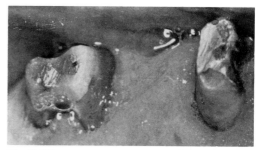

Fig. 20-22b.

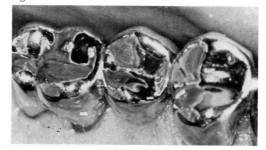

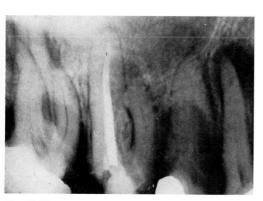

Fig. 20-22a.   *Fig. 20-22c.*

445

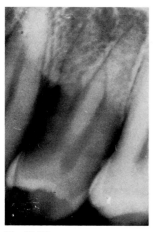

Fig. 20-23a.

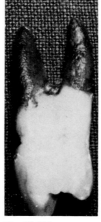

Fig. 20-23b.

position of the various roots in the jaw in relation to neighboring teeth must be considered. The buccal roots, provided they can be subjected to proper endodontic treatment, may be preferred to a palatal root. For example, if the maxillary second premolar (P2) is present (see Fig. 20-24a), one or several of the buccal roots of the molars – later to be used as distal abutments in a cross-arch bridge – should be preserved because of their more favorable position in the dental arch in relation to the premolar in comparison to the palatal roots. In this particular example, the mesiobuccal root of the second molar (arrow) was preserved and used as the distal abutment tooth. Fig. 20-24b demonstrates another case before bridge insertion.

Here the mesiobuccal root of each of the first molars was used as distal abutment in a cross-arch bridge.

Another example of the problems involved in the selection of roots to be retained in a given case is illustrated in Figs. 20-25 a, b. The palatal root was the only root of the maxillary first molar that could be preserved. Following resection of the buccal roots, the palatal root was found to have a high mobility. Due to the fact that the second premolar was palatally displaced in the jaw (cross-bite position; see Fig. 20-25a) and thus located in the same plane as the retained molar root, a splint with proper design could be placed (Fig. 20-25b).

Finally, it should be pointed out that all forms of periodontal surgery, including root resection, result in exposed root dentine surfaces which may be susceptible to carious lesions. Fluoride solutions should routinely be applied to such surfaces after completion of surgery.

Tooth extraction

The extraction of a periodontally involved 2- or multirooted tooth will of course predictably eliminate the disease in this particular area. This therapy is indicated when the destruction of the periodontium has progressed to such a level that no root can be preserved. Extraction may also be performed when the maintenance of the affected tooth will not improve the overall treatment or when treat-

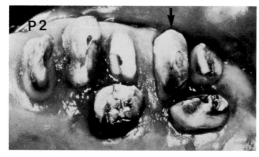

Figs. 20-24a.

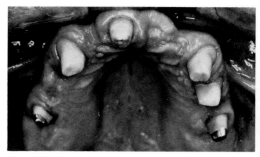

Figs. 20-24b.

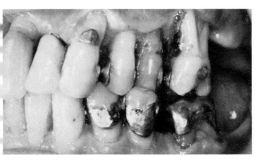

Fig. 20-25a.

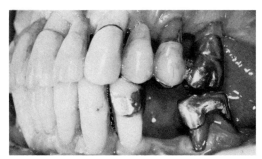

Fig. 20-25b.

ment of the furcation involved tooth will not result in conditions which can be properly maintained by self performed plaque control measures.

In the diagnosis and treatment of furcation involved teeth it should be realized that loss of alveolar bone within the inter-radicular area – besides being caused by periodontal disease – may also be the effect of infection derived from a necrotic pulp. Such a situation is illustrated in Fig. 20-26a. Examination of the affected molar disclosed a nonvital pulp. The tooth was endodontically treated and complete healing of the bony lesion occurred within a few months (Fig. 20-26b). For detailed discussion on interrelationships between periodontics and endodontics, see Chapter 9.

Prognosis

A 5 year follow-up study on the result of treatment of 175 furcation involved, 2- and multirooted teeth was presented by Hamp et al. 1975 (Table 1). The teeth included had been treated in accordance with the principles described in this chapter. Of the 175 teeth, 32 had been treated by scaling and root planing alone. Scaling and root planing in conjunction with furcation plasty including odonto- and/or osteoplasty had been carried out in 49 teeth. 87 furcation involved teeth had been subjected to root resection while a tunnel had been prepared in 7 teeth only. Following the active treatment phase all patients were enrolled in a maintenance care program including recall appointments

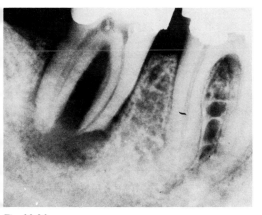

Fig. 20-26a.

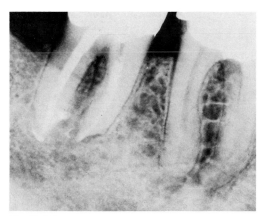

Fig. 20-26b.

447

Table 20-1. Frequency and distribution of various therapeutic procedures in furcation involved teeth (from Hamp et al. 1975)

Therapy	Teeth 36/46	37/47	16/26	17/27	18/28	14/24	Other premolars	Total
Scaling/root planing	8	4	12	6	2	–	–	32
Furcation plasty	12	15	14	8	–	–	–	49
Tunnel preparation	6	–	–	–	–	1	–	7
Root resection	30	14	28	11	–	3	1	87
Total	56	33	54	25	2	4	1	175

once every 3-6 months. At each recall appointment the patients were instructed in oral hygiene measures, and scaling, root planing and polishing of the teeth were performed. *Presence of plaque* and *gingival conditions* at the furcation areas of all teeth were assessed immediately before active treatment and once a year postoperatively using the Plaque- and Gingival Index systems described by Löe & Silness (1963) and Silness & Löe (1964). The mean PlI scores for all types of therapeutic procedures at the final examination varied between 0.2-0.3. The corresponding GI scores were 0.2-0.4.

Pocket depth measurements at the final control revealed that only 16 out of the 175 teeth subjected to furcation treatment had a probing depth exceeding 3 mm. The distribution of these pockets in relation to the different therapeutic procedures is given in Table 2.

Table 20-2. Probing depths in the furcation areas at the final control examination (from Hamp et al. 1975)

Therapy	≤ 3 mm	4-6 mm	> 6 mm	Total
Scaling/ root planing Furcation plasty	77	4	–	81
Tunnel preparation	4	3	–	7
Root resection	78	7	2	87
Total	159	14	2	175

During the observation period (5 years) carious lesions were detected on 12 treated tooth surfaces which had been subjected to scaling, root planing and furcation plasty (3 surfaces), root resection (5 surfaces) and tunnel preparation (4 surfaces).

It should be stressed that different modalities of periodontal surgery, including the various procedures for treatment of furcation involvements described above, constitute only part of the overall treatment of periodontal disease in a given case. The factor which determines success or failure in the long perspective following surgery, is the degree of plaque control that can be obtained and maintained (Hamp et al. 1975, Lindhe & Nyman 1975, Rosling 1976). A successful treatment demands that all tooth surfaces are properly cleaned during the active phase of treatment and that the patients, thereafter, are enrolled in a professionally supervised maintenance program including measures which prevent recurrence of the disease (Nyman et al. 1975, Axelsson & Lindhe 1981, Ravald & Hamp 1981, Westfelt et al. 1983).

In recent years, techniques using acids for demineralization of periodontally involved root surfaces in order to promote regeneration of lost periodontal tissues in furcation areas have been presented. Following mechanical removal of the root cementum from the periodontitis affected parts of the root, citric acid at pH 1 is applied to the denuded dentine surface for 3 min. Such conditioning of the root surfaces with citric acid will promote regeneration of attachment in experimentally induced furcation involvements in dogs (Crigger et al. 1978, Nilvéus 1978), but corresponding treatment in humans has, so far, failed to result predictably in new attachment (La Cuesta 1980). Therefore, at this stage, continued research is required before the introduction of this method in clinical practice is recommended.

(For detailed discussion on new attachment see Chapter 19).

For further reading on the management of teeth with furcation involvements the reader is referred to studies presented by Bergenholtz (1972), Klavan (1975), Ross & Thompson (1978), Waerhaug (1980) and to a recent review article by Newell (1981).

References

Axelsson, P. & Lindhe, J. (1981) The significance of maintenance care in the treatment of periodontal disease. *Journal of Clinical Periodontology* **8**, 281-294.

Bergenholtz, A. (1972) Radectomy of multirooted teeth. *Journal of the American Dental Association* **85**, 870-875.

Crigger, M., Bogle, G., Nilvéus, R., Egelberg, J. & Selvig, K. (1978) The effect of topical citric acid application on the healing of experimental furcation defects in dogs. *Journal of Periodontal Research* **13**, 538-549.

Hamp, S.-E. (1973) On the development and prevention of periodontal disease in the Beagle dog. Thesis. University of Gothenburg, Gothenburg, Sweden.

Hamp, S.-E., Nyman, S. & Lindhe, J. (1975) Periodontal treatment of multirooted teeth. Results after 5 years. *Journal of Clinical Periodontology* **2**, 126-135.

Klavan, B. (1975) Clinical observations following root amputation in maxillary molar teeth. *Journal of Periodontology* **46**, 1-5.

La Cuesta, E. (1980) Repair in furcations of mandibular molar teeth after citric acid treatment. Unpublished research. University of Texas Health Science Center, San Antonio, Texas, U.S.A.

Lindhe, J. & Nyman, S. (1975) The effect of plaque control and surgical pocket elimination on the establishment and maintenance of periodontal health. A longitudinal study of periodontal therapy in cases of advanced disease. *Journal of Periodontology* **2**, 67-79.

Löe, H. & Silness, J. (1963) Periodontal disease in pregnancy. I. Prevalence and severity. *Acta Odontologica Scandinavica* **21**, 533-551.

Newell, D. H. (1981) Current status of the management of teeth with furcation invasions. *Journal of Periodontology* **52**, 559-568.

Nilvéus, R. (1978) Treatment of periodontal furcation pockets. Experimental studies in dogs. Thesis. University of Lund, Malmö, Sweden.

Nyman, S., Rosling, B. & Lindhe, J. (1975) Effect of professional tooth cleaning on healing after periodontal surgery. *Journal of Clinical Periodontology* **2**, 80-86.

Ravald, N. & Hamp, S.-E. (1981) Prediction of root surface caries in patients treated for advanced periodontal disease. *Journal of Clinical Periodontology* **8**, 400-414.

Rosling, B. (1976) Plaque control. A determining factor in the treatment of periodontal disease. Thesis. University of Gothenburg, Gothenburg, Sweden.

Ross, I. F. & Thompson, R. H. (1978) A long-term study of root retention in the treatment of maxillary molars with furcation involvement. *Journal of Periodontology* **49**, 238-244.

Silness, J. & Löe, H. (1964) Periodontal disease in pregnancy. II. Correlation between oral hygiene and periodontal condition. *Acta Odontologica Scandinavica* **22**, 121-135.

Waerhaug, J. (1980) The furcation problem. Etiology, pathogenesis, diagnosis, therapy and prognosis. *Journal of Clinical Periodontology* **7**, 73-95.

Westfelt, E., Nyman, S., Socransky, S. & Lindhe, J. (1983) Significance of frequency of professional tooth cleaning for healing following periodontal surgery. *Journal of Clinical Periodontology* **10**, 148-156.

CHAPTER 21

Occlusal Therapy

Tooth mobility = crown excursion/root displacement

Initial and secondary tooth mobility

A tooth which is surrounded by a normal periodontium may be moved (displaced) in horizontal and vertical directions and may, in addition, be forced to perform limited rotational movements. The mobility (= movability) of a tooth in a horizontal direction is closely dependent on the height of the surrounding bone, the width of the periodontal ligament as well as the shape and number of roots present (Fig. 21-1). Clinically, horizontal tooth mobility is usu-ally assessed by first exposing the crown of the tooth to a certain force and subsequently by determining the distance of crown displacement in buccal and/or lingual direction. The mechanism of tooth mobility was studied in detail by Mühlemann (1954, 1960) who described a standardized method for measuring even minor tooth displacements.

By means of the *"Periodontometer"* a small force (= 100 ponds) was at first applied to the crown of a tooth (Fig. 21-2). The crown started to tip in the direction of the force. The resistance of the tooth supporting structures against displacement of the root is low in the initial phase and the crown was moved 5/100-10/100 mm. This movement of the tooth was by Mühlemann (1954) called "initial tooth mobility – ITM" and is the result of an *intraalveolar* displacement of the root (Fig. 21-3). In the pressure zone there is a 10% reduction in the width of the periodontal ligament and in the tension zone there is a corresponding increase in the width of the ligament. Mühlemann & Zander (1954) stated that "there are good reasons to assume that the initial displacement of the root (initial–TM) corresponds to a reorientation of the periodontal membrane fibers into a position of functional readiness towards tensile strength". The magnitude of the "initial-TM" varies from individual to individual, from tooth to tooth, and is mainly dependent on the structure and organization of the periodontal ligament. The "initial-TM" value of ankylosed teeth is therefore zero.

When a larger force (= 500 ponds) was subsequently applied to the crown, the fiber bundles on the tension side offered resistance to further root displacement and the additional displacement of the crown that was observed in "secondary tooth mobility – secondary-TM" (Fig. 21-3) was enabled by distortion and compression of the entire periodontium. According to Mühlemann

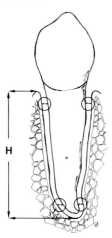

Fig. 21-1. The mobility of a tooth in horizontal direction is dependent on the height of the alveolar bone (H), the width of the periodontal ligament (encircled arrows) and the shape and number of roots.

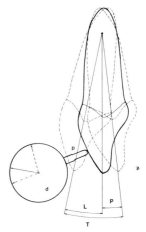

Fig. 21-2. Tooth mobility measurements by means of the Periodontometer. d= dial indicator, p= pointer, L= labial excursion of the crown, P= palatal excursion of the crown, T= L+P= total excursion of the crown.

(1960) the magnitude of "secondary-TM", i.e. the excursion of the crown of the tooth when a force of 500 ponds is applied, 1) varies between different types of teeth (e.g. incisors 10-12/100 mm, canines 5-9/100 mm, premolars 8-10/100 mm and molars 4-8/100 mm), 2) is larger in children than in adults, 3) is larger in females than males and increases during e.g. pregnancy. Furthermore, tooth mobility seems to vary during the course of the day – the lowest value is found in the evening and the largest in the morning.

Clinical measurement of tooth mobility (physiologic and pathologic tooth mobility)

If in the traditional clinical measurement of tooth mobility a comparatively large force ($\approx$ 500 ponds) is placed on the crown of a tooth surrounded by a normal periodontium, the tooth will tip within its alveolus until a close contact has been established between the root and the marginal (or apical) bone tissue. The magnitude of this tipping movement, which is normally assessed using the tip of the crown as a reference point, is referred to as the "physiologic"

tooth mobility. The term "physiologic" implies that "pathologic" tooth mobility may also occur. What then is "pathologic" tooth mobility?

If a similar force ($\approx$ 500 ponds) is applied to a tooth which is surrounded by a periodontal ligament with an increased

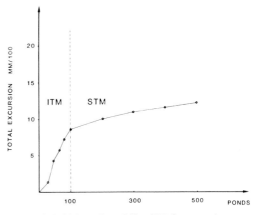

Fig. 21-3. Initial tooth mobility (ITM) means the excursion of the crown of a tooth when a force of 100 ponds is applied to the crown. Secondary tooth mobility (STM) means the excursion of the crown of the tooth when a force of 500 ponds is applied.

width, the excursion of the crown in horizontal direction will become increased; the clinical measurement demonstrates that the tooth has an increased mobility. Should this increased mobility be regarded as "pathologic"?

An increased tooth mobility, i.e. an increased displacement of the crown of the tooth, can also be found in situations where the height of the alveolar bone has been reduced but the remaining periodontal ligament has a normal width. Should this increased mobility be regarded as "pathologic"?

Fig. 21-4a describes a tooth surrounded by alveolar bone with reduced height but normal width of the remaining periodontal ligament. A horizontally directed force (≈ 500 ponds) applied to the coronal portion of the tooth will in this case result in a larger excursion of the crown than if a similar force is applied to a tooth with normal height of the alveolar bone and normal width of the periodontal ligament (Figure 21-4b). The *so-called increased mobility* measured in the case of Fig. 21-4b should, however, also be regarded as *"physiologic"*. The validity of this statement can easily be demonstrated if the displacement of the 2 teeth is assessed not from a reference point on the crown but from a point on the root situated at the level of the bone crest. If a horizontal force is directed to the teeth as indicated in Figs. 21-4a,b the reference points (*) on the root surfaces will be identically displaced in both instances. *Obviously it is not the length of the excursive movement of the crown of the tooth that is important from a biologic point of view, but the displacement of the root within its remaining periodontal ligament.* This means that the "increased" crown mobility observed for teeth with a reduced height of the alveolar bone must not necessarily be regarded as "pathologic".

In plaque associated periodontal disease bone loss is a prominent feature. Increased crown displacement (tooth mobility) assessed by clinical measurements in cases of "horizontal" (i.e. even) bone loss in periodontal disease should, according to the

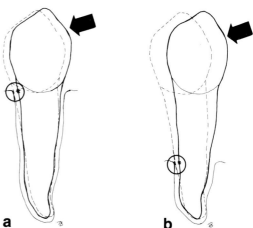

a **b**

Figs. 21-4a, b. (a) illustrates the normal "physiologic" mobility of a tooth with normal height of the alveolar bone and normal width of the periodontal ligament. (b) depicts increased mobility of the crown of a tooth with normal width of the periodontal ligament but reduced height of the alveolar bone. It should be observed that the distance of the horizontal displacement of the reference point (*) on the roots is the same in the 2 situations.

above discussion, also be regarded as physiologic; the root is displaced within the space of its remaining "normal" periodontal ligament.

Increased crown displacement (tooth mobility) may also be detected in a clinical measurement applied to teeth with angular bony defects and/or increased width of the periodontal ligament space. If this mobility is not gradually increasing – from one observation interval to the next – the root is surrounded by a periodontal ligament of increased size but normal composition; further, this mobility should be considered as "physiologic" since the mobility is a function of the height of the alveolar bone and the width of the periodontal ligament. *Only progressively increasing tooth mobility* which occurs during trauma from occlusion characterized by active bone resorption (see Chapter 8) and indicating the presence of inflammatory alterations within the periodontal ligament tissue, *should be considered "pathologic"*.

Clinical symptoms of trauma from occlusion

Angular bony defects

It has often been claimed that *angular bony defects* and *increased tooth mobility* are important symptoms of trauma from occlusion (Glickman 1965, 1967). The validity of this suggestion has, however, been questioned (see Chapter 8). Angular bony defects have been found around teeth affected by trauma from occlusion as well as around teeth with normal occlusal function (Waerhaug 1979). *This means that the presence of angular bony defects per se cannot be regarded as an exclusive symptom of trauma from occlusion.*

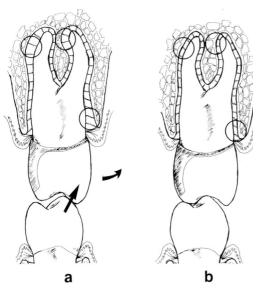

a   **b**

Figs. 21-5a, b. (a) illustrates the contact relationship between a mandibular and a maxillary premolar in occlusion. The maxillary premolar is fitted with an artificial restoration with an improperly designed occlusal surface. Occlusion results in horizontally directed forces which may produce an undue stress concentration within the encircled areas of the periodontium of the maxillary tooth. Resorption of the alveolar bone occurs in these areas. A widening of the periodontal ligament can be detected as well as increased mobility of the tooth. Following adjustment of the occlusion the horizontal forces are reduced. This results in bone apposition and a normalization of the tooth mobility (b).

Increased tooth mobility

Increased tooth mobility, determined by clinical measurements of the amplitude of displacement of the crown of a tooth does not necessarily imply that the "mobile" tooth is subjected to traumatizing forces. Increased tooth mobility can, indeed, be observed in conjunction with trauma from occlusion, but may also be the result of a reduction in the height of the alveolar bone and/or the presence of angular bony defects resulting from plaque associated periodontal disease (see Chapter 8). Increased tooth mobility may further indicate that the periodontal structures have become adapted to an altered functional demand, i.e. a widened periodontal ligament with a normal tissue composition has become the end result of a previous phase of progressive tooth mobility (see Chapter 8) associated with trauma from occlusion.

Progressive (increasing) tooth mobility

In Chapter 8, it was concluded that the diagnosis trauma from occlusion should be used solely in situations where a *progressive mobility* could be observed. This progressive mobility can be identified only through a series of repeated measurements of tooth mobility carried out over a period of days or weeks.

Treatment of increased tooth mobility

A number of situations will be described below which may call for treatment aimed at *reducing an increased tooth mobility.*

Situation I

Increased mobility of a tooth with *increased width* of the periodontal ligament but *normal height* of the alveolar bone

If a tooth (for instance an upper premolar) is

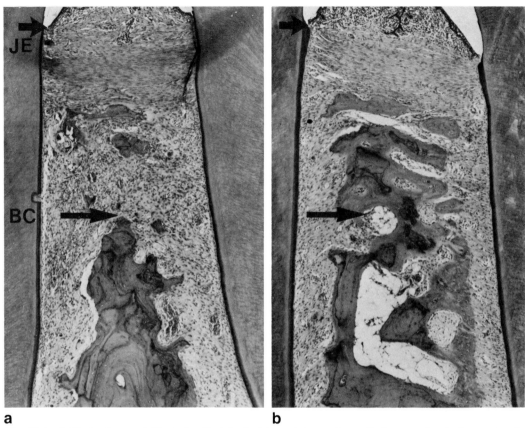

a   b

Figs. 21-6a, b. Photomicrograph illustrating the interdental area between 2 mandibular premolars in the monkey. In (a) the 2 premolars are exposed to jiggling forces. Note the reduction of alveolar bone in the area and the location of the bone crest (arrow; BC). Ten weeks after the elimination of the jiggling forces (b) a considerable regeneration of bone has occurred. Note the increase of the height of the interdental bone and the normalization of the width of the periodontal ligaments. The apical end of the junctional epithelium (JE) is located at the cementoenamel junction. (Courtesy of Dr.Polson; from Polson et al. 1976a).

fitted with an improper filling or crown restoration, occlusal interferences develop and the surrounding periodontal tissues become the seat of inflammatory reactions, i.e. trauma from occlusion (Fig. 21-5). If the restoration is so designed that the crown of the tooth in occlusion is subjected to undue forces directed in a buccal direction, bone resorption phenomena develop in the buccal-marginal and lingual-apical pressure zones with a resulting increase of the width of the periodontal ligament in these zones. The tooth becomes hypermobile or moves away from the "traumatizing" position.

Since such traumatizing forces in teeth with normal periodontium or overt gingivitis cannot result in pocket formation or loss of connective tissue attachment, the resulting increased mobility of the tooth should be regarded as a physiologic adaptation of the periodontal tissues to the altered functional demands. A proper correction of the anatomy of the occlusal surface of such a tooth, i.e. occlusal adjustment will normalize the relationship between the antagonizing teeth in occlusion, thereby eliminating the excessive forces. As a result, apposition of bone will occur in the zones previously exposed to resorption, the width of the periodontal ligament will become normalized and the tooth stabilized, i.e. reassumes its normal mobility (Fig. 21-5). In other words, resorption of alveolar bone which is caused by trauma from occlusion is a reversible process which can be treated by the elimination of occlusal interferences.

The capacity for bone regeneration after resorption following trauma from occlusion has been documented in a number of animal experiments (Waerhaug & Randers-Hansen 1966, Polson et al. 1976a, Karring et al. 1982). In such experiments, the induced bone resorption not only involved the bone within the alveolus but also the alveolar bone crest. When the traumatizing forces were removed, bone tissue was deposited not only in the walls of the alveolus, thereby normalizing the width of the periodontal ligament, but also on the bone crest area whereby the height of the alveolar bone was normalized (Fig. 21-6; Polson et al. 1976a.

In the presence of a maintained, plaque associated lesion in the soft tissue, however, bone regrowth did not occur (Fig. 21-7; Polson et al. 1976b).

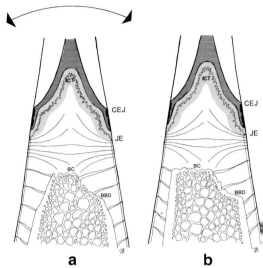

Figs. 21-7a, b. In the presence of an existing marginal inflammation, alveolar bone, lost by jiggling trauma (a), will not regenerate following elimination of the traumatic forces (b). ICT = infiltrated connective tissue; CEJ = cementoenamel junction; JE = apical end of junctional epithelium; BC = alveolar bone crest; BBD = bottom of angular bony defect (From Polson et al. 1976b).

Situation II

Increased mobility of a tooth with *increased width* of the periodontal ligament and *reduced height* of the alveolar bone

When a dentition has been properly treated for plaque associated periodontal disease, gingival health is established in areas of the dentition where teeth are surrounded by periodontal structures of reduced height. If a tooth with a reduced periodontal tissue support is exposed to excessive horizontal forces (trauma from occlusion), inflammatory reactions develop in the pressure zones of the periodontal ligament with accompanying bone resorption. These alterations are similar to those which occur around a tooth with normal height of the supporting structures; the alveolar bone is resorbed, the width of the periodontal ligament is increased in the pressure zones and the tooth becomes

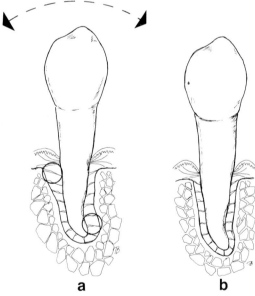

Figs. 21-8a, b. If a tooth with reduced periodontal tissue support (a) has been exposed to excessive horizontal forces a widened periodontal ligament space (encircled areas) and increased mobility (arrow) has resulted. Following reduction or elimination of such forces bone apposition will occur and the tooth will become stabilized (b).

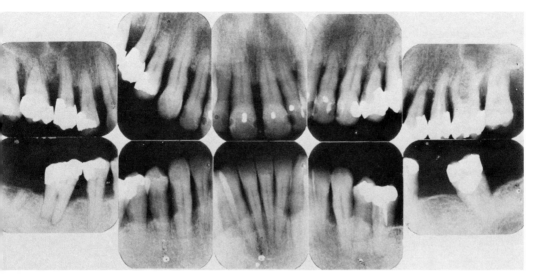

Fig. 21-9. Case A, 64 year old male. Periodontal status and radiographs prior to therapy.

hypermobile (Fig. 21-8a). If the excessive forces are reduced or eliminated by occlusal adjustment, bone apposition to the "pre-trauma" level will occur, the periodontal ligament will regain its normal width and the tooth will become stabilized (Fig. 21-8b).

Conclusion: Situations I and II

Occlusal adjustment is an effective therapy against *increased tooth mobility* when such mobility is caused by an INCREASED WIDTH of the periodontal ligament.

Situation III

Increased mobility of a tooth with *reduced height* of the alveolar bone and *normal width* of the periodontal ligament

The increased tooth mobility which is the result of a reduction in height of the alveolar bone without a concomitant increase in width of the periodontal membrane cannot be reduced or eliminated by occlusal adjust-

Periodontal chart						
Tooth	Pocket depth				Furcation	Tooth
	m	b	d	l	involvement	mobility
17	6	6	8	8	b_2, m_2, d_1	
16	6	6	8	8	m_1, d_2	2
15	8	4	6	7		2
14	7	4	7	4	3	2
13	8	4	8	4		2
12	8	4	8	4		2
11	6	4	7	4		1
21	6	4	6	4		1
22	6	5	7			2
23	6		6	4		2
24	7		8		3	2
25	6	8	8	4		2
26	8		6		b_2, m_2, d_2	
27	6	6	10	8	b_2, d_2	1
46	8	6	6	7	b_1, l_2	
45	6		7	4		1
44	6		6	4		
43	7	7	6	4		
42	4		4	4		1
41	6	4				1
31	6					1
32	4		6	4		1
33	6		6	6		2
34	4		7	4		
35	7		4	6		2
37	8	5	6	4	b_2, l_1	3

ment, since, in teeth with normal width of the periodontal ligament, no further bone apposition on the walls of the alveoli can occur. *If such an increased tooth mobility does not interfere with the patient's chewing function or comfort no treatment is required.* If the patient experiences the tooth mobility as disturbing, however, the mobility can in this situation be reduced only by splinting, i.e. by joining the mobile tooth/teeth together with other teeth in the jaw into a fixed unit – a SPLINT.

A SPLINT is according to the Glossary of Terms (1977) "an appliance designed to stabilize mobile teeth". A splint can be fabricated in the form of joined composite fillings, fixed bridges, removable partial prostheses, etc.

Example: Case A, 64 year old male
The periodontal condition of this patient is illustrated by the probing depth, furcation involvement and tooth mobility data as well as the radiographs from the initial examination in Fig. 21-9. Periodontal disease has progressed to a level where, around the maxillary teeth, only the apical third or less of the roots are invested in supporting alveolar bone. The following discussion is related to the treatment of the maxillary dentition:

In the treatment planning of this case it was decided that the first premolars (teeth 14 and 24) had to be extracted due to advanced periodontal disease and furcation involvement of Degree 3. For the same reasons teeth 17 and 27 were scheduled for extraction. Also 16 and 26 were found to have advanced loss of periodontal tissue support in combination with deep furcation involvements. The most probable definitive treatment should include periodontal and adjunctive therapy in the following parts of the dentition: 15 and 25, and 13, 12, 11, 21, 22, 23. For functional and esthetic reasons, obviously 14 and 24 had to be replaced. The question now arose as to whether these 2 premolars should be replaced by 2 separate unilateral bridges using 13, 15 and 23, 25 as abutment teeth or if the increased mobility of these teeth and also of the anterior teeth

(12, 11, 21, 22; Fig. 21-9) called for a bridge of cross-arch design with the extension 15-25 to obtain a splinting effect. If 14 and 24 are replaced by 2 unilateral bridges, each one of these 3-unit bridges will exhibit the same degree of mobility, in buccolingual direction, as the individual abutment teeth (Degree 2: Fig. 21-9), since a unilateral straight bridge will not provide a stabilizing effect on the abutment teeth in this force direction.

From the radiographs it can be seen that the increased mobility observed in the maxillary teeth of this patient is associated mainly with reduced height of the alveolar bone and not with increased width of the periodontal ligaments. This means that the mobility of the individual teeth should be regarded as normal or "physiologic" for teeth with such a reduced amount (height) of tissue support. This in turn implies that the increased tooth mobility in the present case does not call for treatment unless it interferes with the chewing comfort or jeopardizes the position of the front teeth. This particular patient had not recognized any functional problems related to the increased mobility of his maxillary teeth. Consequently there was no reason to install a cross-arch bridge in order to splint the teeth, i.e. to reduce tooth mobility.

Following proper treatment of the plaque associated periodontal lesions, 2 separate provisional bridges of unilateral design were produced (15, 14, 13; 23, 24, 25, 26 palatal root). The provisional acrylic bridges were used for 6 months during which the occlusion, the mobility of the 2 bridges as well as the position of the front teeth were all carefully monitored. When, after 6 months, no change of position of the lateral and central incisors had occurred and no increase of the mobility of the 2 provisional bridges had been noted, the definitive restorative therapy was performed.

Fig. 21-10 presents radiographs obtained 10 years after initial therapy. The position of the front teeth and the mobility of the incisors and the 2 bridges have not changed during the course of the maintenance

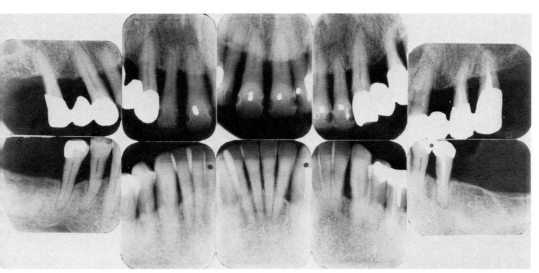

Fig. 21-10. Case A. Radiographs obtained 10 years after periodontal therapy and installation of 2 unilateral bridges in the maxilla.

period. There has been no further loss of periodontal tissue support during the 10 years of observation, no further spread of the front teeth and no widening of the periodontal ligaments around the individual teeth including the abutment teeth for the bridgework.

Conclusion: Situation III

Increased tooth mobility (or bridge mobility) as a result of reduced height of the alveolar bone can be accepted and splinting avoided provided the occlusion is stable (no further migration or further increasing mobility of individual teeth) and provided the degree of mobility existing does not disturb the patient's chewing ability or comfort. Consequently: splinting is indicated when the mobility of a tooth or a group of teeth is so increased that chewing ability and/or comfort are disturbed.

Situation IV

Progressive (increasing) mobility of a tooth (teeth) as a result of gradually *increasing*

width **of the periodontal ligament in teeth with a *reduced height* of the alveolar bone**
Often in cases of advanced periodontal disease the tissue destruction may have reached a level where extraction of one or several teeth cannot be avoided. Teeth which in such a dentition are still available for periodontal treatment may, after therapy, exhibit such a high degree of mobility – or even signs of progressively increasing mobility – that there is an obvious risk that the forces elicited during function may mechanically disrupt the remaining periodontal ligament components and cause extraction of the teeth. Only by means of a splint will it be possible to maintain such teeth. In such patients a fixed splint has 2 objectives namely 1) to stabilize hypermobile teeth and 2) to replace missing teeth.

Example: Case B, 26 year old male
Fig. 21-11 presents radiographs taken prior to therapy and Fig. 21-12 those obtained after periodontal treatment and preparation of the remaining teeth as abutments for 2 fixed splints. All teeth except 13, 12, and 33 have lost around 75% or more of the alveolar bone and widened periodontal ligaments

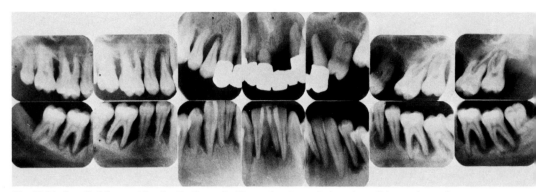

Fig. 21-11. Case B, 26 year old male. Radiographs illustrating the periodontal conditions prior to therapy.

are a frequent finding. The 4 distal abutments for the 2 splints are root separated molars, the remaining roots being the following: the palatal root of 17, the mesio-buccal root of 26 and the mesial roots of 36 and 47. It should be observed tooth 24 is root separated and the palatal root maintained with only minute amounts of periodontium left. Immediately prior to insertion of the 2 splints all teeth except 13, 12 and 33 displayed a mobility varying between Degrees 1 and 3. From the radiographs in Fig. 21-12 it can be noted that there is an obvious risk of extraction in a number of teeth such as 24, 26, 47, 45, 44, 43 and 36 if the patient is allowed to bite with a normal chewing force without the splints in position.

Despite the high degree of mobility of th

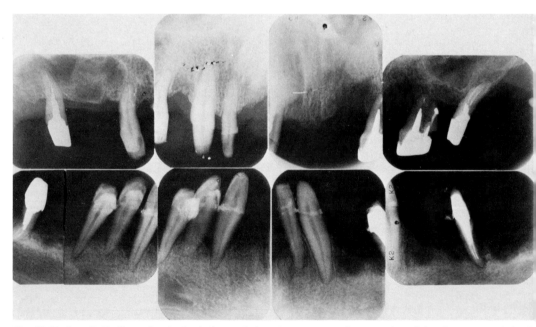

Fig. 21-12. Case B. Radiographs obtained after periodontal treatment and preparation of the abutment teeth for 2 fixed splints.

individual teeth, the splints were, after insertion, entirely stable and have maintained
their stability during a maintenance period
of more than 12 years. Figs. 21-13a, b, c
describe the clinical status and Fig. 21-14
presents the radiographs obtained 10 years
after therapy. From these radiographs it can
be observed (compare with Fig. 21-12) that
during the maintenance period there has
been no further loss of alveolar bone or
widening of the various periodontal ligament spaces.

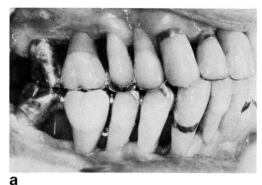

a

Conclusion: Situation IV

Splinting is indicated when the periodontal
support is so reduced that the mobility of the
teeth is progressively increasing, i.e. when a
tooth or a group of teeth during function are
exposed to extraction forces.

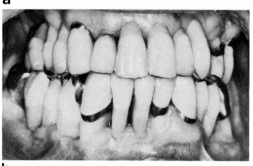

b

Situation V

Increased bridge mobility despite splinting
In a patient with advanced periodontal disease it can often be observed that the destruction of the periodontium has progressed
to varying levels around different teeth and
tooth surfaces in the dentition. Following
proper treatment of the plaque associated
lesions, often including multiple extractions,
the remaining teeth may not only display an
extreme reduction of the supporting tissues
concomitantly with increased or progressive
tooth mobility but they may also be distributed in the jaw in such a way as to make it
difficult, or impossible, to obtain a proper
splinting effect even by means of a cross-arch
bridge. The entire bridge/splint may exhibit
mobility in frontal and/or lateral directions.

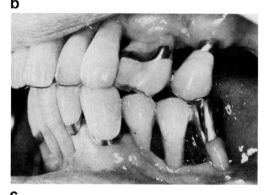

c

Figs. 21-13a-c. Case B. Clinical status 9 years after
therapy.

It was stated above (Situation III) that a
certain mobility of a tooth or a bridge of
unilateral design can be accepted provided
this mobility does not interfere with the
patient's chewing ability or comfort. This is
also valid for a cross-arch bridge/splint.
From a biologic point of view there is no difference between increased tooth mobility on

the one hand and increased bridge mobility
on the other. However, *neither progressive
tooth mobility nor progressive bridge mobility* can be accepted. In cases of extremely
advanced periodontal disease a cross-arch
splint with an increased mobility may be
regarded as an acceptable result of rehabilitation. The maintenance of *status quo* of the
bridge/splint mobility and the prevention of

461

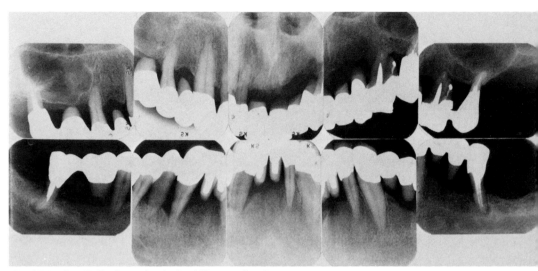

Fig. 21-14. Case B. Radiographs obtained 10 years after therapy.

tipping or orthodontic displacement of the total splint, however, requires particular attention regarding the design of the occlusion. Below a case is reported which may serve the purpose of an interesting illustration to this particular clinical problem.

Example: Case C, 52 year old female
Fig. 21-15 shows radiographs obtained at the initial examination. A 12-unit maxillary bridge was installed 10-15 years prior to the present examination using 18, 15, 14, 13, 12, 11, 21, 22, 23 and 24 as abutments. After a detailed clinical examination it was obvious that 15, 14, 22 and 24 could not be maintained because of severe symptoms of caries and periodontal disease. The remaining teeth were subjected to periodontal therapy and maintained as abutments for a new bridge/splint in the maxilla extending from tooth 18 to the region of 26, i.e. a cross-arch splint was installed which carried 3 cantilever units namely 24, 25 and 26. The mobility of the individual abutment teeth immediately prior to insertion of the splint was the following: Degree 1 (tooth 18), Degree 0 (tooth 13), Degree 2 (teeth 12 and 11), Degree 3 (tooth 21) and Degree 2 (tooth 23).

Radiographs obtained 5 years after therapy are shown in Fig. 21-16. The bridge/splint had a mobility of Degree 1 immediately after its insertion and this mobility was unchanged 5 years later. The radiographs demonstrate that no further widening of the periodontal ligament has occurred around the individual teeth during the maintenance period.

When a cross-arch bridge/splint exhibits increased mobility the center of rotation (the fulcrum) for the movement must be identified. In order to prevent further increase of the mobility and/or to prevent displacement of the bridge, it is essential to design the occlusion in such a way that the bridge/splint when in contact with the teeth of the opposing jaw, is subjected to a balanced load, i.e. equal force on each side of the fulcrum. If this can be achieved the force to which the bridge is exposed in occlusion can be used to retain the fixed prosthesis in proper balance (further increase of the mobility being thereby prevented).

Balanced loading of a mobile bridge/splint has to be established not only in the intercuspal position (IP) and centric occlusion (CP) but also in frontal and lateral excursive movements of the mandible, if the

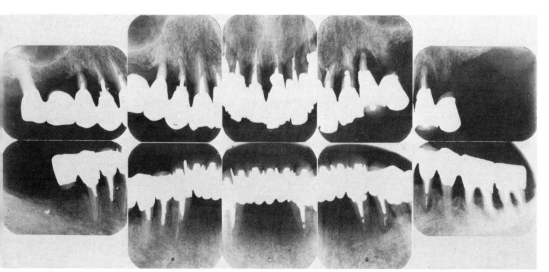

Fig. 21-15. Case C, 52 year old female. Radiographs obtained at the initial examination.

bridge shows mobility or a tendency for tipping in the direction of such movements. In other words, a force which tends to displace the bridge in a certain direction has to be counteracted by the introduction of a balancing force on the opposite side of the rotation center. If, for instance, a cross-arch splint in the maxilla exhibits mobility in frontal direction in conjunction with protrusive movements of the mandible, the load applied to the bridge in the frontal region has to be counterbalanced by a load in the distal portions of the splint; this means that there must be a simultaneous and equal contact relationship between the occluding teeth in both the frontal and the posterior regions of the splint. If the splint is mobile in a lateral direction, the force acting on the working

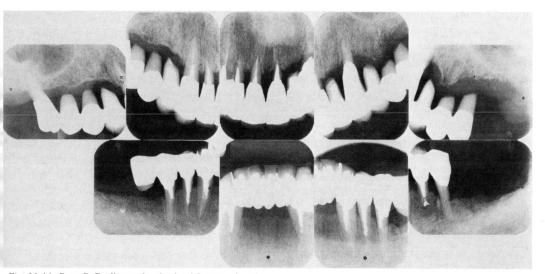

Fig. 21-16. Case C. Radiographs obtained 5 years after therapy.

side of the jaw must be counteracted by a force established by the introduction of balancing contacts in the non-working side of the jaw. The principle for establishing stability of a mobile cross-arch splint is consequently the same as that used to obtain stability in a complete denture. In situations where distal abutment teeth are missing in a cross-arch bridge/splint with increased mobility, balance and functional stability may be obtained by means of cantilever units. *It is in this context important to point out that balancing contacts on the nonworking side should not be introduced in a bridge/splint in which no increased mobility can be observed.*

The maxillary splint in the patient described in Figs. 21-13 to 21-16, exhibited increased mobility in frontal direction. Considering the small amount of periodontal support left around the front teeth, it is obvious that there would be a risk of frontal displacement of the total bridge, had the bridge terminated at the last abutment tooth (23) on the left side of the jaw. The installation of cantilever units in the 24 and 25 region prevented such a displacement of the bridge/- splint by the introduction of a counteracting force against frontally directed forces during protrusive movements of the mandible (Fig. 21-17). In addition, the cantilever units provide bilateral contact relationship towards the mandibular teeth in the intercuspal position, i.e. bilateral stability of the bridge.

In cases similar to the one described above cantilever units can, thus, be used to prevent increasing mobility or displacement of a bridge/splint. It should, however, be pointed out that the insertion of cantilever units increases the risk for failures of technical and biophysical character (fracture of the metal frame, fracture of the abutment teeth, loss of retention, etc). For details regarding the technical aspects of fixed bridgework for patients with advanced periodontal disease, see Chapter 22.

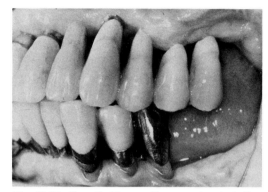

Fig. 21-17. Case C. The cantilever section including teeth 24, 25 and 26.

In cases of severely advanced periodontal disease it is often impossible to anticipate at the planning phase whether a bridge/splint after insertion will show signs of instability and increasing (progressive) mobility. In such cases a provisional splint should always be inserted. Any alterations of the mobility of the bridge/splint can be observed over a prolonged period of time and the occlusion continuously adjusted until after 4-6 months it is known whether stability (i.e. no further increase of the mobility) can be achieved. The design of the occlusion of the provisional acrylic bridge is then reproduced in the permanent bridge construction. *If on the other hand stability cannot be obtained, the rehabilitation of the case cannot be made with a fixed splint.* The alternative treatment then is a complete denture.

Conclusion: Situation V

An increased mobility of a cross-arch bridge/splint can be accepted provided the mobility does not disturb chewing ability or comfort and the mobility of the splint is not progressively increasing.

References

Glickman, I. (1965) Clinical significance of trauma from occlusion. *Journal of the American Dental Association* **70**, 607-618.

Glickman, I. (1967) Occlusion and periodontium. *Journal of Dental Research* **46**, Supplement, 53.

Glossary of Terms (1977) *Journal of Periodontology, Supplement.*

Karring, T., Nyman, S., Thilander, B. & Magnusson, I. (1982) Bone regeneration in orthodontically produced alveolar bone dehiscences. *Journal of Periodontal Research* **17**, 309-315.

Mühlemann, H. R. (1954) Tooth mobility. The measuring method. Initial and secondary tooth mobility. *Journal of Periodontology* **25**, 22-29.

Mühlemann, H. R. (1960) Ten years of tooth mobility measurements. *Journal of Periodontology* **31**, 110-122.

Mühlemann, H. R. & Zander, H. A. (1954) Tooth mobility. III. The mechanism of tooth mobility. *Journal of Periodontology* **25**, 128.

Polson, A. M., Meitner, S. W. & Zander, H. A. (1976a) Trauma and progression of marginal periodontitis in squirrel monkeys. III. Adaption of interproximal alveolar bone to repetitive injury. *Journal of Periodontal Research* **11**, 279-289.

Polson, A. M., Meitner, S. W. & Zander, H. A. (1976b) Trauma and progression of marginal periodontitis in squirrel monkeys. IV. Reversibility of bone loss due to trauma alone and trauma superimposed upon periodontitis. *Journal of Periodontal Research* **11**, 290-298.

Waerhaug, J. (1979) The infrabony pocket and its relationship to trauma from occlusion and subgingival plaque. *Journal of Periodontology* **50**, 355-365.

Waerhaug, J. & Randers-Hansen, E. (1966) Periodontal changes incident to prolonged occlusal overload in monkeys. *Acta Odontologica Scandinavica* **24**, 91-105.

Technical and Biophysical Aspects of Crown and Bridge Therapy in Patients with Reduced Amounts of Periodontal Tissue Support

Introduction

Often in cases of advanced periodontal disease the destruction of the supporting tissues, in one or more parts of the dentition, has progressed to a level which calls for extraction of several teeth (Fig. 22-1). Following treatment of such cases only a few teeth may remain, teeth which not only have a minimum of periodontal tissue support

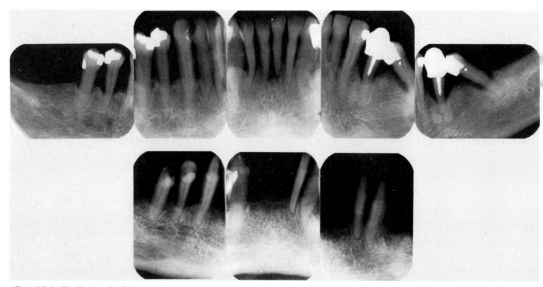

Fig. 22-1. Radiographs illustrating periodontal conditions before (top) and after (bottom) treatment of advanced periodontal disease. The remaining teeth have reduced periodontal tissue support.

466

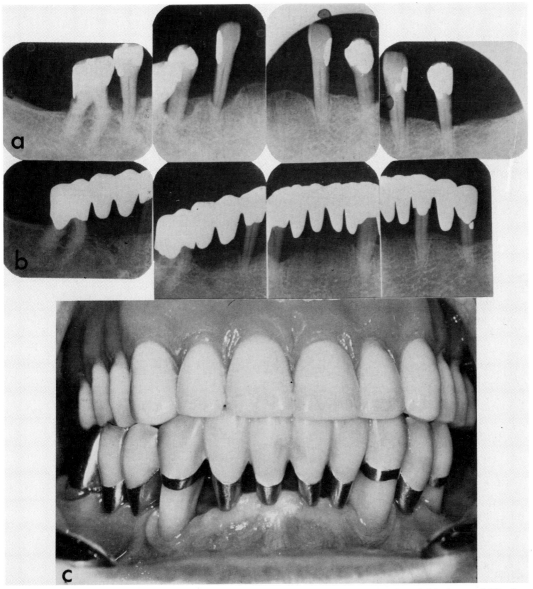

Figs. 22-2a, b, c. Radiographs of a patient with advanced loss of the periodontal tissues (a) before and (b) after combined periodontal and prosthetic treatment. The clinical status 5 years after treatment is shown in (c).

left, but which also frequently show signs of markedly increased mobility. In such cases there is an obvious need for prosthetic treatment in order to 1) restore lost function, 2) improve esthetics and 3) stabilize mobile teeth. The principles of periodontal treatment and the biological rationale for splint-

ing in the treatment of periodontitis are discussed in Chapters 13, 14 and 21.

As a rule, in patients with pronouncd loss of periodontal support, fixed bridges are preferable to removable partial dentures (Fig. 22-2). In contrast to removable partial dentures, fixed bridges provide a degree of

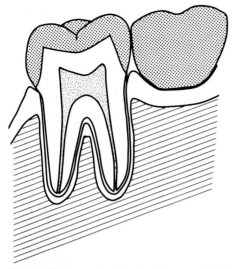

Fig. 22-3. A bridge construction includes not only the metal component and the veneer material of the prosthesis but also the cementing agent, the abutment teeth, the periodontal ligaments and the supporting alveolar bone.

rigidity and a more favorable force distribution to the remaining periodontium (see Chapter 21).

Recently published long-term results of combined periodontal and prosthetic treatment have shown that the limiting criteria for fixed bridgework in patients with few abutment teeth and reduced, but healthy, periodontal tissues around these teeth are related to the technical and biophysical factors involved in the fabrication of the bridges rather than to the biological capacity of the remaining periodontium to support the bridges successfully (Nyman & Lindhe 1979, Nyman & Ericsson 1982). The results showed in fact that it was possible in such patients to prevent recurrence of gingivitis of clinical importance and to arrest further progression of periodontal tissue breakdown by proper periodontal treatment and the institution of a carefully designed postoperative plaque control program. No abutment teeth were lost in these patients as the result of recurrence of periodontal disease during the observation period of more than 10 years. However, technical failures did occur.

These failures were caused 1) by loss of retention of retainers (3.3%), 2) fracture of metal components (2.1%) and 3) fracture of abutment teeth (2.4%). A further analysis revealed that the fundamental principles regarding design and construction of bridgework had often been overlooked in the unsuccessful prostheses. These principles will be discussed in detail in this chapter.

General principles

The basic principles for constructing fixed bridges for patients with few available abutments and reduced periodontal tissue support do not differ from those for patients with many available abutments. The clinical and technical difficulties are, however, more pronounced. Some technical and biophysical factors are discussed here, factors which *per se* have universal applicability in all bridge treatment, but which are of utmost importance when restoring periodontally weak dentitions with fixed bridgework.

It should be emphasized first that the term "bridge" or "bridge construction" is not restricted to the metal component and the veneer material (Fig. 22-3), but refers also to the cementing agent, the abutment teeth, the periodontal ligaments and the supporting alveolar bone.

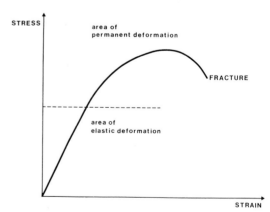

Fig. 22-4. In any object exposed to loading, the created stress will cause strain in the form of elastic/plastic deformation or fracture.

In any object (e.g. a bridge construction) exposed to loading, transferred forces will create stress ($\approx$ force/surface area) which in turn causes strain (Fig. 22-4). It is a fundamental requirement of a bridge construction that in none of the components (i.e. the metal frame, the veneer material, the cementing agent, the abutment teeth, the periodontal ligaments and the alveolar bone) must strain reach such levels during function that permanent deformation or fractures occur. In this context it should be recognized that the different components of a bridge construction have different physical properties. The periodontal ligament and, to a certain degree the alveolar bone, are elastic tissues with good ability to withstand and distribute forces, thereby reducing the risk of adverse stress concentration. On the other hand, dental alloys, ceramics and cementing agents are materials which can withstand only limited amounts of strain without exhibiting permanent deformation or fracture.

Figs. 22-5, 22-6. The magnitudes of loading forces, the proper dimensions of the prosthesis and the threshold values for permanent deformation of the various components of a prosthetic appliance depend on the individual design and extension of the prosthesis and on the distribution of the abutments.

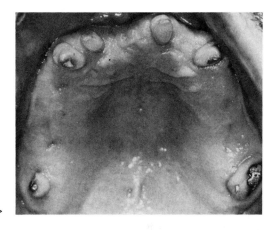

Fig. 22-5. ▷

Fig. 22-6.
▽

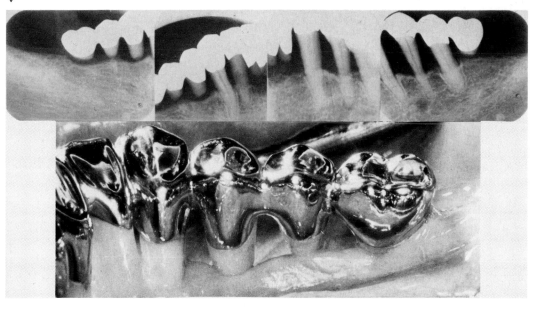

To prevent failures of a technical and biophysical nature in fixed bridgework it is mandatory to locate and define the dimension and shape of each component of a bridge (abutments, cementing agents, retainers, pontics, solderings, etc.) in such a way that not even maximum stress will result in unfavorable strain in any part of the construction. Few available abutments, unfavorably distributed in relation to the extent of the bridge, make it difficult to avoid permanent deformation or fracture. It should be understood, however, that within a bridge construction there are the mechanoreceptors of the periodontal ligaments and the alveolar bone, which possess a controlling effect on the load induced by the masticatory muscles (Hannam 1976). This, in turn, implies that all other bridge components must be located and designed in such a way that they do not exhibit permanent deformation before the mechanoreceptors are activated. The function of the mechanoreceptors is also stress dependent and there is experimental support for the hypothesis that the threshold level of the mechanoreceptor function is lower in teeth with reduced periodontal tissue support than in teeth with normal height of the supporting apparatus (Lundgren et al. 1975). This is an advantage when a fixed bridge is made for a patient with reduced periodontal tissue support since it facilitates the possibilities to give the various components of the bridge sufficient dimensions. Consequently, what can be accomplished in extensive fixed bridges for periodontally involved patients does not apply directly to "normal" patients. It is also important to realize that the threshold level for the mechanoreceptor function is not definite but can be changed, e.g. through adaptation (Öwall & Möller 1974, Goldberg 1976). Therefore, the gap between the threshold level for receptor function and permanent deformation of the other bridge components (prosthetic materials, abutment teeth etc.) should be kept wide. In other words, all other physical components (i.e. prosthetic materials, abutment teeth, etc.) must be capable of withstanding

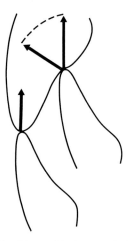

Fig. 22-7. In dentitions with deep vertical overlap the horizontal forces elicited during function are higher than in dentitions with shallow horizontal overlap.

more load than the periodontal tissues.

Depending on the individual design, extension and distribution of abutment teeth, for each bridgework, no formula exists for the relationship between the magnitude of loading forces, the dimensions of the prosthesis, and the threshold values for permanent deformation of the various bridge components (Figs. 22-5, 22-6). When relevant model systems are used, it can be demonstrated that deformation can be kept

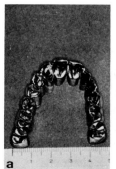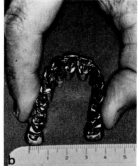

Fig. 22-8. A 13-unit bridge which, evidently, has insufficient rigidity for lateral loading.

within tolerable limits by reducing the length of pontic segments, particularly cantilever segments, and by giving all components sufficient height in all directions of loading which occur during function (Timoshenko & Goodier 1970).

When, as a consequence of a reduced number of available abutment teeth, long pontic spans cannot be avoided or when cantilever pontics must be used to obtain stability of a mobile bridge (see Chapter 21), the increased stress produced by the pontics must be compensated for by a sufficient increase of the height of the prosthesis in the directions of loading (Lindhe & Nyman 1977). Also in this respect the periodontally involved patient offers advantages over the "normal" patient. Resorption of alveolar bone provides abutment teeth with long clinical crowns and a wide distance between the alveolar crest of edentulous areas and the occlusal surfaces of opposing teeth.

To secure a proper design for bridge construction, all functional loading directions must be carefully analysed. For example in a dentition with a deep vertical overlap (Fig. 22-7), the horizontal forces acting on the maxillary teeth during function are large. The horizontal dimensions of the prosthesis must receive special attention to secure rigidity. If rigidity is not obtained in such a case, sooner or later fracture will occur in one or the other of the bridge components (Fig. 22-8).

Selection of retainer crowns

Partial crowns such as inlays, pin-ledges and ¾ crowns often give good esthetic results particularly when the buccal tooth surfaces are intact. It is well known, however, that the rigidity of an intact tube, such as a complete crown, is much higher than that of a tube with a longitudinal opening (Timoshenko & Goodier 1970). This means that, in comparison to a complete crown, a partial

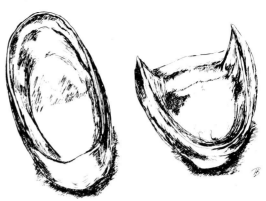

Fig. 22-9. A complete crown has a higher degree of rigidity than a partial crown.

veneer crown has less resistance to deformation. Therefore, complete crowns are preferable as retainers in dentitions with few abutments related to the extension of the bridge (Fig. 22-9).

Preparation design

A fundamental demand, when preparing a tooth for a complete crown, is to ensure "self retention" against horizontally directed forces; that is, the strength of the cement film must not be the sole retentive factor. This demand is met by preparing the abutment teeth with maximum height and minimum taper (Fig. 22-10). *The length of any diagonal of the prepared tooth must exceed the diameter of its base* (for discussion see Hegdahl & Silness 1977).

Fig. 22-11 illustrates a maxilla in which a bridge with a cross-arch design is to be inserted. Assuming that "normal" horizontal and vertical overlaps exist, protrusive movements will produce a force in occluso-anterior direction (arrow, Fig. 22-11) operating on the distal abutment. A dislodging effect of such a force can be prevented if the distal surface of the molar is prepared parallel to the mesial and distal surfaces of the canine and the labial and lingual surfaces

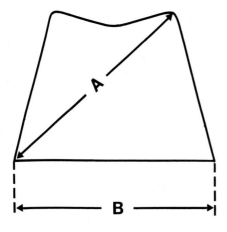

A > B

Fig. 22-10. A complete crown obtains "self retention" to the prepared tooth if the length of the diagonal of the prepared portion of the tooth (A) exceeds the diameter of its base (B).

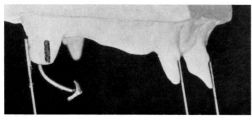

Fig. 22-11. Model of a case in which abutment teeth have been prepared for a maxillary fixed prosthesis. Protrusive contact movements will produce occluso-anteriorly directed forces on the distal abutment.

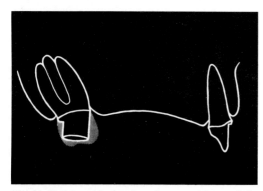

Fig. 22-12. Schematic drawing of a case with a mesially tilted molar abutment. When preparing this tooth the distal surface can be made parallel to the labial surface of the canine by a shoulder preparation.

of the incisor. In addition, the direction of insertion should have a distal angulation in relation to the direction of the dislocating force. To further improve the retention, boxes or grooves which are parallel to the distal surface of the molar can be prepared in the *buccal* (and/or the *lingual*) surfaces.

If a molar abutment tooth has tilted mesially it may no longer be possible, with slice preparation, to obtain parallelism between its distal surface and the opposite surfaces of the front teeth (Fig. 22-12). If this is the case, the distal surface of the molar can often be made parallel to the labial surfaces of anterior teeth by a shoulder preparation. To secure proper retention against laterally dislocating forces, the buccal and lingual surfaces of premolars and molars on each side of the jaw must be parallel to each other and to the proximal surfaces of anterior teeth, if present (Fig. 22-13). If boxes or grooves are added to increase retention they should be prepared on the *proximal* surfaces of posterior teeth.

Pins parallel to the path of insertion and/or horizontal pins can improve retention of cast restorations. Pins can also be used in abutments where the diameter of the base of the preparation is longer than the diagonals. However, pin retention should only be used in a tooth with thick dentine (Fig. 22-14);

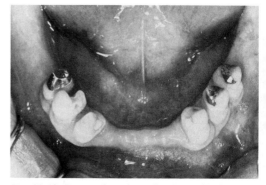

Fig. 22-13. Preparations for a fixed mandibular prosthesis demonstrating how proper retention against dislocating forces in lateral excursion has been secured by preparing the buccal and lingual surfaces of the teeth on each side of the jaw parallel to one another.

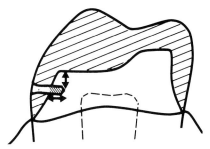

Fig. 22-14. Horizontal pins may be inserted into the preparation to improve retention. Note that the pin is surrounded by a comparatively thick layer of dentine.

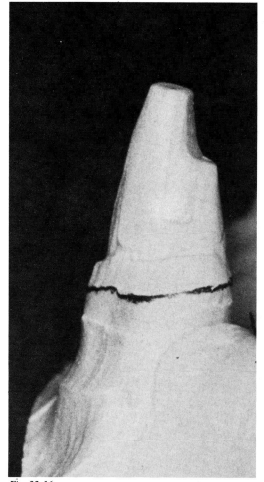

Fig. 22-16.

otherwise, there is an obvious risk of dentine fracture with subsequent loss of retention.

Following periodontal treatment, the remaining teeth may exhibit different degrees of mobility. When these teeth are used as abutments, the most stable tooth (arrow, Fig. 22-15) will act as the fulcrum for rotational and dislocating movements. The establishment of proper retention for this retainer is of critical importance. Therefore, maximum height of the clinical crown should be used when the tooth is prepared. In addition, boxes or grooves may be prepared to further improve retention (Fig. 22-16).

The same demands on parallelism that apply to the design of core preparations,

Fig. 22-15.

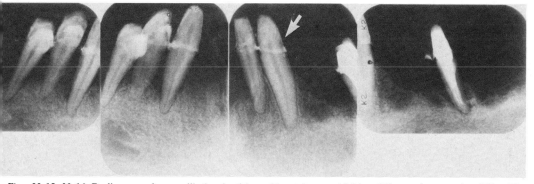

Figs. 22-15, 22-16. Radiogram of a mandibular dentition with retainers exhibiting different degrees of mobility. The most stable retainer (arrow, Fig. 22-15) will act as a fulcrum for dislocating movements. On this retainer optimal retention was established during preparation by using 1) maximum height of the clinical crown and 2) including vertical grooves (Fig. 22-16).

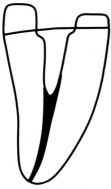

Fig. 22-17. Preparation for insertion of a dowel. The root canal and circumferential bevel are prepared with low angles of convergence.

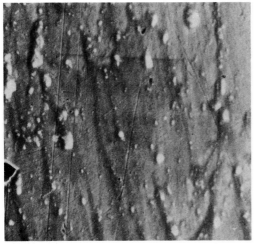

Fig. 22-18. Scanning electron micrograph (× 2500) showing the dentine surface of a prepared tooth coated with foreign material which must be removed before cementation of the crown.

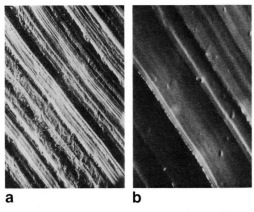

a   b

Figs. 22-19a, b. Prepared dentine surface before (a) and after (b) application of a liner. The liner fills the irregularities in the dentine surface.

must also be met when preparing root canals for insertion of dowels (Fig. 22-17). The root canal and the circumferential bevel should be prepared with as low an angle of convergence as possible.

In summary: if the preparations are given low angles of convergence ($<20°$), the strength of cement films is generally sufficient to prevent loss of retention resulting from forces acting in the opposite direction to the direction of the path of insertion of the bridge. The strength of the cement is not sufficient, however, to withstand horizontally directed forces if the preparations and the retainers do not have sufficient height and correct dimensions.

Surface treatment of prepared teeth

The surfaces of prepared teeth may be coated with various materials such as dentine chips, impression material, temporary cement, adsorbed salivary components, microorganisms and food debris (Fig. 22-18). In order to achieve optimum retention, all such materials must be removed before cementation. Otherwise the necessary close contact between the cement film and the prepared tooth surface will not be obtained. For the maintenance of the microstructure and the quality of the prepared surface, the removal of the foreign materials should be managed with methods and cleaning agents which are non-destructive to the dentine. Effective cleansers such as strong acids and bases should therefore be avoided. Studies by Brännström et al. (1982) indicate that surface active cleaning agents are more effective than the commonly used combination of 3% hydrogen peroxide solution and ethanol. However, considering the wide range of the physical and chemical properties of the various foreign materials, the most effective cleansing procedure includes separate application of 1) an oxidizing agent such as a weak hydrogen peroxide solution, 2) a solvent such as ethanol and 3) a surfactant cleanser.

Following the application of each of these cleansers, the tooth should be rinsed with water to remove loosened material and to prevent the different agents from inhibiting the cleansing effect of the others.

It has been claimed that liners should be applied to prepared dentine before cementation of a crown to protect the pulp. Such treatment drastically reduces the retention of dental cements (Glantz et al. 1978), since the liners fill the irregularities in the dentine (Fig. 22-19) where the cement gains retention.

If the remaining dentine is so thin that the pulp must be protected, the liner should only cover the critical area (Fig. 22-20) and not the entire surface of the preparation. Since liners have chemical and mechanical properties inferior to those of cements, they must not be·applied at or close to crown margins. Low viscous liners are preferred since the retentive capacity of the cement film will decrease with increased viscosity of the liner (Glantz et al. 1978).

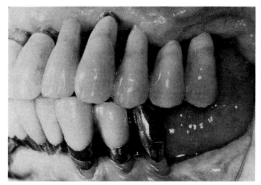

Fig. 22-21. Cantilever pontics used for the stabilization of a mobile bridge.

During cleansing and cementation procedures it is of primary importance to prevent saliva from reaching the prepared tooth surfaces. Even after momentary contact with saliva a thin organic film is adsorbed to the surface, thereby obstructing the direct contact between cement and tooth (Baier & Glantz 1978).

Specific aspects on strength

Fracture of bridgework

Fracture of the metal frame can be prevented by giving the frame adequate dimensions. Cantilever pontics may be used to achieve the balanced loading necessary to obtain stability of a mobile bridge (see Chapter 21). Such a prosthesis (Fig. 22-21) should have increased thickness of the metal frame in the loading directions to compensate for the increased stress produced by the cantilever segment (Nyman et al. 1975). Such compensating increase can, however, only be made in patients with long clinical crowns and a shallow vertical overlap (Fig. 22-22). This implies that cantilever segments should be avoided where the space is not available, such as in patients with short clinical crowns

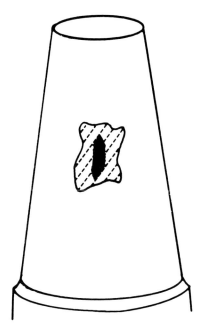

Fig. 22-20. Liner applied to protect the pulp in an area where the covering dentine is thin. Note that the liner covers only the critical area.

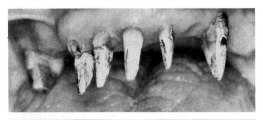

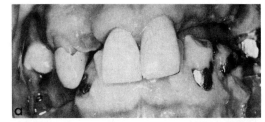

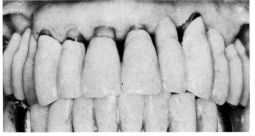

Fig. 22-22. Patient with long clinical crowns (top) and a shallow overlap (bottom). This facilitates proper dimensioning of the metal frame.

Figs. 22-23a, b. Patient with short clinical crowns and a deep overbite (a). In such cases removable restorations or combinations of fixed and removable restorations (b) should be favored at the prosthetic rehabilitation.

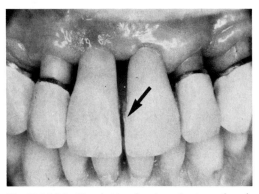

Fig. 22-24. Maxillary bridge showing a fracture of a soldered joint (arrow).

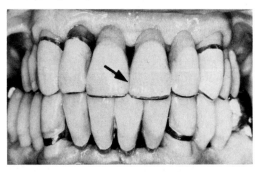

Fig. 22-25. A 10-unit maxillary bridge with 3 retainers (teeth 13, 12 and 23). This bridge has only 1 soldered joint (arrow).

or with deep overbite (Fig. 22-23a). In such individuals, prosthetic treatment with removable restorations or combinations of fixed and removable restorations should be favored (Fig. 22-23b).

Soldered joints are common sites for fractures (Fig. 22-24). The reason is generally poor design and occasionally inferior physical properties in the areas of such joints (Bergman 1976). Solderings should therefore be avoided by casting as many bridge units as possible in one. Soldered joints should not be located in areas subjected to high strain. Examples of such areas are the mesial and distal surfaces of retainers next to cantilever pontics. In the maxillary bridge extending from second premolar to second premolar (Fig. 22-25) there are only 3 abutments (right lateral incisor, canine and left canine). The frame was cast in 2 segments and there is only 1 soldered joint which is located between the central incisors.

The metal frame of all bridges consists of one or several metal alloys. When different metals or alloys are present in the same biological environment, interactions that lower their individual properties occur be-

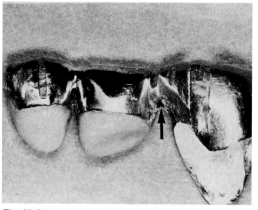

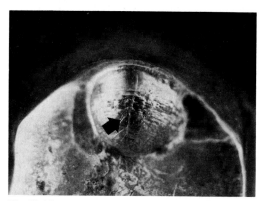

Fig. 22-26.   *Fig. 22-27.*

Figs. 22-26, 22-27. Corrosion products on soldered joints (arrow) (Fig. 22-26), and on the occlusal surface of a complete crown (cast in gold alloy) which for 7 years has been located in contact with a denture frame of a partial removable denture (cast in Co/Cr-alloy) (Fig. 22-27).

tween the materials. Corrosion is the most common reaction and it appears as soon as different metals or alloys are in contact with each other (Figs. 22-26, 22-27). Noble metal alloys should be used whenever possible and the types of alloys to be used in 1 patient should be as few as possible, ideally only 1.

Fracture of luting cement

As already discussed, fracture of the luting agent results in loss of retention of the retainer. In this context it should be stressed

that the larger the area of the cement film, the higher is its total retentive capacity (Fig. 22-28). This fact further strengthens the importance of using the maximum length and maximum surface area of the clinical crown for retention, particularly in bridges with few abutments.

Fracture of abutment teeth

Fracture of abutment teeth has been reported to occur more frequently in root filled (Fig. 22-29) than in vital teeth and

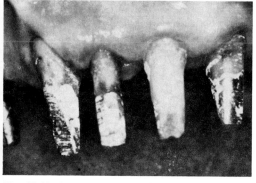

Fig. 22-28. Preparations with large surface areas for maximum cement contact and retention.

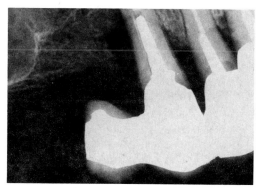

Fig. 22-29. Radiograph showing a cantilever bridge with root fracture in the terminal abutment at the tip of the dowel. Note the bony defect.

477

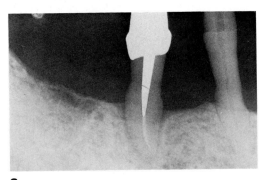

a

Fig. 22-30a. Radiograph and clinical picture of root filled abutment teeth with proper dowel.

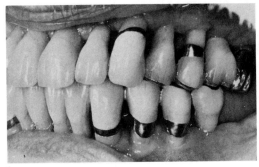

b

Fig. 22-30b. Radiograph and clinical picture of root filled abutment teeth with metal copings.

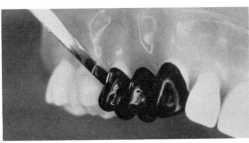

Fig. 22-31. Clinical picture of extensive fixed bridges designed to facilitate proper oral hygiene.

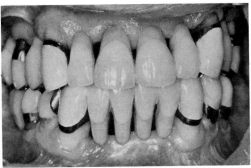

a

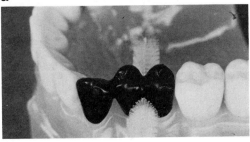

b

Figs. 22-32a,b. Toothpicks and interdental toothbrushes should be used during waxing of bridges (in this case two 3-unit bridges) to ensure a proper outline of the interdental area.

primarily in teeth containing root dowels and serving as terminal abutments for cantilever bridges. To minimize the risk of such fractures the root canal should not be so widened as to undermine the dentine walls (Fig. 22-30a). Furthermore a metal coping should circumscribe the cervix to the tooth (Fig. 22-30b). Using standard model systems, it can be demonstrated that the strength of a root filled tooth with a dowel and a metal coping is about 10 times that of a corresponding root without a coping. The wider the coping, the higher is its retentive capacity.

In addition to these technical and biophysical aspects on fixed bridges in patients with reduced periodontal tissue support, it should be emphasized that all complete crowns, used as retainers and pontics, should be designed to facilitate proper oral hygiene (Fig. 22-31). The margins of the complete crowns should be placed in a supragingival position whenever possible and the buccal and lingual surfaces must not be overcontoured.

In addition, the width of the embrasures should be matched to the size of the particular interdental cleaning device (Figs. 22-32a, b) recommended to the patient.

References

Baier, R. E. & Glantz, P.-O. (1978) Characterization of oral *in vivo* films formed on different types of solid surfaces. *Acta Odontologica Scandinavica* **36**, 289-301.

Bergman, M. (1976) Chemical and thermodynamic studies of dental gold alloys with special reference to homogenization, electrical corrosion and cluster formation. Thesis. University of Umeå, Sweden.

Brännström, M., Glantz, P.-O. & Nordenvall, K.-J. (1982) Cavity cleaners and etchants. In *Biocompatibility of Dental Materials*, vol. II, ed. Smith, D. C. & Williams, D. F. Boca Raton, FL, U.S.A.: CRC Press.

Glantz, P.-O., Gwinnett, A. J. & Jendresen, M. D. (1978) Effects of cavity varnish on surface morphology and retention. *Journal of Dental Research* **57**, Special Issue A, 126.

Goldberg, L. J. (1976) Changes in the excitability of elevator and depressor motoneurons produced by stimulation of intra-oral nerves. In *Mastication,* ed. Anderson, D. J. & Matthews, B. Bristol, U. K.: John Wright & Sons Ltd.

Hannam, A. G. (1976) Periodontal mechanoreceptors. In *Mastication,* ed. Anderson, D. J. & Matthews, B. Bristol, U. K.: John Wright & Sons Ltd.

Hegdahl, T. & Silness, J. (1977) Preparation areas resisting displacement of artificial crowns. *Journal of Oral Rehabilitation* **4**, 201-207.

Lindhe, J. & Nyman, S. (1977) The role of occlusion in periodontal disease and the biological rationale for splinting in treatment of periodontitis. *Oral Sciences Reviews* **10**, 11-43.

Lundgren, D., Nyman, S., Heijl, L. & Carlsson, G. E. (1975) Functional analysis of fixed bridges on abutment teeth with reduced periodontal support. *Journal of Oral Rehabilitation* **2**, 105-116.

Nyman, S. & Ericsson, I. (1982) The capacity of reduced periodontal tissues to support fixed bridgework. *Journal of Clinical Periodontology* **9**, 409-414.

Nyman, S., Lindhe, J. & Lundgren, D. (1975) The role of occlusion for the stability of fixed bridges in patients with reduced periodontal support. *Journal of Clinical Periodontology* **2**, 53-66.

Nyman, S. & Lindhe, J. (1979) A longitudinal study of combined periodontal and prosthetic treatment of patients with advanced periodontal disease. *Journal of Periodontology* **50**, 163-169.

Timoshenko, S. P. & Goodier, J. N. (1970) *Theory of Elasticity*. 3rd ed. New York: McGraw-Hill Book Company.

Öwall, B. & Möller, E. (1974) Oral tactile sensibility during biting and chewing. *Odontologisk Revy* **25**, 327-346.

CHAPTER 23

Orthodontic Tooth Movement in Periodontal Therapy

The continuous migration of teeth is a physiological process caused by alterations in the periodontal tissues initiated by such forces as occlusal and approximal attrition. Loss of teeth and/or periodontal tissues affect physiological tooth migration and can result in malocclusion or malalignment of teeth, changes which can be aggravated by occlusal trauma and/or oral habits, such as tongue thrust and nail biting. Pathological tooth migration can involve a single tooth or a group of teeth, and result in (1) the development of medial diastema or general spacing of the teeth, particularly in the anterior segments of the dentition; (2) in spacing of the teeth combined with proclination of upper incisors; (3) in rotated and tipped bicuspids and molars with collapse of the posterior occlusion and the development of reduced height of the bite. All these symptoms are common in individuals with advanced periodontal disease. Thus, the overall treatment plan for a patient with advanced periodontal disease often involves orthodontic realignment of the teeth to re-establish satisfactory (1) occlusion, (2) esthetic conditions and (3) chewing comfort.

In many cases the orthodontic treatment can be accomplished by comparatively simple measures. All tooth movements, however, must be preceded by a comprehensive orthodontic analysis and treatment planning. Without such an analysis even so-called "minor tooth movements" may produce more problems than they solve.

There are no standardized methods to follow in orthodontic treatment of adult individuals. The biomechanical principles used in orthodontics must be adapted to the individual anatomy of the areas in the dentition where tooth movement is planned. Radiographic examination should be performed at predetermined intervals during the course of orthodontic treatment to ensure early disclosure, and to counteract undesired iatrogenic side effects.

Factors to be considered in orthodontic therapy

Basic differences

It should be remembered that orthodontic treatment in patients with advanced periodontal disease is often performed not in children or adolescents, but in adult individuals. Since growth in such patients is completed, it is not possible by orthodontic measures to influence *zones of growth* and, therefore, treatment in the adult individual is restricted to different types of tooth *alignment*. This limitation of the possibility for orthodontic therapy in an adult patient is important to recognize. One example may illustrate the difficulty discussed.

A deep bite is frequently found in patients with advanced forms of periodontal disease. This deep bite – or reduced height of the bite – is often the result of loss of molar support for the occlusion and may be rehabilitated by means of a bite plane in order to increase the height of the bite. However, if the deep bite is of genuine character and is combined with postnormal malocclusion or occurs in individuals with neutral occlusion with low anterior facial height, an increase of vertical dimension is indeed a doubtful procedure, owing to the risk of development of muscular dysfunction and/or temporomandibular joint (TMJ) problems. Treatment, including intrusion of the incisors in such cases, involves a great risk for root resorption and is, therefore, an orthodontic measure hardly ever indicated in adult patients with periodontal disease.

Patient problems

It is far more difficult for an adult individual to adapt to an orthodontic appliance than for a child. Phonetic adjustment to a removable appliance, for instance, generally requires more time in an adult. In the initial phase of treatment, the patient often has difficulty in fitting the active elements (i.e. springs, elastics) into place, with the risk that the appliance may only be used sporadically. As a consequence the induced orthodontic treatment fails. A fixed appliance is usually better tolerated by adult patients. However, a fixed appliance may for esthetic reasons be difficult to accept by such a patient. The adult patient must thus be very thoroughly prepared for the consequences and implications of orthodontic treatment, and it should

not be initiated unless the patient is in full physical and mental health. As a rule, however, patients with advanced periodontal disease are strongly motivated for orthodontic treatment and will normally cooperate excellently.

Periodontal tissue response

Mesial migration of teeth is dependent on osteoclastic and osteoblastic activity in the periodontium. These are physiological processes that throughout life permit a constant remodeling of bone. With increasing age, however, cellular activity decreases and the tissue becomes richer in collagen. Age *per se* is not a contraindication to orthodontic treatment. But in the elderly the tissue response to orthodontic forces, including both cell mobilization and conversion of collagen fibers, is considerably slower than in children and teenagers. This means that in adults hyalin zones are formed more easily on the pressure side of the orthodontically treated tooth. Such zones may at least temporarily prevent the tooth from moving in the intended direction.

The orthodontic force applied in adults must therefore be *light*. Light forces will result in the desired tooth movement and prevent tissue damage. If the force is strong enough to exceed the capillary blood pressure in the periodontal ligament, local ischaemia occurs, followed by degenerative changes in the ligament tissue, a hyalinization. No osteoclasts can differentiate in this tissue, i.e. tooth movement cannot occur until the hyalinized zones are eliminated through the undermining resorption from the marrow spaces and adjacent areas of the unaffected alveolar bone. Tissue elements invade from the adjacent viable tissue and reorganisation of the posthyalinized area will then occur. Provided there is no invasion of inflammatory elements from the gingival structures, all the changes described above are reversible (see also Chapter 8).

The force applied in the adult patient should preferably be of the *interrupted* type. While the *continuous* force acts for longer periods of time, the *interrupted* force is of comparatively short duration (up to a few weeks). As the magnitude of the force rapidly decreases, the tissue will become properly reorganised before the active elements are reactivated. Thus, if a hyalinized zone is formed in this type of treatment it will be rapidly eliminated. There is also less risk for root resorption and pulpal damage when *interrupted* forces are used.

In the initial stage of orthodontic treatment in adults, an *interrupted* force of 20-30 g is recommended. Later on, the force may be increased (up to 30-50 g in tipping and 50-80 g in bodily movements, corresponding to a distance of movement of 0.5-1 mm per month), depending on the degree of marginal bone loss and the amount of remaining alveolar bone. Clinically, a proper orthodontic force is distinguished by the fact that the treated teeth are tender for not more than 1 or 2 days after reactivation.

Root filled or traumatized teeth which have a normal radiographic appearance may be moved orthodontically provided *light interrupted* forces are used. The selection of proper *anchorage* for the orthodontic tooth movement may present major problems in adult orthodontics, especially in partially edentulous patients and in individuals with reduced amounts of alveolar bone.

The retention period

From observations made in children subjected to orthodontic therapy, Reitan (1959) pointed out that the Sharpey's fibers of the newly formed bundle bone, as well as the principal fibers of the periodontal ligament, will undergo rearrangement even after a retention period of several months. The supraalveolar and transseptal fibers, on the other hand, change very slowly. In order to achieve proper rearrangement of the tissue structures involved in orthodontic therapy and to prevent relapse, the teeth must therefore be retained for a varying period of time.

In adults the retention period is generally long, owing to the decreased ability of the periodontal tissue to react to mechanical

stimuli. Risk for relapse always exists as long as the tissue reorganisation is still in progress. Thus, permanent retainers must often be applied after completion of active orthodontic therapy. It is important to discuss also the duration of the retention period with the patient *before* the orthodontic treatment is initiated.

In orthodontic treatment of children and teenagers it is sometimes recommended to "over-adjust" the orthodontically moved teeth to compensate for relapse. It is difficult, however, to predict the degree of over-correction needed to counteract relapse. In adult orthodontics such over-corrections are not advisable, especially not in

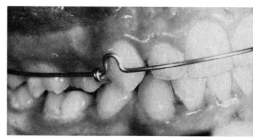

a

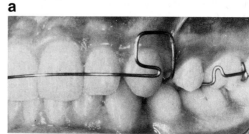

b

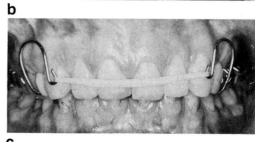

c

Figs. 23-1a-c. Different kinds of removable retainers. a) Hawley plate. b) Plate with Adams clasps and a modification of the labial arch for retaining the cuspids. c) The labial arch is replaced by an elastic (in this case ⅜″ light) for esthetic reasons.

dentitions with reduced periodontal tissue support. The retention after the active orthodontic movement can be achieved with removable or fixed appliances. Different types of removable retainers have been described (Fig. 23-1). A proper retainer should keep each orthodontically treated tooth in the acquired position. The

appliance should be designed to be as inconspicuous as possible, yet strong enough to achieve its objective during the entire period of use. It should also be easy for the patient to clean. Temporary or semi-permanent fixed retainers are often preferred to the removable varieties (Fig. 23-2). When removable retainers are used, the dentist is

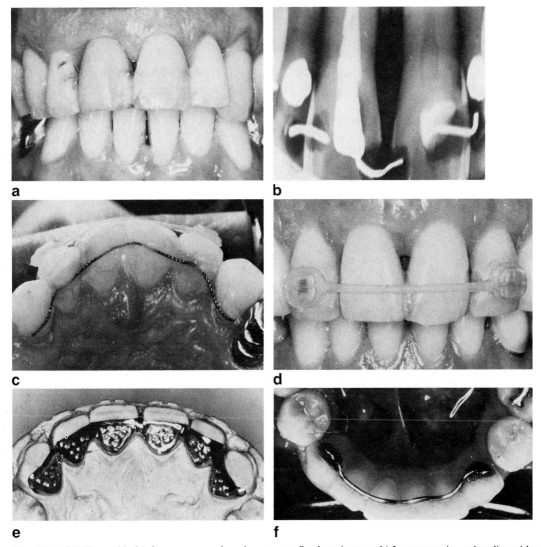

Figs. 23-2a-f. Different kinds of temporary and semipermanent fixed retainers. a, b) Interapproximate bonding with intradental pins in the composite fillings. c, d) Bonded lingual retainer in the upper jaw (Wildcat .0175). The retention is strengthened buccally for 1 month with an Alastic K2. e) Bonded gold skeleton. f) Bonded lingual retainer in the lower jaw (blue Elgiloy .019) strengthened with nets at the cuspids.

often too dependent on the cooperation of the patient. In well documented experiments, Reitan (1967) showed that most relapse following orthodontic tooth movement occurred during the first 5 h after the appliance had been removed. As already mentioned, removable appliances often cause the patient speech problems and inconvenience during chewing. It is therefore understandable that patients often use their removable retainers only in the evening and at night. This, however, results in a daily repeated minor relapse of the tooth movement. This "jiggling" results in alternate bone deposition and resorption and in a further prolongation of the retention period.

Iatrogenic effects associated with orthodontic treatment

Orthodontic treatment may cause injuries to the teeth and periodontium but in most instances this damage is reversible and regeneration or repair of the tooth structures and periodontal tissues occurs. In some cases, however, the changes may get out of control, resulting in irreparable damage. In order to prevent such damage a proper basic knowledge is required of biomechanical principles as well as tissue reactions in orthodontic treatment. Radiography should be performed at regular intervals to disclose any iatrogenic effects during the orthodontic treatment.

Root resorption

This can hardly be avoided during orthodontic tooth movement. The majority of the resorption lacunae which develop are small and insignificant. They generally appear at the border of the hyalinized zone within the marginal and middle thirds of the root and are soon repaired by apposition of cellular

cementum. In contrast, apical root resorption is an irreversible injury, resulting in a permanent shortening of the root. An unfavorable change in the crown-to-root ratio is thereby established. This is particularly alarming in dentitions with marginal bone loss, in which the extraalveolar leverage is already increased. Clinical studies have shown that root resorptions predominantly occur in incisors and that the risk for root resorption is increased in situations where (1) large orthodontic forces are used, (2) prolonged continuous bodily movements and (3) intrusive movements are performed.

It should be remembered that there is also a risk for root resorption in the anchorage teeth, which are often subject to heavy loading. Further, it should be kept in mind that in patients with periodontal disease the resistance of the anchorage unit may be reduced, not only by loss of alveolar bone but also, in many dentitions, by loss of proper anchorage teeth.

Loss of alveolar bone

The possible association between malocclusion and periodontal disease has received much attention in the literature but little support has been found for such an association. Conversely, it has been claimed that orthodontic treatment may have adverse effects on the gingival and periodontal tissues which may hasten or promote periodontal tissue breakdown later in life.

Dentitions with normal height of the attachment apparatus

A number of experiments have demonstrated that in animals with either normal gingiva or overt gingivitis, orthodontic forces cause no damage to the supraalveolar connective tissue and orthodontic treatment will therefore not result in periodontal tissue breakdown and pocket formation.

Some clinical studies, however, report that in children and young adults orthodontic treatment can in fact aggravate a preexisting plaque induced gingival lesion and cause some loss of alveolar bone and periodontal attachment. Recent follow-up studies stressing the importance of the use of light orthodontic forces and proper self performed oral hygiene during the treatment period have reported insignificant or only slight marginal bone loss in orthodontically treated children and teenagers. Compared to subjects who had never received orthodontic therapy, no difference in the general prevalence of periodontal disease was observed.

Dentitions with reduced height of the attachment apparatus

Surprisingly little has been published about adult orthodontics, and most of it in the form of case reports. It is, therefore, understandable that indications for orthodontic treatment in adults have received a subordinate place in the overall treatment of patients with periodontal disease. Only some 10 years ago, very little was known about the effect of orthodontic therapy in patients with advanced periodontal disease. Is it possible to move teeth which have reduced amounts of periodontal tissue support? Will the orthodontic movement cause an aggravation of the periodontal lesions and further promote loss of attachment and bone? Should the orthodontic treatment be performed before or after the cause related or the corrective phase of periodontal therapy? How and for how long should the teeth be stabilized subsequent to orthodontic treatment in patients with reduced amounts of periodontium?

Experiments in beagle dogs

Results were obtained which provided some basic answers to the above questions (Ericsson et al 1977, 1978, Ericsson & Thilander 1978, 1980). In these experiments it was demonstrated that (1) in the absence of plaque, orthodontic forces and tooth movements failed to induce gingivitis. In the presence of plaque, similar forces caused angular

bone defects, and with tipping and intruding movements the forces were capable of converting an overt gingival lesion into a lesion associated with attachment loss. The experiments also demonstrated that (2) orthodontic forces, kept within biological limits, failed to cause gingival inflammation in tooth regions where the periodontal tissue support was markedly reduced but *non*inflammatory, and that (3) the most important factor in initiation, progression and recurrence of periodontal disease in dogs was the microbial plaque present within the gingival pocket.

Reitan (1969) in discussing the prevention of posttreatment orthodontic relapse, pointed out the difference in reaction between the supraalveolar and the periodontal ligament fibers. It has also been shown in man, in the monkey and in the dog, that fibrotomy of the supraalveolar fibers reduces the degree of relapse after orthodontic derotation of teeth. This suggests that periodontal surgery in dentitions with reduced periodontal tissue support should preferably be performed after completion of active orthodontic therapy in order to minimize the risk for and degree of relapse. In the beagle dog experiments described above it was demonstrated, however, that (4) no significant difference existed regarding the tendency for relapse between teeth treated with periodontal surgery before or after orthodontic tipping movements.

Treatment planning

From the experiments in the beagle dog, it was concluded that:
(1) individual teeth can be moved by means of light orthodontic forces in markedly reduced, but healthy periodontal tissue
(2) the connective tissue which regenerated after orthodontic tipping movements was incapable of preventing relapse.

In cases of advanced periodontal disease combined with pathological tooth migration the retention of the orthodontically treated teeth is therefore an important factor, and in many such cases there may be a need for permanent retention using fixed bridges.

Orthodontic treatment of a patient with advanced periodontal disease may follow the protocol described below.

Initial planning

Proper *records* (including casts, photographs, intraoral radiographs) and a thorough *clinical examination* (including Plaque Index, Gingival Index, probing depth and clinical attachment level) are required for the *treatment planning,* in which the following aspects are included: the aim of therapy; the feasibility and means of achieving the aims listed; the periodontal status after cause related and corrective therapy phases; the esthetic and functional improvements required; the expected stability of the dentition; the long-term prognosis.

In simple cases the treatment planning can be performed by the general practitioner, but in more complicated and advanced cases consultation with the orthodontist and the periodontist is necessary. The treatment plan, with its advantages and disadvantages, must be explained in detail to the patient, after which treatment can start.

Treatment of periodontal disease

This includes the elimination of plaque and retention factors for plaque as well as the establishment of a morphology in the dentogingival region which facilitates proper self performed tooth cleaning. Deepened gingival pockets are eliminated and the root surfaces properly debrided before the orthodontic treatment is initiated.

Orthodontic treatment

Light forces of the *interrupted continuous* type are used. The forces are kept within biological limits, and frequent follow-up visits are scheduled for radiographic and clinical assessment of the periodontal status.

The orthodontic appliance has to be properly designed. It must provide stable anchorage without causing tissue irritation from bands, wires, loops, coils and elastics used in fixed appliances or from clasps and springs used in removable appliances. Furthermore, the appliance must be fashioned so as to permit proper self performed plaque control measures.

At each follow-up visit for reactivation (usually every 3-4 weeks) all bands must be checked since loosened bands may stimulate the accumulation of plaque and promote caries. For esthetic reasons bonded plastic brackets are frequently used in adult orthodontics. Excess of bonding material close to the gingival margin promotes plaque accumulation and will rapidly cause gingival inflammation. Loss of bonding material, on the other hand, will result in leakage and risk for demineralization on the buccal tooth surfaces. When elastics are used, the patient must be thoroughly instructed in how they should be applied. There is a risk that elastics may become dislodged into the gingival pocket and cause an inflammatory reaction with additional loss of attachment and bone. It is therefore important to probe the pockets of the anchorage and orthodontically moved teeth at each visit to discover foreign material. In order to facilitate the tooth movements, occlusal adjustment is recommended in appropriate situations during the phase of orthodontic therapy.

In orthodontic treatment the following factors must be considered: a suitable orthodontic appliance must be chosen; proper anchorage teeth must be selected; light and interrupted forces should be used; thorough clinical and radiographic assessments must be made at each follow-up visit; the occlusion should be adjusted if indicated; the oral hygiene technique must be checked. Proper records must be prepared (see under Initial planning) to enable a proper evaluation of the result of the orthodontic treatment.

Final occlusal adjustment and surgical pocket elimination

After the orthodontic treatment, final adjustment of the occlusion is performed to ensure good functional stability. If necessary, additional surgical pocket elimination is also carried out.

Retention

The phase of *retention* is initiated. Appliances of temporary, semipermanent or permanent types are inserted. During this phase assessments must be made regarding esthetics and functional stability of the treatment result. The oral hygiene must be checked and proper recordings and thorough clinical examinations performed

(see Initial planning) to facilitate the evaluation of the final result.

Posttreatment controls

These have to be undertaken to evaluate objectively also the long-term effects of the treatment.

Case presentations

On the following pages are some examples of planned treatment performed according to principles described above.

Case No. 1

A 45 year old woman (Figs. 23-3a-f) had to be treated orthodontically because of tooth migration and rotation of the left central incisor (a, b, c). The periodontal conditions had been treated by a periodontist and the level of plaque control was excellent. The incisor was derotated with a sectional light arch wire (.016 green Elgiloy). Three months later retention was performed by means of a bonded lingual retainer (.0175 Wildcat) together with a temporary buccal elastic retainer for 6 weeks (Alastic K2) (d). Posttreatment control 5 years later (e, f). Note the improvement of the vertical bony pocket mesially to the left central incisor.

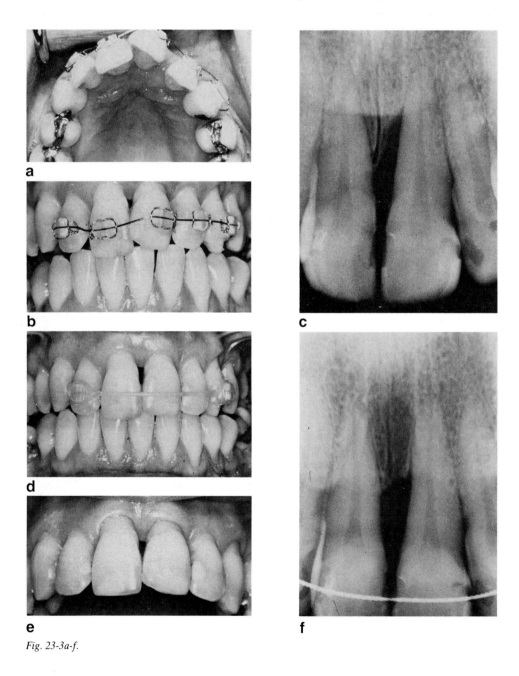

Fig. 23-3a-f.

Case No. 2

A 40 year old woman (Figs. 23-4a-f) had been treated for periodontal disease. The spaces in the upper incisor segment (a, b) were orthodontically closed by means of a light arch wire (.016 green Elgiloy). Four months later semipermanent retention was performed with intradental anchorage pins by refilling the approximal cavities (c, d). Posttreatment control 5 years later with a permanent bridge as retention (e, f). Note the improvement of the vertical bony defect mesially to the left central incisor.

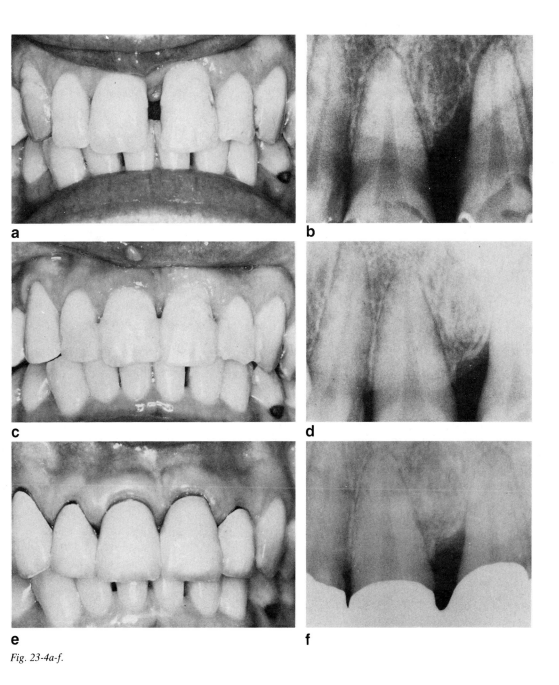

a

b

c

d

e

f

Fig. 23-4a-f.

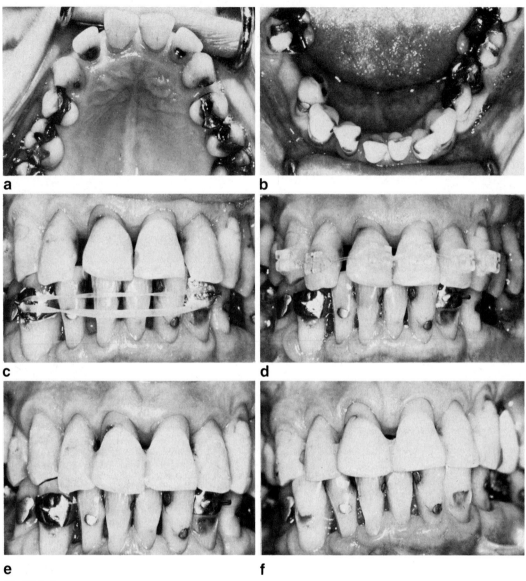

Fig. 23-5a-f.

Case No. 3

A 49 year old woman (Figs. 23-5a-j) had to be treated orthodontically because of tooth migration in the upper and lower frontal segments (a, b, g, h). She had been treated for periodontal disease. Her plaque control was excellent. The incisor spaces were comparatively small and evenly distributed and were closed by means of ³⁄₈″ light latex ligatures in the lower jaw and an Alastic chain in the upper jaw (c, d). After 2 months of treatment, the teeth were retained by interproximal bonding and bonded lingual retainers in both jaws (e). Special care was taken to allow space for cleaning the teeth and for plaque control. Posttreatment control 5 years later (f, i, j).

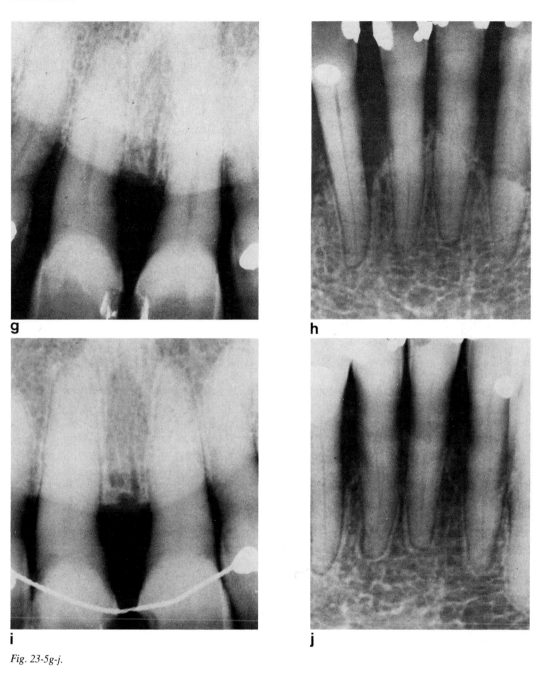

Fig. 23-5g-j.

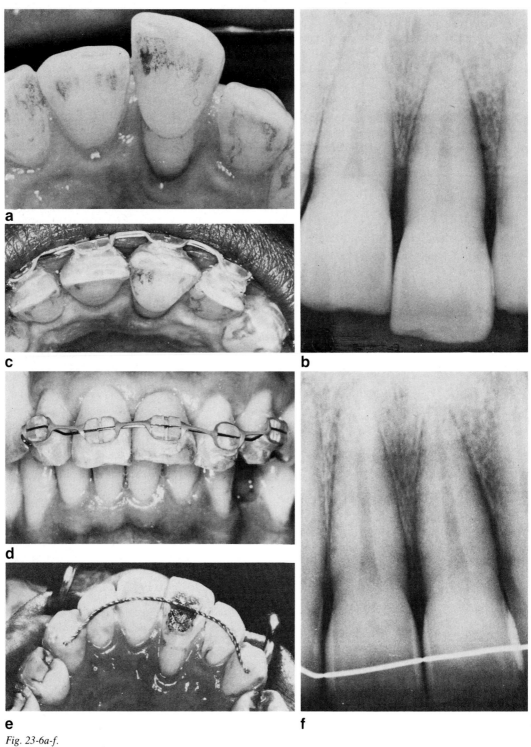

Fig. 23-6a-f.

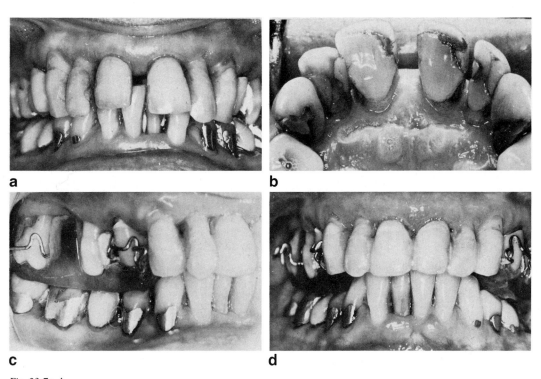

Fig. 23-7a-d.

Case No. 4

A 42 year old man (Figs. 23-6a-f) had been treated for periodontal disease. The buccally tipped and elongated left upper incisor had to be orthodontically realigned (a, b). The incisor was repositioned in the arch by very light forces (c, d). Six months later retention was performed with a bonded lingual retainer (.032 spiral twisted wire, strengthened with a net) (e). Note the improvement of the bone structure around the realigned incisor (f).

Case No. 5

A 52 year old woman (Figs. 23-7a-d) was referred by a general practitioner for excessive overbite and tooth migration in the maxillary frontal segment (a, b). The patient suffered from chronic fissures at the corners of the mouth and discomfort and periodic tenderness of the temporomandibular joint and of the masseter and temporal muscles. The patient tolerated a bite plane well, and the muscle and joint symptoms resolved. Periodontal treatment was carried out and the diastemas in the upper jaw were then closed by means of a fixed appliance. Retention with interproximal bonding and a lingual retainer was inserted after 4 months (c, d). A bite plane was used in the upper jaw until a fixed bridge could be inserted to obtain proper stability of the vertical dimension of the dentition.

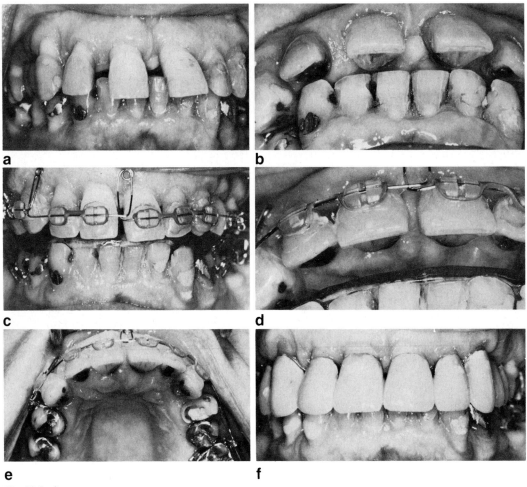

a b

c d

e f

Fig. 23-8a-f.

Case No. 6

A 39 year old woman (Figs. 23-8a-f) was referred by a general practitioner for excessive overbite and tooth migration in the maxillary frontal segment (a, b). An occlusal splint was placed in the lower jaw to raise the bite. The patient tolerated this splint therapy well, periodontal treatment was carried out, after which the diastemas in the upper jaw were closed by means of a fixed appliance (.016 green Elgiloy with contraction loops) (c, d, e). The final result, 4 years after orthodontic treatment and after construction of the crown prosthesis (f).

Case No. 7

A 51 year old woman (Figs. 23-9a-f) was referred to the Dental School for full mouth rehabilitation (a). It was agreed that after endodontic treatment in the frontal segment of the lower jaw and periodontal treatment in both jaws the patient should have orthodontic treatment of the anterior crossbite. The treatment was carried out with a removable appliance which also raised the bite (b, c, d). The clasps were free from occlusal acrylic to permit proper anchorage. The small helical springs and the double, looped spring were reactivated only 1 mm

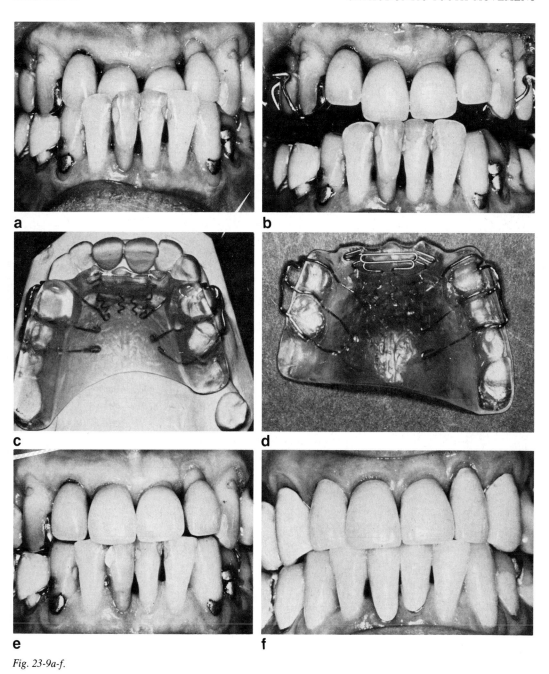

a

b

c

d

e

f

Fig. 23-9a-f.

every third week. The cross-bite was eliminated after 5½ months of treatment (e). After treatment, the periodontal conditions in the frontal segments were good. Note the alignment of the gingival margins. The final result after construction of a crown prosthesis (f).

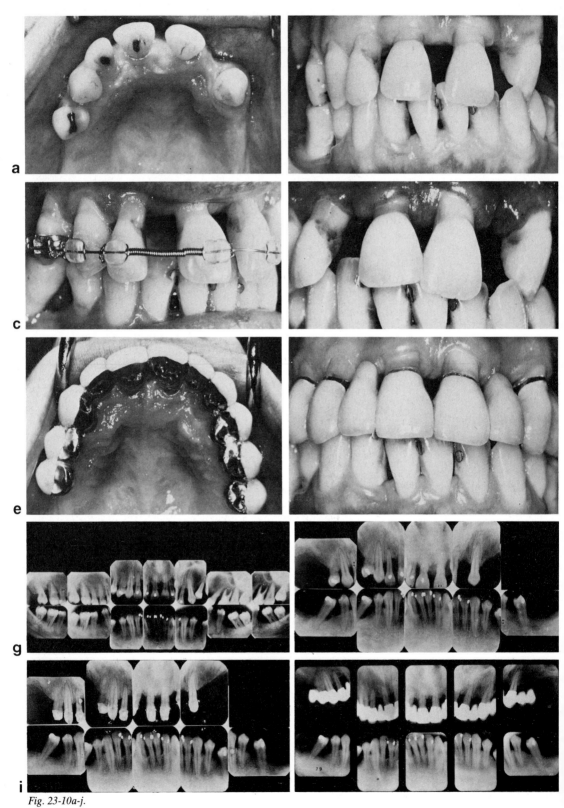

Fig. 23-10a-j.

Case No. 8

A 30 year old woman (Figs. 23-10a-j) had been treated for juvenile periodontitis (a, b). Orthodontic alignment of the teeth was undertaken preparatory to prosthetic reconstruction (c, d). Orthodontic treatment with coiled springs lasted 4 months, after which a bridge was constructed (e, f). Radiographs at the beginning and end of the periodontal treatment (g, h) and at the end of the orthodontic treatment as well as 1 year later (i, j).

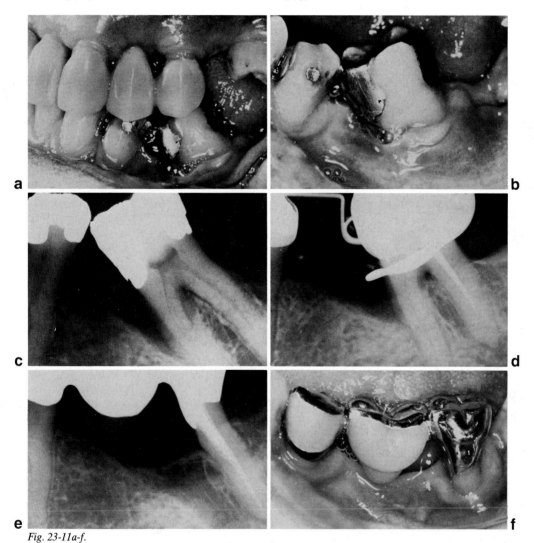

Fig. 23-11a-f.

Case No. 9

A 45 year old woman (Figs. 23-11a-f) was referred by a periodontist for treatment of a mesially tipped left mandibular second molar with a pronounced bony pocket and involvement of the bifurcation (a, b, c). It was considered important to preserve the distal root as abutment for a bridge prosthesis. After periodontal surgery, the tooth was tipped distally with an uprighting spring (.014 Australian) and this was followed by bone regeneration (d). After 7 months of treatment, the distal root was treated endodontically, the tooth was separated, the mesial root was extracted and the bridge prosthesis was constructed (e, f).

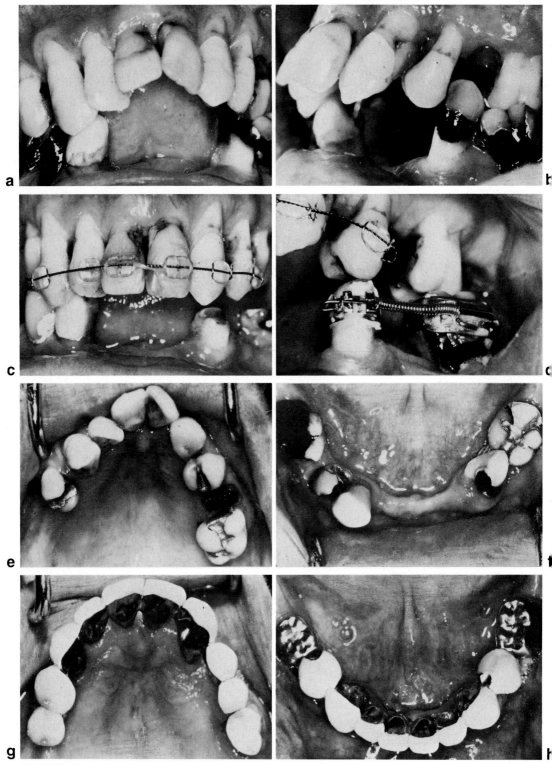

Fig. 23-12a-h.

Case No. 10

A 42 year old man (Figs. 23-12a-h) was referred by a general practitioner for crowding and tipped mandibular teeth following tooth extractions (a, b, e, f). The intention was to use the few lower teeth as abutments for a fixed bridge. Periodontal treatment was carried out. The lower teeth were forced upright (d) with a coiled spring and the upper teeth were aligned (.016 green Elgiloy) (c). After 8 months of orthodontic treatment, bridges were constructed in both jaws (g, h).

References

Ahterton, J. D. (1970) Gingival response to orthodontic treatment. *American Journal of Orthodontics* **58**, 179-186.

Alstad, S. & Zachrisson, B. (1979) Longitudinal study of periodontal condition associated with orthodontic treatment in adolescents. *American Journal of Orthodontics* **76**, 277-286.

Baer, P. N. & Cocarro, P. J. (1964) Gingival enlargement coincident with orthodontic treatment. *Journal of Periodontology* **34**, 436-439.

Chasens, A. I. (1972) Indications and contraindications for adult tooth movement. *Dental Clinics of North America* **16**, 423-437.

Eliasson, L-Å., Hugosson, A., Kurol, J. & Siwe, H. (1982) The effects of orthodontic treatment on periodontal tissues in patients with reduced periodontal support. *European Journal of Orthodontics* **4**, 1-9.

Ericsson, I. & Thilander, B. (1978) Orthodontic forces and recurrence of periodontal disease. *American Journal of Orthodontics* **74**, 41-50.

Ericsson, I. & Thilander, B. (1980) Orthodontic relapse in dentitions with reduced periodontal support. An experimental study in dogs. *European Journal of Orthodontics* **2**, 51-57.

Ericsson, I., Thilander, B. & Lindhe, J. (1978) Periodontal conditions after orthodontic tooth movements in the dog. *Angle Orthodontist* **48**, 210-218.

Ericsson, I., Thilander, B., Lindhe, J. & Okamoto, H. (1977) The effect of orthodontic tilting movements on the periodontal tissues of infected and non-infected dentitions in dogs. *Journal of Clinical Periodontology* **4**, 278-293.

Glickman, I. (1972) *Clinical Periodontology*. 4th ed., Ch. 56. Philadelphia: W.B. Saunders Co.

Goldman, H. M. & Cohen, D. W. (1973) *Periodontal Therapy*. 5th ed., Ch. 23. St. Louis: C.V. Mosby Co.

Goldson, L. & Henrikson, C. O. (1975) Root resorption during Begg treatment. A longitudinal roentgenologic study. *American Journal of Orthodontics* **68**, 55-66.

Hollender, L., Rönnerman, A. & Thilander, B. (1980) Root resorption, marginal bone support and clinical crown length in orthodontically treated patients. *European Journal of Orthodontics* **2**, 197-205.

Iyer, V. S. (1962) Reaction of gingiva to orthodontic force – A clinical study. *Journal of Periodontology* **33**, 26-28.

Kloehn, J. S. & Pfeifer, J. S. (1974) The effect of orthodontic treatment on the periodontium. *Angle Orthodontist* **44**, 127-134.

Kvam, E. (1972) Scanning electron miscroscopy of tissue changes on the pressure surface of human premolars following tooth movement. *Scandinavian Journal of Dental Research* **80**, 357-368.

Linge, B. & Linge, L. (1980) Apikale Wurzelresorptionen der oberen Frontzähne. Eine longitudinelle, röntgenologische Untersuchung in einer kieferorthopädischen Praxis. *Fortschritte Kieferorthopädie* **41**, 276-288.

Morse, P. H. (1971) Resorption of upper incisors following orthodontic treatment. *Dental Practitioner* **22**, 21-35.

Pearson, L. E. (1968) Gingival heights of lower central incisors orthodontically treated and untreated. *Angle Orthodontist* **38**, 337-339.

Pritchard, J. F. (1975) The effect of bicuspid extraction orthodontics on the periodontium. *Journal of Periodontology* **46**, 534-542.

Reitan, K. (1959) Tissue rearrangement during rentention of orthodontically rotated teeth. *Angle Orthodontist* **20**, 106-113.

Reitan, K. (1967) Clinical and histologic observations on tooth movement during and after orthodontic treatment. *American Journal of Orthodontics* **53**, 721-745.

Reitan, K. (1969) Principles of retention and avoidance of post-treatment relapse. *American Journal of Orthodontics* **55**, 776-790.

Reitan, K. (1975) Biomechanical principles and reactions. In *Current Orthodontic Concepts and Techniques,* ed. Graber & Swain, 2nd ed., Ch. 2. Philadelphia: W. B. Saunders Co.

Rönnerman, A., Thilander, B. & Heyden, G. (1980) Gingival tissue reactions to orthodontic closure of extraction sites. Histologic and histochemical studies. *American Journal of Orthodontics* **77**, 620-625.

Rygh, P. (1973) Ultrastructural changes in pressure zones of human periodontium incident to orthodontic tooth movement. *Acta Odontologica Scandinavica* **31**, 109-122.

Rygh, P. (1974) Elimination of hyalinized periodontal tissues associated with orthodontic tooth movement. *Scandinavian Journal of Dental Research* **82**, 57-73.

Sadowsky, C. & BeGole, E. (1981) Long-term effects of orthodontic treatment on periodontal health. *American Journal of Orthodontics* **80**, 156-172.

Schlossberg, A. (1975) *Adult Tooth Movement in General Dentistry.* Philadelphia: W. B. Saunders Co.

Sjölien, T. & Zachrisson, B. (1973) Periodontal bone support and tooth length in orthodontically treated and untreated persons. *American Journal of Orthodontics* **64**, 28-37.

Stuteville, O. H. (1937) Injuries caused by orthodontic appliances and methods of preventing these injuries. *Journal of the American Dental Association* **24**, 1494-1507.

Thilander, B. (1979 a) Ortodontisk behandling i adult ålder. *Tandläkartidningen* **71**, 1036-1046.

Thilander, B. (1979 b) Indications for orthodontic treatment in adults. *European Journal of Orthodontics* **1**, 227-241.

Thilander, B. (1982) Orthodontic treatment in dentitions with reduced periodontal support. *Revue Belge de Médecine Dentaire* **37**, 119-125.

Trosello, V. K. & Gianelly, A. A. (1979) Orthodontic treatment and periodontal status. *Journal of Periodontology* **50**, 665-671.

Zachrisson, B. & Alnaes, L. (1973) Periodontal condition in orthodontically treated and untreated individuals. I. Loss of attachment, gingival pocket depth and clinical crown height. *Angle Orthodontist* **43**, 402-411.

Zachrisson, B. & Alnaes, L. (1974) Periodontal condition in orthodontically treated and untreated individuals. II. Alveolar bone loss: Radiographic findings. *Angle Orthodontist* **44**, 48-55.

CHAPTER 24

An Overview of the Effect of Periodontal Therapy

Objectives and means of therapy
    Plaque control measures to eliminate gingival inflammation
    Scaling and root planing measures to eliminate inflammation
    Periodontal surgery – access for proper debridement
        Curettage/gingivectomy/flap procedures
        Surgical versus nonsurgical approach
        "Critical probing depth"
    Periodontal surgery used to establish conditions which favor regain of supporting tissue
        Keratinized/attached gingiva
        Surgical procedures which favor regrowth of bone, periodontal ligament and root cementum
    Infrabony pockets treated with/without grafts
Occlusal adjustment – splinting to maintain/regain stability of teeth
    References

TREATMENT PLAN

Objectives	Means
I. Eliminate inflammation	I+II. Reduce/eliminate infections
II. Maintain/regain periodontal tissue support	1. Plaque control measures
	2. Scaling and root planing
III. Maintain/regain stability of remaining teeth	3. Periodontal surgery
	A) access for proper debridement
	B) establish conditions which favor regain of supporting tissue
	III. Occlusal adjustment – splinting

Fig. 24-1. Different objectives and procedures available for the treatment of a patient with periodontal disease.

Objectives and means of therapy

The overall objectives of dental therapy in an adult individual include measures to: 1) obtain relief of pain, and 2) satisfy the patient's demands regarding a) esthetics, b) chewing comfort.

Often a patient who suffers from periodontal disease also shows signs of a number of other oral disorders such as caries (primary or recurrent), pulpal disease, mucous membrane disease, temporo-mandibular joint dysfunction, etc. In this chapter we will discuss only procedures which are used in the treatment of periodontal disease. It should be understood, however, that the proper overall therapy of patients with periodontal disease always includes the detailed diagnosis and treatment of other dental and oral disorders present.

Plaque control measures to eliminate gingival inflammation

The efficiency of oral hygiene measures to eliminate infection in deep periodontal pockets has been studied in humans by Tagge et al. (1975), Listgarten et al. (1978) and others.

Tagge et al. (1975) treated 2 supra-bony pockets in each of 22 individuals with periodontal disease in 2 different ways. Three sites (A, B and C) were first examined regarding gingivitis, probing depth and clinical attachment level. Following this examination 1 site (A) was excised and sectioned for histological examination. Site B was subjected to careful scaling and root planing while site C received no professional therapy. The patients were instructed to use meticulous oral hygiene measures for 2 months, following which, sites B and C were reexamined. After a clinical examination the

soft tissue of the 2 sites was excised and prepared for histological examination. The clinical and histological examinations revealed
that oral hygiene measures alone 1) reduced
the overt signs of inflammation, 2) had a
limited effect on the probing depth and 3)
had no effect on the clinical attachment
level. When oral hygiene measures were
combined with scaling and root planing,
however, there was 1) a pronounced reduction in gingival inflammation, 2) a substantial reduction of the probing depth and 3) a
significant gain of clinical attachment.

The authors concluded that scaling and
root planing accompanied by oral hygiene
measures resulted in greater improvement
of the clinical and histopathological parameters describing periodontal disease than oral
hygiene measures alone. In fact, oral
hygiene measures in this study had no obvious effect on the inflammatory lesion in the
deeper parts of the pockets.

Listgarten et al. (1978) studied the effect
of subgingival scaling on periodontal disease
in 6 patients with advanced lesions. Following an examination of a number of gingival
sites for 1) gingival inflammation, 2) probing
depth, 3) attachment level, 4) supragingival
plaque and 5) composition of the subgingival
microbiota, all patients were given detailed
instruction and practice in proper tooth
cleaning measures. This oral hygiene
instruction was repeated at several consecu-
tive sessions. Using a split mouth design of
therapy the teeth in 2 quadrants were carefully scaled while in 2 quadrants no professional tooth debridement was performed.
Eight weeks and 25 weeks after active
therapy the patients were reexamined.

Table 24-1 presents the results from the clinical examinations. The Plaque Index score
representing the nonscaled and scaled sites
revealed that the patients' self performed
oral hygiene was effective in eliminating supragingival deposits (Plaque Index score =
0). But, while in the scaled sites gingival
health was established following therapy
(Gingival Index score = 0) and the probing
depths were reduced from 7.0-4.5 mm, there

Table 24-1

	Examinations	Nonscaled	Scaled
Plaque Index	0 week	2	2
(median)	8	0	0
	25	0	0
Gingival Index	0	2	2
(median)	8	1	0.5
	25	1.5	0
Probing depth	0	7.0±0.9	7.0±0.6
(mm; x̄)	8	6.5±0.9	5.3±1.0
	25	6.5±0.8	4.5±0.9

Listgarten et al. 1978

was in the nonscaled areas no significant
improvement of either gingival conditions or
probing depths.

Table 24-2 describes the alterations that
occurred in the scaled and nonscaled sites
regarding some characteristic features of the
subgingival microbiota, assessed by darkfield microscopy. Scaling and root planing
resulted in a marked increase of the percentage distribution of coccoid cells and straight
rods (bacteria which are associated with
periodontal health) and marked decrease in
the percentage of motile rods and spirochetes (bacteria associated with periodontal
disease). No such alterations of the microbiota occurred in the nonscaled sites. Listgarten et al. (1978) concluded that in
patients with advanced periodontal disease
and deep periodontal pockets supragingival
plaque control without scaling neither elimi-
nates the subgingival infection nor resolves
gingival inflammation.

Table 24-2

	Examinations	Nonscaled	Scaled
Coccoid cells	0 week	41%	42%
+	8	43%	82%
Straight rods	25	39%	75%
Motile rods	0	55%	49%
+	8	48%	13%
Spirochetes	25	51%	8%

Listgarten et al. 1978

Conclusion

From the 2 clinical studies reported it can be concluded that self performed *oral hygiene measures used alone have limited if any effect on the subgingival microbiota and the associated signs of inflammation in deep periodontal pockets*. Oral hygiene measures used alone are therefore *not* effective in the treatment of periodontal disease with deep pockets.

Scaling and root planing measures to eliminate inflammation

The potential of scaling and root planing measures to eliminate inflammation and arrest progression of periodontal disease has been studied in a number of clinical trials, e.g. Lövdal et al. (1961), Suomi et al. (1971), Axelsson & Lindhe (1978, 1981), Hirschfeld & Wasserman (1978), Morrison et al. (1980).

Lövdal et al. (1961) examined around 1.500 individuals in Norway regarding their oral hygiene status, gingival conditions, alveolar bone loss and tooth loss. The patients were subsequently, on an individual basis, given careful oral hygiene instruction including detailed information concerning the proper use of toothbrush, toothpick, dental floss, etc. In addition, their teeth were subjected to meticulous supra- and subgingival scaling and root planing. The oral hygiene instruction as well as the scaling and root planing measures were repeated 2-4 times per year over a 5 year period at the end of which the patients were reexamined. The

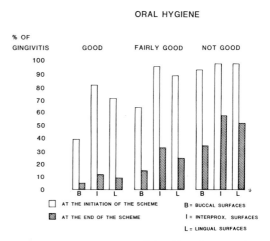

Fig. 24-2. The patients were divided into 3 groups after the initial examination according to their oral hygiene: "good", "fairly good", "not good". During a 5 year period the patients were subjected to scaling and root planing measures 2-4 times per year. The authors noted that in all 3 categories of patients there was a remarkable improvement of gingival conditions after 5 years of repeated plaque control measures. (Data from Lövdal et al. 1961).

authors found (Fig. 24-2; Table 24-3) that "the combined effect of subgingival scaling and controlled oral hygiene definitely reduced the incidence of gingivitis and tooth loss". The improvement was remarkable also in patients whose home-care habits remained improper during the 5 years of trial.

Similar findings were reported by Suomi et al. (1971) from a study comprising 350 individuals in California. A test group of

Table 24-3. Average loss of teeth during the 5 year period and "normal" loss of teeth

	Grade of oral hygiene		
	Good	Fairly good	Not good
"Normal" loss of teeth. Estimate based on the data recorded at the initiation of the period	1.1	1.4	1.8
Actual loss of teeth during the 5 year period	0.4	0.6	0.9
Lövdal et al. 1961			

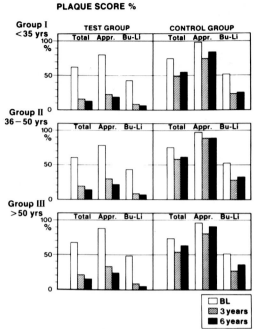

PLAQUE SCORE %

GINGIVITIS SCORE %

Fig. 24-3. Histogram describing the frequency distribution of tooth surfaces harboring plaque at the baseline examination (BL) (open bars) and at the reexaminations 3 (hatched bars) and 6 (black bars) years later. In the control groups, after 3 and 6 years of trial, there was a tendency towards lower plaque scores on buccal-lingual (Bu-Li) surfaces only. In the test groups the individual mean plaque scores were reduced from 60-70% (BL) to around 10-20% (3 and 6 years). (Data from Axelsson & Lindhe 1981).

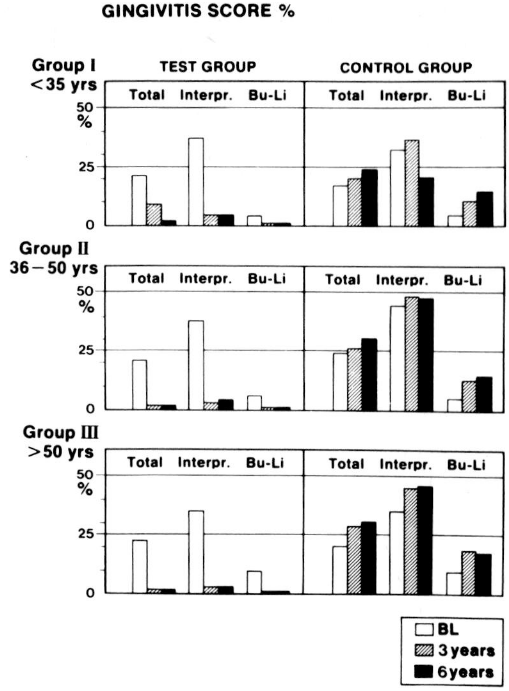

Fig. 24-4. Histogram showing the frequency distribution of inflamed gingival units in the test and control groups at the baseline (open bars) and reexaminations (3 and 6 years; hatched and black bars respectively). The individual mean (Total) figures describe unaltered gingival conditions in the control groups but marked improvements in the test groups during the trial. (Data from Axelsson & Lindhe 1981).

patients received during a 3 year period oral hygiene instruction and scaling 3-4 times per year while a control group during the same period received traditional dental care. At the end of the treatment period the test group patients had significantly less gingivitis and less attachment loss than the controls.

Axelsson & Lindhe (1978, 1981) compared the effect of a prophylactic program including (1) oral hygiene control and (2) scaling and root planing repeated once every 2-3 months over a 6 year period with the effect of traditional dental therapy, i.e. a therapy which was directed towards the

symptoms of dental disorders rather than towards the elimination of the etiological factors. Fig. 24-3 depicts alterations regarding oral hygiene in the test and control groups over the 6 years of observation. In the patients of the control groups there was only a minor improvement in oral hygiene while in the test groups at the reexaminations after 3 and 6 years the mean plaque scores were consistently low (< 20%). In the control groups there was no improvement in gingival conditions (Fig. 24-4) while in the test groups the gingivitis scores had approached 0 values at the reexaminations, meaning gingival health. Fig. 24-5 gives the attachment level alterations between 1972 and 1978. It can be seen that while in the patients of the control groups there was a substantial loss of attachment, in the test patients there was no further breakdown of the attachment apparatus.

Hirschfeld & Wasserman (1978) presented a long-term survey of tooth loss in 600 patients treated for periodontal disease. The patients were reexamined at an average of 23 years after the active treatment which included primarily subgingival scaling and root planing followed by careful maintenance therapy. The authors concluded that "during the posttreatment period 300 patients had lost no teeth from periodontal disease", and "199 had lost 1-3 teeth ..." This means that periodontal therapy directed towards the elimination of the sub-gingival infection by a nonsurgical approach can be effective in preventing tooth loss in most patients and also in those with advanced periodontal disease.

Morrison et al. (1980) studied the *short-term* effect of nonsurgical treatment in 90 subjects with moderately advanced periodontal disease. Following an initial examination the patients were given oral hygiene instruction and the pockets were treated by subgingival scaling and root planing. Reexamination performed 4 weeks after active therapy revealed that 1) the patients had improved their oral hygiene, 2) the gingivitis scores had decreased and 3) the initial depth of the periodontal pockets (Fig. 24-6) was substantially reduced. The authors concluded that already 1 month following the initiation of the hygienic phase of periodontal therapy the clinical severity of periodontal disease can be markedly reduced.

Conclusion

The above review of some important clinical trials demonstrates that *subgingival scaling and root planing are measures which are effective in eliminating inflammation in deep periodontal pockets and in improving clinical attachment levels*. This does not mean that scaling and root planing are always the only measures that are required in order to prop-

erly eliminate subgingival infection. Thus, studies by e.g. Waerhaug (1978) and Rabbani et al. (1981) have revealed that in deep periodontal pockets, residual calculus and plaque may be found even after meticulous scaling and root planing. This means that the clinician has to examine carefully all sites in all his patients and monitor the alterations obtained by the nonsurgical therapy. If, following scaling and root planing, signs of bleeding on probing to the bottom of the pocket persist, and if the clinical attachment level fails to improve, surgical therapy may be indicated.

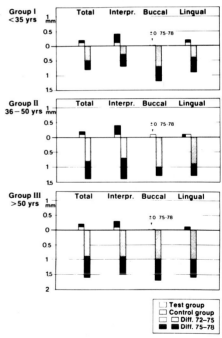

Fig. 24-5. Histogram illustrating alterations of the clinical attachment levels between the baseline (1972) and reexaminations (1975, 1978) in the various test and control groups. The attachment level remained unaltered in the test groups but was reduced in all the control groups (below the 0-line). The average attachment loss per year in control groups was: I=0.13 mm, II=0.23 mm, III=0.26 mm. (Data from Axelsson & Lindhe 1981).

505

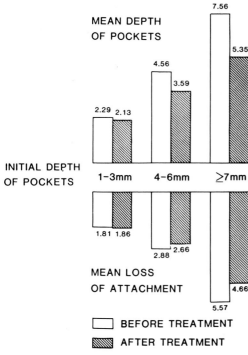

Fig. 24-6. The bars describe reduction of probing depth and some gain of clinical attachment 4 weeks after active therapy comprising subgingival scaling and root planing. (Data from Morrison et al. 1980).

Periodontal surgery – access for proper debridement

Curettage/gingivectomy/flap procedures

The potential of periodontal surgery techniques to enable the operator to get access to the root surfaces for proper debridement and to establish optimal conditions for maintenance therapy has been examined in a number of clinical trials (e.g. Ramfjord et al. 1968, 1973, 1975, Lindhe & Nyman 1975, Rosling et al. 1976 b, Knowles et al. 1979, Nyman & Lindhe 1979, Isidor 1981, Lindhe et al. 1982 a, Pihlstrom et al. 1981).

Ramfjord and coworkers (Knowles et al. 1979) reported on the effect of periodontal treatment in 43 patients with advanced periodontal disease. The patients received a treatment which included oral hygiene

instruction, scaling and root planing followed by either subgingival *curettage, modified Widman flap* surgery or *apically positioned flap* procedures. Following active therapy the patients were, over an 8 year period, recalled once every 3 months for prophylaxis. The annual examinations revealed that periodontal pockets were reduced in depth and stayed reduced and that the clinical attachment levels were improved (Fig. 24-7) over 8 years following either mode of therapy in properly maintained patients.

Lindhe & Nyman (1975) and Nyman & Lindhe (1979) described the long-term effect of treatment on 75 patients who initially suffered from advanced periodontal disease. The patients who were enrolled in the study

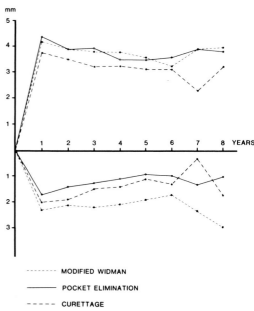

Fig. 24-7. Active therapy including either curettage, modified Widman flap surgery or apically positioned flap procedures (pocket elimination) was carried out during year 0. The patients were maintained by prophylaxis every 3 months over an 8 year period. The probing depths were reduced and stayed reduced and the clinical attachment levels were improved and remained improved in all 3 categories of treatment modalities. (Data from Knowles et al. 1979).

had lost more than 50% of the supporting apparatus. Following an initial therapy which included instruction in oral hygiene measures and scaling, all patients were treated surgically using an *apically positioned flap* technique including bone re-contouring to eliminate angular bony defects. Following active therapy, the patients were, as in the Ramfjord group study described above, for 8 years placed on a maintenance program which included prophylaxis once every 3 months. The reexamination performed immediately after healing revealed that the therapeutic measures used had resulted in low Plaque and Gingival Index scores, markedly reduced probing depths and in the maintenance of the height of the alveolar bone around all remaining teeth. Reexaminations 5 and 8 years later disclosed that the maintenance care delivered prevented recurrence of symptoms of gingivitis and periodontal disease.

In 1976 Rosling et al. (1976b) described the result of treatment of 50 patients who initially suffered from advanced periodontal disease with multiple angular bony defects. Following an initial examination the participants of this trial were distributed into 5 different treatment groups. In 2 groups the periodontal lesions were treated by the *apically positioned flap* technique, in 2 other groups the *modified Widman flap* technique was used and in the fifth group, the periodontal pockets were eliminated by a *gingivectomy* technique. In 1 of each of the 2 flap treatment groups, bone recontouring was carried out to eliminate angular bony defects, while in the remaining groups the infrabony lesions were treated by curettage without osseous surgery. Immediately after treatment the patients were placed on a plaque control regimen which included chlorhexidine mouth rinsing (for 2 months) and professional tooth cleaning once every 2 weeks for 2 years. The re-examinations 2, 6, 12 and 24 months after surgery revealed that all patients had maintained a high standard of oral hygiene (Fig. 24-8). Gingival health was established and maintained for 2 years in most parts of the dentitions. Shallow pockets

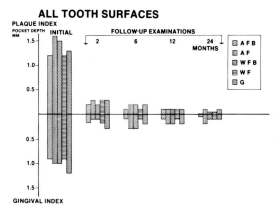

Fig. 24-8. The various treatment modalities (AFB, AF, WFB, WF, and G) are identified in the upper right corner of the diagram. In all 5 categories of patients low Plaque and Gingival Index scores were obtained following active therapy. The low Plaque and Gingival Index scores were maintained during the 24 months of observation. (Data from Rosling et al. 1976).

resulted (Fig. 24-9) and in interproximal sites in which a flap technique without bone recontouring measures had been utilized there was substantial gain of clinical attachment (Fig. 24-10).

Conclusion

The results of the clinical trials described reveal that in patients meeting high requirements of oral hygiene the surgical technique used to get access for proper debridement is of minor importance for the overall result. Since Nyman et al. (1977) demonstrated that in patients who were *not properly* main-

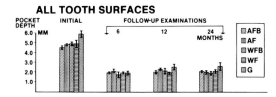

Fig. 24-9. In all 5 groups of patients shallow pockets resulted and remained shallow during the maintenance period. (Data from Rosling et al. 1976; see Fig. 24-8).

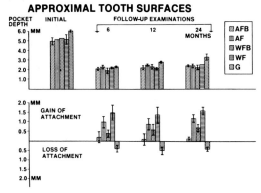

Fig. 24-10. Probing depth and attachment level alterations between the initial examination and the 24 month reexamination are described. During the observation period no loss of clinical attachment occurred in the 5 treatment groups. In patients subjected to flap surgery without additional bone resection there was a substantial gain of clinical attachment. (Data from Rosling et al. 1976; cf. Fig. 24-8).

tained after surgery, signs of recurrence of periodontal disease developed irrespective of surgical technique used for pocket elimination, the findings reported point towards the *quality* of the maintenance system as the discriminating factor between success and failure in surgical treatment of periodontal disease.

Surgical versus nonsurgical approach
Lindhe et al. (1982a) studied healing following 1 surgical and 1 nonsurgical approach of treatment of periodontal disease. Following a baseline examination 15 patients with moderately advanced disease were subjected to treatment using a split mouth technique. In the right or left side of the jaw subgingival scaling and root planing were performed in conjunction with the modified Widman flap procedure (surgery group), while in the contralateral jaw quadrants the treatment was restricted to scaling and root planing (nonsurgery group). Following active therapy the patients were recalled for professional tooth cleaning once every 2 weeks (for 6 months) and thereafter for

prophylaxis once every 3 months (for 18 months). The results demonstrated that scaling and root planing alone were almost equally as effective as their use in combination with surgery for establishing clinically healthy gingiva and in preventing further loss of attachment. Both methods of treatment resulted in a high frequency of sites with probing depth of < 4 mm (Fig. 24-11). The reduction of the probing depth was more pronounced in initially deep than in initially shallow pockets and, for initially deep pockets, more marked in sites subjected to surgery than in sites exposed to scaling and root planing alone. The measurements also showed that sites with initially deep pockets exhibited more gain of clinical attachment than sites with initially shallow pockets (Fig. 24-12). Significant loss of attachment did not occur in sites treated with scaling and root planing alone while attachment loss was found following Widman flap surgery in sites with initial probing depth of < 4 mm.

Similar findings were reported by Isidor (1981) who studied the effect of surgical and nonsurgical methods of periodontal therapy in 17 patients with moderately advanced periodontal disease. Examinations, performed over a 6 year period following treat-

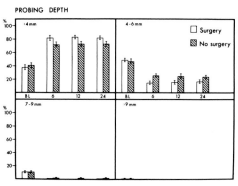

Fig. 24-11. Probing depths. Frequency distribution of probing depths < 4 mm, 4-6 mm, 7-9 mm and > 9 mm calculated from measurements made at the baseline (BL) and reexaminations. At the reexaminations the frequency of probing depths < 4 mm was higher in the Surgery than in the No surgery group. (Data from Lindhe et al. 1982).

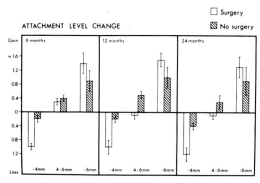

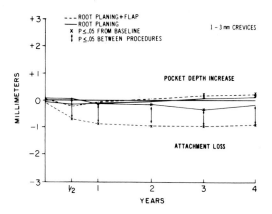

Fig. 24-12. Attachment level change between baseline and the follow-up examinations for probing depths < 4 mm, 4-6 mm and > 6 mm. For sites with probing depths < 4 mm there was loss of attachment while probing depths > 6 mm showed gain of attachment. (Data from Lindhe et al. 1982).

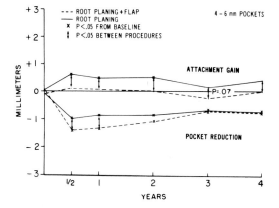

ment, failed to reveal any marked differences in the effect of therapy between the surgical and nonsurgical approaches. In a 4 year study Pihlstrom et al. (1981) compared the effect of a surgical (modified Widman flap) and a nonsurgical mode of therapy and conluded that both procedures were almost equally effective in reducing signs of periodontal disease but that the additional flap procedure tended to result in greater pocket reduction and attachment gain in initially deep pockets (Fig. 24-13).

"Critical probing depth"
The above reported investigations, describing the effect of surgical and nonsurgical therapy in patients with periodontal disease, have demonstrated that while periodontal sites with initially deep pockets tend to gain clinical attachment, sites with initially shallow pockets tend to lose attachment (Ramfjord et al. 1973, 1975, Knowles et al. 1979, Pihlstrom et al. 1981, Lindhe et al. 1982a). In a study by Lindhe et al. (1982b) regression analysis was used to identify so-called "critical probing depths", i.e. initial probing depth values of sites from different groups of teeth and tooth surfaces below which loss of attachment is likely to occur and above

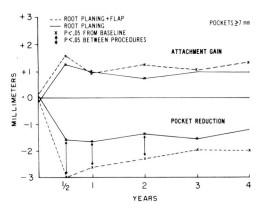

Fig. 24-13. Data from Philstrom et al. (1981).

which clinical attachment gain often results following therapy. By means of this method of analysis it was observed that the "critical probing depth" value for scaling and root planing used as the only measure of therapy

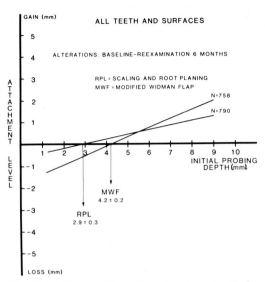

Fig. 24-14. Diagram illustrating alterations in attachment level (gain and loss) between the baseline examination and the reexamination after 6 months. The initial probing depth values are described on the X-axis. The regression lines illustrating the effect of scaling and root planing (RPL) and periodontal surgery (MWF) intersect the X-axis at points representing initial probing depths of 2.9 ± 0.3 (RPL) and 4.2 ± 0.2 (MWF). (Data from Lindhe et al. 1982).

was significantly smaller than the corresponding value for scaling and root planing used in combination with a modified Widman flap technique of surgery. The slope of the regression lines for the 2 modalities (Fig. 24-14) also indicates, however, that in sites with an initial probing depth above the "critical probing depth" more gain of clinical attachment can be expected to occur following Widman flap surgery than following the nonsurgical modality. On the other hand, the surgical approach may result in more attachment loss than scaling and root planing alone, when used in sites with initially shallow pockets. Figs. 24-15 and 24-16 present the "critical probing depth" values for incisors, premolars and molars, as well as buccal, interproximal and lingual sites for a nonsurgical and a surgical method of therapy (Lindhe et al. 1982b).

Conclusion

The findings reported may be interpreted to mean that in patients with a large number of periodontal sites with shallow probing depths, a nonsurgical approach of therapy should be preferred, while in patients with a large number of deep pockets, surgical treatment may result in greater gain of clinical attachment.

Periodontal surgery used to establish conditions which favor regain of supporting tissue

Under this heading methods are discussed which are used to obtain a *zone of keratinized and attached gingiva* and also methods which *favor regrowth of alveolar bone, periodontal ligament* and *root cementum.*

Presence of a zone of keratinized and attached gingiva for the maintenance of gingival health

It has often been claimed that the presence of a zone of keratinized and attached gingiva is necessary for the maintenance of gingival health. Consequently a number of surgical procedures have been developed to maintain or establish a zone of such gingiva or to increase its width as part of the overall treatment of periodontal disease. But what is indeed regarded as an adequate zone, in terms of mm, of keratinized and attached gingiva?

Bowers (1963) stated that it is possible to maintain a clinically healthy gingiva in humans despite a narrow zone of attached gingiva (< 1 mm). However, Bowers also claimed that when there was no attached gingiva present at all, the marginal tissue was usually inflamed.

Lang & Löe (1972) described the results from a clinical trial in humans in which the relationship between the width of keratinized gingiva and gingival health was studied. A group of test subjects without any pathological pockets first went through a preparatory period of 6 weeks during which their oral hygiene was supervised on a daily

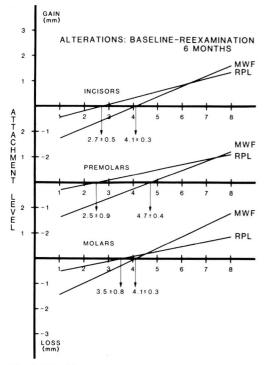

Fig. 24-15. Diagram illustrating the gain and loss of attachment (Y-axis) in *incisors, premolars* and *molars* calculated from measurements made at the baseline examination and the reexamination after 6 months. RPL = scaling and root planing, MWF = modified Widman flap surgery. The initial probing depth values are presented on the X-axis. The nonsurgical approach of therapy (RPL) consistently yielded lower critical probing depth values than the surgical approach of therapy (MWF). (Data from Lindhe et al. 1982).

the attached gingiva for the maintenance of gingival health provided proper plaque control is established.

Wennström et al. (1981) studied the role of keratinized gingiva for gingival health in an experiment in beagle dogs. Cotton floss ligatures were placed around the teeth on the right side (experimental side) of the jaws in 5 dogs and plaque was allowed to accumulate in order to induce periodontal tissue breakdown. After 150 days the inflamed periodontal tissues around the experimental teeth were removed by surgical means using either a "gingivectomy" or a "flap" procedure. In the "gingivectomy" procedure the entire zone of the keratinized gingiva was excised while with the flap procedure the main part of the keratinized tissue was maintained. During 120 days of healing a high standard of plaque control was maintained

basis. Buccal and lingual units were examined at the end of this hygienic phase, for (1) the width of the keratinized gingiva, (2) Gingival Index and Plaque Index scores and (3) the amount of gingival exudate from plaque free units with < 2 mm of keratinized gingiva and with > 2 mm of keratinized gingiva. Lang & Löe concluded that gingival health is compatible with a very narrow zone of the gingiva. In areas with < 2 mm of keratinized gingiva, however, inflammation persisted in spite of effective oral hygiene. A subsequent study by Miyasato et al. (1977), on the contrary, indicated that there may be no requirement at all for a minimum width of

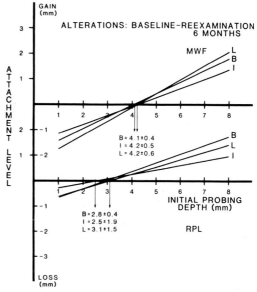

Fig. 24-16. Diagram illustrating gain or loss of attachment between the baseline examination and the reexamination after 6 months following surgical (MWF) and nonsurgical (RPL) modes of therapy. The critical probing depth values for *buccal* (B), *interproximal* (I) and *lingual* (L) surfaces varied between 4.1 and 4.2 mm (MWF) and 2.5 and 3.1 mm (RPL). (Data from Lindhe et al. 1982).

511

by daily professional tooth cleaning. On the left side of the jaw (control side) proper tooth cleaning was performed daily during the entire observation period of 270 days.

The results of this study demonstrated that during a 270 day period of careful plaque control, the width of the keratinized gingiva was maintained unaltered (control side). In comparison, a phase of experimental periodontitis resulted in a substantial decrease in the width of the keratinized gingiva. Subsequent to excision of the inflamed periodontal tissue, which in some areas included the entire zone of the keratinized gingiva, in the majority of the sites a new free gingiva developed. In most respects the structural composition of this regenerated gingival unit was similar to that of a normal noninflamed unit. Furthermore, in the absence of plaque, the regenerated soft tissue was free from signs of inflammation independent of the presence, absence, or width of the keratinized zone.

On day 270 in the dog experiment (Wennström et al. 1982) all tooth cleaning measures were again abolished. After 40 days of plaque accumulation, clinical examination was repeated and biopsies were sampled. The biopsy material was subjected to histometric and morphometric analysis. The results demonstrated that the regenerated free gingiva of sites with a wide as well as with a very narrow (< 1 mm) zone of keratinized gingiva responded to microbial colonization by an inflammatory reaction, the location and extension of which did not vary with the width of the keratinized zone. It was concluded that, in the presence of plaque, a dentogingival unit with a narrow zone of or entirely lacking keratinized gingiva, has an equal capacity for inflammatory response against infection as a unit with a wide zone of keratinized gingiva.

Dorfman & Kennedy (1981) studied the development of gingivitis in 20 patients who in bilateral sites with gingival recession had no attached gingiva present. In one of these bilateral sites an autogenous gingival graft was placed and allowed to heal. The patients were during a subsequent preparatory period placed on a plaque control program until gingival health had been established. At this point all patients ceased oral hygiene measures for 21 days. At the end of the plaque accumulation period an examination revealed that there was no difference between grafted and nongrafted sites regarding the number of gingival units that turned from Gingival Index score = 0 to Gingival Index scores = 1 or 2. Furthermore, there was no difference regarding the net change of gingival fluid flow. Dorfman & Kennedy concluded that recession sites with no attached gingiva are not more susceptible to inflammation than areas with attached gingiva.

Conclusion

The conclusion that can be drawn from the experiments and trials reported above suggests that a certain minimum width of a zone of keratinized and attached gingiva is not necessary for the maintenance of healthy marginal tissue. Furthermore, nonkeratinized dentogingival tissue has a capacity equal to keratinized gingiva to react with an inflammatory lesion to plaque accumulation. The inflammatory lesion in nonkeratinized tissue does not migrate in an apical direction at a more rapid rate than the lesion in keratinized gingiva.

Presence of a zone of keratinized and attached gingiva for the prevention of progressive gingival recession

The claim has been made that a zone of keratinized and attached gingiva is necessary to prevent recession of the gingival margin (e.g. Ochsenbein & Maynard 1974, Gartell & Matthews 1976, Boyd 1978). Results from long-term studies by Dorfman et al. (1980), Hangorsky & Bissada (1980) and Lindhe & Nyman (1980) make it reasonable to question this hypothesis.

Dorfman et al. (1980) presented results regarding the effect of the placement of free autogenous gingival grafts in 107 sites with gingival recession and an inadequate zone of keratinized gingiva. Contralateral sites with corresponding deficiencies served as controls and remained nonoperated. The patients were, following active therapy, recalled for scaling and plaque control at 3 month intervals. After an observation period of 2 years, no further loss of attachment had occurred in either grafted or nonoperated sites. Hangorsky & Bissada (1980) evaluated the long-term effect of gingival grafts on the condition of the periodontium. A total of 43 gingival grafts was placed in 34 patients with nongrafted contralateral sites serving as controls. One to 8 years after treatment, such clinical parameters as width of keratinized gingiva, pocket depth, gingival recession, amount of plaque and degree of gingivitis were examined. The authors concluded that "while the free gingival graft is an effective means to widen the zone of the attached and keratinized gingiva, there is no indication that this increase bears direct influence upon periodontal health".

Lindhe & Nyman (1980) in a retrospective study examined alterations of the position of the marginal soft tissue following periodontal surgery. Forty-three subjects with advanced periodontal disease were in 1969 subjected to periodontal therapy including periodontal surgery using the apically positioned flap technique. After active therapy the patients were placed on a maintenance program which included prophylaxis once every 3 months for 10-11 years. They were examined for the distance in mm between the cementoenamel junction and the gingival margin on buccal surfaces of all teeth, with as well as without, a zone of keratinized gingiva. The examinations were performed prior to surgery, after 2 months of healing and then after 10-11 years of maintenance care. Lindhe & Nyman reported that gingival recession is a common feature of advanced periodontal disease. As a result of periodontal treatment the position of the gingival margin is often further displaced in an apical direction. This displacement, however, is followed by a minor coronal "regrowth" during a 10-11 year period of supervised maintenance. It was further observed that the alterations in the position of the gingival margin followed a

similar pattern in areas with and without a zone of keratinized gingiva.

Conclusion
The results of these studies question the need for a zone of keratinized and attached gingiva to prevent recession of the gingival margin in patients enrolled in a properly designed maintenance care program.

Surgical procedures which favor regrowth of bone, periodontal ligament and root cementum

Regrowth of periodontal tissues has mainly been studied in sites with angular bony defects and infrabony pockets.

Regrowth of periodontal tissues in infrabony pockets treated without grafts
Prichard (1957) and Patur & Glickman (1962) suggested that curettage and root planing of infrabony pockets in conjunction with a flap procedure often resulted in significant gain of periodontal tissue. Ellegaard & Löe (1971) reported the results of a similar modality of treatment of 191 angular bony defects. After a healing period of 2-3 years the patients were re-examined and the authors found that complete healing of the angular defects had occurred in 110 out of 191 sites examined. Partial healing had occurred in an additional 28 sites. Rosling et al. (1976a,b) studied the effect of treatment of 124 angular bony defects in 12 patients. All defects were treated with a modified Widman flap procedure including careful curettage of the bony lesion and proper root debridement. Following surgery, the patients were placed on a maintenance program which included professional tooth cleaning (Axelsson & Lindhe 1974) once every 2 weeks. A control group of 12 patients received an identical initial therapy, but was not enrolled in a corresponding maintenance program. Re-examinations carried out 6, 12 and 24 months after therapy demonstrated that the properly maintained

patients had experienced a mean gain of clinical attachment in the angular bony defects amounting to around 3 mm. Measurements, performed on radiographs or in conjunction with so-called "reentry" procedures, revealed that the test sites had lost 0.4 mm of the bone crest but that the remaining portion of the angular bony defect (2.8 mm) was refilled with bone. In the control patients all sites treated showed signs of recurrent periodontal disease including further loss of clinical attachment and alveolar bone (Fig. 24-17).

Polson & Heijl (1978) described healing in 15 angular bony defects in 9 patients. All defects were treated using a modified Widman flap technique, curettage of the bony defect and proper root planing. Following surgery the patients were during a 6 month period placed on a professional tooth cleaning program. At reentry operations 6-8 months after surgery Polson & Heijl found that "the behaviour of an osseous defect throughout its circumferential extent was characterized by a combination of coronal bone regeneration (77%) and marginal bone resorption (18%)". Infra-bony periodontal defects "may predictably remodel after surgical debridement and establishment of optimal plaque control".

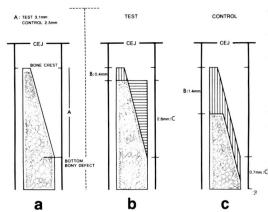

a   **b**   **c**

Figs. 24-17 a-c. Schematic drawings illustrating alterations in the level of the marginal alveolar bone crest and the level of the bottom of the bony defects in the test and control groups. Distance A denotes the distance between the marginal alveolar bone crest and the bottom of the bony defect (a). In the test group patients, this distance was 3.1 mm at the initial examination. The corresponding value in the controls was 2.5 mm. Distance B denotes resorption of the marginal alveolar crest. This distance was 0.4 mm in the test patients and 1.4 mm in the controls (b, c). Distance C denotes gain or loss of bone in the apical portion of the defect. There was a refill of bone in test patients amounting to 2.8 mm, whereas a displacement of 0.7 mm of the bottom of the bony defects in apical direction occurred in the control patients (b, c). (Data from Rosling et al. 1976).

Conclusion

The results from the studies referred to demonstrate that significant bone fill can occur in angular bony defects of single rooted teeth *provided postoperative plaque control is of high standard.* It should be observed, however, that *clinical measures describing bone fill cannot identify the quality of the attachment between the tooth and the newly formed bone tissue,* i.e. whether this attachment is of epthelial or connective tissue nature. It has previously been assumed that bone fill in angular defects was accompanied by the formation of new root cementum and periodontal ligament. However, Caton & Zander (1976) reported from a study in monkeys that "repair of an osseous defect can occur opposite junctional epithelium ... without new attachment of connective tissue". Similar findings were described in a human case report by Moskow et al. (1979). In fact, recently published animal studies (Yukna et al. 1976, Caton et al. 1980) have shown that the dentogingival epithelium during healing consistently migrates to a position close to the presurgical level of the pocket epithelium on the root surface irrespective of the occurrence of suprabony or infrabony pockets, and independent of whether bone fill has resulted from the treatment. For details regarding new attachment, see Chapter 19.

Regrowth of periodontal tissues in infra-bony pockets treated with grafts

The objective of grafts in the treatment of angular and infrabony pockets includes not only the wish to restore the lost alveolar bone but also the desire to improve the conditions for regeneration of a functional attachment apparatus, i.e. regrowth of root cementum and periodontal ligament. The graft materials used so far may according to Schallhorn (1977) be divided into:

I. Autografts (a graft which is transferred from one position to another within the same individual)
 A. Cortical bone ("osseous coagulum")
 B. Combination of cortical and cancellous bone ("bone blend")
 C. Cancellous bone and marrow (intra-oral donor site/extraoral donor site)
II. Allografts (a graft which is transferred between genetically dissimilar members of the same species)
 A. Freeze dried bone
 B. "Viable" cancellous bone and marrow
 C. "Sterilized" cancellous bone and marrow.

Besides autografts and allografts synthetic materials have also been used in attempts to improve healing conditions in angular bony defects.

According to Schallhorn (1977) sufficient information exists on the clinical aspects of osseous grafting therapy to justify the inclusion of osseous grafts into the armamentarium of accepted treatment. A major concern, however, in evaluating the proper benefits of the use of grafts in new attachment procedures rests in the problem of determining whether new connective tissue attachment has in fact occurred or if bone fill is the sole result that has been obtained. In most of the publications so far presented, describing success following various transplantation procedures, the conclusions drawn were based on measurements such as clinical probing, radiographic examination, reentry operations, etc. As discussed in

Chapter 19 such methods cannot be used to identify the formation of new attachment.

Studies in which the effect of bone grafting in new attachment attempts has been evaluated by clinical means can provide information on bone repair ("bone fill") in angular bony defects but may be unreliable in documenting the formation of new attachment.

In some clinical studies attempting to assess the ability of bone grafts to induce new cementum and periodontal ligament formation, the clinical and radiographical methods of examination have been combined with a histological analysis of block sections of the treated areas. Such studies, however, may have a limited value in determining if new attachment has occurred for the following reason: a histological section from biopsy material obtained *after* treatment does not reveal where the coronal level of the connective tissue attachment was located *before* treatment. The pre-operative attachment level in this kind of experiment has most frequently been documented by clinical probing and a reference groove has been prepared in the root surface at this level, but as it is impossible to identify the apical extension of the pocket epithelium by probing *before* therapy, it is equally impossible to verify from a histological section obtained *after* therapy, that connective tissue attachment located coronally to the reference groove is indeed *new attachment*. The problems inherent in the evaluation of results from "new attachment" procedures are further discussed in Chapter 19.

Conclusion

So far no clinical study presented in the literature has provided conclusive evidence that new connective tissue attachment (i.e. the formation of new root cementum and periodontal ligament) may occur following so-called regenerative therapy with or without the use of graft materials. In other words, the potential of bone grafts to induce regeneration of the attachment apparatus including new cementum, alveolar bone and a functionally oriented periodontal ligament *has not so far been unequivocally established.*

Occlusal adjustment – splinting to maintain/regain stability of teeth

Occlusal adjustment and splinting are measures which may be used in order to reduce increased tooth mobility. In a longitudinal study describing the effect of periodontal therapy in patients with advanced periodontal disease (Lindhe & Nyman 1975, Nyman & Lindhe 1979), 676 teeth were treated which initially exhibited not only advanced loss of supporting tissue but also markedly increased mobility. At the initial examination 78 of these teeth were found to establish premature contact either in the intercuspal position (IP) or when the mandible was moved from the IP to the retruded position (RP), or in lateral or frontal excursive movements of the mandible. In these 78 teeth occlusal adjustment was already performed during the presurgical phase of therapy. This therapy resulted, within a few weeks in most cases, in an obvious reduction in tooth mobility. After a few months it was possible to observe in the radiographs that the angular bony defects that were present around some of these teeth were reduced in size, i.e. a narrowing of the periodontal ligament space had occurred. All patients were subsequently surgically treated by means of the apically positioned flap technique. At the termination of the initial 5 year follow-up period, 113 teeth still exhibited a mobility of Degree 1 or 2. In spite of this persisting hypermobility during a 5-8 year period, none of the teeth showed a further breakdown of the attachment apparatus.

Rosling et al. (1976a) studied the effect of periodontal therapy in 12 patients who initially showed signs of advanced periodontal disease combined with multiple angular osseous defects. Of 216 teeth which were subjected to treatment, 37 showed an advanced mobility (Degree 2) at the initial examination. Occlusal adjustment was performed in only 8 of these teeth due to obvious premature contact relationships. Following a presurgical treatment phase, all 216 teeth were subjected to periodontal surgery using the modified Widman flap procedure. In no case was resection of the alveolar bone performed, only curettage of the angular bony defects in combination with scaling and root planing. After completion of active therapy, the patients were enrolled in a careful plaque control program which included maintenance therapy once every 2 weeks. An examination performed 2 years after therapy revealed that all the infrabony defects had healed with almost complete bone fill, despite the fact that 12 of the initially hypermobile teeth still exhibited increased mobility (Degree 2).

It may be concluded from the above that periodontal therapy, directed towards the elimination of plaque and calculus and removal of the chronically inflamed periodontal tissues, also results in proper healing of the periodontal tissues around hypermobile teeth. This conclusion is supported by observations made in animal experiments (Lindhe & Ericsson 1976) showing that trauma from occlusion and resulting tooth hypermobility does not detrimentally influence healing of the supporting tissues following proper treatment of the plaque associated lesion.

In order to understand the overall effect of periodontal therapy on tooth mobility, the following fact should be borne in mind: the vast majority of the initially hypermobile teeth described in the studies by Lindhe & Nyman (1975), Rosling et al. (1976a) and Nyman & Lindhe (1979) showed no signs of increased mobility at the termination of the observation period. Thus, elimination of the chronically inflamed periodontal tissues and establishment of a proper oral hygiene program are in most instances sufficient to normalize the mobility of the teeth.

There are, however, reasons to analyse the occlusion and to eliminate occlusal interferences, if such are present, when teeth, following periodontal treatment, still exhibit permanently increased mobility. This form of occlusal therapy may then result in a narrowing of the periodontal ligament space and a stabilization of the tooth. If such an effort does not diminish the mobility of the tooth (teeth) splinting of the tooth (teeth) may be considered. The mobility of a single tooth is namely dependent not only on the width and quality of the periodontal ligament but also on the height of the remaining supporting bone. This means that teeth invested in a reduced, but healthy, periodontium may exhibit increased mobility even if the remaining periodontal ligament space is not widened. In this context it should be understood that occlusal adjustment and splinting are treatment procedures which are ineffective in the management of plaque associated periodontal disease (Ericsson & Lindhe 1982), but effective in reducing the mobility of hypermobile teeth (Renggli & Mühlemann 1970, Renggli & Schweizer 1974).

References

Axelsson, P. & Lindhe, J. (1974) The effect of preventive programme on dental plaque, gingivitis and caries in schoolchildren. Results after one and two years. *Journal of Clinical Periodontology* **1**, 126-138.

Axelsson, P. & Lindhe, J. (1978) Effect of controlled oral hygiene procedures on caries and periodontal disease in adults. *Journal of Clinical Periodontology* **5**, 133-151.

Axelsson, P. & Lindhe, J. (1981) The significance of maintenance care in the treatment of periodontal disease. *Journal of Clinical Periodontology* **8**, 281-294.

Bowers, G. M. (1963) A study of the width of attached gingiva. *Journal of Periodontology* **34**, 201-209.

Boyd, R. L. (1978) Mucogingival considerations and their relationship to orthodontics. *Journal of Periodontology* **49**, 67-76.

Caton, J., Nyman, S. & Zander, H. (1980) Histometric evaluation of periodontal surgery. II. Connective tissue attachment levels after four regenerative procedures. *Journal of Clinical Periodontology* **7**, 224-231.

Caton, J. & Zander, H. A. (1976) Osseous repair of an infrabony pocket without new attachment of connective tissue. *Journal of Clinical Periodontology* **3**, 54-58.

Dorfman, H. S. & Kennedy, J. (1981) Gingival parameters associated with varying widths of attached gingiva. *Journal of Dental Research* **60**, Special Issue A, Abstract No. 301.

Dorfman, H. S., Kennedy, J. E. & Bird, W. C. (1980) Longitudinal evaluation of free autogenous gingival grafts. *Journal of Clinical Periodontology* **7**, 216-224.

Ellegaard, B. & Löe, H. (1971) New attachment of periodontal tissues after treatment of intrabony lesions. *Journal of Periodontology* **42**, 648-652.

Ericsson, I. & Lindhe, J. (1982) The effect of longstanding jiggling on experimental marginal periodontitis in the beagle dog. *Journal of Clinical Periodontology* **9**, 497-503.

Gartell, J. R. & Matthews, D. P. (1976) Gingival recession, the condition, process and treatment. *Dental Clinics of North America* **20**, 199-213.

Hangorsky, U. & Bissada, N. B. (1980) Clinical assessment of free gingival graft effectiveness on the maintenance of periodontal health. *Journal of Periodontology* **51**, 274-278.

Hirschfeld, L. & Wasserman, B. (1978) A long-term survey of tooth loss in 600 treated periodontal patients. *Journal of Periodontology* **5**, 225-237.

Isidor, F. (1981) Effekt af parodontalkirurgi. Institut for Parodontologi, Århus Tandlæge-højskole. Thesis.

Knowles, J. W., Burgett, F. G., Nissle, R. R., Schick, R. A., Morrison, E. C. & Ramfjord, S. P. (1979) Results of periodontal treatment related to pocket depth and attachment level. Eight years. *Journal of Periodontology* **5**, 225-233.

Lang, N. P. & Löe, H. (1972) The relationship between the width of keratinized gingiva and gingival health. *Journal of Periodontology* **43**, 623-627.

Lindhe, J. & Ericsson, I. (1976) The influence of trauma from occlusion on reduced but healthy periodontal tissues in dogs. *Journal of Clinical Periodontology* **3**, 110-122.

Lindhe, J. & Nyman, S. (1975) The effect of plaque control and surgical pocket elimination on the establishment and maintenance of periodontal health. A longitudinal study of periodontal therapy in cases of advanced disease. *Journal of Clinical Periodontology* **2**, 67-79.

Lindhe, J. & Nyman, S. (1980) Alterations of the position of the marginal soft tissue following periodontal surgery. *Journal of Clinical Periodontology* **7**, 525-530.

Lindhe, J., Socransky, S. S., Nyman, S., Haffajee, A. & Westfelt, E. (1982b) "Critical probing depths" in periodontal therapy. *Journal of Clinical Periodontology* **9**, 323-336.

Lindhe, J., Westfelt, E., Nyman, S., Socransky, S. S., Heijl, L. & Bratthall, G. (1982a) Healing following surgical/non-surgical treatment of periodontal disease. Å clinical study. *Journal of Clinical Periodontology* **9**, 115-128.

Listgarten, M. A., Lindhe, J. & Helldén, L. (1978) Effect of tetracycline and/or scaling on human periodontal disease. Clinical, microbiological, and histological observations. *Journal of Clinical Periodontology* **5**, 246-271.

Lövdal, A., Arno, A., Schei, O. & Waerhaug, J. (1961) Combined effect of subgingival scaling and controlled oral hygiene on the incidence of gingivitis. *Acta Odontologica Scandinavica* **19**, 537-555.

Miyasato, M., Crigger, M. & Egelberg, J. (1977) Gingival condition in areas of minimal and appreciable width of keratinized gingiva. *Journal of Clinical Periodontology* **4**, 200-209.

Morrison, E. C., Ramfjord, S. P. & Hill, R. W. (1980) Short-term effects of initial, non-surgical periodontal treatment (hygienic phase). *Journal of Clinical Periodontology* **7**, 199-211.

Moskow, B. S., Karsh, F. & Stein, S. D. (1979) Histological assessment of bone graft. A case report and critical evaluation. *Journal of Periodontology* **50**, 291-304.

Nyman, S. & Lindhe, J. (1979) A longitudinal study of combined periodontal and prosthetic treatment of patients with advanced periodontal disease. *Journal of Periodontology* **4**, 163-169.

Nyman, S., Lindhe, J. & Rosling, B. (1977) Periodontal surgery in plaque-infected dentitions. *Journal of Clinical Periodontology* **4**, 240-249.

Ochsenbein, C. & Maynard, J. G. (1974) The problem of attached gingiva in children. *Journal Dentistry for Children* **41**, 263-272.

Patur, B. & Glickman, I. (1962) Clinical and roentgenographic evaluation of the post-treatment healing of infrabony pockets. *Journal of Periodontology* **33**, 164-171.

Pihlstrom, B. L., Ortiz-Campos, C. & McHugh, R. B. (1981) A randomized four-year study of periodontal therapy. *Journal of Periodontology* **52**, 227-242.

Polson, A. M. & Heijl, L. C. (1978) Osseous repair in infrabony periodontal defects. *Journal of Clinical Periodontology* **5**, 13-23.

Prichard, J. S. (1957) The infrabony technique as a predictable procedure. *Journal of Periodontology* **28**, 202-216.

Rabbani, G. M., Ash, M. M. & Caffesse, R. G. (1981) The effectiveness of subgingival scaling and root planing in calculus removal. *Journal of Periodontology* **3**, 119-123.

Ramfjord, S. P., Knowles, J. W., Nissle, R. R., Burgett, F. G. & Schick, R. A. (1975) Results following three modalities of periodontal therapy. *Journal of Periodontology* **46**, 522-526.

Ramfjord, S. P., Knowles, J. W., Nissle, R. R., Schick, R. A. & Burgett, F. G. (1973) Longitudinal study of periodontal therapy. *Journal of Periodontology* **44**, 66-77.

Ramfjord, S. P., Nissle, R. R., Schick, R. A. & Cooper Jr., H. (1968) Subgingival curettage versus surgical elimination of periodontal pockets. *Journal of Periodontology* **39**, 167-175.

Renggli, H. H. & Mühlemann, H. R. (1970) Zahnbeweglichkeit, marginale Parodontalentzündung und okklusales Trauma. *Parodontologie* **24**, 39-48.

Renggli, H. H. & Schweizer, H. (1974) Splinting of teeth with removable bridges – Biological effects. *Journal of Clinical Periodontology* **1**, 43-46.

Rosling, B., Nyman, S. & Lindhe, J. (1976a) The effect of systematic plaque control on bone regeneration in infrabony pockets. *Journal of Clinical Periodontology* **3**, 38-53.

Rosling, B., Nyman, S., Lindhe, J. & Jern, B. (1976b) The healing potential of the periodontal tissues following different techniques of periodontal surgery in plaque-free dentitions. A 2-year clinical study. *Journal of Clinical Periodontology* **3**, 233-255.

Schallhorn, R. G. (1977) Present status of osseous grafting procedures. *Journal of Periodontology* **48**, 570-576.

Suomi, J. D., Greene, J. C., Vermillion, J. R., Doyle, J., Chang, J. J. & Leatherwood, E. C. (1971) The effect of controlled oral hygiene procedures on the progression of periodontal disease in adults: Results after third and final year. *Journal of Periodontology* **42**, 152-160.

Tagge, D. L., O'Leary, T. J. & El-Kafrawy, A. H. (1975) The clinical and histological response of periodontal pockets to root planing and oral hygiene. *Journal of Periodontology* **46**, 527-533.

Waerhaug, J. (1978) Healing of the dento-epithelial junction following subgingival plaque control. II. As observed on extracted teeth. *Journal of Periodontology* **49**, 119-134.

Wennström, J., Lindhe, J. & Nyman, S. (1981) Role of keratinized gingiva for gingival health. Clinical and histologic study of normal and regenerated gingival tissue in dogs. *Journal of Clinical Periodontology* **8**, 311-328.

Wennström, J., Lindhe, J. & Nyman, S. (1982) The role of keratinized gingiva in plaque-associated gingivitis in dogs. *Journal of Clinical Periodontology* **9**, 75-85.

Yukna, R. A., Bowers, G. M., Lawrence, J. J. & Fedi Jr., P. F. (1976) A clinical study of healing in humans following the excisional new attachment procedure. *Journal of Periodontology* **47**, 696-700.

CHAPTER 25

The Maintenance Phase of Periodontal Therapy

The primary goal of periodontal therapy is to establish conditions that are conducive to future optimal plaque control and to prevent subgingival bacterial growth so that inflammation and further loss of periodontal attachment can be prevented or reduced to a minimum. The maintenance of periodontal health often requires considerable effort from the patient in retaining a careful and thorough program of oral hygiene. However, it also requires considerable effort on the part of the dental health team. Thus, following the completion of active therapy most patients need professional assistance at regular intervals involving (1) renewed motivation for and instruction in oral hygiene, (2) elimination of calculus and other plaque retentive factors and (3) thorough professional cleaning of the teeth. Without such assistance, periodontal therapy will in many cases eventually and inevitably fail. Obviously, it is also necessary to repeatedly examine the patient's periodontal tissues in order to be able to take proper action at an early stage against possible disease recurrence and further destruction of supporting tissues.

Such professional assistance has been termed *maintenance therapy* or *maintenance care*. The treatment given in this context by the dentist and his auxiliary personnel has also been termed *supportive therapy*.

The rationale for maintenance therapy

Prevention and treatment of gingivitis and periodontitis through plaque control have been practiced for many decades. "Clinical experience" indicates that such treatment may be successful. The extent to which the prevention of supra- and subgingival plaque formation is successful determines the degree of success of the maintenance therapy. If the attempts at plaque control are inadequate or unsuccessful in one or more sites of the dentition, inflammatory changes will ensue in these sites and further loss of periodontal attachment often result. This unfortunately occurs too often, since the continuous maintenance of a sufficiently high level of plaque control is demanding both for the dental health personnel and for the patient.

In recent years the "clinical experience" of the beneficial effect of proper plaque control has been supported by results from clinical trials. The causal relationship between the accumulation of bacterial plaque and the development of gingivitis has been experimentally verified in humans (Löe et al. 1965). In animal experiments it has also been shown that accumulation of bacterial plaque over extended periods of time results in the development of periodontitis with pocket formation, loss of attachment and resorption of alveolar bone (Saxe et al. 1967, Lindhe et al. 1973). Conversely, studies in humans have demonstrated that development of gingivitis and periodontitis can be prevented through measures aimed at preventing or reducing plaque formation (Lövdal et al. 1961, Suomi et al. 1971, Axelsson & Lindhe 1978, 1981a). Considerable knowledge has also been gained regarding the mechanisms through which plaque bacteria produce gingival inflammation and destruction of the attachment apparatus.

In general terms the etiology of gingivitis and periodontitis is therefore fairly well understood. Unfortunately, the causative agents, *i.e.* the microbiota which induce and maintain the inflammatory changes, cannot be eliminated completely from the tooth surfaces for any length of time. The professional treatment can only temporarily reduce the amount of plaque on the tooth surfaces. The microorganisms are still present in the oral cavity and will rapidly recolonize the teeth following professional tooth cleaning. Plaque formation will thus start again and recurrence of the disease will ensue. Controlled, well documented investigations and experiments over extended periods of time have shown that this development can be prevented only through a maintenance program aiming at regularly repeated removal of plaque. Such investigations have furnished us with clinically applicable knowledge and some of them will be briefly reviewed.

Loss of attachment as a result of inadequate plaque control

Investigations by H. Björn (1971), A.-L. Björn (1974) and Håkansson (1978) indicate that loss of periodontal support in population groups of the same age proceeds at

almost the same rate in individuals who receive regular, "traditional dental care" and in individuals who visit the dentist only sporadically (Fig. 25-1). The reason is that "traditional dental care" does not adequately emphasize plaque control, and does not include depuration and periodontal therapy in general (Fig. 25-2).

The rate at which periodontal breakdown and loss of teeth are likely to proceed under such conditions has not been estimated exactly and may vary between different individuals. In patients who had received treatment for advanced periodontitis, but who thereafter had only been examined once a year without special efforts to reinforce plaque control, it was shown that the clinically measurable loss of periodontal support may proceed at an average rate as high as 1 mm per tooth surface per year (Nyman et al. 1975). From other, similar investigations in

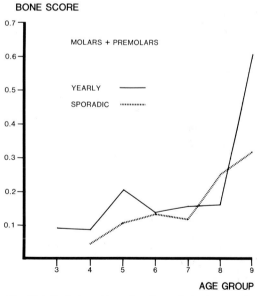

Fig. 25-1. Periodontal bone loss (recorded as increase in "Bone score") over a 6 year period in different age groups in Björn's study (1974). Age group 3 was 25-29 years of age. Age group 9 was 54-59 years of age at the start of the investigation. The loss of bone was more marked in the higher age groups, but there was little difference between those who had seen a dentist regularly at least once per year and those who only visited sporadically.

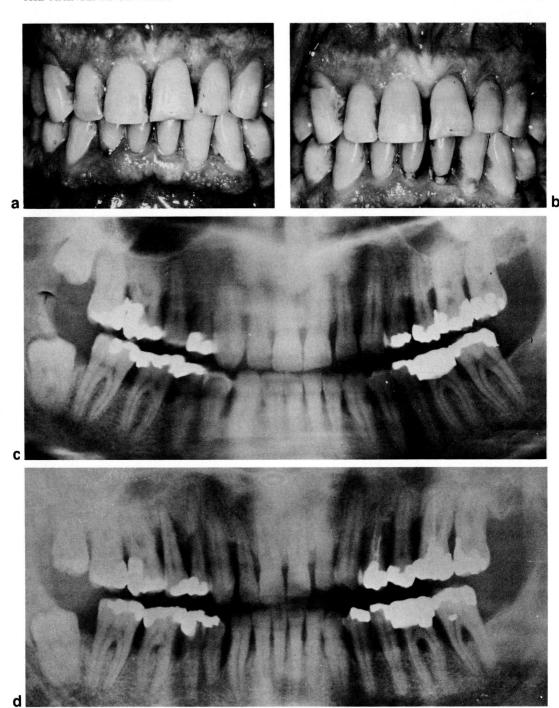

Figs. 25-2a-d. These clinical pictures and radiographs show characteristic changes in one of the subjects included in Björn's investigation (1974). The patient, a 35 year old man, had visited his dentist at least once per year. (a) is a clinical photo and (c), an orthopantomograph taken at the start of the investigation. (b) and (d) are corresponding pictures taken 6 years later. Considerable gingival recession has occurred, particularly in the lower anterior teeth, and tooth 21 shows evidence of migration. Considerable amounts of restorative and endodontic therapy have been given during the 6 year period. The original orthopantomographs also show the presence of considerable amounts of subgingival calculus. The loss of alveolar bone which was already rather advanced at the initial examination (c) has progressed further around all teeth (d), so that the prognosis for several of them was poor at the 6 year examination.

which patients who did not have advanced periodontitis and who received only "traditional" symptomatic dental treatment without adequate emphasis on oral hygiene, Suomi et al. (1971) and Axelsson & Lindhe (1978) reported a somewhat lower annual loss of periodontal support, ranging from 0.1 mm per tooth surface in young adults to 0.3 mm in persons over 50 years of age. Some investigations seem to indicate that with inadequate plaque control and maintenance care, loss of support and bone resorption occur faster with increasing age (Axelsson & Lindhe 1978, Löe et al. 1978). This does not mean, however, that age in itself is a causative factor in the destruction of the periodontal tissues. Plaque retentive factors such as calculus and ill-fitting margins of restorations usually accumulate with age, a process which can be expected to contribute to a more rapid progression of periodontal destruction.

Effect on periodontal conditions of maintenance care including plaque control

The available information indicates that the success or failure of attempts to prevent inflammation and loss of attachment over extended periods of time depends primarily upon the level of oral hygiene but also upon other measures taken to reduce the accumulation of supra- and subgingival plaque. Whether the patient has received proper treatment for any preexisting periodontal disease also seems to be of importance.

The significance of the patient's oral hygiene and of regular control visits including debridement for the maintenance of periodontal health over longer periods of time was studied by Waerhaug and his collaborators (Lövdal et al. 1961). They recorded gingival conditions in 1428 individuals, 20-60 years of age, in an industrial company in Oslo, Norway. Over a period of 5 years, during which the patients were regularly recalled (2-4 times per year) for instruction in oral hygiene and supra- and subgingi-

val scaling, gingival conditions improved by about 60%. Loss of teeth was reduced to about 50% of what would have been expected without these oral hygiene efforts. No surgical treatment of periodontal pockets was performed in this trial, and the investigators found that satisfactory results were very difficult to achieve in areas where pockets were more than 5 mm deep.

Suomi et al. (1971) measured loss of periodontal tissue support in young individuals who only had gingivitis or who had lost only a small amount of the attachment apparatus. An experimental group received scaling and instruction in oral hygiene measures every 3 months over a 3 year period (Fig. 25-3). Plaque accumulation and gingi-

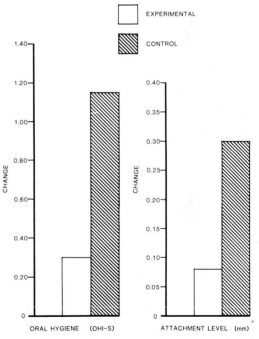

Fig. 25-3. Changes in oral hygiene (plaque scores) and in clinically measured loss of periodontal tissue support over a 3 year period. The experimental group received scaling, polishing and oral hygiene instructions every 3 months. The control group received "traditional dental care", without special measures to improve oral hygiene. The groups were "matched", so that at the start of the experiments they were similar with respect to loss of periodontal support, caries, oral hygiene and in other respects that might be of importance for the comparison. (Adapted from Suomi et al. 1971).

Table 25-1. Mean values for Plaque Index, Gingival Index, pocket depths (mm) and clinical attachment level (mm) registered before treatment and 12 and 24 months after completed periodontal therapy. The test group was given professional cleaning and instructions in oral hygiene every 2 weeks. The control group was only recalled for scaling every 6 months. The average clinically measured loss of periodontal support in the control group over 2 years was 2.2 mm and the pocket depth was almost the same as before treatment. The test group had pockets of less than 3 mm and no further loss of periodontal support. (Adapted from Nyman et al. 1975)

| Parameter | Examination | | | | | |
| | Initial | | 12 months | | 24 months | |
	Test	Control	Test	Control	Test	Control
Plaque Index	1.4	1.3	0.3	1.3	0.1	1.5
Gingival Index	1.5	1.6	0.1	1.1	0.1	1.7
Pocket depth (mm)	4.3	4.7	2.7	3.2	2.5	4.0
Attachment gained (+) or lost (−) (mm)			+0.3	−1.2	+0.1	−2.2

val inflammation were significantly reduced and the clinically measurable loss of attachment was only 0.08 mm per surface over the observation period as compared to 0.30 mm (= 0.10 mm per year) in a control group in which no special measures were instituted to improve oral hygiene.

In longitudinal studies on the effects of various modalities of periodontal therapy in 104 patients, 13-64 years of age, with advanced periodontitis, Ramfjord et al. (1973) recorded an annual loss of attachment amounting to 0.04 mm per tooth surface over a 7 year period. All patients received thorough professional tooth cleaning, polishing and oral hygiene instruction every 3 months. Although there were variations in the effectiveness of the patient's self performed plaque control, this intensive supportive therapy resulted in excellent maintenance of postoperative levels of attachment in all patients. Nevertheless, the results were more favorable in patients with good plaque control than in those with poor oral hygiene (Knowles 1973, Ramfjord et al. 1982).

In an investigation by Nyman et al. (1975) in which 20 patients with advanced periodontitis were surgically treated and where the experimental group subsequently received thorough professional cleaning of the teeth and instruction in oral hygiene every 2 weeks (Table 25-1), no further loss of

attachment could be demonstrated by clinical examination after 2 years (Fig. 25-4). The patients in the control group which received the same initial treatment including surgical pocket therapy were recalled for scaling every 6 months postoperatively, but other measures aiming to maintain plaque control were not instituted. After 2 years these control patients exhibited an average clinical loss of attachment of around 2 mm. This represents a very rapid progression of periodontal destruction and may indicate that in the absence of proper maintenance, surgical periodontal treatment can in fact be more harmful than beneficial. The pocket depths 2 years post-operatively were also approximately the same as before surgical therapy in the patients of the control group, whereas in the experimental group, the pocket depths were maintained at the immediately postoperative level (Fig. 25-5). The results from investigations by Axelsson & Lindhe (1978, 1981a) show that even with somewhat less frequent professional tooth cleaning and oral hygiene instruction, sufficiently low values of plaque scores can be maintained to prevent further pocket formation and loss of attachment (Figs. 25-6a, b). Over a 3 year period when an experimental group of 375 adult persons, aged 20-71 years, received thorough professional prophylaxis and oral hygiene instructions every 2 months for the

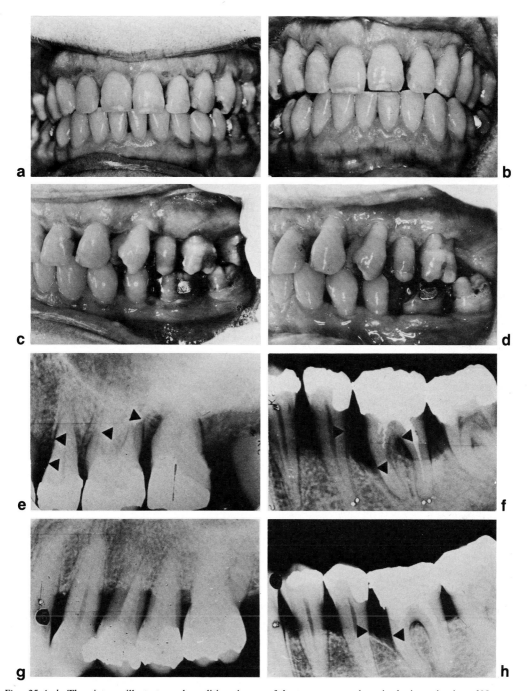

Figs. 25-4a-h. The pictures illustrate oral conditions in one of the test group patients in the investigation of Nyman et al. (1975) (cf. text, Table 25-1). (a) and (b) illustrate the clinical condition immediately before surgical treatment (a) and after 2 years (b). (c) and (d) show the condition around the teeth of the left side before surgical treatment (c) and 2 years later (d). The radiographs are from corresponding segments before treatment (e, f) and after 2 years (g, h). Tooth 27 was extracted during periodontal surgery. Professional tooth cleaning and oral hygiene instruction were given every 2 weeks. The level of the alveolar bone has been maintained very well over the period of observation or there is possibly some regeneration of alveolar bone. Clinically there was no further loss of periodontal support and in no area did the pocket depth exceed 3 mm.

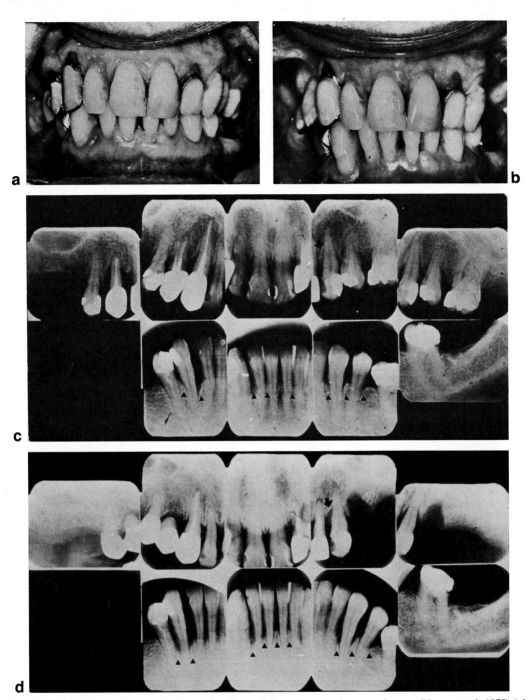

Figs. 25-5a-d. Clinical pictures and radiographs of one of the patients in the control group (Nyman et al. 1975) (cf. text, Table 25-1). The pictures illustrate the conditions before surgical treatment (a, c) and after 2 years (b, d). The patient had been recalled for routine depuration every 6 months but received no oral hygiene instruction. Tooth No. 26 had to be extracted at the start of periodontal therapy. Tooth No. 24 exfoliated spontaneously during the period of observation. The radiographs show that the loss of periodontal support had continued around almost all teeth. Note in particular the rapid loss of alveolar bone around the mandibular teeth.

526

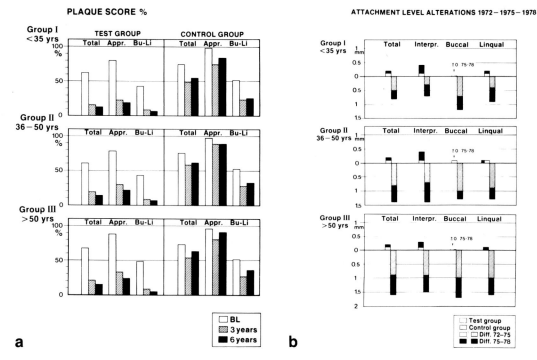

Figs. 25-6a, b. Plaque scores (a) (percentage of tooth surfaces harboring visible plaque) and clinical changes in the level of the supporting tissue (b) in test and control groups in Axelsson & Lindhe's investigation (1978) (cf. explanation in the text). The control group which only received "traditional dental care" once per year for 3 years showed little change in plaque scores. The loss of periodontal support was 0.17-0.30 mm per year in the various age groups. In the test group which received professional cleaning and oral hygiene instructions every 2-3 months, plaque scores were low and no further loss of periodontal support could be demonstrated during the 3 year period of observation.

first 2 years and every 3 months the third year, pocket depths were reduced by approximately 0.5 mm in spite of the fact that they were not originally very deep (on the average 2.0-3.2 mm in the various age groups). Little or no loss of attachment was found in these patients, whereas a control group of patients who were seen annually for "traditional dental care" exhibited a yearly loss of attachment of 0.17-0.30 mm per surface in the various age groups. In the control group pocket depths increased by about 0.5 mm during the experimental period. After 3 more years during which the same regimens were followed, Axelsson & Lindhe (1981a) found that the average annual loss of attachment in the test groups was less than 0.04 mm per tooth surface. In the control groups

the loss of support proceeded at approximately the same rate as during the first 3 years.

Axelsson & Lindhe (1981b) also demonstrated the value of a carefully designed maintenance program for patients who had been treated for advanced periodontal disease. They examined 77 patients before treatment, 2 months after the last surgical procedure, and after 3 and 6 years. Two out of 3 patients (52) were placed on a supervised maintenance program which included oral hygiene instruction, meticulous scaling and professional tooth cleaning every 2 months for the first 2 years and every 3 months for the last 4 years of the observation period (recall group). The remaining patients (25) were sent back to the referring

527

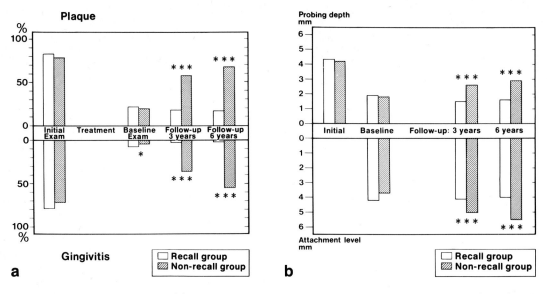

Figs. 25-7a, b. Histograms showing (a) average percentages of tooth surfaces harboring visible plaque (above) and inflamed gingival units (bleeding on probing, below) and (b) average pocket depth (above) and clinically measurable attachment levels (below), at initial, baseline and follow-up examinations in Axelsson & Lindhe's study (1981 b). The recall patients were seen every 2-3 months for oral hygiene instructions, meticulous scaling and professional cleaning. See text for further explanation and details.

dentist, who was informed of the importance of checking their oral hygiene, calculus formation and gingival and periodontal conditions (nonrecall group). The data obtained from the second examination showed that the effect of the initial treatment was good in both groups. Subsequently, the recall patients were able to maintain proper oral hygiene and unaltered attachment levels. In the nonrecall group, plaque scores increased markedly from the baseline values as did the number of inflamed gingival units (Fig. 25-7a). Concomitantly, there were obvious signs of recurrent periodontitis. The mean values for pocket depth and attachment levels at the 3 and 6 year examinations were higher than at baseline (Fig. 25-7b). In the recall group approximately 99% of the tooth surfaces showed either improvement, no change or less than 1 mm loss of attachment, compared to 45% in the nonrecall group (Table 25-2). In the latter patients, 55% of the sites showed 2-5 mm further loss of

attachment at the 6 year examination, and 20% of the pockets were 4 mm deep or more (Tables 25-2; 25-3).

Söderholm (1979) instituted a program of dental care including 3 monthly professional tooth cleaning and oral hygiene instruction

Table 25-2. Percentage of sites showing various changes in clinical attachment level between baseline examination 2 months after completion of periodontal surgery and follow-up examination 6 years later. See text for explanation. (Adapted from Axelsson & Lindhe 1981b)

Change in attachment level	Percentage of surfaces showing change	
	Recall	Non-recall
Attachment level improved	17	1
No change	72	10
Attachment level worse by		
– ≤ 1 mm	10	34
– 2 to 5 mm	1	55

in 443 shipyard employees who had previously been examined by H. Björn (1971) and A.-L. Björn (1974). After 3-4 years, the dental health program had resulted in an improved standard of oral hygiene, and the progressive loss of alveolar bone had been arrested. There was also a decrease in the number of new carious lesions and the need for dental restorations and the rate of tooth mortality had been reduced.

In patients who are well motivated for self performed oral hygiene, the interval between recall sessions may be prolonged according to the observations by Lindhe & Nyman (1975). In 75 such patients who had been treated for very advanced periodontitis with loss of alveolar bone amounting to half the length of the roots or more, and who were seen for professional tooth cleaning and instruction every 3-6 months, no further loss of alveolar bone could be demonstrated radiologically after 5 years. However, for most patients frequent recalls are of utmost importance. The duration of the effects achieved through motivation and oral hygiene instructions in most patients is rather limited (Elliott et al. 1972, Dennison et al. 1974). Without frequent recalls, including renewed oral hygiene instructions, patients tend to revert to their earlier behavior with respect to oral hygiene habits after a relatively short period of time.

In addition to the favorable effects on the periodontal tissues, a systematic thorough maintenance regimen will apparently also significantly reduce the occurrence of caries (Lindhe & Nyman 1975, Axelsson & Lindhe 1978, 1981a, Söderholm 1979), even in patients in whom large areas of the root surfaces have been exposed after treatment of advanced periodontitis (Lindhe & Nyman 1975).

It should be noted that the above results from clinical investigations, carried out under controlled experimental conditions, are supported by a series of documented reviews of patients, treated and maintained for up to 50 years in various dental practices (Oliver 1969, Ross 1971, Hirschfeld & Wasserman 1978). The patients studied had been referred to specialists for treatment of periodontal disease, and the majority of the cases had advanced disease. In all 3 studies the average annual loss of teeth was drastically reduced so that fewer teeth were lost per patient than in the general population. One of the studies (Hirschfeld & Wasserman 1978) reported loss of teeth in 600 patients who had been maintained for 15-53 years (average 22 years). Over the entire observation period the average loss of teeth was 1.8 per individual. Half the number of patients lost no teeth at all, 199 patients lost 1-3 teeth, whereas 25 patients (i.e. 4.2% of the total sample) lost 13.3 teeth per individual. This study therefore not only demonstrates the

Table 25-3. Percentage of pockets of various depths in recall and nonrecall patients at the initial examination, 2 months after treatment and at 3 and 6 year follow-up visits. See text for further explanation. (Adapted from Axelsson & Lindhe 1981b)

| Examinations | Percentage of pockets of various depths | | | | | |
| | ≥ 3 mm | | 4-6 mm | | ≥ 7 mm | |
	Recall	Non-recall	Recall	Non-recall	Recall	Non-recall
Initial	35	50	58	38	8	12
Baseline	99	99	1	1	0	0
3 years	99	91	1	9	0	0
6 years	99	80	1	19	0	1

efficacy of periodontal maintenance therapy but also illustrates the variation in response to such treatment.

Goals for maintenance therapy

Plaque control

Plaque is formed so rapidly and its removal by the patient is so difficult that complete freedom from plaque over extended periods of time is an unrealistic goal. However, although it has been documented that periodontal therapy which is not followed by proper plaque control will inevitably fail (Nyman et al. 1975, Axelsson & Lindhe 1981b), both "clinical experience" and controlled clinical trials have shown that with regular maintenance including professional tooth cleaning, attachment levels can be maintained for several years, even in patients with less than perfect oral hygiene (Axelsson & Lindhe 1978, 1981a,b, Knowles et al. 1979, Ramfjord et al. 1982). For instance, in patients in whom about 5% of the buccal and 25% of the approximal tooth surfaces harbored plaque (average for all surfaces about 16%) there was little or no progression of periodontitis during a 6 year period following active treatment (Axelsson & Lindhe 1981b; cf. Figs. 25-7a,b). One explanation that has been offered (Ramfjord et al. 1982) is that after one episode of proper removal of supra- and subgingival plaque, the complex plaque flora needs some time for reestablishment (Socransky 1977, Listgarten et al. 1978).

It is important, however, to be aware of individual variations, both with respect to the individual patient's ability and motivation to carry out proper oral hygiene procedures and regarding the rate of plaque formation and the response of the tissues to plaque.

Pockets and attachment levels

After pocket elimination, for instance by gingivectomy, Waerhaug (1955) and others have shown that a new dentogingival junction with a clinically measurable pocket of an average depth of 1-3 mm will be established. Under favorable conditions, i.e. with good plaque control and minute signs of gingival inflammation, this pocket is not formed at the expense of periodontal tissue support and should therefore be regarded as a reestablishment of normal anatomical relations. Recurrence of pathologically deepened pockets with loss of attachment, on the other hand, will occur, and may occur relatively rapidly following treatment if plaque control is inadequate (Nyman et al. 1975, Axelsson & Lindhe 1981b). It has been clearly demonstrated that with close to perfect plaque control, recurrence of pockets with loss of attachment can be avoided for at least 5 years (Lindhe & Nyman 1975, Nyman et al. 1975).

Practical routines

Maintenance work should be adjusted to the needs of the individual patient both in order to economize with resources and because such an individual approach is more effective. It is important, however, to institute standardized routines for the maintenance work, routines which can be modified to fit the individual case (Robinson 1980). By following standardized routines, omissions can be avoided and standardized routines in themselves allow the operator to work more efficiently. Routines for maintenance care should include:
1. Examination and evaluation of:
   Periodontal conditions.
   The patient's standard of plaque control.
2. Supportive treatment (as needed):
   Information and motivation.
   Instruction in methods for plaque control.
   Scaling and polishing.
3. Treatment of recurrence of gingivitis and periodontal disease.

Examination and evaluation

Examination during periodontal maintenance care should include:

A. Periodontal conditions:
   1) Gingival inflammation.
   2) Loss of periodontal tissue support.
   3) Furcation involvements and other special problems.

B. The patient's standard of plaque control:
   1) Registration of residual plaque.
   2) Retentive factors.

Periodontal conditions

Loss of periodontal tissue support can be measured in several ways. Usually this is done simply by *probing for pocket depths*, assuming that increased pocket depth reflects progression of the disease and further destruction of the attachment apparatus. *Measurement of clinical attachment levels*, i.e. measurement of the distance from a fixed point on the tooth, usually the cementoenamel junction to the bottom of the clinical pocket is probably a more relevant and precise way to examine alterations in attachment levels. The procedure requires 2 measurements: (1) from the gingival margin to the bottom of the clinical pocket and (2) from the gingival margin to the cementoenamel junction. Many clinicians find this procedure more difficult and time consuming than pocket depth measurements. On the other hand, since the pocket depth is recorded simultaneously, a double set of relevant information is obtained through attachment level measurement.

Assessment of changes in tooth mobility may also yield information concerning possible progression of periodontal breakdown, although increased mobility may have other causes than further progression of marginal periodontitis.

Radiographic examination may give important information concerning possible further progression of periodontal disease. Exposure time, tube angulation and procedures for developing radiographs should be standardized as much as possible. Bite-wing exposures may be useful for examination of marginal osseous contours when bone loss is minimal. In patients who have experienced advanced bone loss, however, periapical exposures, preferably using a paralleling long cone technique, are indispensable.

It is an obvious shortcoming of radiographs that they do not as a rule give information regarding the level and outline of the alveolar bone crest at the labial and lingual-/palatal aspects of the teeth. On the other hand, radiographs give valuable supplementary informationes, *e.g.* of the presence of caries and periapical lesions.

For the registration of *gingival inflammation* one of the indices for scoring of gingivitis may be used. The *Gingival Index system* of Löe & Silness (1963), particularly if combined with the *Plaque Index system* according to Silness & Löe (1964), gives detailed and precise information. Many clinicians, however, find these indices too time consuming for routine clinical use. An index based on the registration of one single characteristic of gingival inflammation, namely "bleeding on probing", has been presented by Ainamo & Bay (1976): *"The Gingival Bleeding Index"*. Gingival bleeding after gentle probing with a blunt periodontal probe strongly indicates inflammation and suggests the presence of sub-gingival plaque and possibly calculus or other retentive factors. (For detailed discussion on examination procedures see Chapter 12).

Tooth brushing trauma or other traumata resulting from faulty oral hygiene practices should be assessed separately.

Furcation involvements are best probed by means of curettes. Radiographs may also give information concerning further progression of periodontal breakdown in furcation areas.

For *scoring and recording of plaque*, a disclosing solution or disclosing tablets should be used, since in this way any remaining plaque is made visible to the operator as well as the patient (Fig. 25-8). This method is helpful both in motivation and instruction in oral hygiene measures. By counting the number of tooth surfaces (mesial, buccal, distal, oral) harboring stained plaque and expres-

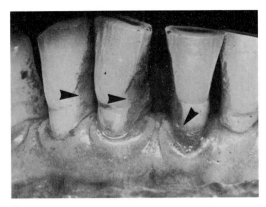
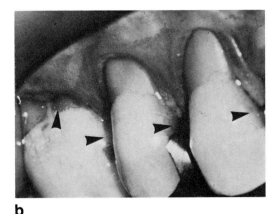

a   **b**

Figs. 25-8a, b. Demonstration of plaque by use of disclosing tablets in recall patients. (a) There is plaque on the interproximal tooth surfaces and the patient has also "missed" the facial surfaces on teeth 41 and 31. Bleeding was provoked by probing facially to tooth No. 31. (b) This patient has maintained relatively good oral hygiene during the 4 months since the last maintenance visit. It is characteristic that plaque can be demonstrated particularly in the interproximal areas and in the concavity coronally to the bifurcation area on tooth No. 36 (arrows).

sing this number as percentage of the total number of tooth surfaces present (4 surfaces per tooth) a numerical expression for the situation with respect to plaque control can be obtained. Scoring and recording of plaque is probably the most important part of the examination, from which both operator and patient will obtain useful information and directives.

Retentive factors such as supra- and subgingival calculus and ill-fitting restoration margins may be assessed merely by recording their localization.

Examination of the periodontium and the patient's plaque control should of course constitute an integral part of the overall examination of the dental conditions, i.e. along with registration of caries and other pathological findings. The findings recorded should give guidelines for the supportive or maintenance therapy. They should also form a basis for evaluation of alterations in the dental and periodontal status of the patient which may occur with time. The findings therefore should be recorded on simple and easy-to-follow charts.

The examination performed during rou-
tine maintenance visits must be repeated several times over the years. They should therefore be as efficient and simple as possible and at the same time as complete and comprehensive as necessary. In patients who have not developed advanced periodontitis, the routine examination can probably be somewhat simplified. Oliver (1977) found that a "screening examination" which included measurements of pocket depths mesiobuccally and distobuccally, registration of bleeding provoked in the same locations through probing, and assessment of mobility in all teeth, would detect 90% of all cases of periodontitis. The cases studied were untreated patients with manifest gingivitis or with established periodontitis. Such simplified examination procedures may be useful for screening of patients on a larger scale, aiming to classify them according to their treatment needs. They can also be used for surveillance after treatment of simple gingivitis without complicating factors such as loss of attachment in furcation areas, etc., but they will probably not be sufficiently exact and thorough when the aim is to monitor alterations in periodontal condi-

tions in individuals who have been treated for advanced forms of periodontitis (see Chapter 2).

Supportive treatment

Information and reinforcement of motivation

Patients expect to be informed about their dental conditions and about the effects of their oral hygiene efforts. If the dentist or the auxiliary personnel does not satisfy the patients' need for information, they may be left with the impression that the dentist is not overly interested or even concerned about their dental health, and both motivation to maintain dental health and confidence in the dentist may suffer. This is particularly true for patients who make great efforts and spend considerable time on oral hygiene procedures, and who may have been subjected to extensive and expensive dental treatment.

Demonstration in the patient's own mouth is usually regarded as being most efficient. Display of bleeding gingival units, deepened pockets and plaque after the use of a disclosing solution is informative and convincing. Many patients need renewal or reinforcement of their motivation for plaque control. To remotivate the patients every time they are seen for control may be tiresome and tedious for the dentist. If such motivating sessions consist primarily of critical remarks they become tiresome and tedious to the patient as well. The effect of this type of motivation is often poor. It is important for both parties that motivation is carried out in a constructive way, so that patients receive the impression that the dentist is genuinely interested in their dental health. Encouragement generally works better than negative criticism (Derbyshire 1980).

During remotivation it is important that the message is varied, so that the patient does not always hear the same "lecture" over again. A program of recalls at regular intervals for control of the periodontal situation

in itself probably serves to maintain the patient's motivation, a fact which constitutes one more reason for frequent regular control visits, particularly for patients with advanced disease.

Instructions for plaque control

Scoring and recording of plaque during recall visits frequently reveals that the patient is in need of renewed instruction in oral hygiene methods. In many instances the patient may not have the manual dexterity necessary to carry out the oral hygiene program that was demonstrated previously, or the patient has not managed to get used to the program and accept it as part of habitual behavior. Undesirable habits which prevent the efficient removal of plaque from certain areas of the dentition may also have been acquired (Fig. 25-8), or the patient may have discontinued the use of one or more of the means or methods of oral hygiene which were introduced. It may become necessary to reevaluate the initial program on the basis of subsequent experience. In any case, the plaque control program should not be made more complicated than is necessary for the maintenance of a healthy periodontium.

Following periodontal surgery, but also as a result of gingival recession or shrinkage, the morphology in the dentogingival region may be changed so that it is necessary to introduce other methods or means of oral hygiene than those recommended during the initial phase. Such changes are frequently seen in interproximal areas where the space between the teeth becomes somewhat wider. Insertion of new restorations such as fillings, crowns or bridges may also necessitate the introduction of new or additional hygiene methods.

During the maintenance phase, the patient should be examined for possible self inflicted trauma due to faulty oral hygiene techniques. Such traumatic lesions may be acute and manifest themselves as epithelial abrasion and varying degrees of ulceration of the gingiva. They can be seen both interdentally, labially and even on the lingual-/palatal gingival surfaces (Figs. 25-9a-c).

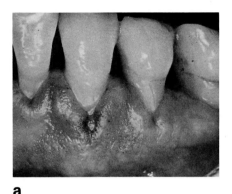
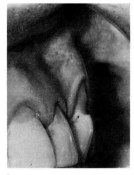
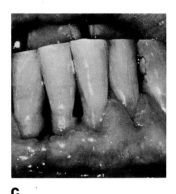

a   b   c

Figs. 25-9a-c. Trauma resulting from faulty oral hygiene habits. (a) Acute tooth brushing trauma on tooth No. 33 and a mild chronic trauma (Y-shaped defect of the "Stillman's cleft" type on tooth 34). Such defects will as a rule heal completely when the method of tooth brushing is corrected. (b) Extensive chronic tooth brushing trauma with defects in hard as well as soft tissues. (c) Hard tissue defects interproximally in the lower incisors caused by long-term energetic use of wooden toothpicks in a 44 year old dentist. Note that denuded root surfaces apically to defects will most likely not be cleaned by the toothpick.

Acute traumata usually heal after a few days when the faulty oral hygiene habits have been corrected. In rare instances it may be necessary to discontinue mechanical cleaning in the affected area for a few days. Daily mouth rinsing with 0.2% chlorhexidine may be useful during such periods.

A special type of acute trauma may arise when the patient fractures a wooden toothpick so that a part of it becomes firmly lodged in an interproximal area. If such a foreign body becomes wedged into close contact with soft tissues, an acute inflammatory condition or even a periodontal abscess with considerable tissue damage may develop. Patients should be instructed to contact their dentist immediately if they notice symptoms indicative of such a situation.

Chronic traumata are usually seen as gingival retractions and wedge shaped defects both on vestibular and lingual/palatal surfaces and occasionally on approximal surfaces (Figs. 25-9b,c). Gingival defects of the "Stillman's cleft" type (Fig. 25-9a) generally disappear after some time when the patient is instructed in correct, gentle but thorough oral hygiene methods in the area. Special techniques for tooth cleansing, for instance use of a single tufted toothbrush, may be indicated. Clinical photographs and casts may be useful adjuncts for monitoring gingival retractions and other chronic defects.

Scaling and professional tooth cleaning

Scaling (depuration) includes removal of supra- and subgingival plaque and calculus, removal of other plaque retentive factors and root planing. Roughness and furrows in the tooth surface should be regarded as retentive factors. Plaque may form more rapidly on rough than on smooth surfaces (Waerhaug 1956, Mörmann et al. 1974). In addition, such areas are difficult for the patient to clean. It is therefore justifiable and desirable to smooth and polish the surfaces of teeth and restorations.

Removal of supragingival plaque and calculus is technically a relatively simple procedure. Subgingival scaling and root planing, on the other hand, are difficult and time consuming. If the patient has many pockets which are deeper than 3 mm, either because they have not been reduced during surgical therapy or new pockets have formed, several appointments may be required to complete the debridement. In deep pockets the complete removal of all accretions is extremely difficult even for the trained and experienced operator. If subgingival calculus is left behind, inflammation with further loss of attachment may result. The choice of treatment mode during planning of the initial treatment as well as thoroughness and meticulous care in its implementation is therefore of utmost importance for the future maintenance work. The choice of instruments for scaling may also have important consequences. Through improper instrumentation, regular scaling over many years may produce furrows and notches in the root surfaces which are extremely difficult to remove and almost impossible to keep clean. Such furrows and notches are most frequently produced by instruments such as hoes and sickles, in which the working edge ends in a sharp corner or a point (Fig. 25-10). Curettes are probably the best and most versatile instruments for scaling and root planing. Rotating instruments such as diamonds produce rough surfaces and considerable loss of tooth substance (Fig. 25-11a). Scaling with ultrasonic instruments is generally considered to be less efficient and produces somewhat rougher surfaces than scaling by means of curettes (Fig. 25-11b). Improper use of ultrasonic instruments easily produces roughness and scratches in metal restorations (see Chapters 16, 17).

The surface structure and marginal fit of restorations made of amalgam change and deteriorate with time, resulting in increased plaque retention. By careful use of small diamond points or wedge shaped EVA diamonds, such fillings can often be properly recontoured. For smoothing and polishing, rubber polishers and abrasive paper strips are useful.

Final polishing of all tooth surfaces should be performed with brushes, rubber cups, dental tape and points as carriers for polishing pastes with decreasing grain size and preferably containing fluoride.

Treatment of recurrent periodontal disease

Choice of treatment for possible recurrences

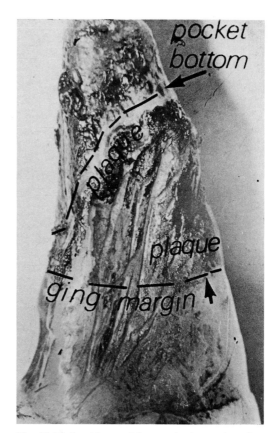

Fig. 25-10. Scratches and furrows in the tooth surface after attempts at subgingival scaling. Such scratches frequently result from the use of hand instruments where the working edge ends in a sharp corner (hoes) or a point (sickles). The pocket was deep. Note that in spite of energetic attempts plaque was still present on the tooth surface. Dental calculus can also be seen, particularly near the bottom of the pocket. (Courtesy of Dr. J. Waerhaug).

of periodontal disease must be based on an analysis of the causes of the recurrence.

Local recurrences are commonly caused by failure of the plaque control in the area. The cause of such failure may be faulty oral hygiene methods or the presence of retentive factors for which the oral hygiene procedures cannot compensate. Not infrequently the cause of the recurrence can be traced back to the initial planning or implementation of the periodontal therapy. Furcation involvements, concavities and root furrows

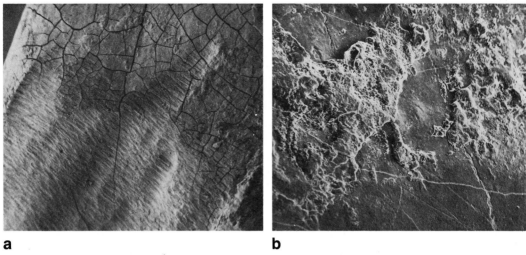

a   **b**

Figs. 25-11a, b. Root surfaces after scaling with a fine diamond (a) or an ultrasonic instrument (b). The pictures are taken in a scanning electron microscope and are from investigations by Lie & Meyer (1977) and Meyer & Lie (1977). The surface which has been treated with a fine grained are flame shaped diamond (a) is uneven and there is considerable loss of tooth substance. (The cracks in the upper part of the picture, due to desiccation during preparation). The surface where attempts were made to scale with an ultrasonic instrument (b) felt entirely smooth upon probing. Nevertheless, remnants of calculus can still be observed.

are common causes of recurrence, in addition to persisting subgingival calculus and subgingival ill-fitting margins of restorations. The possible presence of a root fracture should be considered in endodontically treated teeth, particularly if the tooth carries an artificial crown with a post inserted in the root canal.

Generalized recurrence is most frequently due to deficient maintenance care. Frequent maintenance visits are particularly important in patients who have been treated for advanced periodontitis.

If the recurrence is diagnosed early, it can often be arrested by intensifying maintenance or supportive therapy. Surgical treatment of recurrences should be performed when necessary for the complete removal of subgingival plaque and calculus and when deep pockets or increased pocket depths are accompanied by progressive loss of attachment. If the recurrence is the result of faulty or deficient oral hygiene efforts by the patient, surgical intervention should be postponed until the patient's oral hygiene has been brought to an acceptable level.

Frequency of maintenance visits

General rules regarding frequency of maintenance visits cannot be given. A number of studies have shown that maintenance based on 3 monthly recalls is sufficient for most patients (Suomi et al. 1971, Ramfjord et al. 1973, 1982, Axelsson & Lindhe 1978, 1981a,b, Söderholm 1979). However, some patients may need less frequent visits (Lindhe & Nyman 1975). It is in the interest of both the patient and the health care system to avoid "overtreatment" and still see the patient as often as the individual case requires.

It is often recommended to see the patient relatively frequently during the first period after completion of the initial periodontal treatment and thereafter to adjust the frequency of maintenance care visits as well as the procedures performed during these visits as experience is gained with respect to the needs of the individual patient.

The most important factor to consider when deciding the frequency of recall visits is the patient's level of plaque control (Table

25-4). Most often this reflects the patient's motivation to carry out the oral hygiene program. But the degree of understanding and knowledge as well as the manual dexterity differ from patient to patient (Kenney et al. 1976). The durability of the motivation that the patient has received also varies between patients. In addition, plaque may form at different rates in different individuals. After tooth cleansing, plaque may form less rapidly and probably reaches "mature" composition more slowly if oral hygiene has been proper and the gingiva has been free of inflammation during a period of time preceding the cleansing, than if hygiene has been poor and the gingiva has been inflamed (Hillam & Hull 1977, Socransky 1977, Listgarten et al. 1978). This may be an argument in favor of frequent visits for professional tooth cleaning and oral hygiene instruction, particularly in patients with poor oral hygiene or poor resistance to plaque infection.

Even more important are variations in local conditions which increase plaque retention and complicate plaque removal. Along with calculus, restorations constitute

Table 25-4. Conditions which may influence the frequency of maintenance care visits

Related to plaque control	Patient's motivation Patient's knowledge and ability to carry out oral hygiene procedures. Rate of plaque formation Retentive factors complicating or preventing effective oral hygiene Rate of calculus formation Special periodontal risk factors (furcations, furrows, etc.) Tooth brushing and other oral hygiene trauma

Related to tissue destruction	Tendency for development of gingivitis and for tissue destruction
	   Host tissue resistance
	   Pathogenicity of plaque bacteria

Other	Occlusal relations Caries activity

the most important retention factors, particularly if the margins of the restorations are located subgingivally or close to the gingival margin (Silness 1978). Patients with many such restorations are more exposed to plaque retention and may require more frequent maintenance visits. The position and anatomy of the teeth may further complicate the patient's plaque control (Ainamo 1972). Furrows and concavities in the exposed root surface, frequently found *e.g.* coronally to furcations, may present obstacles to plaque removal. Some patients appear to have a stronger tendency for calculus formation than others. It may be desirable to see such patients more often for this reason.

Patients also respond differently to plaque infection with variations in the rate of development of inflammation and in the tendency to destruction of the supporting tissues (Hirschfeld & Wasserman 1978). This may be due to variations in host resistance or to variations in the composition of the plaque microbiota. Clinically applicable methods for evaluating the pathogenicity of the various bacteria involved in periodontal disease are not as yet available. Only rarely can host tissue resistance to periodontal breakdown be related in practice to well defined systemic conditions which can be diagnosed. One such condition is diabetes mellitus. For the vast majority of patients, however, host tissue response can only be evaluated by recording the loss of periodontal support with time and relating this to the patient's plaque control and other measures taken against the plaque bacteria. However, the clinician may be able to form an opinion about the patient's susceptibility to periodontal disease before treatment by considering the degree of periodontal tissue destruction present in relation to the patient's age. Reduced host tissue response is obvious when there is considerable periodontal breakdown in relatively young patients, as in patients with juvenile periodontitis. Advanced loss of periodontal support in older patients, on the other hand, does not necessarily reflect reduced host tissue resistance, even though the amount of plaque bacteria present at the moment is moderate. Tissue breakdown may have progressed over considerable periods of time and under varying conditions with respect to the amount of plaque and types of bacteria present.

Teeth with reduced periodontal support frequently exhibit increased mobility, even after completion of successful periodontal therapy. Such teeth may also develop hypermobility at a later stage if exposed to unfavorable occlusal forces. Even if unfavorable occlusal relations have been corrected in order to avoid such a development, the situation should be supervised since occlusal relations and habits may change with time (Ramfjord & Ash 1971). Only rarely, however, do such conditions necessitate more frequent recall visits than those required for the maintenance of proper plaque control.

Finally, the question of frequency of maintenance visits has certain practical and economical aspects. Most patients who have been subjected to periodontal treatment should be recalled after a month. Subsequently 3 monthly recalls are instituted. If plaque control continues to be proper and other reasons for more frequent visits do not exist after a year or so, the interval between the appointments can be extended to once every fourth or sixth month. Otherwise, visits every 3 months are continued or the frequency of visits can be increased. For patients who maintain excellent oral hygiene and who show good resistance to periodontal breakdown and low caries activity, yearly controls may be sufficient.

All patients who have received comprehensive periodontal therapy should have a thorough examination with respect to loss of gingival inflammation, furcation involvements, etc., at least once a year. Radiographs should be taken at regular intervals.

Responsibilities of the dental team

The responsibility for periodontal maintenance rests primarily with the patient's general dental practitioner. The patient obviously has a responsibility, but it rests with the dentist to supervise the patient's endeavours to meet the requirements for proper tooth cleaning. It is also the responsibility of the general dental practitioner to diagnose and to treat recurrence of the disease at least as long as the level of severity and difficulty of the particular case do not exceed the dentist's competence. If so, the patient should be referred to a periodontist for treatment.

If the patient has been referred to a periodontist for the initial periodontal therapy, the specialist will frequently supervise the case during the first months following treatment. When the periodontist subsequently sends the patient back to the referring dentist, the latter again assumes responsibility for the maintenance care. The general practitioner may then expect the specialist to submit a written evaluation of the patient's plaque control, prognosis, particular risk areas and preferably also suggestions concerning the future maintenance care and supportive therapy.

Important parts of the supportive therapy such as reinstruction, scaling and professional tooth cleaning can be performed by a dental hygienist. Other specially trained auxiliaries, e.g. "oral hygiene nurses", can also perform such work within the limits of their qualifications and authorization (Söderholm 1979, Hetland et al. 1982). The main responsibility, however, for the treatment that is given by auxiliary personnel still rests with the dentist, who should therefore personally examine the patient at regular intervals and supervise the work he has delegated to the auxiliaries. Firm administrative routines are of great value in this context, particularly with regard to communication between the different members of the dental health team.

References

Ainamo, J. (1972) Relationship between malalignment of teeth and periodontal disease. *Scandinavian Journal of Dental Research* **80**, 104-110.

Ainamo, J. & Bay, I. (1976) Problems and proposals for recording gingivitis and plaque. *International Dental Journal* **25**, 229-235.

Axelsson, P. & Lindhe, J. (1978) Effect of controlled oral hygiene procedures on caries and periodontal disease in adults. *Journal of Clinical Periodontology* **5**, 133-151.

Axelsson, P. & Lindhe, J. (1981a) The effect of controlled oral hygiene procedures on caries and periodontal disease in adults. Results after 6 years. *Journal of Clinical Periodontology* **8**, 239-248.

Axelsson, P. & Lindhe, J. (1981b) The significance of maintenance care in the treatment of periodontal disease. *Journal of Clinical Periodontology* **8**, 281-294.

Björn, A.-L. (1974) Dental health in relation to age and dental care. *Odontologisk Revy,* Supplement 29.

Björn, H. (1971) Tandhälsotillståndet hos manliga anställda vid en svensk industri. *Tandläkartidningen* **63**, 4-21.

Dennison, D., Lucye, H. & Suomi, J. D. (1974) Effects of dental health instruction on university students. *Journal of the American Dental Association* **89**, 1313-1317.

Derbyshire, J. C. (1980) Patient motivation. In *Periodontal Therapy,* ed. Goldman, H. M. & Cohen, D. W., 6th ed., pp. 516-534. St. Louis: C. V. Mosby Co.

Elliott, J. R., Bowers, G. M., Clemmer, B. A. & Rovelstad, G. H. (1972) Evaluation of an oral physiotherapy center in the reduction of bacterial plaque and periodontal disease. *Journal of Periodontology* **43**, 221-224.

Hetland, L., Midtun, N. & Kristoffersen, T. (1982) Effect of oral hygiene instruction given by paraprofessional personnel. *Community Dentistry and Oral Epidemiology* **10**, 8-14.

Hillam, D. G. & Hull, P. S. (1977) The influence of experimental gingivitis on plaque formation. *Journal of Clinical Periodontology* **4**, 56-61.

Hirschfeld, L. & Wasserman, B. (1978) A long-term survey of tooth loss in 600 treated periodontal patients. *Journal of Periodontology* **49**, 225-237.

Håkansson, J. (1978) Tandvårdsvanor, attityder till tandvård samt tandstatus hos 20-60-åringar i Sverige. Thesis. University of Lund.

Kenney, E. B., Saxe, S. R., Lenox, J. A., Cooper, T. M., Caudill, J. S., Collins, A. R. & Kaplan, A. (1976) The relation of manual dexterity and knowledge to performance of oral hygiene. *Journal of Periodontal Research* **11**, 67-73.

Knowles, J. W. (1973) Oral hygiene related to long-term effects of periodontal therapy. *Journal of the Michigan State Dental Association* **55**, 147-150.

Knowles, J. W., Burgett, F. G., Nissle, R. R., Shick, R. A., Morrison, E. C. & Ramfjord, S. P. (1979) Results of periodontal treatment related to pocket depth and attachment level. Eight years. *Journal of Periodontology* **50**, 225-233.

Lie, T. & Meyer, K. (1977) Calculus removal and loss of tooth substance in response to different periodontal instruments. *Journal of Clinical Periodontology* **4**, 250-262.

Lindhe, J., Hamp, S.-E. & Löe, H. (1973) Experimental periodontitis in the Beagle dog. *Journal of Periodontal Research* **8**, 1-10.

Lindhe, J. & Nyman, S. (1975) The effect of plaque control and surgical pocket elimination on the establishment and maintenance of periodontal health. A longitudinal study of periodontal therapy in cases of advanced disease. *Journal of Clinical Periodontology* **2**, 67-79.

Listgarten, M. A., Lindhe, J. & Helldén, L. (1978) Effect of tetracycline and/or scaling on human periodontal disease. Clinical, microbiological and histological observations. *Journal of Clinical Periodontology* **5**, 246-271.

Löe, H. & Silness, J. (1963) Periodontal disease in pregnancy. I. Prevalence and severity. *Acta Odontologica Scandinavica* **21**, 533-551.

Löe, H., Theilade, E. & Jensen, S. B. (1965) Experimental gingivitis in man. *Journal of Periodontology* **36**, 177-187.

Löe, H., Ånerud, Å., Boysen, H. & Smith, M. (1978) The natural history of periodontal disease in man. The rate of periodontal destruction before 40 years of age. *Journal of Periodontology* **49**, 607-620.

Lövdal, A., Arnö, A., Schei, O. & Waerhaug, J. (1961) Combined effect of subgingival scaling and controlled oral hygiene on the incidence of gingivitis. *Acta Odontologica Scandinavica* **19**, 537-553.

Meyer, K. & Lie, T. (1977) Root surface roughness in response to periodontal instrumentation studied by combined use of microroughness measurements and scanning electron microscopy. *Journal of Clinical Periodontology* **4**, 77-91.

Mörmann, W., Regolati, B. & Renggli, H. H. (1974) Gingival reaction to well-fitted subgingival proximal gold inlays. *Journal of Clinical Periodontology* **1**, 120-125.

Nyman, S., Rosling, B. & Lindhe, J. (1975) Effect of professional tooth cleaning on healing after periodontal surgery. *Journal of Clinical Periodontology* **2**, 80-86.

Oliver, R. C. (1969) Tooth loss with and without periodontal therapy. *Periodontal Abstracts* **17**, 8-9.

Oliver, R. C. (1977) Patient evaluation. *International Dental Journal* **27**, 103-106.

Ramfjord, S. P. & Ash, M. M. (1971) *Occlusion.* 2nd ed. Philadelphia, London, Toronto: W. B. Saunders Co.

Ramfjord, S. P., Knowles, J. W., Nissle, R. R., Shick, R. A. & Burgett, F. G. (1973) Longitudinal study of periodontal therapy. *Journal of Periodontology* **44**, 66-77.

Ramfjord, S. P., Morrison, E. C., Burgett, F. G., Nissle, R. R., Shick, R. A., Zann, G. J., Knowles, J. W. (1982) Oral hygiene and maintenance of periodontal support. *Journal of Periodontology* **53**, 26-30.

Robinson, R. E. (1980) Maintenance of the periodontally treated patient. In *Periodontal Therapy,* ed. Goldman, H. M. & Cohen, D. W., 6th ed., pp. 1155-1178. St. Louis: C. V. Mosby Co.

Ross, I.F. (1971) The results of treatment. A long-term study of one hundred and eighty patients. *Parodontologie* **25**, 125-134.

Saxe, S. R., Greene, J. C., Bohannan, H. M. & Vermillion, J. R. (1967) Oral debris, calculus and periodontal disease in the Beagle dog. *Periodontics* **5**, 217-225.

Silness, J. (1978) Placement of margins. In *Prosthodontic treatment for partially edentulous patients,* ed. Zarb, G. A., Bergman, B., Clayton, J. A. & MacKay, H. F. St. Louis: C. V. Mosby Co.

Silness, J. & Löe, H. (1964) Periodontal disease in pregnancy. II. Correlation between oral hygiene and periodontal condition. *Acta Odontologica Scandinavica* **22**, 121-135.

Socransky, S. S. (1977) Microbiology of periodontal disease. Present status and future considerations. *Journal of Periodontology* **48**, 497-504.

Söderholm, G. (1979) Effect of a dental care program on dental health conditions. A study of employees of a Swedish shipyard. Thesis. University of Lund.

Suomi, J. D., Greene, J. C., Vermillion, J. R., Doyle, J., Chang, J. J. & Leatherwood, E. C. (1971) The effect of controlled oral hygiene procedures on the progression of periodontal disease in adults: Results after third and final year. *Journal of Periodontology* **42**, 152-160.

Waerhaug, J. (1955) Depth of incision in gingivectomy. *Oral Surgery, Oral Medecine and Oral Pathology* **8**, 707-718.

Waerhaug, J. (1956) Effect of rough surfaces upon gingival tissue. *Journal of Dental Research* **35**, 323-325.

Index